12th Edition

Nutrition&Diet Therapy

12th Edition
Nutrition&Diet Therapy

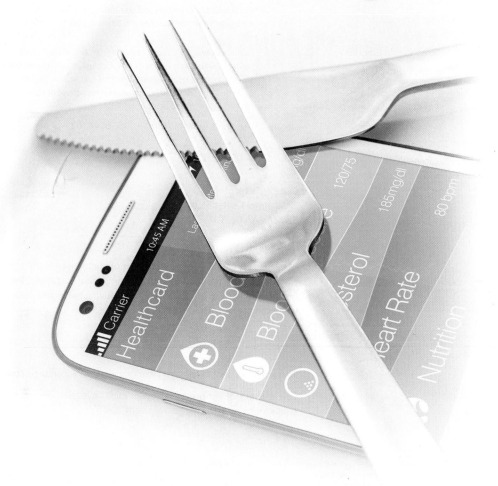

Ruth A. Roth, MS, RDN
&
Kathy L. Wehrle, RDN, CD

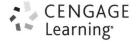

Australia • Brazil • Mexico • Singapore • United Kingdom • United States

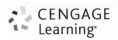
CENGAGE
Learning®

Nutrition & Diet Therapy, **Twelfth Edition**
Ruth A. Roth, Kathy L. Wehrle

SVP, GM Skills & Global Product Management:
Dawn Gerrain

Product Manager: Laura Stewart

Senior Director, Development: Marah
Bellegarde

Product Development Manager: Juliet Steiner

Senior Content Developer: Elisabeth F. Williams

Product Assistant: Deborah Handy

Vice President, Marketing Services: Jennifer
Ann Baker

Senior Marketing Manager: Cassie Cloutier

Senior Production Director: Wendy Troeger

Production Director: Andrew Crouth

Senior Content Project Manager: Kenneth
McGrath

Senior Art Director: Jack Pendleton

Cover image(s): © iStock.com/Chesky_W,
© Shutterstock.com/Spectral-Design

For product information and technology assistance, contact us at
Cengage Learning Customer & Sales Support, 1-800-354-9706

For permission to use material from this text or product,
submit all requests online at **www.cengage.com/permissions.**
Further permissions questions can be e-mailed to
permissionrequest@cengage.com

Library of Congress Control Number: 2016944162

ISBN: 9781305945821

Cengage Learning
20 Channel Center Street
Boston, MA 02210
USA

Cengage Learning is a leading provider of customized learning solutions
with office locations around the globe, including Singapore, the United
Kingdom, Australia, Mexico, Brazil, and Japan. Locate your local office at:
www.cengage.com/global

Cengage Learning products are represented in Canada by Nelson Education, Ltd.

To learn more about Cengage Learning, visit **www.cengage.com**

Purchase any of our products at your local college store or at our preferred
online store **www.cengagebrain.com**

Printed in the United States of America
Print Number: 01 Print Year: 2016

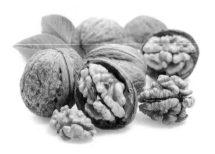

To my family and friends
who love and support me.

Brief Contents

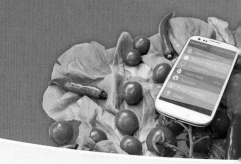

SECTION 1

FUNDAMENTALS OF NUTRITION   1

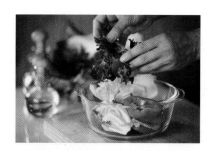

SECTION 2

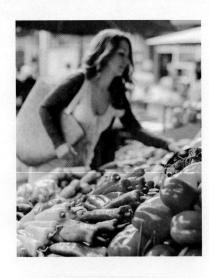

NUTRITION THROUGH THE LIFE CYCLE   169

SECTION 3

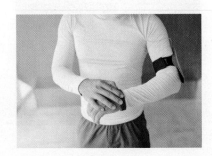

MEDICAL NUTRITION THERAPY   249

Contents

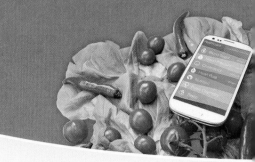

SECTION 1

FUNDAMENTALS OF NUTRITION   1

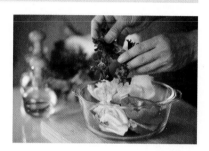

SECTION 2

NUTRITION THROUGH THE LIFE CYCLE   169

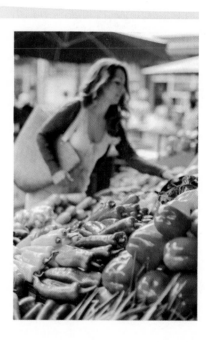

SECTION 3

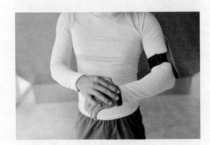

MEDICAL NUTRITION THERAPY 249

Preface

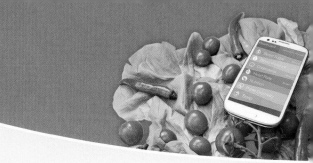

In our health-conscious society, the link between good nutrition and good health is seen everywhere, from magazine and newspaper headlines to television shows, websites, apps, and blogs. The latest diets and stories about foods that claim to prevent certain diseases and health ailments abound. This presents a challenge to nurses working with clients to help them focus on improving both their nutrition and their overall health. *Nutrition & Diet Therapy,* 12th edition, provides sound nutritional information based upon fact. It is important that nurses have a solid foundation in the basic principles and concepts of good nutrition; then they can help clients debunk the myths and help them move toward better health through nutritional awareness.

Section 1, **Fundamentals of Nutrition**, includes chapters on the relationship of nutrition and health; planning a healthy diet; digestion, absorption, and metabolism; as well as chapters on each of the six nutrient groups (carbohydrates, lipids, proteins, vitamins, minerals, and water). Content has been thoroughly revised to embrace the newest MyPlate guidelines.

Section 2, **Nutrition Through the Life Cycle**, includes chapters on nutritional care during the various stages of life, from pregnancy and lactation through infancy, childhood, adolescence, and adulthood. This information provides sound knowledge of the changes in nutritional requirements across the lifespan.

Section 3, **Medical Nutrition Therapy**, includes discussion and research for many nutrition-related disorders. It covers the effects of disease and surgery on nutrition and the appropriate uses of diet therapy in restoring and maintaining health. It includes chapters with specific nutritional information for clients requiring help with weight control, diabetes, cardiovascular disease, renal disease, gastrointestinal problems, and cancer. It also discusses the nutritional needs of surgical clients, clients suffering burns and infections including HIV, and clients requiring enteral and parenteral nutrition. There is also a chapter on foodborne illness, allergies, and intolerances as well as the general nutritional care of clients.

CHAPTER OUTLINE AND FEATURES

Chapters follow a consistent format to help facilitate and enhance learning:

- **Objectives**—learning goals to be achieved upon completion of the chapter

- **Key Terms**—a list of terms used in text and defined in the margin; these are also included in the master glossary

- **In The Media**—boxes highlighting current trends, events, and fads and the potential impact on clients' health
- **Supersize USA**—boxes highlighting information and current events surrounding the national obesity epidemic
- **Exploring the Web**—directions to Internet resources and websites
- **Spotlight on Lifecycle**—boxes focusing on nutritional concerns for the different stages of life
- **Health and Nutrition Considerations**—recommendations for health care professionals to help clients achieve optimal health through the knowledge of nutrition
- **Summary**—a brief narrative overview of the most important chapter highlights
- **Discussion Topics**—critical thinking activities that encourage synthesis and application of new concepts
- **Suggested Activities**—creative suggestions on how to implement the knowledge presented in the chapter
- **Review**—study questions to test understanding of content and to help prepare for examinations
- **Case in Point**—reality-based case studies that apply to the chapter topics, followed up by a "Rate This Plate" challenge that asks for evaluation of a proposed meal plan for a client
- **MyPlate guidelines**—recommended and embraced throughout the text
- **Dietary Guidelines for Americans, 2015–2020**—located in the appendices and throughout the chapters

NEW TO THIS EDITION

- **Chapter 1** *The Relationship of Nutrition and Health* now sheds light on our national targets for health, "Healthy People 2020," and introduces the concept of health disparities, health literacy, and food deserts and their effect on the health of our population. There is new information on the six standard characteristics to diagnose adult malnutrition.
- **Chapter 2** *Planning a Healthy Diet* offers a complete look at the new Dietary Guidelines for Americans 2015–2020, including the five overarching principles in detail. The new proposed food label is compared to the existing label to highlight improvements.
- **Chapter 14** *Weight Management Across the Life Cycle* includes the latest on weight regulation, obesity trends in children and adults, and inflammation as a root cause of obesity. The health consequences of being overweight are discussed as well as the latest prevention and treatment strategies for successful diet therapy. The newer behavioral techniques of motivational interviewing, coaching, mindfulness, and readiness for change are highlighted as well. There is important information on the newer weight loss drugs and a snapshot of surgical treatment for obesity including bariatric surgery, as well as the new gastric balloon placement.

- **Chapter 15** *Diet, Prediabetes, and Diabetes* includes new information on the growing problem of prediabetes. Up-to-date statistics and diagnostic criteria are presented as well as the latest list of oral medications and insulin currently available to treat diabetes. There is a new list of alternative sweeteners and their pros and cons.

- **Chapter 18** *Diet and Gastrointestinal Disorders* includes current information on celiac disease and the growing incidence of gluten sensitivity, as well as new information about irritable and short bowel syndrome.

- **In The Media** boxes have been refreshed throughout the chapters to keep students up to speed on current events and fads in nutrition and health-related topics.

- Updated **Recommended Dietary Allowances (RDA)** and **Daily Recommended Intake (DRI)** can be found in tables throughout the book.

- The **MyPlate** method gives guidelines for intake of nutrients with various calorie levels. Information about the MyPlate method is introduced in Chapter 2, and is referenced throughout the text.

- **Supersize USA** boxes have been refreshed to bring current nutrition concerns to the forefront and to generate discussion in the classroom.

- *Dietary Guidelines for Americans, 2015–2020* has been updated with current recommendations for nutritional intake and exercise.

LEARNING PACKAGE FOR THE STUDENT

MindTap

MindTap is the first of its kind in an entirely new category: the Personal Learning Experience (PLE). This personalized program of digital products and services uses interactivity and customization to engage students, while offering a range of choice in content, platforms, devices, and learning tools. MindTap is device agnostic, meaning that it will work with any platform or learning management system and will be accessible anytime, anywhere: on desktops, laptops, tablets, mobile phones, and other Internet-enabled devices. MindTap can be accessed at http://www.CengageBrain.com. *Nutrition & Diet Therapy,* 12th edition, on MindTap includes:

- An interactive eBook with highlighting, note-taking functions, and more

- Self-quizzes, multiple-choice questions, and exercises

- Client scenarios

- Flashcards for practicing chapter terms

- Video scenarios

- NCLEX-style quizzing

- Diet & Wellness app

TEACHING PACKAGE FOR THE INSTRUCTOR

Instructor Resources

The *Instructor Resources to Accompany Nutrition & Diet Therapy*, 12th edition, contains a variety of online tools to help instructors successfully prepare lectures and teach within this subject area. This comprehensive package provides something for all instructors, from those teaching nutrition for the first time to seasoned instructors who want something new. The following components in the website are free to adopters of the text:

- A downloadable, customizable *Instructor's Manual* containing suggested learning and teaching strategies, additional discussion questions, answers to the text Review Questions, and suggested responses to the Case in Point/Rate This Plate features.

- A *Computerized Test Bank* with several hundred questions and answers, for use in instructor-created quizzes and tests.

- Chapter slides created in PowerPoint® to use for in-class lecture material and as handouts for students.

MindTap

In the new *Nutrition & Diet Therapy,* 12th edition, on MindTap platform, instructors customize the learning path by selecting Cengage Learning resources and adding their own content via apps that seamlessly integrate the MindTap framework with many learning management systems. The guided learning path demonstrates the relevance of basic principles in nutrition through engagement activities, interactive exercises, and real-world scenarios, elevating the study by challenging students to apply concepts to practice. To learn more, visit www.cengage.com/mindtap.

Acknowledgments

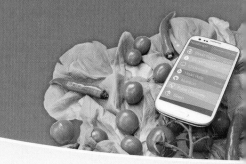

The authors wish to express their appreciation to the following people:

Lauren Mullins
Leigh Ann Brooks
Dayanne Writtenhouse
Mary Tippman Harter
Kyla Zehr
Kylee Bennett
Beth Williams
Jill Ostrem

Contributor to Case in Point Features and Diabetes chapter
Leigh Ann Brooks, RN, RD, CDE
Certified Diabetes Educator

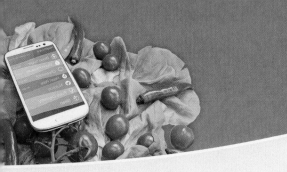

Reviewers

Diane Cohen, RN, MSN
Professor
MassBay Community College
Framingham, Massachusetts

Kelly Collins, MA
Teacher
Tulare Adult School, Tulare Joint Union High School District
Tulare, California

Sarah Darrell, BSN, RN, CNOR
Adjunct Faculty
Ivy Tech
Valparaiso, Indiana

Kathryn P. Jackman-Murphy, RN, MSN
Professor
Naugatuck Valley Community College
Waterbury, Connecticut

Susan Kinney, RN, BSN, CNOR, RMA, COI
Department Head, Health Science
Piedmont Technical College
Greenwood, South Carolina

Jennifer Lipke, RN, MSN
Nursing Faculty
Hibbing Community College
Hibbing, Minnesota

Renee Pilcher, PhD, RN
Assistant Professor of Nursing and Health
Clarke University
Dubuque, Iowa

Monica M. Pusater, RN, MSN
Faculty
Ohio Valley College of Technology
East Liverpool, Ohio

How to Use This Text

OBJECTIVES

Read the chapter Objectives before reading the chapter content to set the stage for learning. Return to the Objectives when the chapter study is complete to see which entries you can respond to with "Yes, I can do that."

KEY TERMS

Glance over this list of terms before you tackle the chapter. Flip through the pages to check the definitions in the margins and make a list of those terms that are unfamiliar.

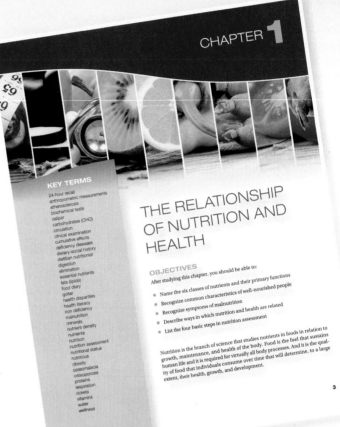

SUPERSIZE USA

Obesity has become a national health epidemic. Read over these boxes to find out why and also for suggestions on what you, as a consumer and as a nurse, can do to help curb this trend.

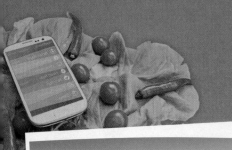

SPOTLIGHT on Life Cycle

Does breastfeeding a child lessen its chances of obesity later in childhood? Several studies have indicated that breastfed infants have a lower risk of childhood obesity than that of formula-fed infants while other studies have not reported a clear association. A large review study was undertaken in 2014 to provide a thorough look at the latest research. Twenty-five studies were reviewed from 1997 to 2014, with over 200,000 participants from 12 countries. This analysis revealed a dose-response effect between breastfeeding duration and reduced risk of childhood obesity and showed in particular that children breastfed for >7 months are significantly less likely to be obese in later childhood.

SPOTLIGHT ON LIFE CYCLE

Nutritional concerns and needs will change at each stage of life. Test your knowledge of the needs of children, adolescents, pregnant women, and the elderly.

In The Media

Sitting Is a Negative Even If You Work Out

According to the World Health Organization, physical inactivity has been identified as the fourth-leading risk factor for death. Sedentary behavior can lead to cardiovascular disease, cancer, and diabetes. Researchers from Toronto analyzed 47 studies of sedentary behavior. Data was adjusted to incorporate the amount someone exercises in a day; however, researchers still found that the amount of sedentary time engaged in outweighed the benefit from exercise. Tactics to help you sit less include taking frequent breaks during the work day to stretch and walk, and decreasing TV time or taking time to stand up during commercial breaks.

IN THE MEDIA

Which of these "hot topics" do you already know something about? Check here for current trends, events, and fads, and understand the potential impact on clients' health.

Exploring THE WEB

Search the Web for information on protein supplements. What are some of the claims of these products? Are they based on solid research and fact? Create fact sheets on protein supplements citing common myths and providing the truth behind the myths. How would you approach a person inquiring about the use of protein supplements?

EXPLORING THE WEB

Be sure to visit these websites for more depth on chapter topics. These are also excellent sources for information to make care plans and teaching guides.

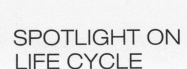

CASE IN POINT

Two case studies conclude each chapter. Read these real-life stories, then look at the sample diet and **Rate This Plate**. Visit CengageBrain.com to see how your answers match up to those of the experts.

CASE IN POINT
JAYDEN: COPING WITH MALNUTRITION

Jayden was living in an apartment with his mother Trina until recently when he was removed and placed in foster care. Jayden's aunt had contacted Child Protective Services because she was concerned about her sister's mental health and ability to care for Jayden. Jayden is only 5 years old and his mother Trina has multiple mental illnesses. Trina was diagnosed as a paranoid schizophrenic and has been on and off her medication depending on whether or not she can afford to purchase it. It was not uncommon for Trina to leave for extended periods of time without thought to Jayden's well-being. He often was without food, sufficient clothing, and clean surroundings. When Trina was home, she was often sleeping and Jayden was still left to fend for himself. When the social worker arrived at the home, she found it to be in disarray. There was very little food in the kitchen and trash and clutter was throughout the home. Jayden was found to be very thin, pale, and unclean. Jayden measured only 40 inches tall and weighed 30 pounds. The social worker noticed sores on his body, and his abdomen appeared to be very swollen. She took an informal diet recall the previous 24 hours and saw poor diet quality and gaps in eating. Jayden was complaining of pain in his legs and was having a difficult time walking. The social worker took Jayden to the emergency room for assessment and arranged for a foster family to be assigned to him.

SUMMARY

This brief narrative overview of the most important chapter highlights is ideal for testing your grasp of the chapter material. Always start your study sessions with a quick glance at the Summary to refresh your memory on the basics of the chapter.

SUMMARY

Nutrition is directly related to health, and its effects are cumulative. Good nutrition is normally reflected by good health. Poor nutrition can result in poor health and even in disease. Poor nutrition habits contribute to atherosclerosis, osteoporosis, obesity, diabetes, and some cancers.

To be well nourished, one must eat foods that contain the six essential nutrients: carbohydrates, fats, proteins, minerals, vitamins, and water. These nutrients provide the body with energy, build and repair body tissue, and regulate body processes. When there is a severe lack of specific nutrients, deficiency diseases may develop. The best way to determine deficiencies is to do a nutrition assessment.

With sound knowledge of nutrition, the health professional will be an effective health care provider and will also be helpful to family, friends, and self.

DISCUSSION TOPICS

Critical thinking is the key to your success as a nurse. Use these activities to synthesize and apply what you have read and learned.

DISCUSSION TOPICS

1. Think about possible health disparities in your area. What have been the contributing factors? What are some solutions?
2. What relationship might nutrition and heredity have to each of the following?
   a. development of physique
   b. ability to resist disease
   c. life span
3. What habits, in addition to good nutrition, contribute to making a person healthy?
4. What are the six classes of nutrients? What are their three basic functions?
5. Why are some foods called low-nutrient-density foods? Give some examples found in vending machines.
6. Explore why it is important to support the nutrition care of a hospitalized patient from a nursing standpoint especially as it relates to malnutrition.
7. What is meant by the saying "You are what you eat"? Give specific examples of how the food we eat can affect our body and long-term consequences.
8. What is meant by the phrase "the cumulative effects of nutrition"? Describe some.
9. How could someone be overweight and at the same time suffer from malnutrition?
10. Discuss why health care professionals should be knowledgeable about nutrition.

SUGGESTED ACTIVITIES

Put your knowledge to the test; see how many of these activities you can successfully complete once you finish studying the chapter. Make a list of any areas needing additional attention.

SUGGESTED ACTIVITIES

1. List 10 signs of good nutrition and 10 signs of poor nutrition.
2. List the foods you have eaten in the past 24 hours. Underline those with low nutrient density.
3. Write a brief description of how you feel at the end of a day when you know you have not eaten
5. Write a brief paragraph discussing the nutrition assessment by a dietitian and its importance.
6. Briefly describe rickets, osteomalacia, and osteoporosis. Include their causes.
7. Ask a registered dietitian to speak to your class about nutrition problems commonly seen in your area.

REVIEW

These study questions are in multiple-choice format, perfect for preparing for your nursing examinations.

REVIEW

Multiple choice. Select the *letter* that precedes the best answer.

1. The result of those processes whereby the body takes in and uses food for growth, development, and maintenance of health is
   a. respiration
   b. diet therapy
   c. nutrition
   d. digestion
2. Nutritional status is determined by
   a. heredity
   b. employment
   c. personality
9. A cumulative condition is one that develops
   a. within a very short period of time
   b. over several years
   c. only in women under 52
   d. in premature infants
10. Malnutrition is assessed by
   a. food records and measurement of vitamin status
   b. how fast weight has been lost and if there is diarrhea
   c. disease progression and blood pressure instability
   d. weight loss, muscle and fat loss, strength of handgrip, and edema

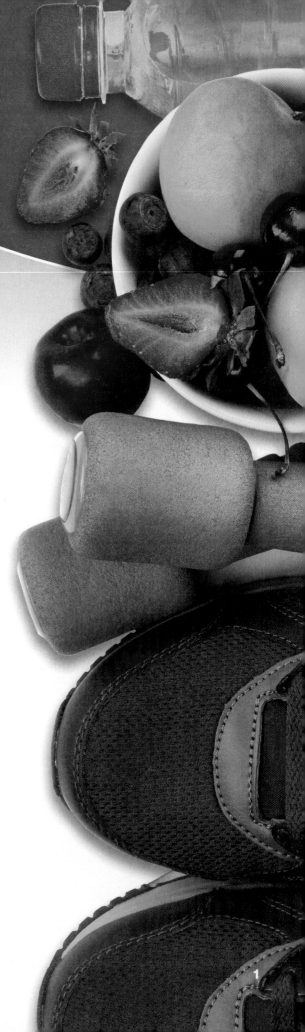

Fundamentals of Nutrition

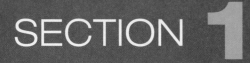

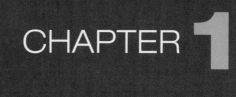

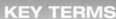

KEY TERMS

24-hour recall
anthropometric measurements
atherosclerosis
biochemical tests
caliper
carbohydrates (CHO)
circulation
clinical examination
cumulative effects
deficiency diseases
dietary-social history
dietitian nutritionist
digestion
elimination
essential nutrients
fats (lipids)
food diary
goiter
health disparities
health literacy
iron deficiency
malnutrition
minerals
nutrient density
nutrients
nutrition
nutrition assessment
nutritional status
nutritious
obesity
osteomalacia
osteoporosis
proteins
respiration
rickets
vitamins
water
wellness

THE RELATIONSHIP OF NUTRITION AND HEALTH

OBJECTIVES

After studying this chapter, you should be able to:

- Name the six classes of nutrients and their primary functions
- Recognize common characteristics of well-nourished people
- Recognize symptoms of malnutrition
- Describe ways in which nutrition and health are related
- List the four basic steps in nutrition assessment

Nutrition is the branch of science that studies nutrients in foods in relation to growth, maintenance, and health of the body. Food is the fuel that sustains human life and it is required for virtually all body processes. And it is the quality of food that individuals consume over time that will determine, to a large extent, their health, growth, and development.

Now more than ever, science has upheld the strong influence diet has on health. Many chronic diseases such as diabetes, heart disease, and stroke are known to be largely preventable and attributed to poor diet and lifestyle habits. As a future clinician, you will likely begin to understand the urgency with which active measures need to be taken to make our social, cultural, political, and economic environment in relation to diet a health-promoting one.

For three decades, national health targets have been set. *Healthy People* is the foundational government platform that provides national objectives every 10 years for improving the health and welfare of all Americans. *Healthy People* serves to empower individuals to make informed decisions, encourages collaboration in communities for health-related behaviors, and serves to measure the impact of such strategies. *Healthy People 2020* has set targets for our nation to reach on leading health indicators that include obesity in children and adults, physical activity, and fruit and vegetable consumption. Growing attention is being given to the environmental and social determinants of health; therefore, the overarching goals of *Healthy People 2020* also include achievement of **health literacy** and equity with an elimination of **health disparities**.

Taking care of one's health is all about prevention. In the past, the focus was on treatment of diseases, with little, if any, attention to prevention. Prevention, however, can often be less costly than treatment and offers a better quality of life for an individual as well as the community. Nutrition and diet choice form a logical starting point for preventive health care measures and education to improve quality of life.

Achieving **wellness** is an active process by which individuals make informed choices toward a more successful existence. Wellness is a state of optimal well-being, not just the absence of disease. It is multidimensional and lends itself to a holistic perspective of the person in terms of mind, body, and spirit. This can be accomplished through lifestyle changes such as focusing on healthy food choices, not smoking, participating in regular physical activity, and maintaining a healthy weight. Expanding one's mind through continued education, in both nutrition and other areas, and finding a source of inner strength to deal with life changes will all contribute to one's sense of wellness.

Living a long life without major health problems is possible. The younger one is when positive changes are made, the healthier one is throughout the life span.

health literacy
the capacity to obtain, process, and understand basic health information needed to make appropriate health decisions

health disparities
a difference in health outcomes among subgroups often linked to social, economic, or environmental disadvantages

wellness
a state of physical, mental, and social well-being

nutrients
chemical substances found in food that are necessary for good health

essential nutrients
nutrients found only in food

NUTRIENTS AND THEIR FUNCTIONS

To maintain health and function properly, the body must be provided with **nutrients**. Nutrients are chemical substances that are necessary for life. They are divided into six classes:

- Carbohydrates (CHO)
- Fats (lipids)
- Proteins
- Vitamins
- Minerals
- Water

The body can make small amounts of some nutrients, but most must be obtained from food in order to meet the body's needs. Those available only in food are called **essential nutrients**. There are about 40 of them, and they are found in all six nutrient classes.

TABLE 1-1 The Six Essential Nutrients and Their Functions

ORGANIC NUTRIENTS	FUNCTION
Carbohydrates	Provide energy
Fats	Provide energy
Proteins	Build and repair body tissues; provide energy
Vitamins	Regulate body processes
INORGANIC NUTRIENTS	**FUNCTION**
Minerals	Regulate body processes
Water	Regulates body processes

The six nutrient classes are chemically divided into two categories: organic and inorganic (Table 1-1). Organic nutrients contain hydrogen, oxygen, and carbon. (Carbon is an element found in all living things.) Before the body can use organic nutrients, it must break them down into their smallest components. Inorganic nutrients are already in their simplest forms when the body ingests them, except for water.

Each nutrient participates in at least one of the following functions:

- Providing the body with energy
- Building and repairing body tissue
- Regulating body processes

Carbohydrates (CHO), proteins, and fats (lipids) furnish energy. Proteins are also used to build and repair body tissues with the help of vitamins and minerals. Vitamins, minerals, and water help regulate the various body processes such as circulation, respiration, digestion, and elimination.

Each nutrient is important, but none works alone. For example, carbohydrates, proteins, and fats are necessary for energy, but to provide it, they need the help of vitamins, minerals, and water. Proteins are essential for building and repairing body tissue, but without vitamins, minerals, and water, they are ineffective. Consuming foods rich in the antioxidant vitamins such as C, E, and beta-carotene may help to enhance your immune system. Foods that contain substantial amounts of nutrients are described as nutritious. Nutrients are discussed in detail in Chapters 4 through 9.

CHARACTERISTICS OF GOOD NUTRITION

Most people find pleasure in eating. Eating allows one to connect with family and friends in pleasant surroundings. This connection creates pleasant memories. Unfortunately, in social situations, it is easy for one to make food choices that may not be conducive to good health.

What determines when one needs to eat? Does one wait until the body signals hunger or eat when one sees food or when the clock says it is time? Hunger is the physiological need for food. Appetite is a psychological desire for food based on pleasant memories. When the body signals hunger, it indicates a decrease in blood glucose levels that supply the body with energy. If one ignores the signal and hunger becomes intense, it is possible to make poor food choices. The choices one makes will determine one's nutrition status. A person who habitually chooses to overeat, or not eat, as a way of coping with life's emotional

carbohydrates (CHO)
the nutrient class providing the major source of energy in the average diet

proteins
the only one of the six essential nutrient classes containing nitrogen

fats (lipids)
highest calorie-value nutrient class

vitamins
organic substances necessary for life although they do not, independently, provide energy

minerals
one of many inorganic substances essential to life

water
major constituent of all living cells; composed of hydrogen and oxygen

circulation
the body process whereby the blood is moved throughout the body

respiration
breathing

digestion
breakdown of food in the body in preparation for absorption

elimination
evacuation of wastes

nutritious
foods or beverages containing substantial amounts of essential nutrients

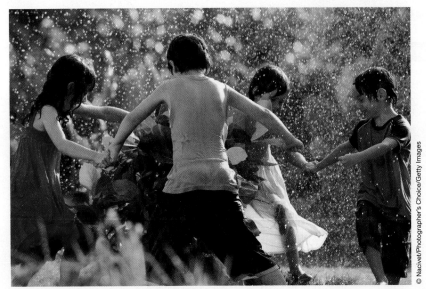
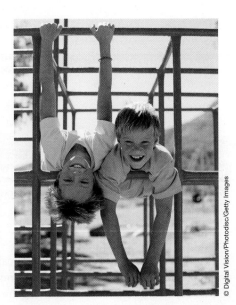

FIGURE 1-1 Good nutrition shows in the happy faces of these children.

struggles may be suffering from an eating disorder. The various eating disorders will be discussed in Chapter 14.

Once food has been eaten, the body must process it before it can be used. **Nutrition** is the result of the processes whereby the body takes in and uses food for growth, development, and the maintenance of health. These processes include digestion, absorption, and metabolism. (They are discussed in Chapter 3.) One's physical condition as determined by diet is called **nutritional status**.

Nutrition helps determine the height and weight of an individual. Nutrition can also affect the body's ability to resist disease, the length of one's life, and the state of one's physical and mental well-being (Figure 1-1).

Good nutrition enhances appearance and is commonly exemplified by shiny hair, clear skin, clear eyes, erect posture, alert expressions, and firm flesh on well-developed bone structures. Good nutrition aids emotional health, provides stamina, and promotes a healthy appetite. It also helps establish regular sleep and elimination habits (Table 1-2).

nutrition
the result of those processes whereby the body takes in and uses food for growth, development, and the maintenance of health

nutritional status
one's physical condition as determined by diet

TABLE 1-2 Characteristics of Nutritional Status

GOOD	POOR
Alert expression	Apathy
Shiny hair	Dull, lifeless hair
Clear complexion with good color	Greasy, blemished complexion with poor color
Bright, clear eyes	Dull, red-rimmed eyes
Pink, firm gums and well-developed teeth	Red, puffy, receding gums and missing or cavity-prone teeth
Firm abdomen	Swollen abdomen
Firm, well-developed muscles and strength	Flaccid, wasted muscle, weakness, and diminished handgrip strength
Well-developed bone structure	Bowed legs, "pigeon" chest
Normal weight for height	Overweight or underweight, recent weight loss
Erect posture	Slumped posture
Emotional stability	Easily irritated; depressed; poor attention span
Good stamina; seldom ill	Easily fatigued; frequently ill
Healthy appetite	Excessive or poor appetite
Healthy, normal sleep habits	Insomnia at night; fatigued during day
Normal elimination	Constipation or diarrhea

MALNUTRITION

Malnutrition is a condition that results when the body does not receive enough nutrients: the body's cells do not receive an adequate supply of the essential nutrients because of poor diet intake or poor utilization of food. It can occur when individuals do not or cannot eat enough of the foods that provide the essential nutrients to satisfy body needs (undernutrition). Even though we think of an individual with malnutrition being at a low body weight, normal weight or even obese individuals can suffer some degree of malnourishment if their diet is of poor nutrition quality. Overweight and obese individuals with overnutrition, who develop a severe acute illness or experience a major traumatic event, are at risk for malnutrition and need intensive nutrition intervention. At other times, people may eat well-balanced diets but they may suffer from diseases of digestion or absorption that prevent normal usage of the nutrients. Malnutrition is critical to identify, as it is a major contributor to increased morbidity and mortality and increased frequency and length of hospital stay.

Nutrient Deficiency

A nutrient deficiency occurs when a person lacks one or more nutrients over a period of time. Nutrient deficiencies are classified as primary or secondary. Primary deficiencies are caused by inadequate dietary intake. Secondary deficiencies are caused by something other than diet, such as a disease condition that may cause malabsorption, accelerated excretion, or destruction of the nutrients. Nutrient deficiencies can result in malnutrition.

INDIVIDUALS AT RISK FROM POOR NUTRITIONAL INTAKE

Individuals of all ages and from all walks of life could be at risk of poor nutrition intake. Persons with recent illness, hospitalizations, or surgery likely experience a disruption in their intake that poses risk. Others may meet or exceed energy intake, but consume foods that are of low nutrient quality. Foods with low **nutrient density** provide an abundance of calories, but the nutrients are primarily carbohydrates (especially added sugars) and fats and, except for sodium, provide very limited amounts of proteins, vitamins, and minerals.

Some individuals may have heightened risk of poor nutritional intake due to budget concerns that preclude them from purchasing nourishing foods. Some lack access to healthy food simply because of their geographic location. It is known that approximately 29 million Americans lack access to healthy, affordable foods. These individuals live in a food desert, which means they do not have a grocery store within 1 mile of their home if they live in an urban area, or within 10 miles if they live in a rural area. Those individuals living in lower-income neighborhoods seem to suffer the most diet-related disease and obesity. The National Health and Nutrition Examination Survey (NHANES), which tracks the health and nutrition status of our population, is a source of information that highlights the sobering disparities in health seen in communities across America.

We think of teenagers as being a generally healthy lot; however, teenagers may eat often but at unusual hours. They may miss regularly scheduled meals, become hungry, and satisfy their hunger with foods that have low nutrient density, such as potato chips, cakes, soda, and candy. Teenagers are subject to peer pressure; that is, they are easily influenced by the opinions of their friends. If friends favor foods with low nutrient density, it can be difficult for a teenager not to go along with them. Fad diets, which unfortunately are common among teens, sometimes

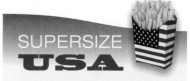

SUPERSIZE USA

Supersizing in the fast food industry and large quantities served in restaurants lead to portion distortion. Those growing up in the supersized world may have no concept of what constitutes a normal portion. Children who are encouraged to, or have been made to, eat everything on their plates may feel compelled to finish their supersized meals, easily contributing to obesity and type 2 diabetes.

malnutrition
any nutrition imbalance

nutrient density
nutrient value of foods compared with number of calories

SPOTLIGHT *on Life Cycle*

Infants, young children, teenage girls, and adults are at risk for iron-deficiency anemia. Full-term infants are born with enough iron stores to last four to six months. A premature infant is at even greater risk for iron-deficiency anemia. Baby foods and cereals are fortified with iron to help prevent iron deficiency in young children. Underweight teens or teenage girls who have heavy monthly periods are at increased risk for iron-deficiency anemia. Women of child-bearing age are also at risk. Pregnant women are prone to anemia due to the increased need for iron during pregnancy. A supplement that is higher in iron may be prescribed for pregnant women. Internal bleeding can lead to iron-deficiency anemia due to blood loss. Clients who have undergone kidney dialysis or gastric bypass surgery are also at an increased risk. Treatments include dietary changes and supplements, medicines, and surgery.

Source: Adapted from "Who Is at Risk for Iron-Deficiency Anemia?" National Heart, Lung, and Blood Institute. U.S. Department of Health and Human Services. 2014. http://www.nhlbi.nih.gov

Exploring THE WEB

Search the Web to find information on osteomalacia and osteoporosis. What are the leading causes? Should you take a calcium plus vitamin D supplement?

result in a form of malnutrition. This condition occurs because some nutrients are eliminated from the diet when the types of foods eaten are severely restricted.

Pregnancy increases a woman's hunger and the need for certain nutrients, especially proteins, minerals, and vitamins. Pregnancy during adolescence requires extreme care in food selection. The young mother-to-be requires a diet that provides sufficient nutrients for the developing fetus as well as for her own still-growing body.

Many factors influence nutrition in the elderly. Depression, loneliness, lack of income, inability to shop, inability to prepare meals, and the state of overall health can all lead to malnutrition.

CUMULATIVE EFFECTS OF NUTRITION

There is an increasing concern among health professionals regarding the **cumulative effects** of nutrition. Cumulative effects are the results of something that is done repeatedly over many years. For example, eating excessive amounts of saturated fats (saturated fats are discussed in Chapter 5) for many years contributes to **atherosclerosis**, which leads to heart attacks. Years of overeating can cause **obesity** and may also contribute to hypertension, type 2 (noninsulin-dependent) diabetes, gallbladder disease, foot problems, certain cancers, and even personality disorders.

Deficiency Diseases

When nutrients are seriously lacking in the diet for an extended period, **deficiency diseases** can occur. The most common form of deficiency disease in the United States is **iron deficiency**, which is caused by a lack of the mineral iron and can cause iron-deficiency anemia, which is discussed further in Chapter 8. Iron deficiency is particularly common among children and women. Iron is a necessary component of the blood and is lost during each menstrual period. In addition, the amount of iron needed during childhood and pregnancy is greater than normal because of the growth of the child or the fetus.

cumulative effects
results of something done repeatedly over many years

atherosclerosis
a form of arteriosclerosis affecting the intima (inner lining) of the artery walls

obesity
excessive body fat and BMI over 30

deficiency diseases
diseases caused by the lack of one or more specific nutrients

iron deficiency
a condition in which the body does not have enough usable iron due to inadequate intake, bleeding, or absorption problems

TABLE 1-3 Nutritional Deficiency Diseases and Possible Causes

DEFICIENCY DISEASE	NUTRIENT(S) LACKING
Iron deficiency	Iron
Iron-deficiency anemia	Iron
Beriberi	Thiamin
Night blindness	Vitamin A
Goiter	Iodine
Kwashiorkor	Protein
Marasmus	All nutrients
Osteoporosis	Calcium and vitamin D
Osteomalacia	Calcium and vitamin D, phosphorus, magnesium, and fluoride
Pellagra	Niacin
Rickets	Calcium and vitamin D
Scurvy	Vitamin C
Xerophthalmia (blindness)	Vitamin A

Rickets is another example of a deficiency disease. It causes poor bone formation in children and is due to insufficient calcium and vitamin D. The same deficiencies cause osteomalacia in young adults and osteoporosis in older adults. Osteomalacia is sometimes called "adult rickets." It causes the bones to soften and may cause the spine to bend and the legs to become bowed. Osteoporosis is a condition that causes bones to become porous and excessively brittle. Too little iodine may cause goiter, and a severe shortage of vitamin A can lead to blindness.

Examples of other deficiency diseases (and their causes) are included in Table 1-3. Information concerning these conditions can be found in the chapters devoted to the given nutrients.

NUTRITION ASSESSMENT

That old saying, "You are what you eat," is true, indeed; but one could change it a bit to read, "You are *and will be* what you eat." Good nutrition is essential for the attainment and maintenance of good health. In a clinical setting, determining whether a person is at risk requires completion of a nutrition assessment, which should be part of a routine examination done by a registered dietitian nutritionist (RDN) or other health care professional specifically trained in the diagnosis of at-risk individuals. A proper nutrition assessment includes anthropometric measurements, clinical examination, biochemical tests, and dietary-social history. Collected data guides the RDN to make the appropriate nutrition diagnosis using the nutrition care model. Interventions are then instituted with follow-up monitoring and evaluation.

Anthropometric measurements include height and weight and measurements of the head (for children), chest, and skinfold (Figure 1-2). The skinfold measurements are done with a caliper. They are used to determine the percentage of adipose and muscle tissue in the body. Measurements out of line with expectations may reveal failure to thrive in children, wasting (catabolism), edema, or obesity, all of which reflect nutrient deficiencies or excesses.

rickets
deficiency disease caused by the lack of vitamin D; causes malformed bones and pain in infants and children

osteomalacia
a condition in which bones become soft, usually in adults because of calcium loss and vitamin D deficiency

osteoporosis
condition in which bones become brittle because there have been insufficient mineral deposits, especially calcium

goiter
enlarged tissue of the thyroid gland due to a deficiency of iodine

nutrition assessment
evaluation of one's nutritional condition

dietitian nutritionist (RDN)
professionals who translate the science of nutrition into practical solutions for improved health

anthropometric measurements
of height, weight, head, chest, skinfold

clinical examination
physical observation

biochemical tests
laboratory analysis of blood, urine, and feces

dietary-social history
evaluation of food habits, including client's ability to buy and prepare food

caliper
mechanical device used to measure percentage of body fat by skinfold measurement

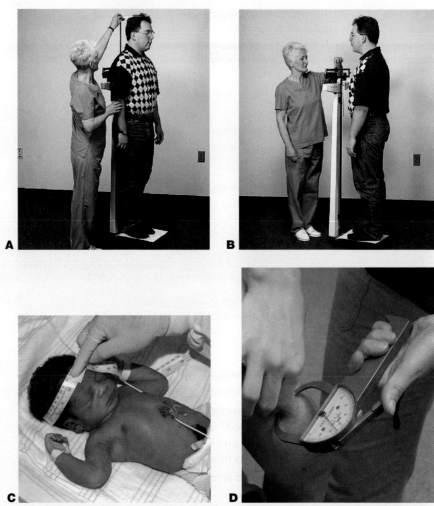

FIGURE 1-2 (A) Height is one anthropometric measurement used in the nutrition assessment. (B) Weight is an anthropometric measurement used in the nutrition assessment. (C) Head circumference is an anthropometric measurement used to assess brain development during the first year of life. (D) Skinfold is an anthropometric measurement used to assess lean muscle mass versus fat.

During the clinical examination, signs of nutrient deficiencies are noted. Some nutrient deficiency diseases, such as scurvy, rickets, iron deficiency, and kwashiorkor, are obvious; other forms of nutrient deficiency can be far more subtle. Table 1-4 lists some clinical signs and probable causes of nutrient deficiencies.

Biochemical tests include various blood, urine, and stool tests. A deficiency or toxicity can be determined by laboratory analysis of the samples. There are a variety of blood tests the registered dietitian nutritionist evaluates when completing the nutrition assessment. Blood urea nitrogen (BUN) may indicate renal failure, insufficient renal blood supply, or blockage of the urinary tract. Serum creatinine is used for evaluating renal function. A 24-hour creatinine excretion test can be used in estimating muscle mass loss. Other evaluations include the hemoglobin (Hgb), hematocrit (Hct), red blood cell (RBC), and white blood cell (WBC) tests. A low Hgb and Hct can indicate anemia. Clients with heart conditions may have a lipid profile ordered, which includes total serum cholesterol, high-density lipoprotein (HDL), low-density lipoprotein (LDL), and serum triglycerides. Urinalysis also can detect protein and sugar in the urine, which can

TABLE 1-4 Clinical Signs of Nutrient Deficiencies

CLINICAL SIGN	POSSIBLE DEFICIENCIES
Pallor; blue half circles beneath eyes	Iron, copper, zinc, B12, B6, biotin
Edema	Protein
Bumpy "gooseflesh"	Vitamin A
Lesions at corners of mouth	Riboflavin
Glossitis	Folic acid
Numerous "black-and-blue"	Vitamin C spots and tiny, red "pinprick" hemorrhages under skin
Emaciation	Carbohydrates, proteins; calories
Poorly shaped bones or teeth	Vitamin D or calcium or delayed appearance of teeth in children
Slow clotting time of blood	Vitamin K
Unusual nervousness, dermatitis	Niacin diarrhea in some client
Tetany	Calcium, potassium, sodium
Goiter	Iodine
Eczema	Fat (linoleic acid)

indicate kidney disease and diabetes. The hemoglobin A1c and/or fasting blood sugar test is used to determine blood glucose control (see Chapter 15).

While the blood tests albumin and prealbumin have long been used as diagnostic indicators of malnutrition, evidence has shown in recent years that these acute phase proteins do not consistently indicate malnutrition but rather are a function of the severity of the inflammatory response. Because of this, these values should be interpreted with caution. In May of 2012, the Academy of Nutrition and Dietetics published a consensus statement in the *Journal of Parenteral and Enteral Nutrition* to offer six standardized characteristics, with parameters, to diagnose adult malnutrition. In sum, they are:

- Insufficient energy intake
- Weight loss
- Loss of muscle mass
- Loss of subcutaneous fat
- Localized or generalized fluid accumulation (that may sometimes mask weight loss)
- Diminished functional status as measured by handgrip strength

The dietary-social history involves evaluation of food habits and is very important in the nutritional assessment of any client. It can be difficult to obtain an accurate dietary assessment. The most common method is the 24-hour recall. In this method, the client is usually interviewed by the dietitian and asked to give the types of, amounts of, and preparation used for all food eaten in the 24 hours prior to admission. Another method is the food diary. The client is asked to list all foods as they are eaten in a three- to four-day period. Neither method is totally accurate because clients forget or are not always truthful about their eating habits. They are sometimes inclined to say they have eaten certain foods because they know they should have done so. Computer analysis of the diet is the best way to determine if nutrient intake is appropriate. It will reveal any nutrient deficiencies or toxicities.

In The Media

Thriving Grocery Chain in Philadelphia Food Deserts

As there are more than 6,500 food deserts in America, innovative approaches are being taken to offer access to healthier foods to curb our nation's obesity epidemic. Brown's Super Stores now have opened seven profitable supermarkets in low-income neighborhoods in and around Philadelphia. The key success factor was getting input from community leaders as to what they wanted in a neighborhood grocery store.

Source: Adapted from "Why One Grocery Store Chain Is Thriving in Philadelphia's Food Deserts." National Public Radio. May 14, 2015. http://www.npr.org

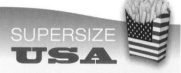

SUPERSIZE USA

Where do you live? Is your state one of the least active in the country? Don't know? Check this list of the 10 least active states, in descending order:

1. Mississippi
2. Tennessee
3. Arkansas
4. Oklahoma
5. Louisiana
6. Alabama
7. West Virginia
8. Indiana
9. Kentucky
10. Texas

Source: State Indicator Report on Physical Activity. 2014. http://www.cdc.gov

24-hour recall
listing the types, amounts, and preparation of all foods eaten in the past 24 hours

food diary
written record of all food and drink ingested in a specified period

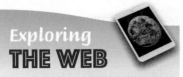
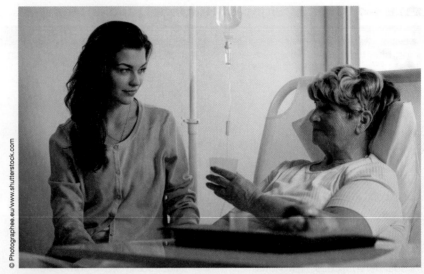

FIGURE 1-3 Nutritional intervention can improve hospital patients' outcomes.

The dietary-social history is important to determine whether the client has the financial resources to obtain the needed food and the ability to properly store and cook food once home. After completing the dietary-social history, the dietitian can assess for risk of food–drug interactions that can lead to malnutrition (see Appendix D). Clients need to be instructed by a dietitian on possible interactions, if any.

When the preceding steps are evaluated together, and in the context of the client's medical condition, the dietitian has the best opportunity of making an accurate nutrition assessment of the client. This assessment can then be used by the entire health care team. The doctor will find it helpful in evaluating the client's condition and treatment. The dietitian can use the information to plan the client's dietary treatment and counseling, and other health care professionals will be able to use it in assisting and counseling the client.

HEALTH AND NUTRITION CONSIDERATIONS

Nutrition is a foundational part of an individual's well-being. Positive diet and lifestyle changes promote vibrant health and can help reduce the risk of chronic disease. During health issues that result in nutrition impairment, timely assessment and quality nutrition intervention can improve outcomes (Figure 1-3). The health professional is obligated to have a sound knowledge of nutrition. Not only do your future clients depend on it, but so does your own personal health, as well as that of your family. Parents must have a good, basic knowledge of nutrition for the sake of their personal health and that of their children. Anyone, in fact, who plans and prepares meals should value, have knowledge of, and be able to apply the principles of sound nutrition practice.

Clients will have questions and complaints about their diets. Their anxieties can be relieved by clear and simple explanations provided by the health professional. Sometimes clients must undergo diet therapy, prescribed by their physicians, which becomes part of their medical treatment in the hospital. In many cases, diet therapy will have to be a lifelong practice for the client. In such cases, eating habits will have to be changed, and the client will need advice or instructions from a registered dietitian nutritionist and support from other health professionals.

Nutrition is currently a popular subject. It is important to recognize that some books and articles concerning nutrition may not be scientifically correct. Also, food ads can be misleading. Nutrition information on websites may not always be accurate or even factual. People with knowledge of sound nutrition practices will be less likely to be misled. They will recognize fad and distinguish it from fact.

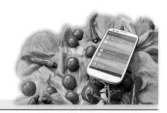

SUMMARY

Nutrition is directly related to health, and its effects are cumulative. Good nutrition is normally reflected by good health. Poor nutrition can result in poor health and even in disease. Poor nutrition habits contribute to atherosclerosis, osteoporosis, obesity, diabetes, and some cancers.

To be well nourished, one must eat foods that contain the six essential nutrients: carbohydrates, fats, proteins, minerals, vitamins, and water. These nutrients provide the body with energy, build and repair body tissue, and regulate body processes. When there is a severe lack of specific nutrients, deficiency diseases may develop. The best way to determine deficiencies is to do a nutrition assessment.

With sound knowledge of nutrition, the health professional will be an effective health care provider and will also be helpful to family, friends, and self.

DISCUSSION TOPICS

1. Think about possible health disparities in your area. What have been the contributing factors? What are some solutions?

2. What relationship might nutrition and heredity have to each of the following?
   a. development of physique
   b. ability to resist disease
   c. life span

3. What habits, in addition to good nutrition, contribute to making a person healthy?

4. What are the six classes of nutrients? What are their three basic functions?

5. Why are some foods called low-nutrient-density foods? Give some examples found in vending machines.

6. Explore why it is important to support the nutrition care of a hospitalized patient from a nursing standpoint, especially as it relates to malnutrition.

7. What is meant by the saying "You are what you eat"? Give specific examples of how the food we eat can affect our body and long-term consequences.

8. What is meant by the phrase "the cumulative effects of nutrition"? Describe some.

9. How could someone be overweight and at the same time suffer from malnutrition?

10. Discuss why health care professionals should be knowledgeable about nutrition.

SUGGESTED ACTIVITIES

1. List 10 signs of good nutrition and 10 signs of poor nutrition.

2. List the foods you have eaten in the past 24 hours. Underline those with low nutrient density.

3. Write a brief description of how you feel at the end of a day when you know you have not eaten wisely.

4. Name the six clinical characteristics of malnutrition.

5. Write a brief paragraph discussing the nutrition assessment by a dietitian and its importance.

6. Briefly describe rickets, osteomalacia, and osteoporosis. Include their causes.

7. Ask a registered dietitian to speak to your class about nutrition problems commonly seen in your area.

8. Investigate *Healthy People 2020* and progress on goals to date with obesity and physical activity. Write a brief summary on this.

REVIEW

Multiple choice. Select the *letter* that precedes the best answer.

1. The result of those processes whereby the body takes in and uses food for growth, development, and maintenance of health is
   a. respiration
   b. diet therapy
   c. nutrition
   d. digestion

2. Nutritional status is determined by
   a. heredity
   b. employment
   c. personality
   d. diet

3. To nourish the body adequately and to maintain health, one must
   a. avoid all low-nutrient-density foods
   b. eat foods containing the six classes of nutrients
   c. include fats at every meal
   d. restrict proteins at breakfast

4. Nutrients used primarily to provide energy to the body are
   a. vitamins, water, and minerals
   b. carbohydrates, proteins, and fats
   c. proteins, vitamins, and fats
   d. vitamins, minerals, and carbohydrates

5. Nutrients used mainly to build and repair body tissues are
   a. proteins, vitamins, and minerals
   b. carbohydrates, fats, and minerals
   c. fats, water, and minerals
   d. fats, vitamins, and minerals

6. Foods such as potato chips, cakes, sodas, and candy are
   a. high-nutrient-density foods
   b. essential nutrient foods
   c. low-nutrient-density foods
   d. nutritious foods

7. Undernutrition of the six classes of nutrients in the diet may result in
   a. increased energy
   b. malnutrition
   c. indigestion
   d. diabetes

8. The cumulative effect of a high-fat diet could be
   a. iron deficiency
   b. blindness
   c. heart disease
   d. diabetes mellitus

9. A cumulative condition is one that develops
   a. within a very short period of time
   b. over several years
   c. only in women under 52
   d. in premature infants

10. Malnutrition is assessed by
    a. food records and measurement of vitamin status
    b. how fast weight has been lost and if there is diarrhea
    c. disease progression and blood pressure instability
    d. weight loss, muscle and fat loss, strength of handgrip, and edema

11. Nutritional status
    a. is determined by heredity
    b. has no effect on mental health
    c. is not reflected in one's appearance
    d. can affect the body's ability to resist disease

12. Infants, young children, adolescents, pregnant adolescents, and the elderly
    a. are commonly overweight
    b. are among those prone to malnutrition
    c. all commonly suffer from osteomalacia
    d. never suffer from primary nutrient deficiencies

13. Organic nutrients are
    a. only found in products grown without pesticides
    b. only sold at health-food stores
    c. substances that cannot be broken down
    d. substances containing a carbon atom

14. Which of the following would be an organic nutrient?
    a. fat
    b. folate
    c. calcium
    d. selenium

15. Anthropometric measures include measures of
    a. iron status
    b. fluid intake
    c. bone density
    d. weight

CASE IN POINT

JAYDEN: COPING WITH MALNUTRITION

Jayden was living in an apartment with his mother Trina until recently, when he was removed and placed in foster care. Jayden's aunt had contacted Child Protective Services because she was concerned about her sister's mental health and ability to care for Jayden. Jayden is only 5 years old and his mother Trina has multiple mental illnesses. Trina has been diagnosed as a paranoid schizophrenic and has been on and off her medication depending on whether she can afford to purchase it. It was not uncommon for Trina to leave for extended periods of time without thought to Jayden's well-being. He often was without food, sufficient clothing, and clean surroundings. When Trina was home, she was often sleeping and Jayden was still left to fend for himself. When the social worker arrived at the home, she found it to be in disarray. There was very little food in the kitchen and trash and clutter was throughout the home. Jayden was found to be very thin, pale, and unclean. Jayden measured only 40 inches tall and weighed 30 pounds. The social worker noticed sores on his body, and his abdomen appeared to be very swollen. She took an informal diet recall the previous 24 hours and saw poor diet quality and gaps in eating. Jayden was complaining of pain in his legs and was having a difficult time walking. The social worker took Jayden to the emergency room for assessment and arranged for a foster family to be assigned to him.

ASSESSMENT

1. List five characteristics of poor nutritional status.
2. Identify characteristics of malnutrition that Jayden is experiencing.
3. Jayden needs to be provided with good nutrition and adequate calories. What would be important to consider in providing meals for Jayden?

DIAGNOSIS

4. Write a nursing diagnosis for Jayden.

PLAN/GOAL

5. What two changes can you predict will occur with the introduction of a good, nutritionally sound diet?
6. Whom can you refer to for assistance?

IMPLEMENTATION

7. Name at least three nursing interventions that could be employed to improve Jayden's nutrition.
8. How might Jayden's dental status impact his nutrition?
9. Would a home visit be beneficial for Jayden and a caregiver?

EVALUATION/OUTCOME CRITERIA

10. What could the doctor assess at the next appointment to see if the plan is working?
11. What observations could the caregiver offer about the success of the plan?

12. What could be an important piece of information from Jayden?

THINKING FURTHER

13. How could the Internet be of benefit to the caregiver?

✔ rate this plate

Jayden has been through a lot of heartache for a child his age. He is placed in a foster home, and his foster mother asks him what he would like to eat for his first dinner with them. He thought and thought and finally decided on the following plate. Rate this plate. Take into consideration that Jayden is malnourished, has not eaten much lately, and is lacking many nutrients.

Fried chicken thigh

½ cup mashed potatoes and 2 Tbsp gravy

½ cup corn with butter

Biscuit with butter

2% milk—8 oz

Can Jayden eat all of this, and should he? Does this plate need to be changed, and how would you change it?

CASE IN POINT

ASNAKU: VITAMIN A DEFICIENCY

Asnaku lives in a small village in Ethiopia. Her family is not wealthy and is unable to travel to see a doctor. There is a nurse who visits the village a few times a year, but that is the extent of the medical care Asnaku's family receives. The last time the nurse visited, she talked to Asnaku's mother about what her family typically eats. The nurse was a little concerned that Asnaku's family eats mostly grains. They rarely get meat, fruit, or vegetables. She spoke with Asnaku's mother about some of the signs and symptoms of vitamin deficiencies that could result from a diet with little access to a wider variety of foods. The nurse told her mother she would return in a few months and would have a mission team with her. These nurses and doctors were coming to provide medical care and assistance to the entire village. She told

Asnaku's mother they would be bringing vitamin supplements that would help prevent nutritional deficiencies as well as other medications. Asnaku's mother has been worried for a while that Asnaku may have a problem with her eyes. Asnaku is 7 years old now and has been fairly independent with her self-care. However, the mother has noticed that Asnaku has gotten lost in the night a couple of times trying to go to the bathroom. Asnaku also has had difficulty with tasks that her mother has asked her to do after the sun goes down. Her mother is worried that she is not able to see very well; however, during the day Asnaku seems fine. The mission team is to return in a couple of weeks, and her mother has requested Asnaku be evaluated to find out what could be wrong.

ASSESSMENT

1. What are the symptoms of vitamin A deficiency?
2. What is Asnaku experiencing that would suggest a vitamin A deficiency?
3. Make a list of foods that are high in vitamin A that should be incorporated into Asnaku's diet.
4. Think about Asnaku's grain-based diet. What other vitamin or mineral deficiencies could she have?

DIAGNOSIS

5. Write a nursing diagnosis for Asnaku.

PLAN/GOAL

6. What change can you predict will occur with the introduction of vitamin A?
7. What can be done to ensure that Asnaku is able to get the vitamin A her body needs?

IMPLEMENTATION

8. If Asnaku was hospitalized under your care, what interventions might you suggest?
9. In the United States, vitamin A deficiency is rare compared to third world countries. There are children in the United States who have diets that do not meet their caloric needs and have little nutritional quality. Why is vitamin A deficiency in the United States so much lower than in other countries?
10. Can you think of other examples of food sources that have been fortified to avoid deficiencies in vitamins or minerals?

EVALUATION/OUTCOME CRITERIA

11. What could the nurse assess at her next visit to Asnaku's village to see if the plan is working?

THINKING FURTHER

12. Access the World Health Organization's web page and read about the programs in place to provide vitamin A supplements to countries worldwide. Briefly discuss this program and the severity of this problem.

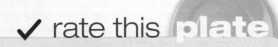

✔ rate this plate

Asnaku's night-blindness sounds like a vitamin A deficiency. As the family does not eat anything grown, such as vegetables and fruit, nutrient deficiencies can result. Having access to biofortified rice can provide Asnaku and her family with nutrients including vitamin A, iron, zinc, and iodine. Asnaku ate the following:

½ cup of fortified rice

¾ cup of vegetable stew

1 slice of flatbread

If Asnaku ate this meal three times a day, would the fortified rice be sufficient to provide her with 100% of her vitamin A and iron needs? What is the role of each nutrient within the biofortified rice?

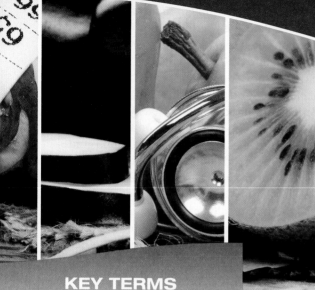

CHAPTER 2

KEY TERMS

balanced diet
daily values
descriptors
Dietary Guidelines for
  Americans
dietary laws
Dietary Reference Intakes (DRIs)
flavonoids
food customs
foodways
fusion
lacto-ovo vegetarians
lactose intolerance
lacto-vegetarians
legumes
masa harina
mirin
miso
MyPlate
vegans
wasabi

PLANNING A HEALTHY DIET

OBJECTIVES

After studying this chapter, you should be able to:

- Define a balanced diet
- List the U.S. government's Dietary Guidelines for Americans and explain the reasons for each
- Identify the food groups and their placement on MyPlate
- Describe information commonly found on food labels
- List some food customs of various cultural groups
- Describe the development of food customs

The statement "eat a balanced diet" has been repeated so often that its importance may be overlooked. The value of this statement is so great, however, that it deserves serious consideration by people of all ages. A **balanced diet** includes all six classes of nutrients and calories in amounts that preserve and promote good health.

Exploring
THE WEB

The *Dietary Guidelines for Americans 2015–2020* (8th edition) offers science-based advice and suggestions for improving health through sound nutrition and physical activity. These guidelines serve as helpful reminders to many Americans that healthy eating and regular physical activity can help people achieve and maintain good health and reduce the risk of chronic disease throughout all stages of the life span. Research the history of the Dietary Guidelines and the rationale for the new standards. Visit http://www.health.gov/dietaryguidelines/2015/.

balanced diet
one that includes all the essential nutrients in appropriate amounts

Dietary Reference Intakes (DRIs)
combines the Recommended Dietary Allowances, Adequate Intake, Estimated Average Requirements, and the Tolerable Upper Intake Levels for individuals into one value representative of the average daily nutrient intake of individuals over time

Dietary Guidelines for Americans
national healthy eating guidelines for disease prevention and optimal health

MyPlate
practical food guidance tool for consumers for making selections based on *Dietary Guidelines for Americans* from the U.S. Department of Agriculture

Daily review of the Dietary Reference Intakes (DRIs) and the Recommended Dietary Allowances (RDAs) would provide enough information to plan balanced diets. However, ordinary meal planning would be cumbersome and time-consuming if that table had to be consulted each time a meal were planned. Fortunately, the U.S. Department of Agriculture (USDA) and the U.S. Department of Health and Human Services (USDHHS) developed an essential resource for health professionals and policymakers as they design and implement food and nutrition programs that influence Americans. It is called the Dietary Guidelines for Americans, now in its 8th edition (2015–2020). In addition, MyPlate, which was released initially in 2010 by the USDA, provides consumer-friendly food guidance and practical tools for daily food choices based on the Dietary Guidelines.

When thinking about helping people shift to healthier intakes, one must factor cultural diversity in food choices. America has historically been referred to as the "melting pot" because of the many nationalities who immigrated to this country in hopes of finding a better life. Individuals with different ethnic backgrounds may continue to favor foods or customs of their country while others may blend in westernized food habits. Regardless of what cuisine is preferred, it is important for a clinician to help clients shift toward healthier choices within those cuisines.

DIETARY GUIDELINES FOR AMERICANS

The Dietary Guidelines provide science-based advice to promote health and to reduce the risk of chronic diseases through diet and physical activity. The guidelines are designed for professionals to help all individuals ages 2 years and older and their families consume a healthy, nutritionally adequate diet. This newest set of guidelines helps Americans focus on their eating patterns over time, encouraging shifts in food intake to a healthier focus. Rather than a rigid prescription, the guidelines seek to help individuals find an adaptable framework with which they can enjoy foods that meet personal, cultural, and traditional preferences while still fitting into their budget.

While previous editions of the Dietary Guidelines focused on changes that need to be made with individual food groups and nutrients, the new guidelines help an individual focus on the big picture so that Americans make choices that add up to an overall healthy eating pattern. There are five overarching guidelines (see Figure 2-1):

- Follow a healthy eating pattern across the life span.
- Focus on variety, nutrient density, and amount.
- Limit calories from added sugars and saturated fats and reduce sodium intake.
- Shift to healthier food and beverages choices.
- Support healthy eating patterns for all.

Follow a Healthy Eating Plan Across the Life Span

This first theme helps individuals understand that food and beverage choices that are made over time do make a difference in someone's health. Chronic diet-related diseases have risen due in part to changes in lifestyle behaviors. A history of poor eating and physical inactivity has a cumulative effect and can lead

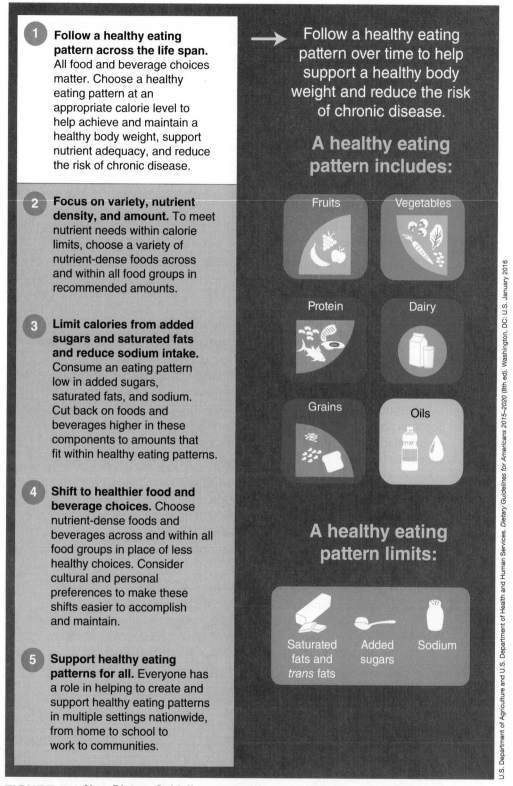

FIGURE 2-1 New Dietary Guidelines summary.

to cardiovascular disease, high blood pressure, type 2 diabetes, some cancers, and poor bone health. In addition, obesity, which has persisted for more than two decades, sets the stage for many chronic diseases to happen and in fact is viewed by some as a chronic disease in itself.

By choosing a healthful diet pattern at the appropriate calorie level, nutrient adequacy is supported, a healthy body weight is achieved, and there is reduced risk for chronic disease. Individuals are guided on consuming a healthy eating pattern that accounts for all food and beverages within an appropriate calorie level.

Key Recommendations

A healthy eating pattern includes:

- A variety of vegetables from all the subgroups—dark green, red, and orange; legumes (beans and peas); starchy; and other
- Fruits (especially whole fruits)
- Grains (at least half of which are whole grains)
- Fat-free or low-fat dairy, including milk, yogurt, cheese, and/or fortified soy beverages
- A variety of protein foods, including seafood, lean meats and poultry, eggs, legumes (beans and peas) and nuts, seeds and soy products
- Oils

MyPlate, found at the ChooseMyPlate.gov site is the consumer-friendly food guidance platform for creating healthy eating solutions. The site offers a plethora of practical advice, tips, and tools for all age groups. You can track your eating, figure out your BMI, look at pediatric growth charts, see meal pattern recommendations, find recipes, watch videos, download educational print materials, and more.

As you will notice on the website, the graphic of MyPlate shows five colored portions representing the five food groups. The divisions within the plate offer a general idea of portions from each specific food group needed to make a balanced diet (Figure 2-2). The five food groups and attributes of each are as follows:

- *Grains*—Any food made from wheat, rice, oats, corn, barley, or other cereal grains is considered a grain product. One half of all our grain servings should be whole grains. Whole grains provide dietary fiber, B vitamins, iron, and magnesium. Enriched products also contain B vitamins and iron, but if they are not made from whole grains, they contain little fiber.
- *Vegetables*—Vegetables provide carbohydrates, some protein, dietary fiber, and a variety of vitamins and minerals such as vitamin A, B-complex, C, E, and K as well as iron, calcium, phosphorus, magnesium, copper, manganese, and sometimes molybdenum. Vegetables are loaded with a vast array of nutrients, including naturally occurring plant

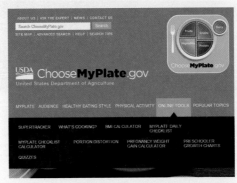
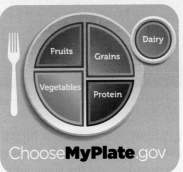

U.S. Department of Agriculture, Center for Nutrition Policy and Promotions. http://www.choosemyplate.gov

FIGURE 2-2 The ChooseMyPlate website offers many consumer friendly tools.

substances such as phytochemicals and **flavonoids** that enhance health. Individuals are encouraged to include all of the subgroups (specific recommendations can be referenced in the guidelines):

- *Dark green vegetables*—Broccoli, spinach, leafy salad greens (including romaine lettuce), collards, bok choy, kale, turnip, and mustard greens and green herbs

- *Red and orange vegetables*—Tomatoes, carrots, tomato juice, sweet potatoes, red peppers, winter squash, and pumpkin

- *Legumes (beans and peas)*—Pinto, white, kidney, and black beans; lentils; chickpeas; lima beans; split peas; and edamame (green soybeans)

- *Starchy vegetables*—Potatoes, corn, green peas, lima beans, plantains, and cassava

- *Other vegetables*—Onions, green beans, cucumbers, celery, green peppers, cabbage, mushrooms, avocado, summer squash, cauliflower, asparagus, snow peas, beets, lettuce (iceberg), and so forth

- *Fruit*—Fruits provide vitamin A and C, potassium, magnesium, carbohydrates, and fiber. Some have iron. It's important to consume more whole fruit, such as oranges, grapefruit, grapes, kiwi, melon, berries, apples, banana, apricots, pineapple, and so forth.

- *Dairy*—Milk, yogurt, and cheese contain excellent sources of calcium, phosphorus, and magnesium. Milk and yogurt contain lactose in greater concentrations than cheese. Riboflavin, vitamin A, vitamin B_{12}, and vitamin D are available in milk. Fat-free or low-fat products are preferred for best health.

- *Protein*—All meats, poultry, fish, eggs, soybeans, dry beans and peas, lentils, and nuts and seeds are included in the protein group. These foods provide not only protein but also iron, copper, phosphorus, zinc, sodium, iodine, and B vitamins, and some have fats and cholesterol. Foods selected should be of a more healthful nature, with less saturated fat and cholesterol.

Refer to Table 2-1 for guidance on healthy U.S. eating patterns.

Focus on Variety, Nutrient Density, and Amount

A diverse and nutrient-dense assortment of food and beverages are needed from all food groups and subgroups to fulfill the health needs in the recommended amounts, without exceeding total calorie limits. When one chooses nutrient-dense foods or beverages, there is an impressive array of vitamins, minerals, and other substances that contribute to positive health effects. Attributes of nutrient-dense foods are that they are in forms that retain naturally occurring components such as dietary fiber and have little or no solid fats, added sugars, refined starches, or sodium. All vegetables, fruits, whole grains, seafood, eggs, beans, peas, unsalted nuts and seeds, fat-free and low-fat dairy products, and lean meat and poultry would be considered nutrient-dense foods.

Key Recommendations for Calorie Balance

Consideration of calorie balance within healthy eating patterns is important. Energy taken "in" (foods, beverages) must balance energy "out" (calories expended from normal metabolic processes and physical activity). Monitoring

flavonoids
naturally occurring water-soluble plant pigments that act as antioxidants

legumes
plant food that is grown in a pod (e.g., beans or peas)

TABLE 2-1 Healthy U.S.-Style Eating Pattern

DAILY AMOUNT OF FOOD FROM EACH GROUP

The Healthy U.S.-Style Pattern includes 12 calorie levels to meet the needs of individuals across the life span. Identify the appropriate calorie level and choose a variety of foods in the recommended amounts that are nutrient dense, are lean or low fat, and are prepared without added fats, sugars, refined starches, or salt. A small number of calories remain within the overall calorie limit of the pattern (i.e., limit on calories for other uses). Calories up to the specified limit can be used for added sugars, added refined starches, solid fats, alcohol, or to eat more than the recommended amount of food in a food group. The overall eating pattern also should not exceed the limits of less than 10% of calories from added sugars and less than 10% of calories from saturated fats.

CALORIE LEVEL[1]

	1,000	1,200	1,400	1,600	1,800	2,000	2,200	2,400	2,600	2,800	3,000	3,200
Fruits	1 cup	1 cup	1.5 cups	1.5 cups	1.5 cups	2 cups	2 cups	2 cups	2 cups	2.5 cups	2.5 cups	2.5 cups
Vegetables	1 cup	1.5 cups	1.5 cups	2 cups	2.5 cups	2.5 cups	3 cups	3 cups	3.5 cups	3.5 cups	4 cups	4 cups
Grains	3 oz–eq	4 oz–eq	5 oz–eq	5 oz–eq	6 oz–eq	6 oz–eq	7 oz–eq	8 oz–eq	9 oz–eq	10 oz–eq	10 oz–eq	10 oz–eq
Meat and beans	2 oz–eq	3 oz–eq	4 oz–eq	5 oz–eq	5 oz–eq	5 1/2 oz–eq	6 oz–eq	6 1/2 oz–eq	6 1/2 oz–eq	7 oz–eq	7 oz–eq	7 oz–eq
Milk	2 cups	2 1/2 cups	2 1/2 cups	3 cups	3 cups	3 cups	3 cups	3 cups	3 cups	3 cups	3 cups	3 cups
Oils (1 tsp=5 g fat)	15 g	17 g	17 g	22 g	24 g	27 g	29 g	31 g	34 g	36 g	44 g	51 g
Limit on calories for other uses -% of calories	150	100	110	130	170	270	280	350	380	400	470	610

ESTIMATED DAILY CALORIE NEEDS

To determine which food intake pattern to use, check this chart for an estimate of individual calorie needs. The calorie range is based on age, gender, and physical activity level. Sedentary: light physical activity associated with typical day-to-day life. Active: physical activity equivalent to walking more than 3 miles per day at 3 to 4 miles per hour, in addition to activity of typical day-to-day life.

CALORIE RANGE		
SEDENTARY	→	ACTIVE
Children		
2–3 years	1,000 →	1,400
Females		
4–8 years	1,200 →	1,800
9–13	1,600 →	2,200
14–18	1,800 →	2,400
19–30	2,000 →	2,400
31–50	1,800 →	2,200

CALORIE RANGE		
SEDENTARY	→	ACTIVE
51+	1,600 →	2,200
Males		
4–8 years	1,400 →	2,000
9–13	1,800 →	2,600
14–18	2,200 →	3,200
19–30	2,400 →	3,000
31–50	2,200 →	3,000
51+	2,000 →	2,800

[1] Calorie levels are set across a wide range to accommodate the needs of different individuals.

Source: Adapted from U.S. Department of Health and Human Services and U.S. Department of Agriculture. *2015–2020 Dietary Guidelines for Americans* (8th ed.). December 2015. http://health.gov/dietaryguidelines/2015/guidelines/.

body weight and adjusting food intake and physical activity help ensure patients are on track for good health maintenance.

All Americans, including children and teens, adults, and older adults, are encouraged to achieve and/or maintain a healthy body weight. Specific recommendations include:

- *Children and adolescents*—Maintain calorie balance to support normal group and development. If overweight or obese, an adjustment should be made to eating and physical activity so as not to affect linear growth.

- *Pregnancy*—Before conceiving, women are encouraged to achieve and maintain a healthy weight. Women who are already pregnant should be encouraged to gain weight within the gestational weight guidelines.

- *Adults*—Obese adults are advised to change eating and activity to prevent additional weight gain and/or promote weight loss. Adults who are overweight should not gain additional weight and those with one or more cardiovascular risk factors (hypertension, hyperlipidemia), should change their lifestyle to lose weight. For a weight loss of 1–1 ½ pounds per week, daily intake should be reduced by 500–750 calories. A level of 1,200–1,500 calories a day for women and 1,500–1,800 calories for men usually is sufficient for weight loss.

- *Older Adults*—Those 65 years and older who are overweight or obese are encouraged to prevent additional weight gain. Those who are obese, especially with cardiovascular risk factors, should consider weight loss, as this can result in improved quality of life and reduced risk of chronic disease and associated disabilities.

Key Recommendations for Physical Activity

In addition to diet, physical activity is one of the most important things Americans can do to improve health and reduce the risk of chronic disease. Only 20% of adults meet the Physical Activity Guidelines for aerobic and muscle-strengthening activity. Adult males are more likely to report regular physical activity versus females (24% and 17%, respectively). Adolescent boys report they engage in exercise 30% of the time whereas their female counterpart only 13% of the time. Thirty percent of adults report no leisure-time physical activity. And, unfortunately, disparities exist in that those with lower income and lower education have lower rates of physical activity in addition to not engaging in leisure-time physical activity.

Diet and physical activity are the main tenets in the calorie balance equation to help manage body weight. The Dietary Guidelines include the key recommendation of meeting the Physical Activity Guidelines for Americans (Table 2-2).

Limit Calories from Added Sugars and Saturated Fats and Reduce Sodium Intake

A healthy eating pattern limits several food components that are of particular public health concern. The recommendations are to:

- *Consume less than 10% of calories per day from added sugars*—The recommendations to limit calories from added sugars is consistent with research examining eating patterns and health. Eating patterns that include lower intake of sources of added sugars are associated with reduced risk of cardiovascular disease in adults as well as obesity, type 2 diabetes, and some types of cancer. Evidence also suggests a relationship between added sugars and dental caries in children and adults. The two main sources of added sugars in the U.S. diet are sugar-sweetened beverages and snacks and sweets. Foods such as these provide few or no essential nutrients or fiber; therefore, they do

TABLE 2-2 National Physical Activity Guidelines

AGE GROUP	GUIDELINES
6 to 17 years	Children and adolescents should do 60 minutes (1 hour) or more of physical activity daily. • Aerobic: Most of the 60 or more minutes a day should be either moderate (a) or vigorous (b) intensity aerobic physical activity and should include vigorous-intensity physical activity at least 3 days a week. • Muscle-strengthening (c): As part of their 60 or more minutes of daily physical activity, children and adolescents should include muscle-strengthening physical activity on at least 3 days of the week. • Bone-strengthening (d): As part of their 60 or more minutes of daily physical activity, children and adolescents should include bone-strengthening physical activity on at least 3 days of the week. • It is important to encourage young people to participate in physical activities that are appropriate for their age, that are enjoyable, and that offer variety.
18 to 64 years	All adults should avoid inactivity. Some physical activity is better than none, and adults who participate in any amount of physical activity gain some health benefits. • For substantial health benefits, adults should do at least 150 minutes (2 hours and 30 minutes) a week of moderate-intensity, or 75 minutes (1 hour and 15 minutes) a week of vigorous-intensity aerobic physical activity, or an equivalent combination of moderate- and vigorous-intensity aerobic activity. Aerobic activity should be performed in episodes of at least 10 minutes and, preferably, should be spread throughout the week. • For additional and more extensive health benefits, adults should increase their aerobic physical activity to 300 minutes (5 hours) a week of moderate-intensity, or 150 minutes a week of vigorous-intensity aerobic physical activity, or an equivalent combination of moderate- and vigorous-intensity activity. Additional health benefits are gained by engaging in physical activity beyond this amount. • Adults should also include muscle-strengthening activities that involve all major muscle groups on 2 or more days a week.
65 years and older	Older adults should follow the adult guidelines. When older adults cannot meet the adult guidelines, they should be as physically active as their abilities and conditions will allow. • Older adults should do exercises that maintain or improve balance if they are at risk of falling. • Older adults should determine their level of effort for physical activity relative to their level of fitness. • Older adults with chronic conditions should understand whether and how their conditions affect their ability to do regular physical activity safely.

a. Moderate-intensity physical activity: Aerobic activity that increases a person's heart rate and breathing to some extent. On a scale relative to a person's capacity, moderate-intensity activity is usually a 5 or 6 on a 0 to 10 scale. Brisk walking, dancing, swimming, or bicycling on a level terrain are examples.

b. Vigorous-intensity physical activity: Aerobic activity that greatly increases a person's heart rate and breathing. On a scale relative to a person's capacity, vigorous-intensity activity is usually a 7 or 8 on a 0 to 10 scale. Jogging, singles tennis, swimming continuous laps, or bicycling uphill are examples.

c. Muscle-strengthening activity: Physical activity, including exercise that increases skeletal muscle strength, power, endurance, and mass. It includes strength training, resistance training, and muscular strength and endurance exercises.

d. Bone-strengthening activity: Physical activity that produces an impact or tension force on bones, which promotes bone growth and strength. Running, jumping rope, and lifting weights are examples.

Source: Adapted from U.S. Department of Health and Human Services. *2008 Physical Activity Guidelines for Americans.* Washington, DC. 2008. Accessed February 2016. http://health.gov/paguidelines

not contribute to diet quality. A swap to artificial sweeteners is not necessarily the answer for those who are overweight. High-intensity artificial sweeteners are not proven to help as a long-term weight management strategy.

• *Consume less than 10% of calories per day from saturated fats*—Replacing saturated fats with unsaturated fats (especially polyunsaturated fats) is associated with reduced blood levels of total cholesterol and low-density lipoprotein (LDL) cholesterol. The main sources of saturated fats in the U.S. diet are mixed dishes containing cheese, meat, or both, such as burgers, sandwiches, tacos, pizza, meat, poultry, and seafood dishes.

- *Consume less than 2,300 milligrams (mg) per day of sodium*—The average sodium intake is 3,440 mg per day. The guidelines note the importance of reduction to 2,300 mg for adults and children ages 14 years and older. A Tolerable Upper Intake Level (UL) of sodium for children younger than 14 years has been established and is available in the Dietary Guidelines. Adults with prehypertension and hypertension would benefit from lowering to 1,500 mg a day. Further evidence shows that adults who would benefit from blood pressure lowering should consider the DASH (dietary approaches to stop hypertension) diet. The DASH eating plan will be described in detail in the cardiovascular chapter. Experts believe 75% of the sodium we consume is already in the food products at consumption.

- *If alcohol is consumed, it should be consumed in moderation*—This translates up to one drink per day for women and up to two drinks per day for men. The Dietary Guidelines do not recommend that individuals who do not drink should start drinking for any reason. Alcohol is not a component of the USDA food patterns.

Shift to Healthier Food and Beverage Choices

The typical eating patterns engaged in by many in the United States do not align with the Dietary Guidelines for Americans. When analysis is done on typical eating patterns, various trends stand out:

- About three-fourths of the population has an eating pattern that is low in vegetables, fruits, dairy products, and oils.

- Over half of the population is meeting or exceeding total grain and protein foods; however, we are not meeting recommendation for the healthier subgroups within each of these food groups.

- Most of us exceed the recommendations for added sugars, saturated fats, and sodium. Further, many in the United States are overconsuming calories, as evidenced by the fact that more than two-thirds of all adults and nearly one-third of all children and youth are either overweight or obese.

Figure 2-3 shows a snapshot of what current dietary intakes are like compared to actual recommendations. This takes into account the percentage of the U.S. population ages 1 year and older who are below, at, or above each dietary goal or limit.

In addition to these food groups or dietary components, it is known that there are underconsumed nutrients of public health concern. They are calcium, potassium, fiber, and Vitamin D. In addition, for young children, women capable of becoming pregnant, and women who are pregnant, low intake of iron is also of public health concern. Choline; magnesium; and vitamins A, E, and C are also nutrients consumed by many individuals in amounts below the Estimated Average Requirement or Adequate Intake levels. The succeeding chapters in this book will offer a deeper look at food sources for each.

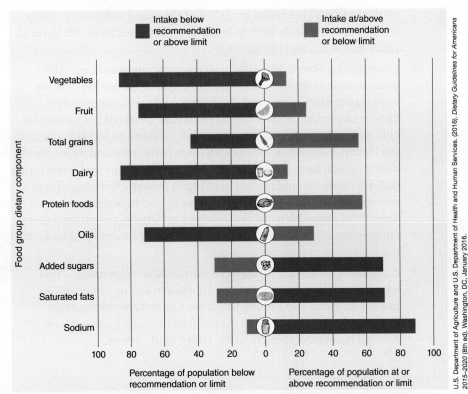

U.S. Department of Agriculture and U.S. Department of Health and Human Services. (2016). *Dietary Guidelines for Americans 2015–2020* (8th ed.) Washington, DC, January 2016.

FIGURE 2-3 Dietary intakes compared to recommendations. Percentage of U.S. population ages 1 year and older who are below, at, or above each dietary goal or limit.

As you will note, shifts are needed to align current intakes to recommendations:

- *Shift to consume more vegetables*—Striving for the healthy meal patterns suggested would increase total vegetable intake for most individuals. Including nutrient-dense forms and an increase in the variety of vegetables would significantly improve health outcomes. Increasing vegetable content of mixed dishes while decreasing amounts of other food components that are often overeaten, such as refined grains or fatty and salty meats, would be advantageous. Also choosing a leafy green salad or a vegetable as a side dish and blending vegetables into most meals and snacks would boost intake significantly.

- *Shift to consume more fruits*—Increasing fruits, mostly in whole form, would benefit most individuals. Shifting to include more fruit as snacks, in salads, as side dishes, and as dessert in place of foods with added sugars, such as cakes, pies, cookies, doughnuts, ice cream, and candies, will yield an increased consumption of fruit.

- *Shift to make half of all grains consumed be whole grains*—Swapping refined grains with whole-grain versions of common foods will help meet recommendations. Going from white to 100% whole wheat breads, white to whole-grain pasta, and white to brown rice would increase whole-grain intakes and lower refined grains. The recommendations discuss selecting foods that have whole grains listed as their first grain ingredient. In addition, cutting back on refined-grain desserts and sweet snacks such as cakes, cookies, and pastries, which are a common source of excess calories, would help meet this goal. Choosing nutrient-dense forms such as plain popcorn increased of buttered, bread instead of croissants, and English muffins instead of biscuits can also help meet guidelines.

- *Shift to consume more dairy products, in nutrient-dense forms*—Shifting toward fat-free or low-fat dairy, yogurt, and cheese or from fortified soy milk would help meet these recommendations. Cheese, however, contains more sodium; saturated fats; and less potassium, vitamin A, and vitamin D than milk or yogurt, so increased intake of dairy products is best served by using more fat-free or low-fat milk and yogurt versus cheese. Choosing yogurt as a snack or in an ingredient in prepared dishes such as salad dressings or spreads would be a positive step.

- *Shift to increase variety in protein foods choices and to make more nutrient-dense choices*—Increasing seafood intake twice per week and use of legumes or nuts and seeds in mixed dishes instead of meat or poultry would be a step in the right direction for meeting this goal. Choosing salmon, a tuna dish, a bean chili or adding almonds to a salad could all increase protein variety. Teen boys and adult men need to reduce overall intake of protein foods; however, the average intake of total protein foods for all others is close to recommendations.

- *Shift from solid fats to oils*—Use of vegetable oils in place of solid fats (butter, stick margarine, shortening, lard, coconut oil) when cooking would be advantageous for health. Shifts could be increasing the intake of foods that naturally contain oils, such as seafood and nuts, in place of some meat and poultry and choosing other foods such as salad dressings and spreads made with oils instead of solid fat.

- *Shift to reduce added sugars consumption to less than 10% of calories*—Shift to choosing beverages with no added sugars such as water in place of sugar-sweetened beverages. Decrease portion size of grain-based and dairy desserts and sweet snacks. Choose unsweetened or no-sugar-added versions of canned fruit, fruit sauces (applesauce), and yogurt.

- *Shift to reduce saturated fats intake to less than 10% of calories*—Choosing lower fat forms of foods and beverages that contain solid fats (lean meat rather than fatty cuts of meat, low-fat cheese in place of regular cheese, etc.) helps meet this goal. Changing ingredients in mixed dishes to increase the amounts of vegetables, whole grains, lean meat, and low-fat cheese in place of fatty meat and/or regular cheese helps with this recommended shift. Reading food labels to choose packaged foods lower in saturated fats and high in polyunsaturated and monounsaturated fats will help consumers as well. Using oil-based dressings and spreads on foods instead of butter, stick margarine, and cream cheese is a move in the right direction.

- *Shift food choices to reduce sodium intake*—Consumers would be wise to use the nutrition facts label to compare sodium content of foods and choose products with less sodium and buy low-sodium, reduced sodium, or no-salt-added versions of products when available. Choose fresh, frozen (no sauce or seasoning), or no-salt-added canned vegetables and fresh poultry, seafood, and lean meat rather than processed meat and poultry. Eating at home more often and cooking from scratch to control sodium makes sense to help uphold this guideline. Limiting sauces, mixes, and "instant" products including flavored rice, instant noodles, and ready-made pasta is also a logical health step toward lower sodium. Flavoring foods with herbs and spices instead of salt can help as well.

See Figure 2-4 for a practical representation of how food choices can shift to become healthier.

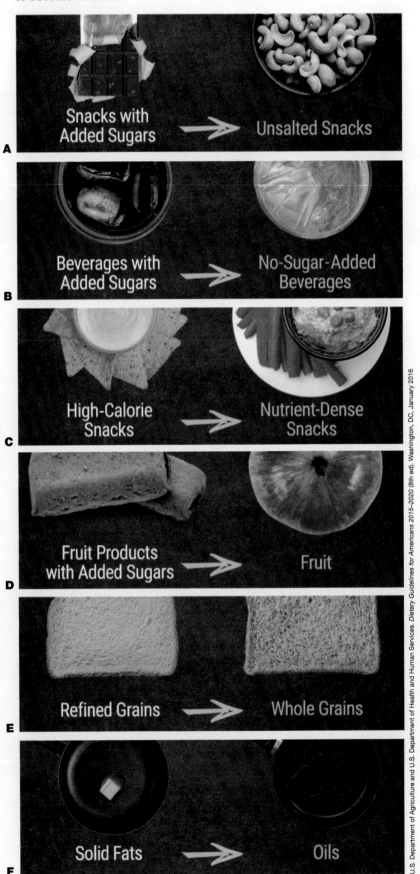

FIGURE 2-4 Examples of food shifts to make to meet dietary guidelines.

U.S. Department of Agriculture and U.S. Department of Health and Human Services. *Dietary Guidelines for Americans 2015–2020* (8th ed). Washington, DC, January 2016

MyPlate, MyWins

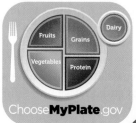

Find your healthy eating style
and maintain it for a lifetime. This means that
everything you eat and drink over time matters.
The right mix can help you be healthier now and in the future.

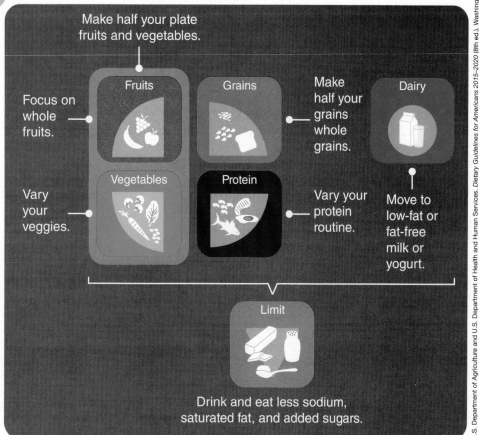

Make half your plate fruits and vegetables.

Focus on whole fruits.

Fruits

Grains

Make half your grains whole grains.

Dairy

Vary your veggies.

Vegetables

Protein

Vary your protein routine.

Move to low-fat or fat-free milk or yogurt.

Limit

Drink and eat less sodium, saturated fat, and added sugars.

FIGURE 2-5 Key messaging from MyPlate, MyWins.

U.S. Department of Agriculture and U.S. Department of Health and Human Services. *Dietary Guidelines for Americans 2015–2020* (8th ed.). Washington, DC, January 2016

Shifting to eating more vegetables, fruits, whole grains, and dairy will increase nutrients of public health concern. Low intakes of fiber are due to low intakes of vegetables, fruits, and whole grains. Americans' low intake of potassium is due in large part to low intakes of vegetables, fruits, and dairy. Lower intakes of calcium are related to low intakes of dairy. If more fatty fish such as salmon, herring, and tuna were eaten, along with more foods fortified with vitamin D, higher levels of vitamin D would be seen in our population.

MyPlate, My Wins is a new section of the ChooseMyPlate website that helps consumers learn how to implement needed shifts in eating in a practical way to meet the Dietary Guidelines. This section of food guidance emphasizes the importance of starting with small changes to make healthier choices (Figure 2-5).

Support Healthy Eating Patterns for All

Everyone has a role in supporting healthier eating patterns as we go about daily life. Healthy lifestyle choices need to be easy, accessible, and affordable wherever we choose food—home, school, work, and in communities and food retail outlets. Our policy makers know there needs to be collective action to create new ways of doing things to support American's health. Delivery of information that is compelling and empowering and most of all adaptable will be a concrete step in changing our nation's health.

Layers of influence shape a person's eating choices and styles and physical activity. What you believe to be true—your family traditions and heritage and for some, your religion—influences your decisions. Some give health priority, others do not make the connection readily between what we eat and how we move our body, and ultimate health outcomes.

Where we live can affect our access to healthy food and our opportunities to be physically active. Changes to sectors—education, health care, organizations and business, and industries—can have a huge role in influencing the degree to which people have access to healthy food and physical activity. The settings, whether they be early childcare and education (day care, preschools), schools, worksites, community centers, grocery stores, and restaurants, are all places where strategies to align with the Dietary Guidelines can and need to be carried out. Here are some strategies we can think about:

- *In the home setting*—Try small changes such as cutting down screen time by going on a walk every evening. Add more vegetables to family meals. Try your hand at cooking more at home and eating out less. Pack your lunch for work.

SPOTLIGHT on Life Cycle

Two Important Nutrients—Calcium and Iron

Adequate calcium intake and weight-bearing activity are important components in optimizing bone mass and decreasing the risk of osteoporosis. Calcium consumption is especially important during the preteen and teen years, when bones are growing at the fastest rate. By age 17, most teens have finished their growth spurts and have established 90% of their adult bone mass. Unfortunately, the majority of teens do not meet the recommended intake for calcium (1,300 mg/day). Rich sources of calcium include low-fat or fat-free milk, cheese, and yogurt; dark green leafy vegetables; calcium-fortified foods such as orange juice, cereal, bread, and tofu products; and nuts such as almonds. Adequate weight-bearing activity is also important in achieving and maintaining peak bone mass. Activities such as walking, playing tennis or basketball, jumping rope, dancing, and weightlifting can be incorporated into any exercise plan to keep bones healthy.

The most common nutrient deficiency in the world is lack of iron. This is particularly prevalent among infants, adolescents, and pregnant and menstruating women. It can result in iron-deficiency anemia. The health care provider can help by:

- Identifying those clients at risk (e.g., children under 2 years of age, adolescents, women with heavy menstrual flow, pregnant women, individuals with malabsorption syndromes, gastrointestinal bleedings, and gross dietary deficiencies).
- Performing complete nutritional assessments on high-risk clients.
- Encouraging clients to eat foods high in iron. These include lean meats, poultry, fish, enriched breads, legumes, leafy green vegetables, dried fruits, and nuts.

Exploring THE WEB

Explore the Web to learn how much sodium the average American is consuming on a daily basis and how this amount compares to the recommendation set by the 2015 Dietary Guidelines for Americans. What foods are high in sodium? What are some strategies to help reduce the amount of sodium intake in the American diet? What are some health risks associated with increased sodium intake? Research the CDC and/or FDA for more information.

Exploring THE WEB

The Wheat Foods Council website (http://www.wheatfoods.org) provides an abundance of information on grains and nutrition. Visit the Resources section to find slide shows and information to share with clients. Create fact sheets from the information found at this site that can be distributed to clients.

- *In the school setting*—Advocate for improving the selection of healthy food choices in cafeterias, vending machines, and so forth. Help support nutrition education programs and school-based gardening, as well as more physical activity during the day. Encourage parents to begin healthy changes at home.

- *In the work setting*—Workplaces can offer healthier options in the cafeteria and their vending machines. They can institute policies for healthy meeting food choices. They can offer places where employees can exercise or walk or take active breaks. They can support employees' participation in health and wellness programs and nutrition counseling.

- *In the community setting*—A variety of organizations can help increase access to affordable, healthy food choices by supporting community gardens, farmer's markets, shelters, and food banks. City and county governments can create walkable communities by maintaining safe places to move and exercise. Grocery stores can help support healthy decisions at a point of purchase. More and more large grocery chains can employ dietitians. Restaurants can improve menu items as more and more of us are looking for healthier choices when eating out.

There are many strategies that can result in shifts to improve intake and physical activity. If we have a concerted effort among professionals within communities, business and industry, organizations, governments, and other segments of society, we can get the needle to change on public health. And the call to action needs to be underway now as this will have a meaningful impact on the health of current and future generations.

FOOD LABELING

As a result of the passage by Congress of the Nutrition Labeling and Education Act (NLEA) in 1990, nutrition labeling regulations became mandatory in May 1994 for nearly all processed foods. The primary objective of the changes was to ensure that labels would be on most foods and would provide consistent nutrition information. The resulting food labels provide the consumer with more information on the nutrient contents of foods and how those nutrients affect health than former labels provided. Health claims allowed on labels are limited and set by the Food and Drug Administration (FDA). Serving sizes are determined by the FDA and not by the individual food processor. Descriptive terms used for foods are standardized. For example, *low fat* means that each serving contains 3 g of fat or less.

The nutrition label has a formatted space called Nutrition Facts. Currently, the food label includes information on the following components: total calories, calories from fat, total fat, saturated fat, trans fat, cholesterol, sodium, total carbohydrates, dietary fiber, sugars, protein, vitamin A, calcium, and iron.

A new, easier-to-understand food label is nearing FDA approval (see Figure 2-6). As it had been 20 years since the food label had been updated, the FDA and a variety of health experts believed that changes needed to be made based on new public health and nutrition science information. The new label has updated information on serving-size requirements to reflect amount of foods and beverages people are actually consuming. The format is refreshed to be easier to read; in particular, serving sizes, calories, and percent daily value are more clearly prominent.

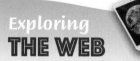

Exploring THE WEB

The website for the Center for Food Safety and Applied Nutrition, of the U.S. Food and Drug Administration (http://www.fda.gov), has an abundance of information on using the food label. Visit the website and create fact sheets on how to use the food label to lose weight, lower salt intake, control diabetes, and prevent heart disease. These sheets can also be used to aid in client teaching.

Nutrition Facts

Serving Size 2/3 cup (55g)

Servings Per Container About 8

Amount Per Serving

Calories 230	Calories from Fat 72

	% Daily Value*
Total Fat 8g	12%
Saturated Fat 1g	5%
Trans Fat 0g	
Cholesterol 0mg	0%
Sodium 160mg	7%
Total Carbohydrate 37g	12%
Dietary Fiber 4g	16%
Sugars 1g	
Protein 3g	
Vitamin A	10%
Vitamin C	8%
Calcium	20%
Iron	45%

* Percent Daily Values are based on a 2,000 calorie diet. Your daily value may be higher or lower depending on your calorie needs:

		Calories:	2,000	2,500
Total Fat	Less than		65g	80g
Sat Fat	Less than		20g	25g
Cholesterol	Less than		300mg	300mg
Sodium	Less than		2,400mg	2,400mg
Total Carbohydrate			300g	375g
Dietary Fiber			25g	30g

Nutrition Facts

8 servings per container

Serving size   2/3 cup (55g)

Amount per 2/3 cup

Calories   **230**

% DV*

12%	**Total Fat** 8g
5%	**Saturated Fat** 1g
	Trans Fat 0g
0%	**Cholesterol** 0mg
7%	**Sodium** 160mg
12%	**Total Carbs** 37g
14%	**Dietary Fiber** 4g
	Sugars 1g
	Added Sugars 0g
	Protein 3g
10%	**Vitamin D** 2mcg
20%	**Calcium** 260mg
45%	**Iron** 8mg
5%	**Potassium** 235mg

* Footnote on Daily Values (DV) and calories reference to be inserted here.

U.S. Health and Human Services, Food and Drug Administration.

FIGURE 2-6 Food label comparison—current (left) versus proposed (right).

There is an additional line on the proposed food label for "added sugars" as the addition of sugar to our foods is a growing public health concern. The FDA is considering proposal of a percent daily value for added sugars based on the recommendations for added sugars not to exceed 10% of total calories.

The calcium and iron content of the food will be listed as well as the daily value this product would contribute. Vitamin C and vitamin A information will be removed from the food label but will be replaced with information on nutrients of growing importance in the American diet: vitamin D and potassium. The FDA is proposing an easy-to-understand footnote to help consumers understand the daily value.

The food processor can voluntarily include additional information on food products. If a health claim is made about the food or if the food is enriched or fortified with an optional nutrient, then nutrition information about that nutrient becomes required. The standardized serving size is based on amounts of the specific food commonly eaten, and it is given in both English and metric measurements (Table 2-3).

Daily values on the label give the consumer the percentage per serving of each nutritional item listed, based on a daily diet of 2,000 calories. For example, total fat in Figure 2-6 shows 8 g, which represents 12% of the amount of fat someone on a 2,000-calorie diet should have.

daily values

represent percentage per serving of each nutritional item listed on food labels based on a daily intake of 2,000 calories

TABLE 2-3 Household and Metric Measures

HOUSEHOLD	METRIC
1 teaspoon (tsp) =	5 milliliters (mL)
1 tablespoon (Tbsp) =	15 milliliters (mL)
1 cup (C) =	240 milliliters (mL)
1 fluid ounce (fl oz) =	30 milliliters (mL)
1 ounce (oz) =	28 grams (g)

The ingredient list is just below the nutrition facts panel. The ingredient list includes each ingredient in descending order of predominance (Figure 2-6).

Health Claims

Because diet has been implicated as a factor in heart disease, stroke, birth defects, and cancer, the following *health claims* linking a nutrient to a health-related condition are allowed on labels. They are intended to help consumers choose foods that are the most healthful for them and to avoid being deceived by false advertisements on the label. The allowed claims are for the relationship between the following:

- Calcium and *osteoporosis*
- Sodium and *hypertension*
- Diets low in saturated fat and cholesterol and high in fruits, vegetables, and grains containing dietary fiber and *coronary heart disease*
- Diets low in fat and high in fruits and vegetables containing dietary fiber and the antioxidants, and vitamins A and C and *cancer*
- Diets low in fat and high in fiber-containing grains, fruits, and vegetables and *cancer*
- Folic acid and *neural tube defects*
- Soy protein and *coronary heart disease*

Two additional criteria must also be met:

1. A food whose label makes a health claim must be a naturally good source (containing at least 10% of the daily value) of at least one of the following nutrients: protein, vitamin A, vitamin C, iron, calcium, or fiber.
2. Health claims cannot be made for a food if a standard serving contains more than 20% of the daily value for total fat, saturated fat, cholesterol, or sodium.

Terminology

The FDA has also standardized **descriptors** (terms used by manufacturers to describe products) on food labels to help the consumer select the most appropriate and healthful foods. The following are examples:

- *Low calorie* means 40 calories or less per serving.
- *Calorie free* means less than 5 calories per serving.
- *Low fat* means a food has no more than 3 g of fat per serving or per 100 g of the food.

descriptors
terms used to describe something

- *Fat free* means a food contains less than 0.5 g of fat per serving.

- *Low saturated fat* means 1 g or less of saturated fat per serving.

- *Low cholesterol* means 20 mg or less of cholesterol per serving.

- *Cholesterol free* means less than 2 mg of cholesterol per serving.

- *No added sugar* means that no sugar or sweeteners of any kind have been added at any time during the preparation and packaging. When such a term is used, the package must also state that it is not low calorie or calorie reduced (unless it actually is).

- *Low sodium* means less than 140 mg of sodium per serving.

- *Very low sodium* means less than 35 mg of sodium per serving.

Obviously, the information on food labels is useful to all consumers and especially to those who must select foods for therapeutic diets. Health care professionals should become thoroughly knowledgeable about the labeling law. On request, many food manufacturers will provide the consumer with additional detailed information about their products.

It can be a challenge for many consumers to cut through the haze in selecting food products at the grocery store. The average grocery store is said to have over 600,000 products. Many food manufacturers make the front packages look enticing and as though their product is full of healthy ingredients. Sometimes that may not be the case. One must be knowledgeable about looking at the ingredient list and the nutrition facts, as that is where the *real* information lies. Overall, choosing foods that have shorter ingredient lists made up of nutritious items is the best bet. Avoiding long, complicated food additives, fillers, and preservatives is best. Nutrition Detectives™ is an innovative online teaching tool for elementary students and others wanting easy ways to decipher the food label.

FOOD CUSTOMS

MyPlate and Nutrition Facts labels (if available) are useful in planning a nutritionally sound diet, but dietary and religious customs must also be taken into consideration. People from each country have favorite foods. Frequently, there are distinctive food customs originating in just a small section of a particular country. People of a particular area favor the foods that are produced in that area because they are available and economical. Some religions have dietary laws that require particular food practices. Because most people prefer the foods they were accustomed to while growing up, food habits are often based on nationality and religion.

One's economic status and social status also contribute to food habits. For example, the poor do not grow up with a taste for prime rib, whereas the wealthy may at least be accustomed to it—whether or not they like it. Those in a certain social class will be apt to consume the same foods as others in their class. And the foods they choose will probably depend on the work they do. For example, people doing hard, physical labor will require higher-calorie foods than will people in sedentary jobs.

When people move from one country to another or from one area to another, their economic status may change. They will be introduced to new foods and new food customs. Although their original food customs may have been nutritionally adequate, their new environment may cause them to change their eating habits. For example, if milk was a staple (basic) food in their diet before moving and is unusually expensive in the new environment, milk may be replaced by a cheaper, nutritionally inferior beverage such as soda, coffee, or tea. Candy, possibly a luxury in their former environment, may be inexpensive and popular in their new environment. As a result, a family might increase consumption of soda or candy and reduce purchases of more nutritious foods. Someone who is not familiar with the nutritive values of foods can easily make such mistakes in food selection.

The meal patterns of national and religious groups different from one's own may seem strange. However, the diet may well be nutritionally adequate. When a client's eating habits need to be corrected, such corrections are most easily made if the food customs of the client are known and understood. The health care professional can gain this knowledge by talking with the client and learning about her or his background. A dietitian can use that knowledge to plan nourishing menus consisting of foods that appeal to the client. The necessary adjustments in the diet can then be made gradually and effectively.

U.S. CULTURAL DIETARY INFLUENCES

American cuisine (cooking style) is a marvelous composite of countless national, regional, cultural, and religious food customs. Consequently, categorizing a client's food habits can be difficult. Nevertheless, it is sometimes helpful to be able to do so to a certain extent. People who are ill commonly have little interest in food. Sometimes comfort foods (foods that were familiar to them during their childhood) are more apt to tempt them than other types. The following section briefly discusses some food patterns typical of various cultures, regions, and countries. Of course, there can be and usually are enormous variations within any one classification.

Native American Influence

It is thought that approximately half of the edible plants commonly eaten in the United States today originated with the Native Americans. Examples are corn, potatoes, squash, cranberries, pumpkins, peppers, beans, wild rice, sunflower seeds, sweet potatoes, avocados, papayas, and cocoa beans. In addition,

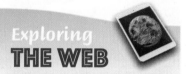

Exploring THE WEB

Search the Web for sources of information on the nutritional values of food patterns related to different cultures and economic levels. Choose cultures and economic levels that are represented in the community where you live. You will also find valuable resources at the USDA's website (http://www.usda.gov). What additional resources were you able to find?

food customs
food habits

dietary laws
rules to be followed in meal planning in some religions

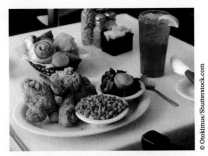

FIGURE 2-7 A traditional southern meal has foods like fried chicken, black-eyed peas, collard greens, cornbread and biscuits, and sweet tea.

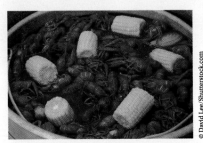

FIGURE 2-8 Crawfish are widely used in Cajun and Creole cooking.

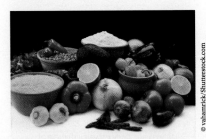

FIGURE 2-9 Ingredients used in Mexican cuisine include avocados, peppers, rice, and tomatoes.

foodways
the food traditions or customs of a group of people

fusion
a style of cooking that combines ingredients and techniques from different cultures or countries

masa harina
traditional flour made from field corn

lactose intolerance
inability to digest lactose because of a lack of the enzyme lactase; causes abdominal cramps and diarrhea

wild fruits, game, and fish are also popular. Foods are commonly prepared as soups and stews or are dried. The original Native American diets were probably more nutritionally adequate than are current diets, which frequently consist of too high a proportion of sweet and salty, snack-type low-nutrient-dense foods. Native American diets today may be deficient in calcium, vitamins A and C, and riboflavin.

U.S. Southern Influences

The foods of the South are as diverse as the people who settled in the southern United States. Food influenced by the South is so much a part of our national food culture that you probably have eaten many of these foods without even realizing their origin.

African American Influence

Down-home breads such as cornbread, biscuits, and cracklin' bread are served with most meals. Collard, turnip, and mustard greens are prepared with fatback (a cut along the back of pigs) for flavor. Black-eyed peas, okra, sweet potatoes, peanuts, corn, green beans, hot and sweet peppers, lima beans, and rice are an important part of African American heritage (Figure 2-7). Pork, chicken, and fried fish are served often. The term *soul food* was created in the 1960s to put emphasis on African American **foodways** (the food traditions or customs of a group of people) and preparation styles. Too much fat and sodium are consumed. This diet has too many carbohydrates but could be deficient in iron, calcium, fiber, potassium, and vitamin C.

French American Influence

Cajun and Creole cuisine is native to the "bayou" country in Louisiana and is a **fusion** of French and Spanish cooking. Cajuns lived off the land and waterways. Cajun cooks use wild game, seafood, vegetables, herbs, rice, tomatoes, sausage, hot peppers, and crawfish (resembling small lobsters) (Figure 2-8). Cajuns usually make their meals in one pot. Creole cooking uses many of the same foods but adds rich sauces that increase calories. Calcium and vitamins D, E, and C could be lacking in their diets, so the addition of fruit is needed.

Spanish Influences

The Spaniards were great seafaring explorers. They were responsible for finding and naming most of the islands in the Caribbean, along with Mexico and the west coast of South America. The Spanish and the natives who inhabited these countries have also greatly influenced our cuisine.

Mexican Influence

Mexican food is a combination of Spanish and Native American. Beans, rice, tomatoes, onions, jalapeños, other chilies, and **masa harina** (traditional flour made from field corn) are staples for Hispanics. Corn tortillas are made from masa harina and are used as bread as well as stuffed with cheese, beef, pork, and other ingredients to make enchiladas. Pork, goat, garlic, wheat and frijoles refritos (refried beans), avocados, and cheese are common foods (Figure 2-9). Flan, a custardlike pudding with caramel sauce, is a favorite dessert. The diet is lacking in vitamin C as well as green and yellow vegetables and fruits. Cheese supplies some calcium in the diet, but calcium intake may be low because of **lactose intolerance.**

Puerto Rican Influence

Puerto Rican cuisine has been influenced by the Spanish, African, and Taino Indians (first inhabitants). This cuisine uses corn, wheat, seafood, beef, pork, rice, olive oil, chicken, pinto beans, and okra. Plantains, green bananas, white and yellow sweet potatoes, chayote squash, taro, and breadfruit are starchy vegetables and are eaten often. Tropical fruits such as pineapple, mango, papayas, guava, and coconut are used often in desserts. Traditional desserts include flan, sweet potato balls with cinnamon, cloves and coconut, and guava jelly served with white cheese. Milk is not consumed often enough. Increased consumption of nonstarchy vegetables would add variety and eliminate some carbohydrates.

Mediterranean Influences

The Mediterranean diet is the healthiest in the world (Figure 2-10). The most important aspects of the Italian Mediterranean diet are the use of olive oil and the eating of small portions. The Italians on the Mediterranean have the lowest incidence of heart disease because of their eating habits.

Italian Influence

Italians consume a healthy mix of pasta, rice, beans, olives, fruits, vegetables, and seafood (Figure 2-11). Beef is seldom eaten on the Mediterranean side

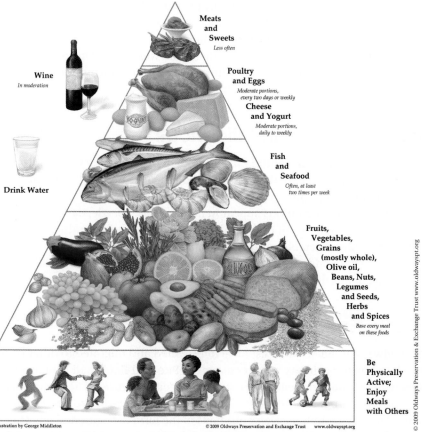

FIGURE 2-10 Follow the Mediterranean Food Guide Pyramid, and you will be eating the healthiest diet in the world.

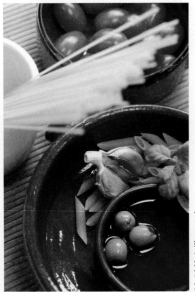

FIGURE 2-11 Olive oil, herbs, garlic, pasta, and tomatoes are ingredients commonly used in Italian cooking.

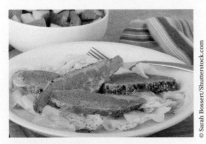

FIGURE 2-12 Countries in northern and western Europe have traditional "meat and potatoes" dishes like corned beef, cabbage, and potatoes.

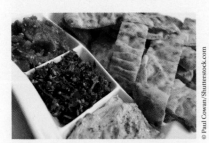

FIGURE 2-13 In Middle Eastern cuisine, flat bread is often eaten with hummus, tabouleh, or baba ganoush.

of Italy. Meats such as prosciutto salami, veal, and pork are favored. Cheese is important in Italian cooking but is often eaten by itself. Small portions are the norm. The primary fat used is olive oil. Dessert is usually fresh fruit. The Italians eat their main meal at lunch. Dinner is a light meal and could be pizza (not the Americanized version). Adding fat-free milk and low-fat meat would improve their already nutritious diet.

Greek Influence

In the past and even today in remote villages, the Greeks eat only what is in season at the time. Broccoli and cauliflower were first grown in Greece. Greeks eat salads of wild greens, artichokes, fava beans, green beans, eggplant, legumes, home-cured olives, yogurt, and feta cheese. Bread is the basis of a Greek meal, and fruity olive oil is the primary fat in the Greek diet. Fresh or cured fish and seafood are abundant and eaten regularly. Meats such as lamb, goat, and pork are also included in their diet. Dessert usually consists of fresh fruit. The Greeks have always eaten (and many continue to eat) a Mediterranean diet, but Western influence in the larger cities has changed the eating habits of younger generations.

Northern and Western European Influences

There are 20 countries in northern and western Europe that have influenced the foods we eat. These countries gave us our "meat and potato" mentality (Figure 2-12). The northern European diet consists of large servings of meat, poultry, or fish with small side dishes of vegetables and starch. Most countries use locally grown foods, such as greens, potatoes, beets, mushrooms, barley, plums, and rye. Sausages (including blood sausage), head cheese, dark breads, and dairy products are essential food in their diets. Pickled herring is favored in many countries. Some countries in northern and western Europe are extremely cold, limiting the growing season. The addition of fresh fruit and vegetables would add fiber and many vitamins and minerals.

Central European Influences

There are 16 countries in central Europe, and all of them have very similar cuisines. Pork and chicken are the most common meats eaten, but beef, sausages, fish, and game are popular too. Cabbage, sauerkraut, carrots, turnips, potatoes, beans, lentils, and onions appear in many meals. Spatzle, dark breads, and muesli are main sources of carbohydrates. Eggs and dairy products are used abundantly. Raw vegetables and fruits would increase vitamins, minerals, and fiber. Fewer eggs and the use of low-fat or fat-free dairy products would help to decrease fat in this diet.

Middle Eastern Influences

The foodways of the Middle East have intertwined and migrated to other countries. Lamb is the primary meat consumed. Pita and flat bread (unleavened) along with sourdough breads are eaten with meals (Figure 2-13). Legumes are an important part of the diet; these include chickpeas (garbanzo beans), which are used to make hummus. Dairy products in the form of yogurt and feta cheese are used extensively. Fortunately, fresh fruit is eaten for snacks and dessert. For centuries, dates and figs have been a staple in this diet. Pistachios are used to make baklava, a very sweet dessert. At the end of a meal, a dense, sweet coffee is served. The addition of fresh vegetables would be desirable to increase vitamins, minerals, and fiber.

Asian Influences

Each Asian country has its traditional foods. Most familiar is Chinese, but Japanese cuisine is becoming more available, as are the foods of Southeast Asia. Even though there may not be a wok in every kitchen, the art of stir-frying has become common practice. Cutting vegetables in small pieces and cooking them quickly preserves nutrients. Read the common foods consumed from each country and check how many you have eaten either at home or at a restaurant.

Chinese Influence

The Chinese believe that the five essential grains of life are rice, soybeans, barley, wheat, and millet. Their diet uses many vegetables, such as bean sprouts, shitake and other varieties of mushrooms, broccoli, peppers, snow peas, onions, green beans, bok choy, Napa cabbage, asparagus, chili peppers, seaweed, and cucumber (Figure 2-14). Protein is obtained from seafood, eggs, pork, chicken, beef, and tofu (soybean curd). Peanut oil for stir-frying and corn oil for deep frying are used extensively. Water chestnuts, walnuts, almonds, cashews, and sesame seeds are used in desserts and stir-fried dishes. Vegetarianism has expanded since the discovery of tofu. Some of the preferred seasonings are soy sauce, garlic, and fresh ginger along with various spices. The use of soy sauce and MSG (monosodium glutamate) may contribute to high blood pressure. Calcium sources are lacking in this diet, perhaps because of lactose intolerance in the Asian populations.

Japanese Influence

In ancient times, much of the traditional Japanese cuisine was influenced by the Chinese and Koreans. The medieval period triggered a gradual transformation with new tastes and flavors. The Japanese strive to use only the freshest ingredients. Essential ingredients include bamboo shoots, tofu, cucumbers, eggplant, enoki and other mushrooms, spinach, ginger, seaweed, rice, sesame, and green onions. Their protein is from seafood (both raw and cooked), eggs, and chicken. Seasonings used extensively are **mirin** (rice wine with 40–50% sugar), soy sauce, **miso** (a thick fermented paste made from soybeans), and **wasabi** (Japanese horseradish). Sushi is a well-known food item (Figure 2-15). The Japanese drink green tea rather than milk. Lactose intolerance plays an important role in their choices. Fresh fruit is a needed addition.

Southeast Asian Influence

India and China have influenced much cooking. Many vegetables are eaten because 75% of the population is agricultural-based. Rice is the staple food, but noodles are used often (Figure 2-16). Two times as much fish is consumed compared with other meats; pork, chicken, and beef are eaten less often. Southeast Asians prefer coconut milk to any dairy products. They, like other Asians, use soybean milk, soybean paste, soy sauce, and ginger. Fruits are part of the meals. The inhabitants of Southeast Asia, with the exception of Vietnam, eat with their fingers, but this is changing. High blood pressure caused by a high-sodium diet could be an issue. Cow's milk alternatives such as soy or rice milk are favored because of lactose intolerance.

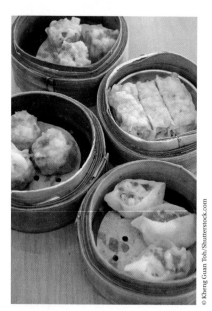

FIGURE 2-14 Steamed, baked, and fried dim sum is part of traditional Chinese cuisine.

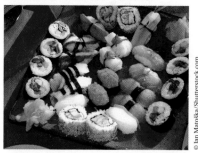

FIGURE 2-15 Sushi is a popular type of Japanese cuisine.

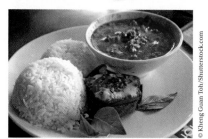

FIGURE 2-16 This Thai dish of spicy curry-steamed fish pudding and rice is an example of traditional Southeast Asian cuisine.

mirin
rice wine with 40–50% sugar

miso
a thick fermented paste made from soybeans

wasabi
Japanese horseradish

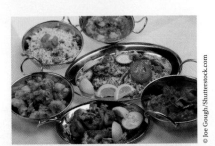

FIGURE 2-17 A sample of traditional Indian curry dishes.

Indian Influences

Religion and climate are two factors in the development of food habits in India. Vegetarianism is prevalent (over 80%) because of religious beliefs. Lentils, beans, and milk and milk products supply protein to their diet. The rest of the population eats small quantities of meat and fish for their protein. Vegetables grown locally are combined with rice in the south and wheat products in the north (Figure 2-17). Garlic and eggplants are native to India. Curry is a spice but also denotes Indian dishes. Eating with your fingers is acceptable. Sunflower, coconut, and mustard oils are used in cooking. Calcium could be a problem if consumption of milk is inadequate.

New Immigrant Influences

The United States is made up of immigrants who bring with them an interesting variety of foods that are native to their country. Immigrants will always prepare their native foods and enjoy sharing with others. Have you ever thought about what traditional foods your family eats and where they originated?

Somali Influence

No pork is eaten because of religious doctrine; however, Somalis consume lamb, goat, chicken, and some beef. They prefer to fry their foods. They use rice, flat bread, teff, and corn flour, and they eat some vegetables and fruit. They make meat sauces and curries. Unfortunately, some drink sweet tea and soda, and children may be given too much fruit juice. Some may not get enough calcium. The adaption of the westernized diet has led to the consumption of fast foods and high-fat snacks food.

Haitian Influence

African, Spanish, and French culinary influences have shaped Haitian foodways. The diet is based on starch staples, such as rice, corn, millet, yams, and beans. Only the wealthy can afford meat, lobster, shrimp, duck, and sweet desserts. The country's national dish is rice and beans. They fry their meals in lard for enhanced flavor. Tropical fruits, such as avocados, mangoes, pineapples, coconuts, and guava, grow abundantly in Haiti. Lack of dairy products in the diet means that there will be a deficiency of calcium.

Korean Influence

In Korea, the growing of rice dates back to 2000 BC. Millet, soybeans, red beans, and other grains were also produced. Red meat is scarce, but chicken and seafood are abundant. Rice is eaten with every meal, along with vegetables. The national dish of Korea is kimchi, a fermented cabbage with spices, green onions, and radishes. Korean food is very spicy with the use of red pepper paste, green onion, ginger, garlic, and bean paste (Figure 2-18). Soy sauce is used extensively. Fresh fruits, such as apples, pears, persimmons, and melons, or dried fruits, are eaten for snacks and dessert. Almost all South Koreans receive adequate nutrition.

Dominican Republic Influence

Dominican Republic cuisine is a mix of Spanish and Taino Indian. Goat and chicken are the meats eaten most often. Fresh seafood, such as shrimp, mahi-mahi, rock lobster, and marlin is served often in seaside towns. Tropical fruits such as bananas, papayas, pineapples, mangoes, and avocados are eaten often.

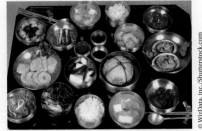

FIGURE 2-18 A traditional Korean meal, served with kimchi, rice, spicy pastes, and sauces.

Plantains, yuca (cassava), chayote, and rice are starchy foods in the diet. Salad is usually eaten with the midday meal.

Burmese Influence

The Burmese people consume many tropical fruits, such as pineapples, papayas, oranges, bananas, and mangoes. Cabbage, cucumbers, cauliflower, beets, carrots, bean sprouts, and tomatoes are just some of the vegetables eaten. Carbohydrate sources are rice, noodles, red lentils, and mung peas (Figure 2-19). Protein sources are pork, beef, lamb, chicken, duck, fish or prawns (large shrimp), tofu, and eggs. Fresh fruits are served for dessert, but sweets are eaten as snacks or at breakfast.

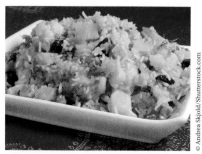

FIGURE 2-19 The Burmese version of biryani is often made with rice, chicken, cashew nuts, yogurt, raisins, peas, cloves, cinnamon, saffron, and bay leaves.

FOOD PATTERNS BASED ON RELIGION OR PHILOSOPHY

Jewish

Interpretations of the Jewish dietary laws vary. Persons who adhere to the Orthodox view consider tradition important and always observe the dietary laws. Foods prepared according to these laws are called *kosher* (Figure 2-20). Conservative Jews are inclined to observe the rules only at home. Reform Jews consider their dietary laws to be essentially ceremonial and so minimize their significance. Essentially the laws require the following:

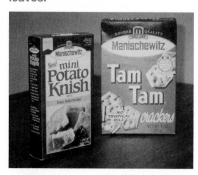

FIGURE 2-20 Kosher food labels.

- Slaughtering must be done by a qualified person in a prescribed manner. The meat or poultry must be drained of blood, first by severing the jugular vein and carotid artery, then by soaking in brine before cooking.
- Meat and meat products may not be prepared with milk or milk products.
- The dishes used in the preparation and serving of meat products must be kept separate from those used for dairy foods.
- Dairy products and meat may not be eaten together. At least six hours must elapse after eating meat before eating dairy products, and 30 minutes to one hour must elapse after eating dairy products before eating meat.
- The mouth must be rinsed after eating fish and before eating meat.
- There are prescribed fast days: Passover Week, Yom Kippur, and the Feast of Purim.
- No cooking is done on the Sabbath, from sundown Friday to sundown Saturday.

Jewish dietary laws forbid the eating of the following:
- The flesh of animals without cloven (split) hooves or that do not chew their cud
- Hindquarters of any animal
- Shellfish or fish without scales or fins
- Birds of prey
- Creeping things and insects
- Leavened (contains ingredients that cause it to rise) bread during Passover

In general, the food served is rich. Chicken and fresh-smoked and salted fish are popular, as are noodles, eggs, and flour dishes. These diets can be deficient in fresh vegetables and milk.

Roman Catholic

Although the dietary restrictions of the Roman Catholic religion have been liberalized, meat is not allowed on Ash Wednesday and Good Friday, and the Pope requests adherents to abstain on the other Fridays during Lent.

Eastern Orthodox

The Eastern Orthodox religion includes Christians from the Middle East, Russia, and Greece. Although interpretations of the dietary laws vary, meat, poultry, fish, and dairy products are restricted on Wednesdays and Fridays and during Lent and Advent.

Seventh-Day Adventist

In general, Seventh-Day Adventists are **lacto-ovo vegetarians,** which means they use milk products and eggs but no meat, fish, or poultry. They may also use nuts, legumes, and meat analogues (substitutes) and tofu. They consider coffee, tea, and alcohol to be harmful.

Mormon (Latter-Day Saints)

The only dietary restriction observed by the Mormons is the prohibition of coffee, tea, and alcoholic beverages.

Islamic

Adherents of Islam are called Muslims. Their dietary laws prohibit the use of pork and alcohol, and other meats must be slaughtered according to specific laws. During the month of Ramadan, Muslims do not eat or drink during daylight hours.

Hindu

To the Hindus, all life is sacred, and animals contain the souls of ancestors. Consequently, most Hindus are vegetarians. They do not use eggs because eggs represent life.

OTHER FOOD PATTERNS

Vegetarians

lacto-ovo vegetarians
vegetarians who will eat dairy products and eggs but no meat, poultry, or fish

There are several vegetarian diets. The common factor among them is that they do not include meat. Some include eggs, milk, and cheese, and some do not. When carefully planned, these diets can be nutritious. They can even contribute to a reduction of obesity and a reduced risk of high blood pressure, heart disease, some cancers, and possibly diabetes. They must be carefully planned so that they include all the needed nutrients.

Lacto-ovo vegetarians use dairy products and eggs but no meat, poultry, or fish. **Lacto-vegetarians** use dairy products but no meat, poultry, or eggs. **Vegans** avoid all animal foods. They use soybeans, chickpeas, meat analogues, and tofu. It is important that their diets be carefully planned to include appropriate combinations of the essential amino acids. For example, beans served with corn or rice or peanuts eaten with wheat are better in such combinations than any of them would be if eaten alone. Vegetarians need to focus on ensuring they get enough calcium, vitamin D, vitamin B_{12}, iron, zinc, and proteins. ChooseMyPlate has eating tips for vegetarians and the *Dietary Guidelines for Americans 2015–2020* offers a healthy vegetarian eating plan.

Zen-Macrobiotic Diets

The macrobiotic diet is a system of 10 diet plans, developed from Zen Buddhism. Adherents progress from the lower number diet to the higher, gradually giving up foods in the following order: desserts, salads, fruits, animal foods, soups, and ultimately vegetables, until only cereals—usually brown rice—are consumed. Beverages are kept to a minimum, and only organically grown foods are used. Foods are grouped as yang (male) or yin (female). A ratio of 5:1 yang to yin is considered important. Most macrobiotic diets are nutritionally inadequate. As the adherents give up foods according to plans, their diets become increasingly inadequate. These diets can be especially dangerous because avid adherents promise medical cures from the diets that cannot be attained, and so medical treatment may be delayed when needed.

HEALTH AND NUTRITION CONSIDERATIONS

The Dietary Guidelines provide current evidence-based recommendations to improve the health of our populous. Learning and understanding the tools they offer will help guide diet and physical activity recommendations for all health care professionals so that they can help their clients. All clients should be viewed as individuals whose food customs, which may be different from those of the health care professional, must be respected. A registered dietitian will help with a specific diet plan for a hospitalized client. The dietitian will take into account the client's likes, dislikes, and food customs.

lacto-vegetarians
vegetarians who eat dairy products

vegans
vegetarians who avoid all animal foods

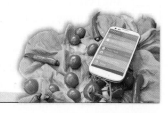

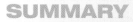
SUMMARY

Many Americans are not meeting food and activity guidelines set out by the Dietary Guidelines; as a result, chronic disease rates remain high. Professionals need to help support our nation in making shifts in eating and exercise to significantly improve health. Using the user-friendly ChooseMyPlate platform from the USDA helps individuals apply simple tools and concepts to their eating and exercise.

Food habits have many diverse origins. Nationality, religion, and economic and social status all affect their development. When food customs result in inadequate diets, corrections should be made gradually. Corrections are easier to make and are more effective when the reasons for the food habits are understood.

DISCUSSION TOPICS

1. Should health care professionals practice the rules of good nutrition themselves?

2. How do food habits originate?

3. What effects do environment have on particular food habits? When do the effects of a new environment improve diets, and when do they impair them?

4. From personal experience, explain why certain foods are enjoyed more than others that are commonly available in the local area.

5. Why might Scandinavians like fish more than Hungarians do?

6. Pick a cultural diet that reflects your likes and dislikes. If you were to move to this country, could you adapt to the food habits? Why or why not?

7. Discuss vegetarian diets. Are they safe? Explain.

8. Why is it difficult to convince someone to change her or his food habits? Discuss.

9. Define a balanced diet.

10. Describe the U.S. healthy eating pattern, including number of servings or portion size recommended for each group

11. How might one include milk in the diet of a 4-year-old who refuses to drink it?

12. Why would yogurt be a good snack or dessert for a pregnant woman?

13. What would be five examples of shifts in eating that someone could make to uphold the main tenets of the Dietary Guidelines?

14. Why should "crash" or "fad" diets be avoided? What is a better alternative? Why?

15. Discuss the sale of foods with low-nutrient density in school cafeterias. Is it a good practice? If so, why? If not, why not? What would your position be on this subject if you were principal of an elementary school? Of a middle or senior high school?

SUGGESTED ACTIVITIES

1. Assign a series of short reports on food customs. Each student should select a different country or area within a country for study. After the reports have been presented, hold a class discussion on whether climate, availability of food, or economic or other factors determine the food customs of the countries studied. Include answers to the following questions: What is the climate of the country? What types of crops are grown there? Are modern methods of agriculture used? Does the country depend on imports for much of its food supply? If so, what foods are imported? Are the majority of the citizens poor? What types of foods are popular? What types are expensive? Which of these foods are produced in the country? Which are imported? What is the prevalent religion?

2. Plan a diet for a client who adheres to no meat on Friday during Lent.

3. Investigate farmer's markets in your area. Are they accessible to those that are underserved or live in food deserts? What is being done in your area to improve access to healthy foods?

4. Buy some fruits and vegetables that are new to you. Bring them to class and sample them. Share ideas about their potential uses. Perhaps these might be added to family menus.

5. Using a restaurant menu, choose breakfast, lunch, and dinner. Check the selection of foods against MyPlate. Are they balanced meals? Discuss the problems that people who eat all their meals in restaurants might have in maintaining a well-balanced diet.

6. Using the following table, fill in the "Menus" column with the foods eaten in the past two days. In the "Food Groups Used" column, list the group to which each food belongs. To evaluate personal dietary habits, fill in the "Food Groups Not Used" column. Compare the table with those of the rest of the class and discuss how your eating habits could be improved.

Menus	Food Groups Used	Food Groups Not Used
Breakfast		
Lunch		
Dinner		
Snacks		

7. As you've analyzed what types of foods you eat, and some possible gaps in eating, address nutrients in your diet that are of special public

health concern. How is your diet consumption for calcium, vitamin D, potassium, and fiber? Use appendices or the Internet for more information as you investigate their nutrient levels in your diet.

8. Adapt the following menu for a person of the Orthodox Jewish faith.

   Baked ham

   Scalloped potatoes

   Buttered peas

Bread and butter

Fresh fruit

Milk or coffee

9. Keep a food journal, writing down everything you eat for three days. Visit http://www. choosemyplate.gov and use the diet analysis tool called "Supertracker" to determine if your nutrient needs are met. For the nutrients that are deficient, what are you willing to add to your diet to improve your health?

REVIEW

Multiple choice. Select the *letter* that precedes the best answer.

1. Food customs mean one's
   a. food nutrients
   b. food habits
   c. food requirements
   d. all of the above

2. Food customs
   a. may be based on religion or nationality
   b. are always nutritious
   c. are easily changed
   d. are not affected by one's social status

3. Moving to a new environment or experiencing a change in salary
   a. rarely changes established food habits
   b. usually influences established food habits
   c. always reduces the amount of food eaten
   d. never reduces the quality of food eaten

4. Rice is a popular carbohydrate food in
   a. Puerto Rico
   b. central Europe
   c. northern Europe
   d. all of the above

5. The new proposed food label will
   a. appear on the front cover of all products
   b. include information on vitamins D, E, and C
   c. list added sugars as a separate line
   d. no longer list protein, as most Americans meet this nutrient

6. How many Americans do not meet their vegetable requirements?
   a. Nearly 25%
   b. Nearly 75%
   c. Just under 50%
   d. We all meet our requirements

7. A balanced diet is one that includes
   a. equal amounts of carbohydrates and fats
   b. only corn, green beans, and potatoes as vegetables
   c. all six classes of nutrients
   d. more vegetables than fruits

8. Fruits and vegetables are rich sources of
   a. vitamins
   b. fats
   c. protein and fiber
   d. only B vitamins

9. Teenagers should have a serving of milk (or its substitute)
   a. not more than twice a day
   b. three times a day
   c. not more than four times a week
   d. not at all if they are overweight

10. How many adults meet the physical activity guidelines for aerobic and muscle-strengthening activities?
    a. 15%
    b. 20%
    c. 30%
    d. 60%

11. Milk and its products are the best dietary source of
    a. proteins and fats
    b. calcium and vitamin D
    c. carbohydrates
    d. all of the above

12. Breads, cereals, rice, and pasta are rich sources of
    a. vitamin D
    b. fats
    c. carbohydrates
    d. all of the above

13. Daily intake from the protein (meat) group for a 2,000-calorie diet should be
    a. 2 oz
    b. 5.5 oz
    c. 8 oz
    d. 11 oz

14. High-fat meats and egg yolks contain large amounts of
    a. sodium
    b. fiber
    c. fat and cholesterol
    d. carbohydrates and sodium

15. An example of a breakfast with high-nutrient density is
    a. pancakes and cocoa
    b. melon, bran muffin, and cocoa made with fat-free milk
    c. fruit-flavored beverage, cinnamon bun, and coffee
    d. fried eggs, bacon, and coffee

16. Excessive amounts of salt in the diet
    a. raise cholesterol levels substantially
    b. are thought to contribute to hypertension
    c. cause cirrhosis of the liver
    d. have no relevance to one's nutritional status

17. MyPlate
    a. food groups are nutritionally interchangeable
    b. is an outline for meal planning for adults only
    c. advises that fruits and vegetables be eaten in moderation
    d. recommends portion ranges for the five food groups

18. The Nutrition Labeling and Education Act of 1990
    a. requires that descriptive words used for foods be standardized
    b. sets maximum amounts of cholesterol allowed for each food serving
    c. permits no health claims on food containers
    d. does not require the food manufacturer or processor to list the total amounts in each serving of calories, sodium, or dietary fiber

19. Foods rich in complex carbohydrates, such as whole-grain breads and cereals, are also excellent sources of
    a. calcium and phosphorus
    b. vitamins C and D
    c. dietary fiber and B vitamins
    d. proteins and fats

20. When choosing foods from the meats, poultry, and fish food group, one should be careful to select foods that
    a. are rich in calcium and phosphorus
    b. provide at least one-half of one's daily need for carbohydrates
    c. have limited amounts of protein and iron
    d. are low in saturated fats and cholesterol

21. The two new nutrients on the proposed food label that will be required to be included as amounts per serving on food labels are
    a. vitamin A and thiamine
    b. niacin and folic acid
    c. vitamin D and potassium
    d. vitamins D and K

22. Consuming alcoholic beverages
    a. by pregnant women can cause birth defects
    b. can cause cirrhosis of the liver only in men
    c. has little or no effect on one's nutritional status
    d. has no effect on one's appetite

23. People of the Jewish faith eat Kosher foods because
    a. they only like meat
    b. they believe it makes them live longer
    c. they adhere to strict dietary laws
    d. the diet contains more sodium

CASE IN POINT

MARA: MAINTAINING A HEALTHY DIET WHILE GAINING INDEPENDENCE

Mara's parents immigrated to the United States from Mexico when she was young. She has lived with her parents who have worked for farmers since moving to the United States. They have been able to enjoy many of the fresh vegetables and fruits grown by the farmers. They also have access to a local farmer's market where her parents deliver produce from the farmers. They purchase fresh meats and seafood at the market as well. Her mother loves to cook and therefore they have rarely eaten at restaurants. Now that Mara has finished high school, she has received a scholarship to college. The college is nearby; however, Mara will be living on campus and not with her parents. Her mother is concerned about her health and nutrition as she goes away to college. She is concerned she will make poor nutritional choices if she is not educated on nutrition. She would like her to be aware of the consequences of fast foods and alcohol consumption. Mara and her parents will be traveling to college to get her registered for classes soon. Mara's mother has made an appointment with a dietitian at the local hospital before they leave. She would like the dietitian to review healthy nutrition for Mara. She would like her to discuss with Mara how to incorporate American foods and eating out while still maintaining a healthy diet. Mara is currently 5 ft 4 in and 119 lb. She is happy with her current body weight and feels good about herself. She tells the dietitian she is interested in becoming more aware of what she is eating. She knows that in her new independence it will be easier to prepare healthy meals if she has the knowledge she needs to accomplish this task.

ASSESSMENT

1. What factors will be influencing Mara as she attends college?
2. List the subjective information that can be obtained from Mara and her mother about her eating habits.
3. What can you caution Mara regarding her introduction into the college world of nutrition?
4. How significant are these problems?
5. Is Mara currently at a healthy weight for her height?

DIAGNOSIS

6. Write a nursing diagnosis for Mara.

PLAN/GOAL

7. What changes will Mara expect to see if she decides to eat less healthily?
8. What situations will be most stressful to Mara?
9. What could Mara do to help keep her nutrition and food consumption on track?
10. What goals could Mara set to also help maintain her weight and her health?

IMPLEMENTATION

11. List some strategies Mara can use to help keep healthy.
12. What substitutes could Mara make to be able to fit in with the crowd and still be eating well?
13. What would you caution Mara about in regard to stressful situations?

EVALUATION/OUTCOME CRITERIA

14. How will Mara be able to determine her success for healthy eating?
15. How well will Mara be able to associate body changes with poor food choices?
16. How could the dietitian evaluate Mara's progress?

THINKING FURTHER

17. Who else will benefit from Mara's food choices?
18. What resources could help Mara achieve her goals?

✔ rate this plate

Analyze the meal that Mara has prepared for dinner. Are the portions the right size for Mara? How would you change the portion sizes you feel are not correct? Rework this plate.

2 chicken tacos with lettuce, tomato, cheese, and onion

1 cup rice

¾ cup refried beans made with lard

12 oz regular soda

CASE IN POINT

THOMAS: CONSIDERING A VEGAN LIFESTYLE

Thomas has always been an athlete. He played a wide variety of sports throughout his high school years. He continued to be very active even in college. He has done some bodybuilding and has always consumed a high percentage of his calories from protein and meat sources. Thomas is 26 years old and Caucasian. He is currently 5 ft 9 in tall and 215 lb. Recently he has been dating a woman with whom he is really in love. His only concern is that she is of Indian decent and due to her cultural and religious beliefs, she is a vegan. She has not tried to persuade him to adopt the vegan lifestyle; however, he knows that meals at home with her would never contain animal proteins. He is not sure that he would ever be able to give up his meat sources for a different protein source. He is primarily concerned he would not get the adequate protein he needs for his weightlifting and bodybuilding activities. He has decided it may be in his best interest to discuss his concerns with his doctor. His doctor suggested meeting with a registered dietitian to review his calorie and protein needs and to discuss his options for alternative protein sources.

ASSESSMENT

1. Thomas is 5 ft 9 in tall. What is the ideal body weight for him?
2. Is Thomas at a healthy body weight for his height?
3. Using Table 2-1, what would you expect an appropriate calorie range for Thomas to be?
4. What would be important to discuss with Thomas when considering a vegan diet plan?

DIAGNOSIS

5. Write a nursing diagnosis for Thomas.

PLAN/GOAL

6. What could Thomas do to help ensure he is receiving adequate nutrition and meeting his macro- and micronutrient needs?

IMPLEMENTATION

7. Name food sources Thomas could consume that are high in calcium.
8. Name food sources Thomas could consume that are high in vitamin B12.
9. Name food sources Thomas could consume that are high in iron.
10. Name food sources that Thomas could consume that are high in omega-3 fatty acids.

EVALUATION/OUTCOME CRITERIA

11. How would you determine the success of Thomas's transition to his new vegan lifestyle?

THINKING FURTHER

12. What other types of vegetarian lifestyles are options for Thomas if he would like to incorporate some animal food sources?

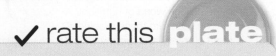

✔ rate this **plate**

Thomas is concerned about getting enough protein on a vegan diet. Will this meal provide Thomas with enough protein? What vegan protein sources could Thomas include in the meal or as a snack to meet his protein needs? Rate this plate.

Tofu stir-fry with broccoli, snow peas, carrots, and onion

   ½ **cup brown rice**

   1/6 of a cantaloupe, sliced

   Carbonated fruit beverage

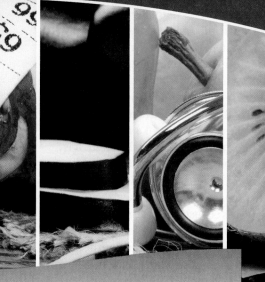

CHAPTER 3

KEY TERMS

absorption
adipose tissue
aerobic metabolism
anabolism
anaerobic metabolism
basal metabolism rate (BMR)
bile
bolus
bomb calorimeter
calorie
capillaries
cardiac sphincter
catabolism
catalyst
chemical digestion
cholecystokinin (CCK)
chyme
colon
digestion
duodenum
energy balance
energy requirement
enzymes
esophagus
feces
fundus (of stomach)
gastric juices
gastrin
gastrointestinal (GI) tract
hormones
hydrolysis
ileum
jejunum
kilocalorie (kcal)
Krebs cycle
lactase
lacteals
lean body mass

DIGESTION, ABSORPTION, AND METABOLISM

OBJECTIVES

After studying this chapter, you should be able to:

- Describe the processes of digestion, absorption, and metabolism
- Name the organs in the digestive system and describe their functions
- Name the enzymes or digestive juices secreted by each organ and gland in the digestive system
- Calculate your basal metabolic rate

Although the body is infinitely more complex than the automobile engine, it may be compared to the engine because both require fuel to run. The body's fuel is, of course, food. For the body to use its fuel, it must first prepare the food and then distribute it appropriately. It does this through the processes of digestion and absorption. The actual use of the food as fuel, resulting in energy, is called **metabolism**.

KEY TERMS *(Continued)*

lymphatic system
maltase
mechanical digestion
metabolism
pancreas
pancreatic amylase
pancreatic lipase
pancreatic proteases
pepsin
peptidases
peristalsis
pylorus
resting energy expenditure (REE)
saliva
salivary amylase
secretin
sucrase
villi

metabolism
the use of the food by the body after
digestion, which results in energy

digestion
breakdown of food in the body in preparation
for absorption

gastrointestinal (GI) tract
pertaining to the digestive system

DIGESTION

Digestion is the process whereby food is broken down into smaller parts, chemically changed, and moved through the gastrointestinal system. The **gastrointestinal (GI) tract** consists of the body structures that participate in digestion. Digestion begins in the mouth and ends at the anus. Along the entire GI tract, secretions of mucus lubricate and protect the mucosal tissues. As the process of digestion is discussed, refer to Figure 3-1 and note the locations and function of the digestive structures.

Digestion occurs through two types of action—mechanical and chemical. During **mechanical digestion**, food is broken into smaller pieces by the teeth. It is then moved along the GI tract through the esophagus, stomach, and intestines. This movement is caused by a rhythmic contraction of the muscular walls of the tract called **peristalsis**. Mechanical digestion helps to prepare food for chemical digestion by breaking it into smaller pieces. Several small pieces collectively have more surface area than fewer large ones and thus are more readily broken down by digestive juices.

During **chemical digestion**, the composition of carbohydrates, proteins, and fats is changed. Chemical changes occur through the addition of water and the resulting splitting, or breaking down, of the food molecules. This process is called **hydrolysis**. Food is broken down into nutrients that the tissues can absorb and use. Hydrolysis also involves digestive **enzymes** that act on food substances, causing them to break down into simple compounds. An enzyme can also act as a **catalyst**, which speeds up the chemical reactions without itself being changed in the process. Digestive enzymes are secreted by the mouth, stomach, **pancreas**, and small intestine (see Table 3-1). An enzyme is often named for the substance on which it acts. For example, the enzyme sucrase acts on sucrose, the enzyme maltase acts on maltose, and lactase acts on lactose.

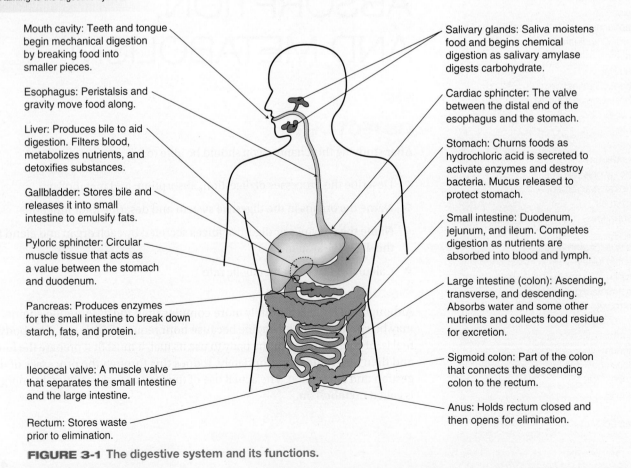

Mouth cavity: Teeth and tongue begin mechanical digestion by breaking food into smaller pieces.

Esophagus: Peristalsis and gravity move food along.

Liver: Produces bile to aid digestion. Filters blood, metabolizes nutrients, and detoxifies substances.

Gallbladder: Stores bile and releases it into small intestine to emulsify fats.

Pyloric sphincter: Circular muscle tissue that acts as a value between the stomach and duodenum.

Pancreas: Produces enzymes for the small intestine to break down starch, fats, and protein.

Ileocecal valve: A muscle valve that separates the small intestine and the large intestine.

Rectum: Stores waste prior to elimination.

Salivary glands: Saliva moistens food and begins chemical digestion as salivary amylase digests carbohydrate.

Cardiac sphincter: The valve between the distal end of the esophagus and the stomach.

Stomach: Churns foods as hydrochloric acid is secreted to activate enzymes and destroy bacteria. Mucus released to protect stomach.

Small intestine: Duodenum, jejunum, and ileum. Completes digestion as nutrients are absorbed into blood and lymph.

Large intestine (colon): Ascending, transverse, and descending. Absorbs water and some other nutrients and collects food residue for excretion.

Sigmoid colon: Part of the colon that connects the descending colon to the rectum.

Anus: Holds rectum closed and then opens for elimination.

FIGURE 3-1 The digestive system and its functions.

TABLE 3-1 Enzymes and Foods Acted Upon

SOURCE	ENZYME	FOOD ACTED UPON
Mouth	Salivary amylase	Starch
Stomach	Pepsin	Proteins
	Rennin	Proteins in milk
	Gastric lipase	Emulsified fat
Small intestine	Pancreatic amylase	Starch
	Pancreatic proteases	Proteins
	(trypsin)	
	(chymotrypsin)	
	(carboxypeptidases)	
	Pancreatic lipase	Fats
	(steapsin)	
	Lactase	Lactose
	Maltase	Maltose
	Sucrase	Sucrose
	Peptidases	Proteins

Exploring THE WEB

Visit the website of the American College of Gastroenterology (http://www.acg.gi.org). Browse around the website and become familiar with common problems related to digestion and the GI tract. Create fact sheets for the common disorders and include tips for combating them. Choose one topic from the website for class discussion.

Digestion in the Mouth

Digestion begins in the mouth, where the food is broken into smaller pieces by the teeth and mixed with saliva. At this point, each mouthful of food that is ready to be swallowed is called a **bolus**. **Saliva** is a secretion of the salivary glands that contains water, salts, and a digestive enzyme called **salivary amylase** (also called ptyalin), which acts on complex carbohydrates (starch). Food is normally held in the mouth for such a short time that only small amounts of carbohydrates are chemically changed there. The salivary glands also secrete a mucous material that lubricates and binds food particles to help in swallowing the bolus. The final chemical digestion of carbohydrates occurs in the small intestine.

The Esophagus

The **esophagus** is a 10-in muscular tube through which food travels from the mouth to the stomach. When swallowed, the bolus of food is moved down the esophagus by peristalsis and gravity. At the lower end of the esophagus, the **cardiac sphincter**, also known as the lower esophageal sphincter, opens to allow passage of the bolus into the stomach. The cardiac sphincter prevents the acidic content of the stomach from flowing back into the esophagus. When this sphincter malfunctions, it causes acid reflux disease.

Digestion in the Stomach

The stomach consists of an upper portion known as the **fundus**, a middle area known as the body of the stomach, and the end nearest the small intestine called the **pylorus**. Food enters the fundus and moves to the body of the stomach, where the muscles in the stomach wall gradually knead the food, tear it, and mix it with gastric juices and with the intrinsic factor necessary for the absorption of

mechanical digestion
the part of digestion that requires certain mechanical movements, such as chewing, swallowing, and peristalsis

peristalsis
rhythmical movement of the intestinal tract; moves the chyme along

chemical digestion
chemical changes in foods during digestion caused by hydrolysis

hydrolysis
the addition of water, resulting in the breakdown of the molecule

enzymes
organic substances that cause changes in other substances

catalyst
a substance that causes another substance to react

pancreas
gland that secretes enzymes essential for digestion and insulin, and that is essential for glucose metabolism

bolus
food in the mouth that is ready to be swallowed

saliva
secretion of the salivary glands

salivary amylase
also called ptyalin; the enzyme secreted by the salivary glands to act on starch

esophagus
tube leading from the mouth to the stomach; part of the gastrointestinal system

cardiac sphincter
the muscle at the base of the esophagus that prevents gastric reflux from moving into the esophagus

fundus (of the stomach)
upper part of the stomach

pylorus
the end of the stomach nearest the intestine

chyme
the food mass as it has been mixed with gastric juices

gastrin
hormone released by the stomach

gastric juices
the digestive secretions of the stomach

pepsin
an enzyme secreted by the stomach that is essential for the digestion of proteins

duodenum
first (and smallest) section of the small intestine

jejunum
middle section comprising about two-fifths of the small intestine

ileum
last part of the small intestine

secretin
hormone causing the pancreas to release sodium bicarbonate to neutralize acidity of the chyme

cholecystokinin (CCK)
hormone that triggers the gallbladder to release bile

bile
secretion of the liver, stored in the gallbladder, essential for the digestion of fats

pancreatic proteases
enzymes secreted by the pancreas that are essential for the digestion of proteins

pancreatic amylase
the enzyme secreted by the pancreas that is essential for the digestion of starch

pancreatic lipase
enzyme secreted by the pancreas that is essential for the digestion of fats

lactase
enzyme secreted by the small intestine for the digestion of lactose

vitamin B_{12}, before it can be propelled forward in slow, controlled movements. The food becomes a semiliquid mass called **chyme** (pronounced "kime"). When the chyme enters the pylorus, it causes distention and the release of the hormone **gastrin**, which increases the release of gastric juices.

Gastric juices are digestive secretions of the stomach. They contain hydrochloric acid, **pepsin**, and mucus. Hydrochloric acid activates the enzyme pepsin, prepares protein molecules for partial digestion by pepsin, destroys most bacteria in the food ingested, and makes iron and calcium more soluble. As the hydrochloric acid is released, a thick mucus is also secreted to protect the stomach from this harsh acid. In children, there are two additional enzymes: rennin, which acts on milk protein and casein, and gastric lipase, which breaks the butterfat molecules of milk into smaller molecules.

In summary, the functions of the stomach include the following:

- Temporary storage of food
- Mixing of food with gastric juices
- Regulation of a slow, controlled emptying of food into the intestine
- Secretion of the intrinsic factor for vitamin B_{12} (to be discussed in Chapter 7)
- Destruction of most bacteria inadvertently consumed

Digestion in the Small Intestine

Chyme moves through the pyloric sphincter into the **duodenum**, the first section of the small intestine. It subsequently passes through the **jejunum**, the midsection of the small intestine, and the **ileum**, the last section of the small intestine.

When food reaches the small intestine, the hormone **secretin** causes the pancreas to release sodium bicarbonate to neutralize the acidity of the chyme. The gallbladder is triggered by the hormone **cholecystokinin (CCK)**, which is produced by intestinal mucosal glands when fat enters, to release **bile**. Bile is produced in the liver but stored in the gallbladder. Bile emulsifies fat after it is secreted into the small intestine. This action enables the enzymes to digest the fats more easily.

Chyme also triggers the pancreas to secrete its juice into the small intestine. Pancreatic juice contains the following enzymes:

- Trypsin, chymotrypsin, and carboxypeptidases split proteins into smaller substances. These are called **pancreatic proteases** because they are protein-splitting enzymes produced by the pancreas.
- **Pancreatic amylase** converts starches (polysaccharides) to simple sugars.
- **Pancreatic lipase** reduces fats to fatty acids and glycerol.

The small intestine itself produces an intestinal juice that contains the enzymes **lactase**, **maltase**, and **sucrase**. These enzymes split lactose, maltose, and sucrose, respectively, into simple sugars. The small intestine also produces enzymes called **peptidases** that break down proteins into amino acids.

The Large Intestine

The large intestine, or **colon**, consists of the cecum, colon, and rectum. The cecum is the blind, pouch-like beginning of the colon in the right lower quadrant of the abdomen. The appendix is a diverticulum that extends off the cecum. The cecum is separated from the ileum by the ileocecal valve and is considered to be the beginning of the large intestine (colon). Its primary function is to absorb water and salts from undigested food. It has a muscular wall that can knead the contents to enhance absorption. One of the end products of fermentation in the cecum is volatile fatty acids. The major volatile fatty acids are acetate, propionate, and butyrate. These are absorbed from the large intestine and used as sources of energy. The digested food then enters the ascending colon and moves through the transverse colon and on to the descending colon, the sigmoid colon, the rectum, and, finally, the anal canal.

ABSORPTION

After digestion, the next major step in the body's use of its food is absorption. **Absorption** is the passage of nutrients into the blood or **lymphatic system** (the lymphatic vessels carry fat-soluble particles and molecules that are too large to pass through the capillaries into the bloodstream).

To be absorbed, nutrients must be in their simplest forms. Carbohydrates must be broken down to the simple sugars (glucose, fructose, and galactose), proteins to amino acids, and fats to fatty acids and glycerol. Most absorption of nutrients occurs in the small intestine, although some occurs in the large intestine. Water is absorbed in the stomach, small intestine, and large intestine.

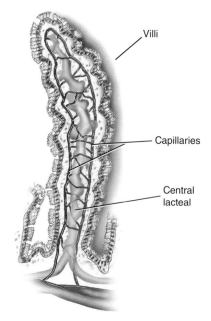

FIGURE 3-2 Wall of the small intestine.

Absorption in the Small Intestine

The small intestine, the longest digestive structure at approximately 20 ft in length, has mucosal folds, villi, and microvilli on its inner surface to increase the surface area for maximum absorption. The fingerlike projections called **villi** have hundreds of microscopic, hairlike projections called microvilli. The microvilli are very sensitive to the nutrient needs of our bodies (see Figure 3-2). Each villus contains numerous blood **capillaries** (tiny blood vessels) and **lacteals** (lymphatic vessels). The villi absorb nutrients from the chyme by way of these blood capillaries and lacteals, which eventually transfer them to the bloodstream. Glucose, fructose, galactose, amino acids, minerals, and water-soluble vitamins are absorbed by the capillaries. Fructose and galactose are subsequently carried to the liver, where they are converted to glucose. Lacteals absorb glycerol and fatty acids (end products of fat digestion) in addition to the fat-soluble vitamins.

Absorption in the Large Intestine

When the chyme reaches the large intestine, most digestion and absorption have already occurred. The colon is roughly 5 ft long and 3 in in diameter. Its walls secrete mucus as a protection from the acidic digestive juices in the chyme, which is coming from the small intestine through the ileocecal valve.

The major tasks of the large intestine are to absorb water, to synthesize some B vitamins and vitamin K (essential for blood clotting), and to collect food residue. Food residue is the part of food that the body's enzyme action cannot digest and consequently the body cannot absorb. Such residue is commonly called dietary fiber. Examples include the outer hulls of corn kernels and grains of wheat, celery strings, and apple skins. It is important that the diet contains adequate fiber because it promotes the health of the large intestine by helping to produce softer stools and more frequent bowel movements (see Chapter 4).

maltase
enzyme secreted by the small intestine essential for the digestion of maltose

sucrase
enzyme secreted by the small intestine to aid in digestion of sucrose

peptidases
enzymes secreted by the small intestine that are essential for the digestion of proteins

colon
large intestine

absorption
passage of nutrients into the blood or lymphatic system

lymphatic system
transports fat-soluble substances from the small intestine to the vascular system

villi
tiny, hairlike structures in the small intestines through which nutrients are absorbed

capillaries
tiny blood vessels connecting veins and arteries

lacteals
lymphatic vessels in the small intestine that absorb fatty acids and glycerol

feces
solid waste from the large intestine

aerobic metabolism
combining nutrients with oxygen within the cell; also called oxidation

anaerobic metabolism
reduces fats without use of oxygen

Krebs cycle
a series of enzymatic reactions that serve as the main source of cellular energy

anabolism
the creation of new compounds during metabolism

catabolism
the breakdown of compounds during metabolism

hormones
chemical messengers secreted by a variety of glands

kilocalorie (kcal)
the unit used to measure the fuel value of foods

calorie
represents the amount of heat needed to raise the temperature of 1 kg of water by 1 degree Celsius (°C)

ELIMINATION

Undigested food is excreted as **feces** by way of the rectum. The urge to defecate happens when the rectum becomes distended because of accumulating waste residue. Body waste comprises a variety of substances, including dietary fibers, connective tissue from meat that was undigestible, fats bound to minerals, bacteria, pigments, mucus, and water. In healthy people, 99% of carbohydrates, 95% of fats, and 92% of proteins are absorbed. Overall transit time from food ingestion to elimination can range from 16 to 27 hours, though this can vary widely.

METABOLISM

After digestion and absorption, nutrients are carried by the blood to the cells of the body. Within the cells, nutrients are changed into energy through a complex process called metabolism. During **aerobic metabolism**, nutrients are combined with oxygen within each cell. This process is known as oxidation. Oxidation ultimately reduces carbohydrates to carbon dioxide and water; proteins are reduced to carbon dioxide, water, and nitrogen. **Anaerobic metabolism** reduces fats without the use of oxygen. The complete oxidation of carbohydrates, proteins, and fats is commonly called the **Krebs cycle**.

As nutrients are oxidized, energy is released. When this released energy is used to build new substances from simpler ones, the process is called **anabolism**. An example of anabolism is the formation of new body tissues. When released energy is used to reduce substances to simpler ones, the process is called **catabolism**. This building up (anabolism) and breaking down (catabolism) of substances is a continuous process (metabolism) within the body and requires a continuous supply of nutrients.

Metabolism and the Thyroid Gland

Metabolism is governed primarily by the **hormones** secreted by the thyroid gland. These secretions are *triiodothyronine* (T_3) and *thyroxine* (T_4). When the thyroid gland secretes too much of these hormones, a condition known as hyperthyroidism may result. In such a case, the body metabolizes its food too quickly, resulting in weight loss. When too little T_4 and T_3 are secreted, the condition called hypothyroidism may occur. In this case, the body metabolizes food too slowly, and the client tends to become sluggish and accumulates fat.

ENERGY

Energy is constantly needed for the maintenance of body tissue and temperature and for growth (involuntary activity), as well as for voluntary activity. Examples of voluntary activity include walking, running, swimming, and gardening. The three groups of nutrients that provide energy to the body are carbohydrates, proteins, and fats. Carbohydrates are and should be the primary energy source (see Chapter 4).

Energy Measurement

The unit used to measure the energy value of foods is the **kilocalorie (kcal)**, commonly known as the large calorie, or **calorie**. In the metric system, it is known as the kilojoule. One kilocalorie is equal to 4.184 kilojoules, but this may be rounded off to 4.2 kilojoules. One calorie is the amount of heat needed to raise the temperature of 1 kg of water by 1 degree Celsius (°C).

The number of calories in a food is its energy value, or caloric density. Energy values of foods vary a great deal because they are determined by the types and amounts of nutrients each food contains.

One gram of carbohydrate yields 4 calories; 1 g of protein yields 4 calories; and 1 g of fat yields 9 calories. One gram of alcohol yields 7 calories.

The energy values of foods are determined by a device known as a **bomb calorimeter**. The inner part of a calorimeter holds a measured amount of food, and the outer part holds water. The food is burned, and its caloric value is determined by the increase in the temperature of the surrounding water. The number of calories in average servings of common foods is listed in Appendix B.

Basal Metabolic Rate

One's basal metabolism is the energy necessary to carry on all involuntary vital processes while the body is at rest. These processes are respiration, circulation, regulation of body temperature, and cell activity and maintenance. The rate at which energy is needed only for body maintenance is called the **basal metabolism rate (BMR)**. The BMR may be referred to as the **resting energy expenditure (REE)**.

Medical tests can determine one's BMR (or REE). When such a test is given, the body is at rest and performing only the essential, involuntary functions. Voluntary activity is not measured in a BMR test. Factors that affect one's BMR are lean body mass, body size, sex, age, heredity, physical condition, and climate.

Lean body mass is muscle, as opposed to fat tissue. Because there is more metabolic activity in muscle tissue than in fat or bone tissue, muscle tissue requires more calories than does fat or bone tissue. People with large body frames require more calories than do people with small frames because the former have more body mass to maintain and move.

Men usually require more energy than women. They tend to be larger and to have more lean body mass than women.

Children require more calories per pound of body weight than adults because they are growing. As people age, the lean body mass declines, and the basal metabolic rate declines accordingly. Heredity is also a determining factor. Like appearance, one's BMR may resemble that of a parent. One's physical condition also affects the BMR. For example, women require more calories during pregnancy and lactation than at other times. The basal metabolic rate increases during fever and decreases during periods of starvation or severely reduced calorie intake. People living and working in extremely cold or warm climates require more calories to maintain normal body temperature than they would in a more temperate climate.

Thermic Effect of Food

The body requires energy to process food (digestion, absorption, transportation, metabolism, and storage); this requirement represents 10% of daily energy (calorie) intake. Multiply BMR by 0.10 and add to the BMR (REE) before an activity factor is calculated.

Estimating BMR

Dietitians commonly use the Harris-Benedict equation to determine the BMR (REE) of persons above the age of 18. This equation uses height, weight, and age as factors and results in a more individualized estimate of the REE than some other methods (see Figure 3-3).

bomb calorimeter
device used to scientifically determine the kcal value of foods

basal metabolism rate (BMR)
the rate at which energy is needed for body maintenance; also referred to as resting energy expenditure (REE)

resting energy expenditure (REE)
same as basal metabolism rate (BMR)

lean body mass
percentage of muscle tissue

Female: **REE = 655 + (9.6 × weight in kg) + (1.8 × height in cm) − (4.7 × age)**

Male: **REE = 66 + (13.7 × weight in kg) + (5 × height in cm) − (6.8 × age)**

W = weight in kilograms (kg) (weight in pounds ÷ 2.2 = kg)
H = height in centimeters (cm) (height in inches × 2.54 = cm)
A = age in years

FIGURE 3-3 Harris-Benedict equation.

Another method used to estimate one's BMR, or REE, is the following:

1. Convert body weight from pounds to kilograms (kg) by dividing pounds by 2.2 (2.2 lbs equal 1 kg).
2. Multiply the kilograms by 24 (hours per day).
3. Multiply the answer obtained in step 2 by 0.9 for a woman and by 1.0 for a man.

For example, assume that a woman weighs 110 lbs. Divide 110 by 2.2 for an answer of 50 kg. Multiply 50 kg by 24 hours in a day for an answer of 1,200 calories. Then multiply 1,200 calories by 0.9 for an answer of 1,080 calories. This is the estimated basal metabolic energy requirement for that particular woman.

SUPERSIZE USA

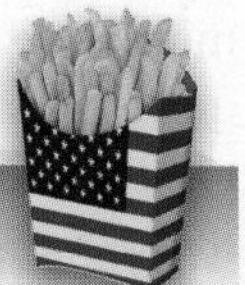

When you drive through the fast food restaurant, keep in mind the following worst fast food choices:

Order	Calories	Fat	Carbs	Protein	Sodium
McDonald's Angus Chipotle BBQ Bacon Burger	830	41 g	67 g	48 g	2,060 mg
Burger King Tendercrisp Chicken Caesar Garden Salad with Dressing	650	43 g	39 g	30 g	1,670 mg
Denny's Country Fried Steak with Gravy	1,010	69 g	64 g	33 g	2,490 mg
Burger King Sausage, Egg, & Cheese Croissan'wich	500	33 g	32 g	19 g	930 mg
Wendy's Chocolate Frosty Shake, Large	580	15 g	96 g	16 g	270 mg
Applebees Oriental Chicken Salad	1,400	99 g	92 g	40 g	1,630 mg
Pizza Hut Meat Lover's Pan Pizza (3 Slices)	930	51 g	81 g	39 g	2,250 mg

Source: Data retrieved from website for each fast food restaurant, 2015

Calculating Total Energy Requirements

An individual's average daily **energy requirement** is the total number of calories needed in a 24-hour period. Energy requirements of people differ, depending on BMR (REE) and activities. More energy is burned playing soccer than playing the piano. Refer to Table 3-2 for calorie guidelines according to MyPlate.

Table 3-3 shows suggested weights for adults according to height.

energy requirement
number of calories required by the body each day

TABLE 3-2 ESTIMATED DAILY CALORIE NEEDS

The calorie range for each age and gender is based on physical activity level, from sedentary to active. Sedentary means a lifestyle that includes only the light physical activity associated with typical day-to-day life. Active means a lifestyle that includes physical activity equivalent to walking more than 3 miles per day at 3–4 miles per hour, in addition to the light physical activity associated with typical day-to-day life.

	CALORIE RANGE				CALORIE RANGE		
	SEDENTARY	→	ACTIVE		SEDENTARY	→	ACTIVE
Children				**Males**			
2–3 years	1,000	→	1,400	4–8 years	1,400	→	2,000
Females				9–13	1,800	→	2,600
4–8 years	1,200	→	1,800	14–18	2,200	→	3,200
9–13	1,600	→	2,200	19–30	2,400	→	3,000
14–18	1,800	→	2,400	31–50	2,200	→	3,000
19–30	2,000	→	2,400	51+	2,000	→	2,800
31–50	1,800	→	2,200				
51+	1,600	→	2,200				

Source: Adapted from U.S. Department of Health and Human Services and U.S. Department of Agriculture. (December 2015). *2015–2020 Dietary Guidelines for Americans* (8th ed.). Available at http://health.gov/dietaryguidelines/2015/guidelines/

TABLE 3-3 Suggested Weights for Adults

HEIGHT (WITHOUT SHOES)	WEIGHT IN POUNDS WITHOUT CLOTHES 19–34 YEARS	35 YEARS AND OVER
5'0"	97–128	108–138
5'1"	101–132	111–143
5'2"	104–137	115–148
5'3"	107–141	119–152
5'4"	111–146	122–157
5'5"	114–150	126–162
5'6"	118–155	130–167
5'7"	121–160	134–172
5'8"	125–164	138–178
5'9"	129–169	142–183
5'10"	132–174	146–188
5'11"	136–179	151–194
6'0"	140–184	155–199
6'1"	144–189	159–205
6'2"	148–195	164–210
6'3"	152–200	168–216
6'4"	156–205	173–222
6'5"	160–211	177–228
6'6"	164–216	182–234

Note: The higher weights in the ranges generally apply to men, who tend to have more muscle and bone; the lower weights more often apply to women, who have less muscle and bone.

Source: U.S. Department of Health and Human Services and U.S. Department of Agriculture. *Dietary Guidelines for Americans* (3rd ed.). Washington, DC. Accessed August 31, 2015. http://www.cnpp.usda.gov

SPOTLIGHT *on Life Cycle*

Maintaining energy, or calorie, balance can be achieved by balancing "energy in" with "energy out." What you eat and drink is "energy in." Through daily activities and physical activity, energy is expended and can be considered as "energy out." When "energy in" equals "energy out" over time, body weight will stay the same. When there is more "in" than "out" over time, weight gain can result. When there is more "out" than "in" over time, weight loss can result. Eating an additional 150 calories per day for a year can result in a 10-lb weight gain. Reducing "energy in" or increasing "energy out" can help a person lose unwanted weight. Here are a few ways to cut 150 calories ("energy in"):

- Drink water instead of a 12-oz regular soda.
- Order a small serving of French fries instead of a medium serving.
- Eat an egg-white omelet instead of whole eggs.
- Use tuna canned in water instead of oil.

Here are a few ways to burn 150 calories ("energy out") in just 30 minutes (for a 150-lb person):

- Shoot hoops
- Walk 2 miles
- Do yard work
- Go for a bike ride
- Dance with family or friends

Source: Adapted from the National Heart Lung and Blood Institute. "Balance Food and Activity." Accessed August 30, 2015. http://www.nhlbi.nih.gov

Energy Balance

A person who takes in fewer calories than she or he burns usually loses weight. If someone takes in more calories than she or he burns, the body stores them as **adipose tissue** (fat). Some adipose tissue is necessary to protect the body and support its organs. Adipose tissue also helps regulate body temperature, just as insulation helps regulate the temperature of a building. An excess of adipose tissue, however, leads to obesity, which can endanger health because it puts extra burdens on body organs and systems. For the healthy person, the goal is **energy balance**. This means that the number of calories consumed matches the number of calories required for one's BMR (REE) and activity.

HEALTH AND NUTRITION CONSIDERATIONS

The health care professional will find that clients may make broad statements concerning the way their bodies work. An example would be: "Milk doesn't agree with me." This is when the appropriate questions need to be asked, such as "Does it cause flatulence (gas)?" or "Do you have to go to the bathroom immediately?" The first is a classic symptom of lactose intolerance, whereas the latter

adipose tissue
fatty tissue

energy balance
occurs when the caloric value of food ingested equals the calories expended

could indicate an allergy or other serious problems that would require further workup. Clients needing education about metabolism and energy requirements may tell you that they don't eat anything but keep gaining weight or that they exercise all the time but don't lose an ounce. Clients deserve current and correct health information; therefore, health care professionals must continually educate themselves in order to provide the most accurate information to their clients.

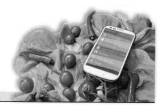

SUMMARY

The body is comparable to an automobile engine because both require fuel. Food acts as fuel, but to be usable, it must undergo a series of processes that include digestion, absorption, and metabolism. Digestion is the process whereby food is broken down into smaller parts, chemically changed, and moved along the gastrointestinal tract. Mechanical digestion refers to that part of the process performed by the teeth and muscles of the digestive system. Chemical digestion refers to that part of the process wherein food is broken down to molecules that the blood can absorb. Enzymes are essential for chemical digestion. After digestion, nutrients are transported by the blood and lymphatic system, primarily in the small intestine, and then carried to all body tissues. After absorption, food is metabolized. During metabolism, carbohydrates and proteins are combined with oxygen in a process called oxidation. Energy released during oxidation is measured by the calorie. Caloric values of foods vary, as do people's energy requirements. Requirements depend on age, body size, sex, lean body mass, physical condition, climate, and activity.

DISCUSSION TOPICS

1. Describe the process of digestion.
2. Of what value are enzymes to digestion? Name five enzymes and the nutrients on which they act.
3. Describe absorption of nutrients.
4. Describe metabolism.
5. Explain why the body requires fuel even during sleep.
6. Explain the differences between the terms *energy value* and *energy requirement*.

SUGGESTED ACTIVITIES

1. Using the method given in this chapter, calculate your total energy requirement.
2. Prepare a brief description of the processes of digestion and absorption that could be presented to a fourth-grade class.
3. Role-play a situation where the client asks the health care provider to explain *metabolism*.
4. Compare your total energy requirement with your intake from your three-day food analysis in Chapter 2.

REVIEW

Multiple choice. Select the *letter* that precedes the best answer.

1. Digestion begins in the
   a. mouth
   b. stomach
   c. liver
   d. small intestine

2. Most of the digestive processes occur in the
   a. mouth
   b. stomach
   c. small intestine
   d. colon

3. The small intestine is divided into three segments. They are, in descending order,
   a. ileum, jejunum, duodenum
   b. jejunum, ileum, duodenum
   c. duodenum, ileum, jejunum
   d. duodenum, jejunum, ileum

4. The fluid mixture that moves from the stomach through the pyloric sphincter is called
   a. bolus
   b. chyme
   c. food
   d. gastrin

5. A muscular movement that moves food down the GI tract is called
   a. GI pump
   b. peristalsis
   c. lymphatic circulation
   d. circular propulsion

6. What body system transports fat throughout the body?
   a. lymphatic system
   b. circulatory system
   c. digestive system
   d. blood system

7. An organic substance that causes changes in other substances is a/an
   a. hormone
   b. bacterium
   c. enzyme
   d. acid

8. Maltase, sucrase, and lactase are produced in the
   a. stomach
   b. small intestine
   c. colon
   d. pancreas

9. Bile is needed to digest
   a. fats   c. proteins
   b. fiber   d. carbohydrates

10. When energy intake is greater than energy output, the body weight will
    a. remain the same
    b. decrease
    c. increase and then decrease
    d. increase

11. What is the BMR for a 170-lb male?
    a. 1,854   c. 1,720
    b. 2,010   d. 1,400

CASE IN POINT

JANEESHA: WEIGHT MAINTENANCE AFTER SMOKING CESSATION

Janeesha has been smoking cigarettes for almost 10 years. Both of her parents were smokers, so she started smoking at about 15 years old. She began with just a few here and there, but gradually worked her way up to about a pack per day. When she first started smoking, she was not concerned about the health risks to her body. She thought it was cool, and many of her friends were also smoking. Now that she's older, she has seen first-hand what smoking can do. Her mother has been diagnosed with lung cancer and her father is now on oxygen to aid his breathing difficulties caused by his emphysema. In addition, Janeesha was married last year and her new husband is not a smoker. He has encouraged her to stop smoking. He is concerned for her health, and if they choose to have children, he would not want her to smoke during the pregnancy. Janeesha has decided she is ready to stop smoking. She has been attending a smoking cessation class. She has also discussed medication options for smoking cessation with her doctor. One of Janeesha's concerns about quitting is the weight gain that many people experience. Janeesha is African American, and she is currently 5 ft 2 in tall and 140 lbs. She knows she is already slightly overweight, but likes her fuller figure. Her husband thinks she is beautiful at her current weight. However, she does not want to gain more weight and create additional health problems as she stops smoking. In discussing her concerns with her doctor, he suggests that Janeesha make an appointment with a dietitian to have some nutritional education as well as her calorie needs calculated. Janeesha is hopeful that the dietitian may also give her some suggestions for healthier meals and snacks.

ASSESSMENT

1. Identify the significant data in this case study.
2. Calculate Janeesha's REE using the Harris-Benedict equation and account for the thermic effect of food (TEF).
3. What does Janeesha need to discuss with her doctor to assist with her smoking cessation?
4. What questions or concerns might Janeesha want to discuss with the dietitian?

DIAGNOSIS

5. Write a nursing diagnosis for Janeesha.

PLAN/GOAL

6. What changes can Janeesha implement to help prevent weight gain?
7. Set two measurable realistic goals for Janeesha during this process to prevent further weight gain.
8. How could information on exercise be helpful to Janeesha?

IMPLEMENTATION

9. What strategies can be used to help Janeesha become aware of her food consumption and the time it takes her to eat?
10. What actions would help Janeesha carry out these goals?
11. Who can help her?

EVALUATION/OUTCOME CRITERIA

12. What will Janeesha be able to identify if the plan is successful?

13. What will she be able to measure as evidence of her success?

THINKING FURTHER

14. Janeesha's husband is concerned about her smoking. He would like her to quit not only for her own health but also his (exposure to secondhand smoke) and for their potential children if Janeesha were to become pregnant. What are some of the risks associated with smoking and some of the added benefits of quitting?

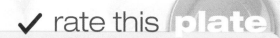 ✔ rate this **plate**

With smoking cessation, Janeesha needs to realize that her hands are going to miss the smoking since it's such a habit. Most people will eat something to fill the temptation. Rate this plate to see if Janeesha will be able to maintain her current weight.

Cheeseburger with lettuce, tomato, and onion

Medium French fries

Side salad with low-fat ranch dressing

32 oz regular soda

Calculate the calories that are in this meal and determine if it's one-third of the calories she needs in a day. What can be eliminated from this meal to reduce fat and calories?

CASE IN POINT

ED: CONTROLLING SYMPTOMS OF CROHN'S DISEASE

Ed was diagnosed with Crohn's disease when he was 16. Now that he is 28 years old, he is having increased difficulty controlling his symptoms. His disease is primarily affecting his large intestine. Ed is 6 ft 1 in tall and weighs 223 lbs. He knows he is prone to flare-ups and must be careful about what he eats. His triggers can be malabsorption of any of the macronutrients: carbohydrate, protein, and fat. Ed and his wife recently took a trip to El Salvador to visit her family. He thoroughly enjoyed the food his mother-in-law prepared. She is a fabulous cook. During their visit, the symptoms began to flare up. He couldn't stop eating all the delicious foods. The cuisine was such a mix of spicy, salty, and sweet flavors, and he loved it all. For the last two weeks since returning home, he has been having mainly diarrhea and loose stools. He has lost 8 lbs. He has wanted to lose weight, however, he knows this is not the way to achieve weight loss. His wife feels terrible that the spicy foods may have caused his problem. She has encouraged Ed to go see his doctor. He makes an appointment with his physician. His physician orders a CBC, albumin, folic acid, and B_{12} levels to be drawn. She also would like Ed to see a dietitian. She would like for him to begin a low-lactose, low-fat, low-fiber, and high-protein diet.

ASSESSMENT

1. What are the pertinent objective and subjective data related to Ed's problem?
2. Calculate Ed's target caloric intake and weight range according to Tables 3-2 and 3-3.

DIAGNOSIS

3. Write a nursing diagnosis for Ed.
4. What is the cause of Ed's problem with elimination?

PLAN/GOAL

5. Write a measurable goal for controlling Ed's diarrhea.
6. Write a goal to help Ed adapt to his new diet. Incorporate Ed's desire to lose weight.
7. Where could the dietitian direct Ed to obtain information to increase his understanding of his disease and the related nutrition issues?

IMPLEMENTATION

8. List at least one action to help Ed meet each goal.
9. List two foods Ed should avoid.
10. List three things Ed needs to include in his diet.
11. How could the website http://www.ccfa.org for Crohn's and ulcerative colitis be helpful to Ed?

EVALUATION/OUTCOME CRITERIA

12. What will Ed report when your plan for his Crohn's disease is effective?
13. How will Ed know his new diet is successful?
14. What can the doctor measure when all the goals are successful?

15. If the plan were not successful, what would Ed be experiencing?
16. What could be an unplanned, undesirable outcome of this diet change?

THINKING FURTHER

17. What challenges does Ed face with chronic progressive disease?

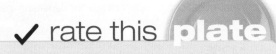

✔ rate this **plate**

Ed's doctor recommends a low-lactose, low-fat, high-fiber, and high-protein diet to begin treating his symptoms. Ed ate the following meal for dinner. Rate this plate.

- **10 oz ribeye steak**
- **Baked potato with sour cream, bacon bits, and butter**
- **½ cup of lima beans**
- **Whole wheat rolls with butter**
- **10 oz of whole milk**
- **Whole wheat fruit crumble**

What foods on this plate might give Ed continued symptoms of Crohn's disease? How might you adjust this meal to fit the diet prescribed by the physician?

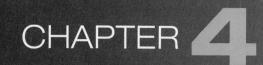

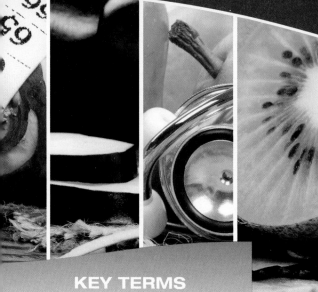

bran
cellulose
dietary fiber
disaccharides
endosperm
flatulence
fructose
galactose
germ
glucagon
glucose
glycogen
hemicellulose
hyperglycemia
hypoglycemia
insulin
intact grains
islets of Langerhans
ketosis
ketones
lactose
lignins
maltose
monosaccharides
mucilage
pectin
polysaccharides
refined grains
starch
sucrose
whey

CARBOHYDRATES

OBJECTIVES

After studying this chapter, you should be able to:

- Identify the functions of carbohydrates
- Name the primary sources of carbohydrates
- Describe the classification of carbohydrates

Carbohydrates are considered energy foods that can be rapidly oxidized by the body to release energy and its by-product, heat. Carbohydrates, fats, and proteins provide energy for the human body, but carbohydrates are the primary source. They are somewhat inexpensive compared to the other food groups and most abundant of the energy nutrients. Foods rich in carbohydrates such as fruit, vegetables, legumes, and grains grow easily in most climates.

Carbohydrates provide the major source of energy for people all over the world. They provide approximately half the calories for people living in the United States. In some areas of the world, where fats and proteins are scarce and expensive, carbohydrates provide as much as 80–100% of calories. Carbohydrates are named for the chemical elements they are composed of—carbon (C), hydrogen (H), and oxygen (O).

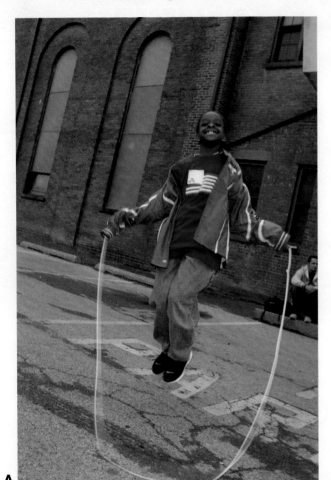
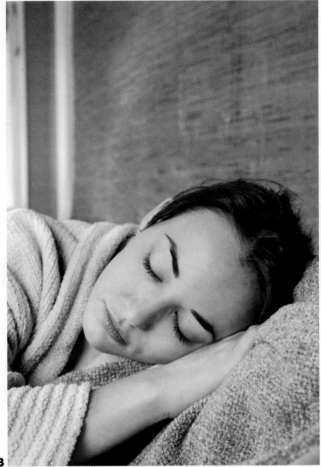

FIGURE 4-1 The need for carbohydrates is constant, whether you are active (A) or at rest (B).

FUNCTIONS

Providing energy is the major function of carbohydrates. Each gram of carbohydrate provides 4 calories. The body needs to maintain a constant supply of energy (see Figure 4-1). Therefore, it stores approximately half a day's supply of carbohydrate in the liver and muscles for use as needed. In this form, it is called glycogen.

Protein-sparing action is also an important function of carbohydrates. When enough carbohydrates (at least 50–100 g/day) are ingested to supply a person's energy needs, they spare proteins for their primary function of building and repairing body tissues.

Normal fat metabolism requires an adequate supply of carbohydrates. If there are not enough carbohydrates to fulfill the energy requirement, the body will resort to an alternative method to fuel itself. Excess fat is broken down in order to provide a source of glucose. During such an emergency need for energy, fat oxidization in the cells is not complete and substances called ketones are produced. **Ketones** are acids that accumulate in the blood and urine and **ketosis** results.

In individuals with sound health who are not pregnant, ketosis occurs after three to four days of eating less than 50 g of carbohydrate. With ketosis, you feel less hungry; therefore, some adopt the low-carbohydrate eating plan as a popular weight loss strategy. Ketoacidosis, however, is a serious condition whereby the levels of ketones reach an abnormally high level; this usually happens to diabetic

ketones
substances to which fatty acids are broken down in the liver

ketosis
condition in which ketones collect in the blood; caused by insufficient glucose available for energy

patients when they don't take enough insulin or become ill or dehydrated. This is addressed in Chapter 15.

When sufficient carbohydrates are eaten, the body is protected against ketones. This is sometimes called the antiketogenic effect of carbohydrates.

Providing fiber in the diet is another important function of carbohydrates. Dietary fiber is found in grains, vegetables, and fruits. Fiber creates a soft, bulky stool that moves quickly through the large intestine.

FOOD SOURCES

The principal sources of carbohydrates are plant foods: cereal grains, legumes (starchy beans), vegetables, fruits, and sugars (see Figure 4-2). The only substantial animal source of carbohydrates is milk.

Cereal grains and their products are dietary staples in nearly every part of the world. Rice is the basic food in Latin America, Africa, Asia, and many sections of the United States. Wheat and, increasingly, corn are used in various foods such as bread, cereal, pasta, and snack foods common to American and European diets. Rye and oats are commonly used in breads and cereals in the United States and Europe. Cereals also contain vitamins, minerals, and some proteins. During processing, some of these nutrients are lost. To compensate for this loss, food producers in the United States commonly add the B vitamins—thiamine, riboflavin, and niacin—plus the mineral iron to the final product. The product is then called *enriched*. When a nutrient that has never been part of a grain is added, the grain is said to be *fortified*. An example of fortification is the addition of folic acid to cereal grains to prevent neural tube defects (see Chapter 7).

Vegetables such as potatoes, beets, peas, starchy beans such as lima beans, and corn provide substantial amounts of carbohydrates (in the form of starch). Green leafy vegetables provide dietary fiber. All of them also provide vitamins and minerals.

Fruits provide fruit sugar, fiber, vitamins, and minerals.

Sugars such as table sugar, syrup, and honey and sugar-rich foods such as desserts and candy provide carbohydrates in the form of sugar with few other nutrients except for fats. Therefore, the foods in which they predominate are commonly called low-nutrient-dense foods.

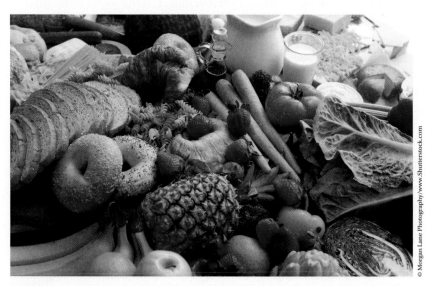

FIGURE 4-2 Fruits, vegetables, grains, and some dairy products are good sources of carbohydrates.

SPOTLIGHT *on Life Cycle*

Many adults can benefit from consuming quality fiber in their meals, as diets high in fiber have been shown to be beneficial in disease prevention. The possible benefits are decreased weight and decreases in the risks of colon cancer, rectal cancer, heart disease (decreases serum cholesterol levels), dental caries, constipation, and diverticulosis.

To follow a fiber-rich diet, counsel the adult as follows:

- Eat fresh foods instead of processed foods.
- Consume more starchy beans (legumes) and fruits and vegetables.
- Eat whole grains, especially intact ones such as brown rice, quinoa, barley, cracked wheat, and oats.
- Increase water intake; minimum is 6–8 glasses per day.
- Obtain fiber from the diet rather than from supplements.

CLASSIFICATION

Carbohydrates are divided into three groups: monosaccharides, disaccharides, and polysaccharides (Table 4-1).

Monosaccharides

Monosaccharides are the simplest form of carbohydrates. They are sweet, require no digestion, and can be absorbed directly into the bloodstream from the small intestine. They include glucose, fructose, and galactose.

Glucose, also called dextrose, is the form of carbohydrate to which all other forms are converted for eventual metabolism. It is found naturally in corn syrup and some fruits and vegetables. The central nervous system, the red blood cells, and the brain use only glucose as fuel; therefore, a continuous source is needed.

Fructose, also called levulose or fruit sugar, is found with glucose in many fruits and in honey. It is the sweetest of all the monosaccharides.

Galactose is a product of the digestion of milk. It is not found naturally.

Disaccharides

Disaccharides are pairs of the three sugars just discussed. They are sweet and must be changed to simple sugars by hydrolysis before they can be absorbed. Disaccharides include sucrose, maltose, and lactose.

Sucrose is composed of glucose and fructose. It is the form of carbohydrate present in granulated, powdered, and brown sugar and in molasses. It is one of the sweetest and least expensive sugars. Its sources are sugar cane, sugar beets, and the sap from maple trees.

Maltose is a disaccharide that is an intermediary product in the hydrolysis of starch. It is produced by enzyme action during the digestion of starch in the body. It is also created during the fermentation process that produces alcohol. It can be found in some infant formulas, malt beverage products, and beer. It is considerably less sweet than glucose or sucrose.

Lactose is the sugar found in milk. It is distinct from most other sugars because it is not found in plants. It helps the body absorb calcium. Lactose is less sweet than monosaccharides or other disaccharides.

---

monosaccharides
simplest carbohydrates; sugars that cannot be further reduced by hydrolysis; examples are glucose, fructose, and galactose

glucose
the simple sugar to which carbohydrate must be broken down for absorption; also known as *dextrose*

fructose
the simple sugar (monosaccharide) found in fruit and honey

galactose
the simple sugar (monosaccharide) to which lactose is broken down during digestion

disaccharides
double sugars that are reduced by hydrolysis to monosaccharides; examples are sucrose, maltose, and lactose

sucrose
a double sugar or disaccharide; examples are granulated, powdered, and brown sugar

maltose
the double sugar (disaccharide) occurring as a result of the digestion of grain

lactose
the sugar in milk; a disaccharide

Many adults are unable to digest lactose and suffer from bloating, abdominal cramps, and diarrhea after drinking milk or consuming a milk-based food such as processed cheese. This reaction is called lactose intolerance. It is caused by insufficient lactase, the enzyme required for digestion of lactose. There are special low-lactose milk products that can be used instead of regular milk. Lactase-containing products are also available.

TABLE 4-1 Carbohydrates

TYPE	SOURCE	FUNCTIONS	DEFICIENCY SYMPTOMS
Monosaccharides (Simple Sugars)			
Glucose	Berries Grapes Sweet corn Corn syrup	Furnish energy Spare proteins Prevent ketosis	Fatigue Weight loss
Fructose	Ripe fruits Honey Soft drinks	Fruits provide vitamins, minerals, and fiber	
Galactose	Lactose		
Disaccharides			
Sucrose	Sugar cane Sugar beets 　Granulated sugar 　Confectioner's sugar 　Brown sugar Molasses Maple syrup Candy Jams and jellies	Furnish energy Spare proteins Prevent ketosis	Fatigue Weight loss
Maltose	Digestion of starch		
Lactose	Milk		
Polysaccharides (Complex Carbohydrates)			
Starch	Cereal grains and their products: cereals, breads, rice, flour, pasta, crackers Potatoes Corn Lima beans Yams Navy beans Green bananas Sweet potatoes	Furnish energy Prevent ketosis Vegetables provide vitamins, minerals, and fiber	Fatigue Weight loss
Dextrins	Starch hydrolysis		
Glycogen	Glucose stored in liver and muscles		
Cellulose	Wheat bran, whole grain cereals, green and leafy Vegetables, fruits, especially apples, pears, oranges, grapefruit, grapes	Provide fiber	Constipation Colon cancer Diverticulosis

During the process of making hard cheese, milk separates into curd (solid part from which hard cheese is made) and **whey** (liquid part). Lactose becomes part of the whey and not the curd. Therefore, lactose is not a component of natural cheese. However, manufacturers can add milk or milk solids to processed cheese, so it is important that persons who are lactose intolerant check the labels on cheese products.

If eating dairy products consistently produces symptoms of flatulence, diarrhea, and abdominal pain, the doctor may recommend eliminating dairy products from the diet and adding them back after a period of time to ascertain the client's reaction. If the symptoms persist, the client is lactose intolerant. Doctors can order a hydrogen breath test to measure lactose intolerance (which is considered the most reliable) or a lactose intolerance test in which the blood sugar is measured after a specific quantity of lactose is consumed.

Polysaccharides

Polysaccharides are commonly called *complex carbohydrates* because they are compounds of many monosaccharides (simple sugars). Three polysaccharides are important in nutrition: starch, glycogen, and fiber.

Starch is a polysaccharide found in grains and vegetables. It is the storage form of glucose in plants. Vegetables contain less starch than grains because vegetables have a higher moisture content. Legumes (dried beans and peas) are another important source of starch as well as of dietary fiber and protein. Starches are more complex than monosaccharides or disaccharides, and it takes the body longer to digest them. Thus, they supply energy over a longer period of time. The starch in grain is found mainly in the **endosperm** (center part of the grain). This is the part from which white flour is made. The tough outer covering of grain kernels is called the **bran** (see Figure 4-3). The bran is used in coarse cereals and whole-wheat flour. The **germ** is the smallest part of the grain and is a rich source of B vitamins, vitamin E, minerals, and protein. Wheat germ is included in products made of whole wheat. It also can be purchased and used in baked products or as an addition to breakfast cereals.

whey
liquid part of milk that separates from the curd (solid part) during the making of hard cheese

polysaccharides
complex carbohydrates containing combinations of monosaccharides; examples include starch, dextrin, cellulose, and glycogen

starch
polysaccharide found in grains and vegetables

endosperm
the inner part of the kernel of grain; contains the carbohydrate

bran
outer covering of grain kernels

germ
embryo or tiny life center of each kernel of grain

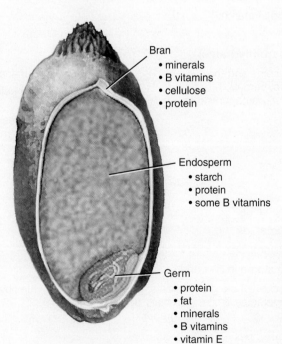

Bran
• minerals
• B vitamins
• cellulose
• protein

Endosperm
• starch
• protein
• some B vitamins

Germ
• protein
• fat
• minerals
• B vitamins
• vitamin E

FIGURE 4-3 A grain of wheat has three parts. All parts are used in whole-wheat flour; only the endosperm is used in white flour.

Whole grains contain 100% of the original kernel, which includes the bran, germ, and endosperm. When these three layers are present, they are referred to as **intact grains**. The processing method used determines the final product's nutrition profile. Whole grains that are processed just enough to improve taste and digestibility and still have the bran and germ layers partially intact (not ground into flour) are nutritionally superior to refined grains. It takes longer for digestion to occur, which slows the conversion of starch to sugar, keeping you fuller longer and preventing a surge in blood sugar.

Refined grains have the bran and germ layers removed, leaving only the endosperm, which is mostly refined starch. These tend to be less healthful, as they are rapidly digested, producing a quicker blood sugar response. Refined grain products are used to a large degree in the U.S. food supply; however, the Dietary Guidelines recommend we consume at least one-half of our grains as whole grains.

Glycogen is the storage form of glucose in the body. In the healthy adult, approximately one-half day's supply of energy is stored as glycogen in the liver and muscles. The hormone **glucagon** helps the liver convert glycogen to glucose as needed for energy. (See Chapter 12 for information on glycogen loading.)

The Fibers

Dietary fiber, also called roughage, is indigestible because it cannot be broken down by digestive enzymes. Some fiber is insoluble (it does not readily dissolve in water), and some is soluble (it partially dissolves in water) (see Figure 4-4). Insoluble fibers include cellulose, some hemicellulose, and lignins. Soluble fibers are gums, pectins, some hemicellulose, and mucilages. See Table 4-2 for food sources. **Cellulose** is a primary source of dietary fiber. It is found in the skins of fruits, the leaves and stems of vegetables, and legumes. Highly processed foods such as white bread, pasta (other than whole wheat), and pastries contain little if any cellulose because it is removed during processing. Because humans cannot digest cellulose, it has no energy value. It is useful because it provides bulk for the stool.

Hemicellulose is found mainly in whole-grain cereal. Some hemicellulose is soluble; some is not. **Lignins** are the woody part of vegetables such as carrots and asparagus or the small seeds of strawberries; they are not a carbohydrate.

Pectin, some hemicellulose, gums, and **mucilage** are soluble in water and form a gel that helps provide bulk for the intestines. They are useful also because they bind cholesterol, thus reducing the amount the blood can absorb.

Fiber is considered helpful to clients with diabetes mellitus because it can help lower blood glucose levels. It may prevent some colon cancers by moving waste materials through the colon faster than would normally be the case, thereby reducing the colon's exposure time to potential carcinogens. Fiber helps prevent constipation, hemorrhoids, and diverticular disease by softening and increasing the size of the stool.

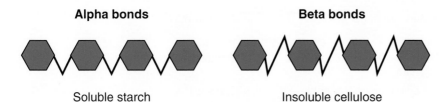

Alpha bonds — Soluble starch

Beta bonds — Insoluble cellulose

FIGURE 4-4 The alpha bonds that link glucose molecules together can be broken down during digestion. The beta bonds in cellulose cannot be broken by digestive enzymes and are eliminated without being digested.

intact grain
grains that contain all three layers intact—the bran, germ, and endosperm

refined grain
grains that have had the bran and germ removed through grinding and sifting

glycogen
glucose as stored in the liver and muscles

glucagon
hormone from alpha cells of the pancreas; helps cells release energy

dietary fiber
indigestible parts of plants; absorbs water in large intestine, helping to create soft, bulky stool; some are believed to bind cholesterol in the colon, helping to rid cholesterol from the body; some are believed to lower blood glucose levels

cellulose
indigestible carbohydrate; provides fiber in the diet

hemicellulose
dietary fiber found in whole grains

lignins
dietary fiber found in the woody parts of vegetables

pectin
edible thickening agent

mucilage
gel-forming dietary fiber

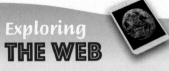
TABLE 4-2   Water-Soluble and Water-Insoluble Sources of Fiber

WATER-SOLUBLE FIBER		WATER-INSOLUBLE FIBER
Fruit (pectin)	**Grains**	All vegetables
Apples	Oats	Fruit
Peaches	Barley	Whole grains
Plums and prunes	**Legumes**	Brown rice
Bananas	Dried peas	Wild rice
	Beans	Wheat bran
	Lentils	Nuts
		Seeds

The optimal recommendation for fiber intake is 20–35 g/day. The normal U.S. diet is thought to contain approximately 11 g. In general, Americans do not consume sufficient amounts of fruits and vegetables. The CDC reports that in 2013, only 13.1% met the recommended amount of fruit intake and only 8.9% met the recommended vegetable intake. The recommended fruit intake is 2 cups a day and vegetables at 2 ½ cups a day for someone who needs to consume 2,000 calories a day. Fiber intake should be increased gradually and should be accompanied by an increased intake

SUPERSIZE USA

Portion distortion is an enormous contribution to overweight and obesity. Having a realistic visual image of portion size is helpful when preparing meals and choosing foods. Did you know . . .

Portion	Visualization of Size or Amount
3 oz meat, poultry, or fish	Deck of playing cards, or the palm of a woman's hand
1 oz meat, poultry, fish, or cheese	1 in. cube or rolling dice
1 pat butter or margarine (1 serving)	Scrabble tile
2 Tbsp peanut butter	Ping-pong ball
1 oz salad dressing	Small restaurant ladle
1 cup fresh greens	Tennis ball
1 Tbsp mayonnaise	Woman's thumb
1 oz chips or pretzels	One handful—not heaping
1 medium potato	Computer mouse
1 standard bagel	Hockey puck
1 cup mashed potatoes, rice, or pasta	Person's fist or tennis ball
1 medium orange or apple	Baseball
1/2 cup cooked vegetable	1/2 a baseball or 7–8 baby carrots, 1 ear corn, 3 spears of broccoli
1 oz nuts, raisins, candy	Small handful, 2 Tbsp

Nutrition Facts

Serving Size 2/3 cup (55g)
Servings Per Container About 8

Amount Per Serving

Calories 230	Calories from Fat 72

	% Daily Value*
Total Fat 8g	**12%**
Saturated Fat 1g	**5%**
Trans Fat 0g	
Cholesterol 0mg	**0%**
Sodium 160mg	**7%**
Total Carbohydrate 37g	**12%**
Dietary Fiber 4g	**16%**
Sugars 1g	
Protein 3g	

Vitamin A 10%	•	Vitamin C 8%
Calcium 20%	•	Iron 45%

* Percent Daily Values are based on a 2,000 calorie diet.
  Your daily value may be higher or lower depending on
  your calorie needs:

	Calories	2,000	2,500
Total Fat	Less than	65g	80g
Sat Fat	Less than	20g	25g
Cholesterol	Less than	300mg	300mg
Sodium	Less than	2,400mg	2,400mg
Total Carbohydrate		300g	375g
Dietary Fiber		25g	30g

FIGURE 4-5 Refer to the Nutrition Facts Label to determine how many grams of fiber an item contains.

of water. Eating too much fiber in a short time can produce discomfort, **flatulence** (abdominal gas), and diarrhea. It also could obstruct the GI tract if intake exceeds 50 g. Insoluble fiber has binders (phytic acid or phytate), which are found in the outer covering of grains and vegetables. These can prevent the absorption of minerals such as calcium, iron, zinc, and magnesium, so excess intake should be avoided.

Because Americans know they should be consuming more fiber, food companies have begun to add isolated fiber to manufactured foods. Inulin (from chicory root), maltodextrin, and methylcellulose are just a few types of fibers added. Ideally the type of fiber consumed should be from natural food sources rather than from commercially prepared fiber products because the foods contain vitamins, minerals, and phytochemicals as well as fiber. Figure 4-5 shows where the amount of fiber per serving is listed on the Nutrition Facts panel. Foods labeled "high in fiber" must contain at least 5 g of fiber per serving. In terms of the percent daily value listed on the nutrition facts panel, 5% or less is considered low and 20% or more is considered high (or a good source) of that nutrient. Table 4-3 lists the dietary fiber content of selected foods.

DIGESTION AND ABSORPTION

Monosaccharides—glucose, fructose, and galactose—are simple sugars that may be absorbed from the intestine directly into the bloodstream. They are subsequently carried to the liver, where fructose and galactose are changed to glucose. The blood then carries glucose to the cells.

Disaccharides—sucrose, maltose, and lactose—require an additional step of digestion. They must be converted to the simple sugar glucose before they can be

flatulence
gas in the intestinal tract

TABLE 4-3 Dietary Fiber Content of Selected Foods

FOOD GROUP	ITEM	PORTION	FIBER (GMS)
Fruit	Apple	1 medium	3
	Banana	1 medium	3
	Blackberries	1 cup	8
	Blueberries	1 cup	4
	Cantaloupe	1 cup cubes	1
	Grapefruit	1 large	2
	Grapes	1 cup	1
	Kiwi	1 large	3
	Nectarine	1 large	3
	Orange	1 large	4
	Pear	1 medium	5
	Pineapple	1 cup, diced	2
	Plums	2 small	2
	Prunes	3 whole	2
	Raspberries	1 cup	8
	Strawberries	1 cup, sliced	3
	Watermelon	1 cup balls	1
Vegetables	Asparagus	1 cup	4
	Beets, cooked	1 cup	3
	Broccoli, cooked	1 cup	5
	Brussels sprouts	1 cup	4
	Cabbage, cooked	1 cup	3
	Carrots, cooked	1 cup	5
	Carrots, raw	1 cup	4
	Cauliflower, cooked	1 cup	3
	Celery, diced	1 cup, diced	2
	Collard greens, cooked	1 cup	4
	Corn	1 cup	5
	Cucumber	1 cup	1
	Green beans, cooked	1 cup	4
	Green peas	1 cup	9
	Kale, cooked	1 cup	3
	Mushrooms, cooked	1 cup	2
	Peppers, chopped	1 cup	2
	Potatoes, with skin	1 cup	3
	Romaine lettuce	1 cup	1
	Spinach, raw	1 cup	1
	Sweet potato	1 cup	8
	Tomato, raw, chopped	1 cup	2
	Winter squash, baked	1 cup	9
	Zucchini, cooked with skin	1 cup	2
Grains, Legumes, Seeds, and Nuts	Barley, cooked	1 cup	6
	Bran flakes	1 cup dry	7
	Bread, white	1 slice	1

(continues)

TABLE 4-3 *(continued)*

FOOD GROUP	ITEM	PORTION	FIBER (GMS)
	Bread, whole wheat	1 slice	3
	Corn flakes	1 cup dry	1
	Corn tortilla	1 medium	2
	Crackers, whole wheat	5	1
	Legumes: cooked Beans, average of all	½ cup	7
	Oatmeal, cooked	1 cup	4
	Pasta (refined)	1 cup	2
	Quinoa, cooked	½ cup	2
	Sunflower seeds, peanuts or almonds	¼ cup	3
	Wheat tortilla	6 inch	3
	Whole wheat pasta	1 cup	4

Source: Adapted from *USDA National Nutrient Database for Standard Reference* Release 28. http://ndb.nal.usda.gov/ndb/foods

absorbed into the bloodstream. This conversion is accomplished by the enzymes sucrase, maltase, and lactase, which were discussed in Chapter 3 (see Table 3-1).

Polysaccharides are more complex, and their digestibility varies. After the cellulose wall is broken down, starch is changed to the intermediate product dextrin; it is then changed to maltose and finally to glucose. Cooking can change starch to dextrin. For example, when bread is toasted, it turns golden brown and tastes sweeter because the starch has been changed to dextrin.

The digestion of starch begins in the mouth, where the enzyme salivary amylase begins to change starch to dextrin. The second step occurs in the stomach, where the food is mixed with gastric juices. The final step occurs in the small intestine, where the digestible carbohydrates are changed to simple sugars by the enzyme action of pancreatic amylase and are subsequently absorbed into the blood.

METABOLISM AND ELIMINATION

All carbohydrates are changed to the simple sugar glucose before metabolism can take place in the cells. After glucose has been carried by the blood to the cells, it can be oxidized. Frequently, the volume of glucose that reaches the cells

In The Media

Sugar High?

We love our sweet foods here in America. Evidence continues to mount that sugar is not only wreaking havoc on our waistlines but is a contributing factor to the development of cardiovascular disease, hypertension, type 2 diabetes, and even kidney disease and fatty liver. So why can't we leave the stuff alone? It's in approximately 75% of packaged food now and Americans' intake of added sugars has never been higher. Turns out sugar stimulates brain pathways and offers a "high" and pleasurable feelings just as a drug would. Studies have shown lab rats would rather choose sugar over cocaine. The fix? We need to start with awareness and a call to action to lobby for changes in our food supply. In the end, we need to purport consumption of whole, natural foods.

Source: Adapted from "Sugar Season. It's Everywhere and Addictive." *New York Times.* December 23, 2014. http://www.nytimes.com

exceeds the amount the cells can use. In these cases, glucose is converted to glycogen and is stored in the liver and muscles. (Glycogen is subsequently broken down only from the liver and released as glucose when needed for energy.) When more glucose is ingested than the body can either use immediately or store in the form of glycogen, it is converted to fat and stored as adipose (fatty) tissue.

The process of glucose metabolism is controlled mainly by the hormone **insulin**, which is secreted by the **islets of Langerhans** in the pancreas and that maintains normal blood glucose at 70–110 mg/dl. When the secretion of insulin is impaired or absent, the glucose level in the blood becomes excessively high. This condition is called **hyperglycemia** (blood glucose more than 126 mg/dl) and is usually a symptom of diabetes mellitus. If control by diet is ineffective, an oral hypoglycemic or insulin injections must be used to control blood sugar. When insulin is given, the diabetic client's intake of carbohydrates must be carefully controlled to balance the prescribed dosage of insulin (see Chapter 15). When blood glucose levels are unusually low, the condition is called **hypoglycemia** (blood glucose less than 70 mg/dl). A mild form of hypoglycemia may occur if one waits too long between meals or if the pancreas secretes too much insulin. Symptoms include fatigue, shaking, sweating, and headache.

Oxidation of glucose results in energy. With the exception of cellulose, the only waste products of carbohydrate metabolism are carbon dioxide and water. It is a very efficient nutrient.

DIETARY REQUIREMENTS

Although there is no specific daily dietary requirement for carbohydrates, the Food and Nutrition Board of the National Research Council recommends that half of one's energy requirement come from carbohydrates, preferably complex carbohydrates. For example, assume that one's total energy requirement is 2,000 calories. One half of this is 1,000. Divide 1,000 calories by 4 (the number of calories in each gram of carbohydrate) for an estimated carbohydrate requirement of 250 g/day. Due to the high sugar intake of Americans, it is recommended than no more than 10% of calorie intake come from simple sugars. For an average American, that equates to about 12 teaspoons per day. The American Heart Association has taken a stronger stand and recommends men consume no more than 9 teaspoons of added sugar a day and women no more than 6 teaspoons a day.

A mild deficiency of carbohydrates can result in weight loss and fatigue. A diet seriously deficient in carbohydrates could cause ketosis, a stage in metabolism occurring when the liver has been depleted of stored glycogen and switches to a fasting mode. At this point, energy from fat is mobilized to the liver and used to synthesize glucose. The by-products of fat breakdown are ketones that build up in the bloodstream and are then released through the kidneys. To prevent these effects, one needs a minimum of 50–120 g of carbohydrates each day.

Obesity constitutes a major health problem in the United States, and some believe eating excess carbohydrates is driving this phenomenon. Although surplus carbohydrates are changed to glycogen, the major part of any surplus becomes adipose tissue. One could argue, however, based on unfolding science, that it is the quality and type of carbohydrate consumed that may be the underlying factor. Many health experts now believe that it is the refined carbohydrates and especially the simple sugar fructose that is driving obesity. These rapidly digested carbohydrates lead to precipitous swings in blood sugar, which can lead to insulin resistance, which is a major driver of obesity, high blood pressure, and type 2 diabetes. In addition, some experts feel these types of carbohydrate are appetite-stimulating and may fuel cravings.

insulin
secretion of the islets of Langerhans in the pancreas gland; essential for the proper metabolism of glucose

islets of Langerhans
part of the pancreas from which insulin is secreted

hyperglycemia
excessive amounts of glucose in the blood

hypoglycemia
subnormal levels of blood glucose

HEALTH AND NUTRITION CONSIDERATIONS

The role of the health care professional in teaching about carbohydrates may be complicated. Some patients will have to be taught the nutritional differences between a baked potato and potato chips, between whole-wheat toast and Danish pastry, and between a fresh peach and canned fruit cocktail. Many will need to learn what dietary fiber is, where it can be found, and why it is needed. Some will need to learn that sugar should be used in moderation; others that it cannot be used in excess. All will require acceptance, understanding, and patience on the part of the health care professional.

SUMMARY

Energy foods are those that can be rapidly oxidized by the body to release energy. Carbohydrates are and should be the major source of energy. They are composed of carbon, hydrogen, and oxygen. One gram of carbohydrate provides 4 calories. Carbohydrates are the least expensive and most abundant nutrient. The principal sources of carbohydrates are plant products such as grains and their products, vegetables, fruits, legumes, and sugars. In addition to providing energy, carbohydrates spare proteins, maintain normal fat metabolism, and provide fiber. Digestion of carbohydrates begins in the mouth, continues in the stomach, and is completed in the small intestine. Although they are obviously essential to the health and well-being of the body, eating an excess of the wrong type of carbohydrates can cause dental caries, digestive disturbances, and obesity.

DISCUSSION TOPICS

1. What are the three basic groups of carbohydrates? Name several foods in each group.

2. Discuss the effects of excessive intake of carbohydrates.

3. Why should one's diet contain dietary fiber? Name three sources of dietary fiber.

4. Describe the digestion and metabolism of carbohydrates.

5. Discuss the following menus. Which foods contain simple sugars and/or complex carbohydrates? Which foods would be considered intact grains?

Orange juice	Baked chicken	Cheese sandwich
Steel cut oats	Wild rice	on whole-wheat
Milk and sugar	Green beans	bread with
Toast	Coleslaw	lettuce and tomato
Butter and jelly	Bread and	Carrot and
Coffee	Butter	celery sticks
	Raspberry	Fresh fruit
	sherbet	Cookies
	Milk	Milk

6. Why are complex carbohydrates preferable to simple sugars?

7. Discuss *enrichment*. What does it mean to enrich foods and what nutrients are returned? Why is it done? Which foods are typically enriched in the United States? Would you recommend that one purchase enriched foods? Why or why not?

8. Is it true, as many people say, that "carbs are fattening"? Explain your answer.

SUGGESTED ACTIVITIES

1. Hold a soda cracker in your mouth until you notice the change in flavor as the starch changes to dextrin. What causes this to happen?

2. Make a list of the foods you have eaten in the past 24 hours. Circle the carbohydrate-rich foods and underline the complex carbohydrates. Approximately what percentage of your calories were in the form of carbohydrates? In the form of complex carbs? How much added sugar did you consume? Could your diet be improved? If so, how?

3. Role-play a situation between a diet counselor and a teenage girl who has placed herself on an extremely low–calorie diet. She refuses to eat anything that she thinks contains carbohydrates. Explain to her the functions of carbohydrates in the human body.

REVIEW

Multiple choice. Select the *letter* that precedes the best answer.

1. The three main groups of carbohydrates are
   a. fats, proteins, and minerals
   b. glucose, fructose, and galactose
   c. monosaccharides, disaccharides, and polysaccharides
   d. sucrose, cellulose, and glycogen

2. Intact grains
   a. are hard to digest and should not be included in diet
   b. stick together when cooked
   c. have all three layers of the seed relatively intact (bran, germ, and endosperm)
   d. should make up 10% of our calorie needs daily

3. The simple sugar to which all forms of carbohydrates are ultimately converted is
   a. sucrose
   b. glucose
   c. galactose
   d. maltose

4. A fibrous form of carbohydrate that cannot be digested is
   a. glucose   c. cellulose
   b. glycogen   d. fat

5. Glycogen is stored in the
   a. heart and lungs
   b. liver and muscles
   c. pancreas and gallbladder
   d. small and large intestines

6. Glucose, fructose, and galactose are
   a. polysaccharides
   b. disaccharides
   c. enzymes
   d. monosaccharides

7. How do we get lactose?
   a. bread
   b. honey
   c. grains
   d. yogurt

8. The only form of carbohydrate that the brain uses for energy is
   a. glycogen
   b. galactose
   c. glucose
   d. glucagon

9. When insufficient carbohydrates are eaten, the liver produces
   a. galactose
   b. estrogen
   c. thyroxin
   d. ketones

10. Starch is
    a. the form in which glucose is stored in plants
    b. a monosaccharide
    c. an insoluble form of dietary fiber
    d. found only in grains

11. Insoluble dietary fiber
    a. can increase blood glucose
    b. can decrease blood cholesterol
    c. commonly causes diverticular disease
    d. is preferably provided by commercially prepared fiber products

12. The enzyme in the mouth that begins the digestion of starch is
    a. salivary ptyalin
    b. salivary amylase
    c. sucrase
    d. lipase

13. The optimal recommendation for fiber intake is:
a. 1 g for every year of age
b. 9–11 g a day
c. 20–35 g a day
d. 40–50 g a day

14. Carbohydrates
a. are rich in fat
b. are generally expensive
c. should provide approximately half of the calories in the U.S. diet
d. frequently are an excellent substitute for proteins in the human diet

15. Glucose metabolism is
a. controlled mainly by the hormone insulin
b. not affected by any secretion of the islets of Langerhans in the pancreas
c. managed entirely by glucagon
d. not related to human energy levels

CASE IN POINT

ANGELA: STEROIDS IMPACTING DIABETES CONTROL

Angela has been having problems for a couple of years with her left hip and has decided it is time to have it replaced. Her arthritis in combination with her lupus has made the pain in her hip intolerable. She is a 62-year-old Hispanic woman who is 5 ft 6 in tall and her current weight is 198 lb. The day of her surgery she arrives at the hospital early. She has not taken anything by mouth, including her medications, in preparation for her surgery. Angela follows up with her surgeon one week after the surgery. He is concerned that the incision is not healing as well as it should. He decides since Angela takes prednisone routinely for her lupus that it would be wise to recheck her blood sugar levels. In his office, her blood sugar is 342 mg/dl. He diagnoses Angela with steroid-induced diabetes. He requests that she follow up with her family physician as soon as possible. He refers her to the local diabetes center to review meal planning as well as other aspects of diabetes care.

ASSESSMENT

1. The dietitian can help Angela regulate her diet and in so doing lose weight. Calculate Angela's ideal caloric intake and weight using Tables 3-2 and 3-3, the Harris–Benedict equation, and thermic effect of food (TEF).
2. What does the dietitian need to know about Angela's meal choices?
3. What does the dietitian need to know about Angela's lifestyle?
4. What information will be helpful once Angela is discharged and at home?
5. What sources of carbohydrates would be most helpful in weight loss?

DIAGNOSIS

6. Write a nursing diagnosis for Angela.

PLAN/GOAL

7. Write a goal related to weight loss that Angela should achieve at the end of diabetic classes.
8. State two goals for Angela related to her diet and blood sugar.

IMPLEMENTATION

9. List the topics that you would teach Angela to achieve her goals.
10. What agencies or community resources can you provide to help Angela achieve her goals?

EVALUATION/OUTCOME CRITERIA

11. What can you expect from Angela to show she understands what you have taught?

12. What should Angela's fasting blood sugar read?
13. How long do you think it would take Angela to learn a new diet plan, check her blood sugar, learn a new exercise plan, and demonstrate integration into her everyday life?

THINKING FURTHER

14. What blood test could the doctor order to see if Angela had maintained her blood sugar at a normal level over the past few months?
15. What are some of the serious health consequences if Angela does not manage her diabetes well?

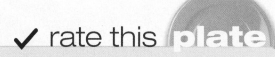
✔ rate this plate

While at the diabetes center, Angela was educated about the diabetic meal plan. She continues to learn about how medications, along with her eating habits, can affect her blood sugar levels. Rate this plate to see how she has done with planning breakfast on her 1,600–1,800 calorie meal plan.

2 pieces of French toast

2 strips of bacon

1 cup of mixed fruit

Coffee with cream and sugar

CASE IN POINT

JEROME: COPING WITH GASTROPARESIS

Jerome has had type 1 diabetes since he was 6 years old. After being diagnosed at such a young age, his parents assisted with his insulin, blood sugar checks, and meal planning. Once he was grown and on his own, he began to slack off in caring for himself. He ate whatever he wanted, rarely monitored his sugar, and took his insulin only when he remembered. He has not seen his doctor in nearly three years, but now at age 41, he is starting to notice certain problems. Jerome is beginning to have difficulty with his vision. He has also had tingling and burning sensations in his feet and legs. Lately, he has even felt nauseated more often than not after he eats and has even vomited a few times after meals. He has decided it is time to see his doctor. His doctor is very concerned about his complications. He discusses with

Jerome that it is extremely important he start caring for himself more aggressively. He tells Jerome that his nausea and vomiting are related to a diabetes complication known as gastroparesis. This is damage to the nerves surrounding the stomach. It causes paralysis of the stomach and delayed emptying of foods. It is going to require more focus on his meal planning to control the symptoms. He refers him to a registered dietitian for this instruction. The dietitian discusses with Jerome the key points to meal planning for gastroparesis. He is going to have to consume small but frequent (4–6) meals daily, and follow a low-fat, low-fiber diet. Jerome needs to chew his food thoroughly before swallowing and avoid foods that are difficult to digest, such as broccoli, corn, popcorn, nuts, and seeds.

ASSESSMENT

1. What has caused the gastroparesis that Jerome is now experiencing?
2. What symptoms did Jerome have?
3. How will the disease alter his life?
4. How significant is this disease?

DIAGNOSIS

5. Write a diagnostic statement for Jerome's potential alteration in nutrition.
6. Write a diagnosis for Jerome's deficient knowledge related to the new diet.

PLAN/GOAL

7. What dietary goals are measurable and appropriate for Jerome?
8. What education goals are specific and measurable for Jerome?

IMPLEMENTATION

9. What major topics about gastroparesis does Jerome need to understand to make necessary dietary changes?
10. What dietary changes does Jerome need to learn to control his symptoms?

EVALUATION/OUTCOME CRITERIA

11. At his follow-up doctor's appointment, what is his doctor likely to ask to determine if the plan was successful?

THINKING FURTHER

12. Can gastroparesis be cured?
13. What medications are typically used to help manage this disease?

✔ rate this plate

Jerome has been instructed to consume a diet low in fat and fiber in order to make digestion easy and rest his gut. How did he do in planning the following meal according to the dietitian's recommendations? Rate his plate:

4 oz beef roast with cooked potatoes, carrots, celery, and onions

¾ cup apple Waldorf salad

1 whole-wheat roll

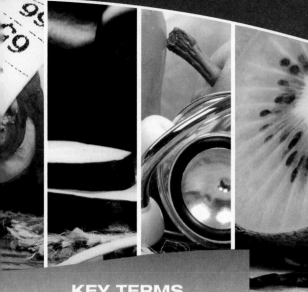

CHAPTER 5

KEY TERMS

cholesterol
chylomicrons
fatty acids
glycerol
high-density lipoproteins (HDLs)
hydrogenation
hypercholesterolemia
invisible fats
lecithin
linoleic acid
linolenic acid
lipids
lipoproteins
low-density lipoproteins (LDLs)
monounsaturated fats
omega-3 fatty acids
plaque
polyunsaturated fats
satiety
saturated fats
trans-fatty acids (TFAs)
triglycerides
very-low-density lipoproteins
   (VLDLs)
visible fats

LIPIDS (FATS)

OBJECTIVES

After studying this chapter, you should be able to:

- State the functions of fats in the body
- Identify sources of dietary fats
- Explain common classifications of fats
- Describe disease conditions with which excessive use of fats is associated

Fats belong to a group of organic compounds called **lipids**. The word *lipid* is derived from *lipos*, a Greek word for fat. Forms of this word are found in several fat-related health terms such as blood *lipids* (fats in the blood), hyper-*lipid*emia (high levels of fat in the blood), and *lipo*proteins (carriers of fat in human blood).

Fats are greasy substances that are not soluble in water. They are soluble in some solvents such as ether, benzene, and chloroform. They provide a more concentrated source of energy than carbohydrates; each gram of fat contains 9 calories. This is slightly more than twice the calorie content of carbohydrates. Fat-rich foods are generally more expensive than carbohydrate-rich foods. Like carbohydrates, fats are composed of carbon, hydrogen, and oxygen but with a substantially lower proportion of oxygen.

FUNCTIONS

In addition to providing energy, fats are essential for the functioning and structure of body tissues (see Table 5-1). Fats are a necessary part of cell membranes (cell walls). They contain essential fatty acids and act as carriers for fat-soluble vitamins A, D, E, and K. The fat stored in body tissues provides energy when one cannot eat, as may occur during some illness and after abdominal surgery. Adipose (fatty) tissue protects organs and bones from injury by serving as protective padding and support. Body fat also serves as insulation from cold. In addition, fats provide a feeling of satiety (satisfaction) after meals. This is due partly to the flavor fats give other foods and partly to their slow rate of digestion, which delays hunger.

FOOD SOURCES

Fats are present in both animal and plant foods. The animal foods that provide the richest sources of fats are red meats; higher-fat poultry cuts with skin such as the thigh and wing; whole, low-fat, and reduced-fat milk; cream; butter; cheeses made with cream; egg yolks (egg white contains no fat; it is almost entirely protein and water); and fatty fish such as tuna and salmon. In general, the saturated fat consumed from animal foods raises serum cholesterol, which could contribute to heart disease.

The plant foods containing the richest sources of fats are cooking oils made from olives; from sunflower, safflower, or sesame seeds; or from corn, peanuts, canola oil; or soybeans, margarine, salad dressing; or mayonnaise (which is made from vegetable oils), nuts, seeds, avocados, coconut, and cocoa butter. Plant fats do not raise cholesterol and are therefore more heart healthy.

TABLE 5-1 **Fats**

FUNCTIONS	DEFICIENCY SIGNS	SOURCES
Provide energy	Eczema	Animal
Carry fat-soluble vitamins	Weight loss	Meat and poultry
Supply essential fatty acids	Retarded growth	Milk
Protect and support organs and bones		Butter
		Cheese
Insulate from cold		Cream
Provide satiety after meals		Egg yolk
		Fatty fish such as salmon
		Plant
		Vegetable oils
		Nuts and seeds
		Chocolate
		Avocados
		Olives
		Margarine, salad dressing, and mayonnaise

lipids
fats

satiety
feeling of satisfaction; fullness

Visible and Invisible Fats in Food

Sometimes fats are referred as visible or invisible, depending on their food sources. Fats that are purchased and used as fats, such as butter, margarine, lard, and cooking oils, are called **visible fats**. Hidden or **invisible fats** are those found in other foods, such as meats, cream, whole milk, cheese, egg yolk, fried foods, pastries, avocados, and nuts.

It is often the invisible fats that can make it difficult for clients on limited-fat diets to regulate their fat intake. For example, one 3-in doughnut may contain 12 g of fat, whereas one 3-in bagel contains only 2 g of fat. One fried chicken drumstick may contain 11 g of fat, whereas one roasted drumstick may contain only 2 g of fat.

It is essential that the health care professional confirm that clients on limited-fat diets are carefully educated about sources of hidden fats.

CLASSIFICATION

Triglycerides, *phospholipids*, and *sterols* are all lipids found in food and the human body. Most lipids in the body (95%) are triglycerides. They are in body cells and circulate in the blood.

Triglycerides are composed of three (*tri*) fatty acids attached to a framework of **glycerol**, hence their name (see Figure 5-1). Glycerol is derived from a water-soluble carbohydrate. **Fatty acids** are organic compounds of carbon atoms to which hydrogen atoms are attached. They are classified in two ways: essential or nonessential. *Essential fatty acids (EFAs)* are necessary fats that humans cannot synthesize; EFAs must be obtained through diet. EFAs are long-chain polyunsaturated fatty acids derived from **linoleic acid** and **linolenic acid**. There are two families of EFAs: omega-3 and omega-6. The omega-9 fatty acids are necessary but nonessential because the body can manufacture a modest amount, provided EFAs are present. (Also see the later section on polyunsaturated fats.)

The other method of classification of fatty acids is by their degree of saturation with hydrogen atoms. In this method, they are described as *saturated*, *monounsaturated*, or *polyunsaturated*, depending on their hydrogen content (Figure 5-2).

Saturated Fats

With **saturated fats**, each of the fatty acid's carbon atoms carries all the hydrogen atoms possible. In general, animal foods contain more saturated fatty acids than unsaturated. Examples include meat, poultry, egg yolks, whole milk, whole-milk cheeses, cream, ice cream, and butter. Although plant foods generally contain more polyunsaturated fatty acids than saturated fatty acids, chocolate, coconut, palm oil, and palm kernel oils are exceptions. They contain substantial amounts of saturated fatty acids. Foods containing a high proportion of saturated fats are usually solid at room temperature. It is recommended that one consume no more than 10% of total daily calories as saturated fats. The American Heart Association takes a stronger stance and recommends we consume no more than 7% of our calories from saturated fat, with a further reduction to 5–6% of total calories if lipids are high and there is concern for heart disease.

Monounsaturated Fats

In the case of **monounsaturated fats**, there is one place among the carbon atoms of its fatty acids where there are fewer hydrogen atoms attached than in saturated

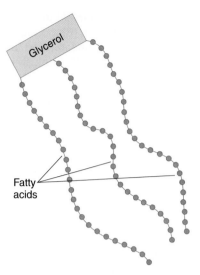

FIGURE 5-1 A triglyceride is composed of three fatty acids attached to a framework of glycerol.

visible fats
fats in foods that are purchased and used as fats, such as butter or margarine

invisible fats
fats that are not immediately noticeable, such as those in egg yolk, cheese, cream, and salad dressings

triglycerides
three fatty acids attached to a framework of glycerol

glycerol
a component of fat; derived from a water-soluble carbohydrate

fatty acids
a component of fat that determines the classification of the fat

linoleic acid
fatty acid essential for humans; cannot be synthesized by the body

linolenic acid
fatty acid essential for humans; cannot be synthesized by the body

saturated fats
fats whose carbon atoms contain all of the hydrogen atoms they can; considered a contributory factor in atherosclerosis

monounsaturated fats
fats that are neither saturated nor polyunsaturated and thought to play little part in atherosclerosis

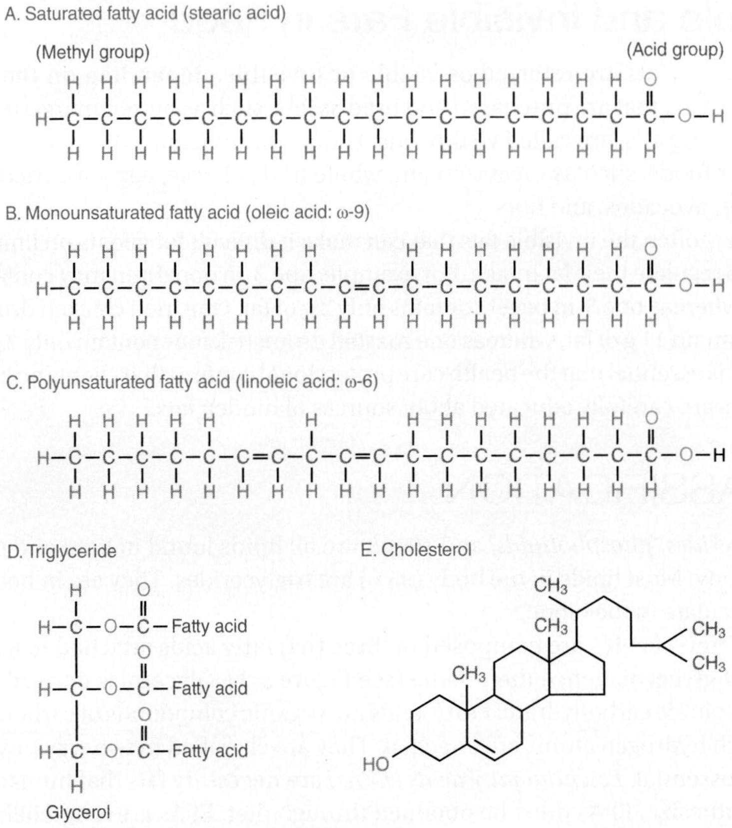

FIGURE 5-2 Chemical formula for **(A)** saturated fatty acid, **(B)** monounsaturated fatty acid, **(C)** polyunsaturated fatty acid, **(D)** triglyceride, and **(E)** cholesterol.

A. Saturated fatty acid (stearic acid)

(Methyl group)   (Acid group)

B. Monounsaturated fatty acid (oleic acid: ω-9)

C. Polyunsaturated fatty acid (linoleic acid: ω-6)

D. Triglyceride

E. Cholesterol

fats. Examples of foods containing monounsaturated fats are olive oil, peanut oil, canola oil, avocados, and cashew nuts. Research indicates that monounsaturated fats lower the amount of low-density lipoprotein (LDL) ("bad cholesterol") in the blood, but only when they replace saturated fats in one's diet. They have no effect on high-density lipoproteins (HDLs) ("good cholesterol"). It is recommended that one consume 20% of total daily calories as monounsaturated fats (Figure 5-3).

Polyunsaturated Fats

In the case of **polyunsaturated fats**, there are two or more places among the carbon atoms of its fatty acids where there are fewer hydrogen atoms attached than in saturated fats. The point at which carbon-carbon double bonds occur in a polyunsaturated fatty acid is the determining factor in how the body metabolizes it. The two major fatty acids denoted by the placement of their double bonds are the omega-3 and omega-6 fatty acids. **Omega-3 fatty acids** have been reported to help lower the risk of heart disease. Because omega-3 fatty acids are found in fish oils, an increased intake of fatty fish is recommended. Omega-6 (linoleic acid) has a cholesterol-lowering effect. The use of supplements of either of these fatty acids is not recommended. Examples of foods containing polyunsaturated fats include cooking oils made from sunflower, safflower, or sesame seeds or from corn or soybeans; soft margarines whose major ingredient is *liquid* vegetable oil; and fish. Foods containing high proportions of polyunsaturated fats are usually soft or oily. Polyunsaturated fats should not exceed 10% of total daily calories.

polyunsaturated fats
fats whose carbon atoms contain only limited amounts of hydrogen

omega-3 fatty acids
help lower the risk of heart disease

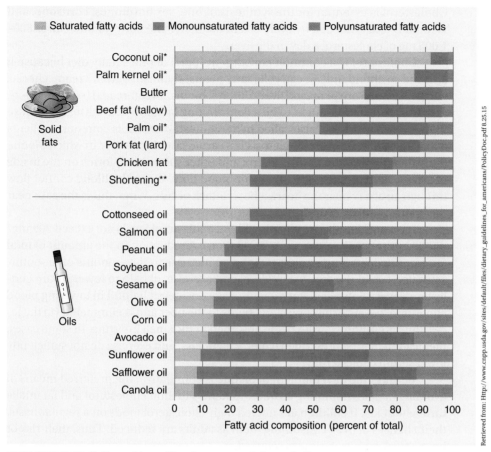

FIGURE 5-3 Fatty acid profile of common fats and oils.

Retrieved from: Http://www.cnpp.usda.gov/sites/default/files/dietary_guidelines_for_americans/PolicyDoc.pdf 8.25.15

Trans-Fatty Acid

Trans-fatty acids (TFAs) are produced when hydrogen atoms are added to monounsaturated or polyunsaturated fats to produce a semisolid product like margarine and shortening. A product is likely to contain a significant amount of TFAs if partially hydrogenated vegetable oil is listed in the first three ingredients on the label. The major source of TFAs in the diet is baked goods and foods eaten in restaurants. Trans-fatty acids were required to be listed on the food label in 2006. TFAs raise LDLs but decrease HDLs. Eating trans fats can increase your risk of developing heart disease and stroke. Trans fats are also associated with a higher risk of developing type II diabetes.

Hydrogenated Fats

Hydrogenated fats are polyunsaturated vegetable oils to which hydrogen has been added commercially to make them solid at room temperature. This process, called **hydrogenation**, turns polyunsaturated vegetable oils into saturated fats. Margarine is made in this way. (Soft margarine contains less saturated fat than firm margarine.)

CHOLESTEROL

Cholesterol is a sterol (see Figure 5-2). It is not a true fat but a fatlike substance that exists in animal foods and body cells. It does not exist in plant foods.

trans-fatty acids (TFAs)
produced by adding hydrogen atoms to a liquid fat, making it solid

hydrogenation
the combining of fat with hydrogen, thereby making it a saturated fat and solid at room temperature

cholesterol
fatlike substance that is a constituent of body cells, is synthesized in the liver, also available in animal foods

Exploring THE WEB

Search the Web for cholesterol-lowering products. What claims do these products make? Are food–drug interactions mentioned? Are the claims based on scientific research and facts? What advice would you give a client who is inquiring about such products? Create a fact sheet that lists the myths regarding fats and cholesterol and present the facts that dispel these myths.

Cholesterol is essential for the synthesis of bile, sex hormones, cortisone, and vitamin D and is needed by every cell in the body. The body manufactures 800–1,000 mg of cholesterol a day in the liver.

Cholesterol is a common constituent (part) of one's daily diet because it is found so abundantly in egg yolk, fatty meats, shellfish, butter, cream, cheese, whole milk, and organ meats (liver, kidneys, brains, sweetbreads) (see Table 5-2).

Cholesterol is thought to be a contributing factor in heart disease because high serum cholesterol, also called **hypercholesterolemia**, is common in clients with atherosclerosis. Atherosclerosis is a cardiovascular disease in which **plaque** (fatty deposits containing cholesterol and other substances) forms on the inside of artery walls, reducing the space for blood flow. When the blood cannot flow through an artery near the heart, a heart attack occurs. When this is the case near the brain, a stroke occurs (see Chapter 16).

It is considered advisable that blood cholesterol levels not exceed 200 mg/dL (200 mg of cholesterol per 1 dL of blood). A reduction in the amount of total fat, saturated fats, and cholesterol and an increase in the amounts of monounsaturated fats in the diet, weight loss, and exercise all help to lower serum cholesterol levels. Soluble dietary fiber is also considered helpful in lowering blood cholesterol because the cholesterol binds to the fiber and is eliminated via the feces, thus preventing it from being absorbed in the small intestine. In some cases, medication may be prescribed if diet, weight loss, and exercise do not sufficiently lower serum cholesterol.

Because the development of plaque is cumulative, the preferred means of avoiding or at least limiting its development is to limit cholesterol and fat intake throughout life. If children are not fed high-cholesterol foods on a regular basis, their chances of over-consuming them as adults are reduced. Thus, their risk of heart attack and stroke is also reduced.

SUPERSIZE USA

Taco Bell® is a favorite place to eat for the younger generation. My son would come home with three soft tacos, three crunchy tacos, nachos bellgrande, and a large cola. Let us look at the calories, fat, and sodium content of his meal.

Food Item	Calories	Fat/Sat Fat (g)	Sodium (mg)
Soft Beef Taco	210	9/4	530
Crunchy Beef Taco	170	10/3.5	290
Nachos BellGrande	770	42/7	1,020
Large Cola	200		13
Totals for son's meal:			
3 Soft Beef Tacos	630	27/12	1,590
3 Crunchy Beef Tacos	510	30/10.5	870
Nachos Bellgrande	770	42/7	1,020
Large Cola	200		40
Grand Total	**2,110**	**99/29.5**	**3,520**

What a tasty meal! Because it is his favorite place to eat and it fits within his budget, should he continue to eat there? As a mother and dietitian, I tried to tell him the cons for his body, but like all kids he knows everything. He doesn't exercise much and worries about his weight. He should—he is on the way to supersizing himself.

Source: Accessed October 2011. http://www.tacobell.com/nutrition/information

hypercholesterolemia
unusually high levels of cholesterol in blood; also known as high serum cholesterol

plaque
fatty deposit on interior of artery walls

TABLE 5-2   Fat and Cholesterol Content of Some Common Foods

FOOD	AMOUNT	SATURATED FAT (g)	CHOLESTEROL (mg)	TOTAL FAT (g)	TOTAL KILOCALORIES
Dairy					
Creamed cottage cheese (4% fat)	1 cup	6.4	34	10	235
Uncreamed cottage cheese (0.5% fat)	1 cup	0.4	10	1	125
Cream cheese	1 oz	6.2	31	10	100
Swiss cheese	1 oz	5.0	24	8	105
American processed cheese	1 oz	5.6	27	9	105
Half and half	1 Tbsp	1.1	6	2	20
Heavy cream	1 Tbsp	3.5	21	6	54
Nondairy creamer	1 Tbsp	1.4	0	1	20
Whole milk	1 cup	5.1	33	8	150
Reduced-fat milk	1 cup	2.9	18	5	120
Low-fat milk	1 cup	1.6	10	3	100
Fat-free milk	1 cup	0	4	0	90
Chocolate milk shake	10 oz	4.8	30	8	335
Ice cream (11% fat)	½ cup	8.9	59	14	270
Egg (large)	1	1.6	213	5	75
Oils					
Butter	1 Tbsp	7.1	31	11	100
Margarine	1 Tbsp	2.2	0	11	100
Corn oil	1 Tbsp	1.8	0	14	125
Seafood					
Crabmeat (canned)	1 cup	0.5	135	3	135
Salmon (canned)	3 oz	0.9	34	5	120
Shrimp (canned)	3 oz	0.2	128	1	100
Tuna					
Water-packed	3 oz	0.3	48	1	135
Oil-packed	3 oz	1.4	55	7	165
Vegetable					
Avocado	½	2.2	0	15	150
Bread					
Bagel	1	0.3	0	2	200
Doughnut	1	2.8	20	12	210
English muffin	1	0.3	0	1	140
Nuts					
Peanuts (dry roasted)	1 oz	2.0	0	15	170
Meat					
Ground beef (lean)	3 oz	6.2	74	16	230
Roast beef (lean)	4.4 oz	7.2	100	18	300
Leg lamb (lean)	5.2 oz	4.8	130	12	280
Leg lamb (lean and fat)	6 oz	11.2	156	26	410
Bacon	3 slices	3.3	16	9	110
Pork chop (lean)	5 oz	5.2	142	16	330
Frankfurter	1.5 oz	4.8	23	13	145
Chicken leg, fried (meat and skin)	5 oz	6.0	124	22	390
Chicken leg, roasted (meat only)	3.2 oz	1.4	82	4	150

Source: U.S. Department of Agriculture. "Nutritive Values of Foods." *Home and Garden Bulletin*, No. 72. 2002 (rev. ed.). Revised 2011

DIGESTION AND ABSORPTION

Although 95% of ingested fats are digested, it is a complex process. The chemical digestion of fats occurs mainly in the small intestine. Fats are not digested in the mouth. They are digested only slightly in the stomach, where gastric lipase acts on emulsified fats such as those found in cream and egg yolk. Fats must be mixed well with the gastric juices before entering the small intestine. In the small intestine, bile emulsifies the fats, and the enzyme pancreatic lipase reduces them to fatty acids and glycerol, which the body subsequently absorbs through villi (see Figure 5-4).

Lipoproteins

Fats are insoluble in water, which is the main component of blood. Therefore, special carriers must be provided for the fats to be absorbed and transported by the blood to body cells. In the initial stages of absorption, bile joins with the products of fat digestion to carry fat. Later, protein combines with the final products of fat digestion to form special carriers called **lipoproteins**. The lipoproteins subsequently carry the fats to the body cells by way of the blood.

Lipoproteins are classified as **chylomicrons, very-low-density lipoproteins (VLDLs), low-density lipoproteins (LDLs)**, and **high-density lipoproteins (HDLs)**, according to their mobility and density. Chylomicrons are the first lipoprotein identified after eating. They are the largest lipoproteins and the lightest in weight. They are composed of 80–90% triglycerides. Lipoprotein lipase acts to break down the triglycerides into free fatty acids and glycerol. Without this enzyme, fat could not get into the cells.

Very-low-density lipoproteins are made primarily by the liver cells and are composed of 55–65% triglycerides. They carry triglycerides and other lipids to all cells. As the VLDLs lose triglycerides, they pick up cholesterol from other lipoproteins in the blood, and they then become LDLs. Low-density lipoproteins are approximately 45% cholesterol with few triglycerides. They carry most of the blood cholesterol from the liver to the cells. Elevated blood levels greater than 130 mg/dL of LDL are thought to be contributing factors in atherosclerosis. LDL is sometimes termed *bad cholesterol*.

High-density lipoproteins carry cholesterol from the cells to the liver for eventual excretion. The level at which low HDL becomes a major risk factor for

lipoproteins
carriers of fat in the blood

chylomicrons
the largest lipoprotein; transport the lipids after digestion into the body

very-low-density lipoproteins (VLDLs)
lipoproteins made by the liver to transport lipids throughout the body

low-density lipoproteins (LDLs)
carry blood cholesterol to the cells

high-density lipoproteins (HDLs)
lipoproteins that carry cholesterol from cells to the liver for eventual excretion

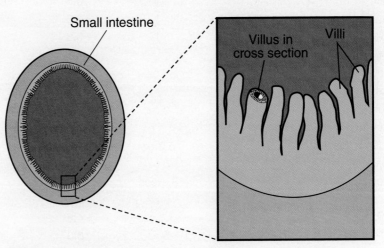

FIGURE 5-4 The body absorbs fatty acids and glycerol through the villi of the small intestine.

heart disease has been set at 40 mg/dL. Research indicates that an HDL level of 60 mg/dL or more is considered protective against heart disease. High-density lipoproteins are sometimes called *good cholesterol*. Exercising, maintaining a desirable weight, and giving up smoking are all ways to increase one's HDL.

METABOLISM AND ELIMINATION

The liver controls fat metabolism. It hydrolyzes triglycerides and forms new ones from this hydrolysis as needed. Ultimately, the metabolism of fats occurs in the cells, where fatty acids are broken down to carbon dioxide and water, releasing energy. The portion of fat that is not needed for immediate use is stored as adipose tissue. Carbon dioxide and water are by-products that are used or removed from the body by the circulatory, respiratory, and excretory systems.

FATS AND THE CONSUMER

Fats continue to be of particular interest to the consumer. Most people know that fats are high-calorie foods and that they are related to heart disease. But people who are not in the health field may not know *how* fats affect health. Consequently, they may be easily duped by clever ads or salespersons marketing nutritional supplements or new "health food" products.

It is important that the health care professional carefully evaluate any new dietary "supplement" for which a nutrition claim is made. For example, supplements for omega-3 fatty acids, fish oil, and vitamin E should be approved by your physician before taking. If the item is not included in the RDA, DRI, or AI, it is safe to assume that medical research has not determined that it is essential. Ingestion of dietary supplements of unknown value could, ironically, be damaging to one's health.

Lecithin

Lecithin is a fatty substance classified as a phospholipid. It is found in both plant and animal foods and is synthesized in the liver. It is a natural emulsifier that helps transport fat in the bloodstream. It is used commercially to make food products smooth.

Lecithin supplements have been promoted by some health food salespersons as being able to prevent cardiovascular disease. To date, this has not been scientifically proven.

Fat Alternatives

Research into fat alternatives has been in progress for decades. Olestra is an example of a fat alternative made from sugar and fatty acids. The FDA has approved olestra for use only in snack foods such as potato chips, tortilla chips, and crackers. The government requires that food labels indicate that olestra "inhibits the absorption of some vitamins and other nutrients." Therefore, the fat-soluble vitamins A, D, E, and K have been added to foods containing olestra. Olestra contains no calories, but it can cause cramps and diarrhea. The products manufactured with olestra should be used in moderation.

Simplesse is made from either egg white or milk protein and contains 1.3 kcal/g. It can be used only in cold foods such as ice cream because it becomes thick or gels when heated. It is not available for home use.

lecithin

fatty substance found in plant and animal foods; a natural emulsifier that helps transport fats in the bloodstream; used commercially to make food products smooth

Oatrim is carbohydrate-based and derived from oat fiber. Oatrim is heat-stable and can be used in baking but not in frying. Manufacturers have used carbohydrate-based compounds for years as thickeners. Oatrim does provide calories, but significantly less fat.

The long-term effects these products may have on human health and nutrition are unknown. If they are used in the way the U.S. population uses artificial sweeteners, they probably will not reduce the actual fat content in the diet. They may simply be additions to it. One concern among nutritionists is that they will be used in place of nutritious food that, in addition to fat, also provides vitamins, minerals, proteins, and carbohydrates.

DIETARY REQUIREMENTS

Although no specific dietary requirement for fats is included in the RDA and DRIs, deficiency symptoms do occur when fats provide less than 10% of the total daily calorie requirement. When gross deficiency occurs, eczema (inflamed and scaly skin condition) can develop. This has been observed in infants who were fed formulas lacking the essential fatty acid linoleic acid and in clients maintained for long periods on intravenous feedings that lack linoleic acid. Also, growth may be retarded and weight loss can occur when diets are seriously deficient in fats.

On the other hand, excessive fat in the diet can lead to obesity or heart disease. In addition, studies point to an association between high-fat diets and cancers of the colon, breast, uterus, and prostate.

The Food and Nutrition Board's Committee on Diet and Health recommends that people reduce their fat intake to 30% of total calories. The American Heart Association's newest recommendation is to consume less or no more than 7% of saturated fats, 10% polyunsaturated fats, and 20% monounsaturated fats. According to the Mayo Clinic, currently 35% of calories in U.S. diets are derived from solid fats and sugar.

In The Media

Eating Southern Fare Comes with Risks

A new study has shown that regularly eating southern-style dishes may increase your risk for a heart attack. The study, carried out for 6 years in more than 17,000 people, was linked to a 56% increased risk for heart attack. The hallmarks of a southern diet such as fried meat and chicken, rich gravies, biscuits, sweet tea, and greens cooked in bacon fat offer saturated fats, nitrates, and sugar, which increase cholesterol, insulin resistance, and body weight subsequently increasing risk for heart disease. New shifts in cooking variations of these foods are being taught by nutrition professionals in southern state health systems.

Source: Adapted from "Southern Diet Linked to Big Increases in Heart Diseases." CBS News. August 11, 2015. http://www.cbsnews.com

SPOTLIGHT on Life Cycle

When we think about exercise activities for adults, we think of running on a treadmill or joining a gym; however, for children, exercise consists of playing with friends, being physically active in school, and participating in extracurricular activities. Sadly, studies have shown that children are becoming more sedentary, with the average child spending 4.5 hours a day watching television. Television, video games, and computer time have replaced the time that children should be spending riding their bikes, playing outside, and being physically active. The American Academy of Pediatrics recommends that children under the age of 2 years watch no TV at all and that quality programming should be limited to one to two hours for children 2 years and older. Parents need to ensure that their child is getting enough exercise in order to positively influence bone and muscle growth and prevent childhood overweight or obesity. Keeping physical activity fun and embracing a healthier lifestyle will encourage children, as well as their families, to participate in regular exercise.

Source: Adapted from KidsHealth. "Kids and Exercise." Accessed August 30, 2015. http://www.kidshealth.org

HEALTH AND NUTRITION CONSIDERATIONS

To accomplish dietary change, the health care professional should review clients' usual diets *with* them. Changes can then be introduced clearly and sensitively and with the clients' active participation. Unless clients understand *why* dietary changes are needed and want to make them, they are unlikely to change their diets.

SUMMARY

In addition to providing an important source of energy, fats carry essential fatty acids and fat-soluble vitamins, protect organs and bones, insulate from cold, and provide satiety to meals. They are composed of carbon, hydrogen, and oxygen and are found in both animal and plant foods. Each gram of fat provides 9 calories. Digestion of fats occurs mainly in the small intestine, where they are reduced to fatty acids and glycerol. An excess of fat in the diet can result in obesity and possibly heart disease or cancer.

DISCUSSION TOPICS

1. Why are fats considered a more concentrated source of energy than carbohydrates?

2. Of what value are fats to the body? List some foods rich in fats.

3. Discuss adipose tissue. Is it good? Is it bad? Explain.

4. Describe atherosclerosis. Its effects are said to be cumulative. Explain.

5. Describe the digestion and metabolism of fats. What are the end products of fat digestion?

6. Why might a client on a low-fat diet complain? How might the health care professional be helpful in such a case?

7. What are hydrogenated fats? Are they polyunsaturated? Explain.

8. Why is there a greater danger of excess fat in the U.S. diet than a deficiency of fat?

9. Discuss invisible fats and their potential impact on low-fat diets.

10. What are the probable reasons that omega-3 fatty acid capsules and lecithin have become so popular with the general public?

SUGGESTED ACTIVITIES

1. List the foods you ate yesterday. Circle those containing visible fats. Underline those containing invisible fats. Explain why some foods are both circled and underlined. Revise your list, making it appropriate for someone on a limited-fat diet.

2. Using a cookbook, review recipes for baked products and answer the following questions about them.
   a. Why do bagels contain no cholesterol?
   b. Why does angel food cake contain no cholesterol?
   c. Why does a doughnut contain cholesterol when an English muffin does not?
   d. Why does French toast contain cholesterol when the white bread it is made from may not?
   e. Why does lemon meringue pie filling contain cholesterol when apple pie filling does not?
   f. Why does a cheeseburger contain more cholesterol than a hamburger?

3. Write down five typical meals in your family's diet—one breakfast, one lunch, one dinner, and two snacks. How could you modify them to reduce the fat content?

4. Visit a fast food restaurant and review the menu. How many items are high in fat? How many are not? Is there any invisible fat in the more "healthy" items? Share your findings with the class.

REVIEW

Multiple choice. Select the *letter* that precedes the best answer.

1. Fats provide the most concentrated form of
   a. carbon
   b. oxygen
   c. lipase
   d. energy

2. Adipose tissue is useful because it
   a. protects and insulates
   b. prevents eczema
   c. provides satiety
   d. can synthesize triglycerides

3. Atherosclerosis is thought to increase the risk of
   a. cancer
   b. plaque
   c. heart attacks
   d. hypercholesterolemia

4. A diet grossly deficient in fats may be deficient in
   a. lipase
   b. linoleic acid
   c. cholesterol
   d. triglycerides

5. Invisible fats can be found in
   a. cake and cookies
   b. orange and tomato juice
   c. egg white and skim milk
   d. lettuce and tomatoes

6. Plant foods that contain saturated fats are
   a. olives and avocados
   b. coconut and chocolate
   c. corn and soybeans
   d. cashew nuts and canola oil

7. When a polyunsaturated vegetable oil is changed to a saturated fat, the process is called
   a. hydrolysis
   b. hypercholesterolemia
   c. hydrogenation
   d. hyperlipidemia

8. Linoleic acid is one of the fatty acids that is known to be
   a. a triglyceride
   b. saturated
   c. monounsaturated
   d. essential to the human diet

9. Cholesterol is
   a. not essential to the human diet
   b. thought to contribute to atherosclerosis
   c. not found in animal foods
   d. classified as a mineral

10. I work at an ice cream factory and am responsible for choosing a fat alternative for the ice cream. Which product should I use?
    a. oatrim
    b. truvia
    c. simplesse
    d. olestra

11. Three groups of lipids found naturally in the human body and in food are triglycerides, phospholipids, and
    a. cortisone
    b. steroids
    c. sterols
    d. hydrogenated fats

12. Fatty acids are organic compounds of carbon atoms and
    a. hydrogen atoms
    b. arachidonic acids
    c. triglycerides
    d. glycerol

13. Cholesterol
    a. is found in both plants and animals
    b. is found only in plants
    c. does not contribute in any way to heart disease
    d. is a sterol

14. HDL (high-density lipoprotein)
    a. is sometimes called good cholesterol
    b. carries lipids to the cells
    c. is the same as lipase
    d. levels should be less than 40 mg/dL of human blood

15. For digestion, fats require the help of gastric lipase,
    a. bile, and fatty acids
    b. bile, and pancreatic lipase
    c. pancreatic lipase, and glycerol
    d. cholesterol, and bile

16. How many calories are in 13 g of fat?
    a. 117
    b. 130
    c. 210
    d. 155

17. Which would be the healthiest fat to use when frying a chicken?
    a. lard
    b. olive oil
    c. solid shortening
    d. canola oil

CASE IN POINT

MURALI: FAMILY HISTORY AND ELEVATED CHOLESTEROL

Murali is from Sri Lanka. He moved to the United States when he was 19 years old. His family has a history of heart disease and high cholesterol. Murali's father and brother both died of heart attacks in their 40s. Murali is now 52 years old. His wife Annika is worried about his health. Annika has tried to be careful in preparing his meals. For many years, Murali's cholesterol has been in the high-normal range and he has not needed medication. He has recently landed a new contract with a *Fortune* 500 company at work. He has been very busy with luncheons and dinner meetings. He has been taking clients to many of the classy restaurants in town for four-course meals that always include dessert. He has been working on this contract for several months. Due to the added stress of this new lifestyle, he is rarely taking time to eat healthy. He also has resumed his old habit of smoking. He is so busy that rarely has time for any exercise. Annika is worried and convinces Murali to see his physician. His physician orders blood work that reveals a total cholesterol of 428 mg/dL, an LDL of 263 mg/dL, and an HDL of 28 mg/dL. Due to his family history his physician orders a cholesterol-lowering medication. However, he stresses to Murali that this is no replacement for good nutrition and exercise. He refers Murali to a cardiac education class for both nutrition and fitness information. He also refers Murali to a smoking-cessation program.

ASSESSMENT

1. What data do you have about Murali?
2. As a nurse, what conclusion can you draw from Murali's lab results?
3. What do you need to know about his current eating habits? Could foods with unknown fat content have a bearing on his current diet? How could a 24-hour food diary help?
4. Should his health habits, like smoking and alcohol use, be of concern?
5. What is Murali doing that is healthy for his heart?

DIAGNOSIS

6. What is the cause of Murali's imbalanced nutrition, more than body requirements?
7. Complete this statement: Murali's change of lifestyle is related to ___.

PLAN/GOAL

8. What are two possible goals you have for Murali?

IMPLEMENTATION

9. What topics do you need to cover related to dietary fats?
10. Name three things Murali can do to help him recognize hidden fats in fast food restaurants.
11. Who else should be in class with Murali?
12. What agencies or resources could you provide to support Murali at home?
13. How could the information on the American Heart Association website (http://www.americanheart.org) be helpful to Murali?

EVALUATION/OUTCOME CRITERIA

14. What can the physician measure to determine the effectiveness of the plan?
15. What can Murali provide to demonstrate his compliance with the plan?

THINKING FURTHER

16. What is the worst consequence if Murali does not reduce his cholesterol?
17. What does family history have to do with Murali's results?
18. What are the challenges of maintaining a diet and exercise plan for life?

✔ rate this plate

Murali attended the nutrition class to learn how to choose healthy foods while eating out. He attended a dinner meeting with his clients and ordered the following meal. Rate this plate for foods that contain large amounts of cholesterol and fat.

4 oz shrimp cocktail appetizer

2 cups chicken Caesar salad with 2 Tbsp light vinaigrette dressing

2 hot dinner rolls with creamy butter

1 slice of cheesecake with strawberries

20 oz iced tea

CASE IN POINT

CECELIA: ELEVATED CHOLESTEROL AND TRANS FATS

Cecelia moved to New York City from Italy with her mother and father when she was a young girl. Her parents opened an Italian bakery and Cecelia spent much of her time there growing up. Her parents are now ready to hand the bakery over to Cecelia so they can retire. At 42 years old, she is very excited about taking charge of the bakery. She has always enjoyed baking and has learned so much through the years about running a business. Her parents recently had physicals and they both had elevated cholesterol. They were concerned for Cecelia and asked her to see her doctor and have her cholesterol tested as well. Cecelia has always been in pretty good health, but decides this wouldn't be a bad idea. When Cecelia sees her doctor, he informs her that she, too, has elevated cholesterol. Her total cholesterol is 282. Her LDL is 186 and her HDL is 27. He discusses with her the

importance of weight loss. She is currently 5-ft 4-in tall and 173 lb. He also refers her to a dietitian for an assessment of her diet. The dietitian discusses with her the foods that can affect her cholesterol level. In addition to saturated fats, she mentions trans fats. Cecelia has heard this term before, but never understood its meaning. The dietitian explains that trans fats are created from hydrogenating (solidifying) vegetable oils. The dietitian tells Cecelia that trans fats are usually present in baked goods. She also discusses with Cecelia that New York City passed a law banning trans fats in restaurants. She educates Cecelia on the importance of not just eliminating the trans fats from her diet, but making sure that her parents adjusted the recipes for their bakery items to remove all trans fats as well.

ASSESSMENT

1. Why were Cecelia's parents concerned about her cholesterol levels?
2. Cecelia's doctor shares with her the results of her lipid panel. What are the recommendations for total cholesterol, LDL, and HDL levels for Cecelia?
3. What is Cecelia's ideal body weight range? Is her current weight within her ideal range?
4. What is trans fat and what are the impacts of trans fats on the body?

DIAGNOSIS

5. Write a nursing diagnosis for Cecelia.

PLAN/GOAL

6. Cecelia should be educated on what foods will elevate her cholesterol. What are some of these foods?
7. Cecelia should understand that cholesterol comes not only from foods but also from what other source?
8. What goals would you set for Cecelia?

IMPLEMENTATION

9. What is important for Cecelia to understand about trans fats?
10. How often should Cecelia have her cholesterol assessed?

EVALUATION/OUTCOME CRITERIA

11. How will Cecelia and her doctor know if she has been successful with her goals?

THINKING FURTHER

12. Search guidelines on the National Cholesterol Education Program website (http://www.nhlbi.nih.gov) for cholesterol levels and take the 10-year risk assessment at the bottom of the page. Are you at risk for a cardiac event in the next 10 years? Are there changes in your diet that could help to decrease your risk?

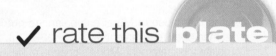

✔ rate this **plate**

Cecelia would like to modify the following recipe for dark chocolate cake in order to make it healthier for her family and customers. What ingredient could be adjusted to make it more healthful?

2 cups boiling water

1 cup unsweetened cocoa powder

2¾ cups all-purpose flour

2 teaspoons baking soda

½ teaspoon baking powder

½ teaspoon salt

1 cup butter, softened

2¼ cups white sugar

4 eggs

1½ teaspoons vanilla extract

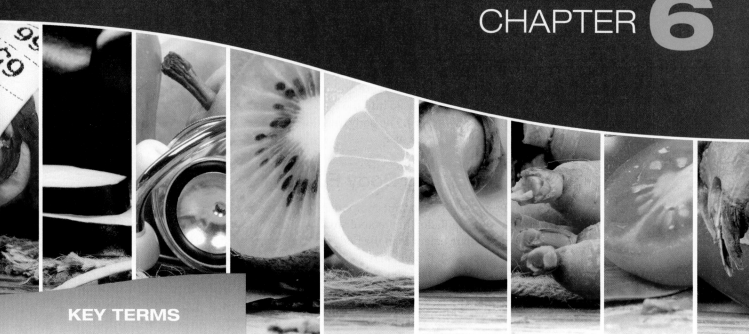

CHAPTER 6

KEY TERMS

albumin
amino acids
bioavailable
carboxypeptidase
chymotrypsin
complementary proteins
complete proteins
incomplete proteins
kwashiorkor
marasmus
mental retardation
negative nitrogen balance
nitrogen
nitrogen balance
physical trauma
polypeptides
positive nitrogen balance
protein energy malnutrition
    (PEM)
trypsin

PROTEINS

OBJECTIVES

After studying this chapter, you should be able to:

- State the functions of proteins in the body
- Identify the elements of which proteins are composed
- Describe the effects of protein deficiency
- State the energy yield of proteins
- Identify at least six food sources of complete proteins and six food sources of incomplete proteins

Proteins are the basic material of every body cell. By the age of 4, body protein content reaches the adult level of about 18% of body weight. An adequate supply of proteins in the daily diet is essential for normal growth and development and for the maintenance of health. Proteins are appropriately named. The word *protein* is of Greek derivation and means "of first importance."

FUNCTIONS

Proteins build and repair body tissue, play major roles in regulating various body functions, and provide energy if there is insufficient carbohydrate and fat in the diet.

Building and Repairing Body Tissue

The primary function of proteins is to build and repair body tissues. This is made possible by the provision of the correct type and number of amino acids in the diet. Also, as cells are broken down during metabolism (catabolism), some amino acids released into the blood are recycled to build new and repair other tissue (anabolism). The body uses the recycled amino acids as efficiently as those obtained from the diet.

Regulating Body Functions

Proteins are important components of hormones and enzymes that are essential for the regulation of metabolism and digestion. Proteins help maintain fluid and electrolyte balances in the body and thus prevent edema (abnormal retention of body fluids). Proteins are also essential for the development of antibodies and, consequently, for a healthy immune system.

Providing Energy

Proteins can provide energy if and when the supply of carbohydrates and fats in the diet is insufficient. Each gram of protein provides 4 calories. This is not a good use of proteins, however. In general, they are more expensive than carbohydrates, and most of the complete proteins also contain saturated fats and cholesterol.

FOOD SOURCES

Proteins are found in both animal and plant foods (Table 6-1). The animal food sources provide the highest quality of complete proteins. They include meats, fish, poultry, eggs, milk, and cheese.

Despite the high biologic value of proteins from animal food sources, they also provide saturated fats and cholesterol. Consequently, complete proteins should be carefully selected from healthfully prepared, low-fat animal foods such as fish, poultry, lean meats, and low-fat dairy products. Whole eggs should be limited to two or three a week if hyperlipidemia is a problem.

Healthful protein swaps for a meat eater could look as follows:

- Instead of fried fish, baked salmon is chosen.
- Instead of a double cheeseburger, a grilled turkey burger is chosen.
- Instead of barbeque ribs, a broiled center-cut boneless pork chop is chosen.

Proteins found in plant foods are incomplete proteins and are of a lower biologic quality than those found in animal foods. Even so, plant foods are important sources of protein when a variety are consumed within a given day. Examples

TABLE 6-1   Rich Sources of Proteins

COMPLETE PROTEINS		INCOMPLETE PROTEINS	
Meats	Eggs	Soybeans	Grains
Fish	Milk	Peanuts	Nuts
Poultry	Cheese	Peas	Sunflower seeds
		Navy beans	Sesame seeds

SPOTLIGHT *on Life Cycle*

As we age, there is a gradual and progressive loss of muscle mass, which results in lowered strength and physical stamina. Population studies show that around age 50, muscle mass loss averages 1–2% per year. Muscle strength declines by an average of 3% per year once we hit 60 and by 70, we may have lost an estimated 20–40% of our muscle strength. Protein intake may be the key to preventing age-related muscle loss. The adequacy of the RDA for protein of 0.8 g/kg/day for older folks has been questioned. The recent review has proposed that there is good and consistent evidence that a recommended level of 1.0–1.3 g/kg/day for older people is more appropriate, though the government has not changed the RDA to date. This higher level of protein along with twice weekly strength training seems to be the best tools to combat muscle mass and strength losses.

Source: (2015, Aug 14). *Nutrients*, 7(8), pp. 6874-6899.

of plant foods containing protein are nuts, sunflower seeds, sesame seeds, and legumes such as soybeans, navy beans, pinto beans, split peas, chickpeas, and peanuts. Grain such as wheat, barley, corn and rice also provide some incomplete protein to the diet.

Plant proteins can be used to produce textured soy protein and tofu, also called analogues. Meat alternatives (analogues) made from soybeans contain soy protein and other ingredients mixed together to simulate various kinds of meat. Meat alternatives may be canned, dried, or frozen. Analogues are excellent sources of protein, iron, and B vitamins.

Tofu is a soft, cheese-like food made from soy milk. Tofu is a bland product that easily absorbs the flavors of other ingredients with which it is cooked. Tofu is rich in high-quality proteins and B vitamins and is low in sodium. Textured soy protein and tofu are both economical and nutritious meat replacements.

Because of their inclusion of either dairy products and eggs or dairy products alone, most individuals who follow lacto-ovo vegetarian or lacto-vegetarian diets will be able to meet their protein requirements through a balanced diet that includes milk and milk products, enriched grains, nuts, and legumes. Strict vegetarians who consume no animal products will need to be more careful to include other protein-rich food sources such as soybeans, soy milk, and tofu.

Healthful protein swaps for a vegetarian could look as follows:

- Instead of macaroni and cheese, a vegetable tofu stir-fry with brown rice is chosen.

- Instead of a processed vegetable hot dog, lentil soup with whole grain bread is chosen.

- Instead of a frozen cheese pizza, a vegetable pizza on thin whole-grain crust with light cheese is chosen.

The subject of food sustainability is gaining international momentum, as concern continues to mount on the environmental effects of industrial food production, especially that of livestock. With American's voracious appetite for meat (mostly beef), characteristically most U.S. farming is devoted to growing commodity crops to be used for animal feed. Raising cattle, especially on factory farms, is further problematic, as cattle emit significant greenhouse gases and in turn require significant resources such as water as well as create significant solid waste. Shifting the American diet away from meat, with more inclusion of fruits, vegetables, and plant proteins is important for the health of our planet as well as ourselves. The dietary guidelines clearly offer the impetus to eat less red and processed meats.

CLASSIFICATION

The classification and quality of a protein depends on the number and types of amino acids it contains. There are 20 amino acids, but only 10 are considered essential to humans (Table 6-2). Two additional amino acids are sometimes incorporated into proteins during translation: selenocysteine and pyrrolysine. Essential amino acids are necessary for normal growth and development and must be provided in the diet. Proteins containing all the essential amino acids are of high biologic value; these proteins are called **complete proteins** and are extremely **bioavailable**. The nonessential amino acids can be produced in the body from the essential amino acids, vitamins, and minerals.

Incomplete proteins are those that lack one or more of the essential amino acids. Consequently, incomplete proteins cannot build tissue without the help of other proteins. The value of each is increased when it is eaten in combination with another incomplete protein, not necessarily at the same meal but during the same day. In this way, one incomplete protein food can provide the essential amino acids the other lacks. The combination may thereby provide all the essential amino acids (Figure 6-1). When this occurs, the proteins are called **complementary proteins** (Table 6-3). Gelatin is the only protein from an animal source that is an incomplete protein.

COMPOSITION

Like carbohydrates and fats, proteins contain carbon, hydrogen, and oxygen, but in different proportions. In addition, and most important, they are the only nutrient group that contains **nitrogen**, and some contain sulfur. Figure 6-1 is an example of an amino acid with a nitrogen (N) molecule.

Proteins are composed of chemical compounds called **amino acids** (Figure 6-2). Amino acids are sometimes called the building blocks of protein because they are combined to form the thousands of proteins in the human body. Heredity determines the specific types of proteins within each person.

DIGESTION AND ABSORPTION

The mechanical digestion of protein begins in the mouth, where the teeth grind the food into small pieces. Chemical digestion begins in the stomach.

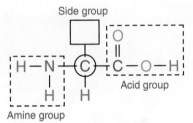

Side group

Amine group

Acid group

FIGURE 6-1 Two different foods (e.g., grains and dairy products) alone may not provide all the essential amino acids. Combined, however, they form a complete protein and therefore are considered complementary.

complete proteins
proteins that contain all the essential amino acids

bioavailable
ability of a nutrient to be readily absorbed and used by the body

incomplete proteins
proteins that do not contain all of the essential amino acids

complementary proteins
incomplete proteins that when combined provide all 10 essential amino acids

nitrogen
chemical element found in protein; essential to life

amino acids
nitrogen-containing chemical compounds of which protein is composed

TABLE 6-2 Amino Acids

ESSENTIAL		NONESSENTIAL	
Arginine*	Phenylalanine	Alanine	Glutamine
Histidine*	Threonine	Arginine*	Glycine
Isoleucine	Tryptophan	Asparagine	Histidine*
Leucine	Valine	Aspartic acid	Proline
Lysine		Cysteine	Serine
Methionine		Glutamic acid	Tyrosine

*Essential during childhood only.

TABLE 6-3 Examples of Complementary Protein Foods

PROTEIN 1	WITH	PROTEIN 2
Rice		Beans
Bread		Peanut butter
Bread		Split pea soup
Bread		Cheese
Rice		Tofu
Macaroni		Cheese
Cereal		Milk

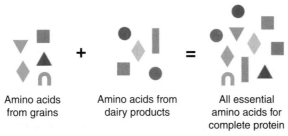

Amino acids from grains **+** Amino acids from dairy products **=** All essential amino acids for complete protein

FIGURE 6-2 All amino acids have a chemical backbone of a carbon atom; an amine group, which contains nitrogen; an acid group; and a side group. It is the chemical structure of the side group that gives each amino acid its unique identity.

Hydrochloric acid prepares the stomach so that the enzyme pepsin can begin its task of reducing proteins to **polypeptides**.

After the polypeptides reach the small intestine, three pancreatic enzymes (**trypsin**, **chymotrypsin**, and **carboxypeptidase**) continue chemical digestion. Intestinal peptidases finally reduce the proteins to amino acids.

After digestion, the amino acids in the small intestine are absorbed by the villi and are carried by the blood to all body tissues. There, they are used to form needed proteins.

METABOLISM AND ELIMINATION

All essential amino acids must be present to build and repair the cells as needed. When amino acids are broken down, the nitrogen-containing amine group is stripped off. This process is called deamination. Deamination produces ammonia, which is released into the bloodstream by the cells. The liver picks up the ammonia, converts it to urea, and returns it to the bloodstream for the kidneys to filter out and excrete. The remaining parts are used for energy or are converted to carbohydrate or fat and stored as glycogen or adipose tissue.

DIETARY REQUIREMENTS

One's protein requirement is determined by size, age, sex, and physical and emotional conditions. A large person has more body cells to maintain than a small person. A growing child, a pregnant woman, or a woman who is breastfeeding needs more protein for each pound of body weight than the average adult. Athletes and active individuals require more protein.

polypeptides
ten or more amino acids bonded together

trypsin
pancreatic enzyme; helps digest proteins

chymotrypsin
pancreatic enzyme necessary for the digestion of proteins

carboxypeptidase
pancreatic enzyme necessary for protein digestion

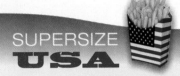

When digestion is inefficient, fewer amino acids are absorbed by the body; consequently, the protein requirement is higher. This is sometimes thought to be the case with the elderly and is addressed further in Chapter 13. Extra proteins are usually required after surgery, severe burns, or during infections in order to replace lost tissue and to manufacture antibodies. In addition, emotional trauma can cause the body to excrete more nitrogen than it normally does, thus increasing the need for protein foods.

The National Research Council of the National Academy of Sciences considers the average adult's daily requirement to be 0.8 g of protein for each kilogram of body weight. To determine your requirement, do the following:

1. Divide body weight by 2.2 (the number of pounds per kilogram).

2. Multiply the answer obtained in step 1 by 0.8 (gram of protein per kilogram of body weight).

In 2002, the Dietary Reference Intakes (DRIs) for protein were published by the National Academy of Sciences (see Table 6-4). An Adequate Intake (AI) was established for infants 0–6 months, with all other recommendations based on the RDA. The RDAs for children are higher on a gram-per-body

TABLE 6-4   Recommended Dietary Allowances for Protein

LIFE STAGE GROUP	AGE	PROTEIN (GRAMS/DAY)
Infants	0–6 mo	9.1*
	7–12 mo	11*
Children	1–3 y	13
	4–8 y	19
Males	9–13 y	34
	14–18 y	52
	19–30 y	56
	31–50 y	56
	51–70 y	56
	> 70 y	56
Females	9–13 y	34
	14–18 y	46
	19–30 y	46
	31–50 y	46
	51–70 y	46
	> 70 y	46
Pregnancy	14–18 y	71
	19–30 y	71
	31–50 y	71
Lactation	14–18 y	71
	19–30 y	71
	31–50 y	71

*Infant values are Adequate Intakes (AI); all other values are Recommended Dietary Allowances (RDA).

Source: Reprinted with permission from the National Academies Press, Copyright © 2006, National Academy of Sciences. *Dietary Reference Intakes: The Essential Guide to Nutrient Requirements.*

weight basis than for adults. RDAs are also greater for women who are pregnant or lactating; otherwise, all recommendations are based on 0.8 g/kg of body weight.

It is helpful to note that the "Choose My Plate" website has a useful daily protein foods chart that lists the "ounce equivalents" of protein by age group. In general, 1 oz of meat, poultry or fish; ¼ cup cooked beans; 1 egg; 1 tablespoon of peanut butter; or ½ oz of nuts or seeds can be considered as 1 oz-equivalent from the Protein Foods Group. Table 6-5 provides an idea of the amount of protein in an average day's diet.

Protein Excess

It is easy for people living in the developed parts of the world to ingest more protein than the body requires. There are a number of reasons why this should be avoided. The saturated fats and cholesterol common to complete protein foods may contribute to heart disease and provide more calories than desirable. Some studies seem to indicate a connection between long-term high-protein

TABLE 6-5 Protein in an Average Diet for One Day

	SERVING SIZE	PROTEIN (g)	CALORIE
Breakfast			
Orange juice	½ cup	1	45
Oatmeal	1 cup	6	165
with sugar	2 tsp		30
Whole wheat toast	1 slice	4	75
Peanut butter	1 Tbsp	4	95
1% milk	½ cup	4	50
Lunch			
Grapefruit juice	½ cup	1	50
Tuna salad	⅔ cup	20	220
in whole wheat pita	1 large	6	170
Lettuce			
Carrot sticks	1 carrot	1	25
Canned pears	½ cup	1	100
Oatmeal cookies	2	1	160
1% milk	1 cup	8	100
Dinner			
Chicken breast	3 oz	26	160
Baked red potato	1 medium	4	150
Asparagus	½ cup		25
Sliced tomato salad	1 tomato	1	25
Roll	1	2	100
with butter	1 Tbsp		100
Fresh apple	Medium		80
1% milk	1 cup	8	100
		98	2,025

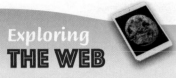

Exploring
THE WEB

Search the Web for information on protein supplements. What are some of the claims of these products? Are they based on solid research and facts? Create fact sheets on protein supplements that cite common myths and provide the truth behind the myths. How would you approach a person inquiring about the use of protein supplements?

diets and colon cancer and high calcium excretion, which depletes the bones of calcium and may contribute to osteoporosis. People who eat excessive amounts of protein-rich foods may ignore the also essential fruits and vegetables, and excess protein intake may put more demands on the liver (which converts nitrogen to urea) and the kidneys to excrete excess urea than they are prepared to handle. Therefore, the Centers for Disease Control and Prevention recommends that protein intake represent no more than 10–35% of one's daily calorie intake and not exceed double the amount given in the table of DRIs (see Table 6-4).

Protein and Amino Acid Supplements

Protein and amino acid supplements are taken for a number of reasons. Often, information in the media may lead consumers to think that specific protein and amino acid supplements should be taken for fueling workouts and building muscle for "bulking up." While it is now generally accepted that athletes do require more protein, most often, protein needs can easily be met through the diet. Some athletes who don't have access to a normal healthy diet may choose to supplement. Some individuals may physically need to supplement with additional protein due to illness or surgery.

Whatever the reason, consumers are searching out protein and amino acid supplements with great vigor. Protein shakes, bars, and powders are available at nearly every health food store, pharmacy, fitness center, and grocery. The protein may come from whey (most common), casein, soy, bean, or pea protein. The amount of protein varies greatly in these supplements. An average scoop of protein powder has 20 g of protein. Some protein powders offer as much as 80 g per serving. The danger is that too much protein is inherently hard on your kidneys and liver.

High-quality protein foods are more bioavailable than expensive supplements. Single amino acids can be harmful to the body and never occur naturally in food. The body was designed to handle food, not supplements. If a single amino acid has been recommended, it is very important that a physician be consulted before the amino acid is used.

Nitrogen Balance

Protein requirements may be discussed in terms of **nitrogen balance**. This occurs when nitrogen intake equals the amount of nitrogen excreted. **Positive nitrogen balance** exists when nitrogen intake exceeds the amount excreted. This indicates that new tissue is being formed, and it occurs during pregnancy, during children's growing years, when athletes develop additional muscle tissue, and when tissues are rebuilt after **physical trauma** such as illness or injury. **Negative nitrogen balance** indicates that protein is being lost. It may be caused by fevers, injury, surgery, burns, starvation, or immobilization.

Protein Deficiency

When people are unable to obtain an adequate supply of protein for an extended period, muscle wasting will occur, and arms and legs become very thin. At the same time, **albumin** (protein in blood plasma) deficiency will cause edema, resulting in an extremely swollen appearance. The water is excreted when sufficient protein is eaten. People may lose appetite, strength, and weight, and

nitrogen balance
when nitrogen intake equals nitrogen excreted

positive nitrogen balance
nitrogen intake exceeds outgo

physical trauma
extreme physical stress

negative nitrogen balance
more nitrogen lost than taken in

albumin
protein that occurs in blood plasma

wounds may heal very slowly. Clients suffering from edema become lethargic and depressed. These signs are seen in grossly neglected children or in the elderly, poor, or incapacitated. It is essential that people following vegetarian diets, especially vegans, carefully calculate the types and amount of protein in their diets so as to avoid protein deficiency.

Protein Energy Malnutrition

People suffering from **protein energy malnutrition (PEM)** lack both protein and energy-rich foods. Such a condition is not uncommon in developing countries, where there are long-term shortages of both protein and energy foods. Children who lack sufficient protein do not grow to their potential size. Infants born to mothers eating insufficient protein during pregnancy can have permanently impaired mental capacities.

Two deficiency diseases that affect children are caused by a grossly inadequate supply of protein or energy, or both. **Marasmus**, a condition resulting from severe malnutrition, afflicts young children and adults who lack both energy and protein foods as well as vitamins and minerals. The infant with marasmus appears emaciated but does not have edema. Hair is dull and dry, and the skin is thin and wrinkled (Figure 6-3). The other protein-deficiency disease that affects children as well as adults is kwashiorkor (Figure 6-4). **Kwashiorkor** appears when there is a sudden or recent lack of protein-containing food (such as during a famine). This disease causes fat to accumulate in the liver, and the lack of protein and hormones results in edema, painful skin lesions, and changes in the pigmentation of skin and hair. The mortality rate for kwashiorkor clients is high.

Those who survive these deficiency diseases may suffer from permanent **mental retardation**. The ultimate cost of food deprivation among young children is high, indeed. Table 6-6 lists some signs that help distinguish marasmus from kwashiorkor.

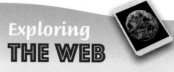

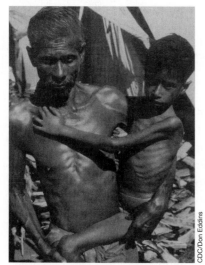

FIGURE 6-3 Visible signs of marasmus include extreme wasting, wrinkled skin, and irritability.

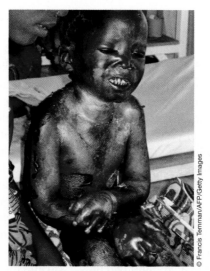

FIGURE 6-4 Edema, skin lesions, and hair changes are common signs of kwashiorkor.

protein energy malnutrition (PEM)
malnutrition resulting from inadequate intake of protein and energy-rich foods; marasmus and kwashiorkor

marasmus
severe wasting caused by lack of protein and all nutrients or faulty absorption; PEM

kwashiorkor
deficiency disease caused by extreme lack of protein

mental retardation
below-normal intellectual capacity

TABLE 6-6 Differentiating Marasmus and Kwashiorkor

MARASMUS	KWASHIORKOR
Total surface fat (TSF)* and mid-arm circumference (MAC) decreased	TSF and MAC within normal limits
Weight decreased	Weight possibly within normal limits
Visceral proteins (albumin) within normal limits or decreased	Visceral proteins decreased
Immune function within normal limits	Immune function decreased
Dull, dry hair	Reddish-color hair
Emaciated, wrinkled appearance	Puffy appearance
Lack of protein and total energy	Edema

*TSF and MAC can be determined by anthropometric measurements (see Chapter 1), which are done by a dietitian. The results are then compared with standard values obtained from measurement of a large number of people.

HEALTH AND NUTRITION CONSIDERATIONS

Proteins have acquired an unfairly high value among the general public in the United States. Also, many people think that proteins are found only in animal food sources. As a result, complete proteins tend to be overused in most diets.

Research about the cumulative effects of the overuse of proteins in the diet is beginning to suggest that excessive use of protein could damage kidneys, possibly contribute to osteoporosis and cancer, and cause overweight and heart disease.

The health care professional may find that reeducating clients about the need to reduce their protein intake to 10–35% of total calories is a challenging task.

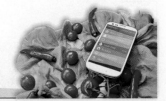

SUMMARY

Proteins contain nitrogen, an element that is necessary for growth and the maintenance of health. In addition to building and repairing body tissues, proteins regulate body processes and can supply energy. Each gram of protein provides 4 calories. Proteins are composed of amino acids, 10 of which are essential for growth and repair of body tissues.

Complete proteins contain all of the essential amino acids and can build tissues. The best sources of complete proteins are animal foods such as meat, fish, poultry, eggs, milk, and cheese. Incomplete proteins do not contain all of the essential amino acids, and two or more of these proteins must be combined in order to

build tissues. The best sources of incomplete proteins are legumes, corn, grains, and nuts. The nutritional value of incomplete protein foods can be increased by eating two or more incomplete protein foods during the day. Chemical digestion of proteins occurs in the stomach and small intestine. Proteins are reduced to amino acids and ultimately are absorbed into the blood through the villi in the small intestine.

A severe deficiency of protein in the diet can cause kwashiorkor and can contribute to marasmus in children and adults. Both conditions can result in impaired physical and mental development.

DISCUSSION TOPICS

1. Why are proteins especially important to children, pregnant women, and people who are ill?

2. Of which elements are proteins composed?

3. What functions do proteins perform in the body?

4. Discuss why it may be unwise to use protein foods as energy foods.

5. Discuss the effects of protein deficiency in both children and adults.

6. Describe the digestion of proteins.

7. Describe the metabolism of proteins.

8. Tell what amino acids are and explain their importance. Tell where they are found.

9. Describe complete and incomplete protein foods and name several of each type.

10. How does one determine protein requirements? Calculate your mother's or father's protein requirements.

11. Why might someone with a broken hip develop negative nitrogen balance in the hospital?

SUGGESTED ACTIVITIES

1. Keep a record of the foods you eat in a 24-hour period. Using the Internet or the diet analysis software at MyPlate, compute the grams of protein consumed. Did your diet provide the recommended amount of protein as indicated in Table 6-4?

2. Plan a day's menu for yourself. Include foods especially rich in complete proteins.
   a. Alter your planned menu by replacing some of the complete protein foods with those containing incomplete proteins.
   b. Visit a local supermarket and compute the cost of the menu that contains complete proteins. Compute the cost of the menu that contains incomplete proteins. Which is less expensive? Why?

REVIEW

Multiple choice. Select the *letter* that precedes the best answer.

1. The building blocks of proteins are
   a. ascorbic acids
   b. amino acids
   c. nitrogen and sulfur only
   d. meat and fish

2. Proteins are essential because they are the only nutrient that contains
   a. nitrogen
   b. niacin
   c. hydrochloric acid
   d. carbon

3. Corn, peas, and beans
   a. are complete protein foods
   b. are incomplete protein foods
   c. contain no protein
   d. lose proteins during cooking

4. Protein deficiency may result in
   a. beriberi
   b. goiter
   c. edema
   d. leukemia

5. Good sources of complete protein foods are
   a. eggs and chicken
   b. breads and cereals
   c. butter and margarine
   d. legumes and nuts

6. One gram of protein provides
   a. 4 calories
   b. 9 calories
   c. 7 calories
   d. 19 calories

7. Proteins are broken down in the body into
   a. peptides
   b. ascorbic acids
   c. amino acids
   d. calories

8. The *primary* function of protein is to
   a. build and repair body cells
   b. provide energy
   c. digest minerals and vitamins
   d. none of the above

9. Once proteins reach the small intestine, chemical digestion continues through the action of
   a. rennin
   b. pancreatic enzymes
   c. bile
   d. hydrochloric acid

10. It is unwise to regularly ingest excessive amounts of protein because
    a. it can cause positive nitrogen balance
    b. it may reduce the work of the kidneys
    c. it can contribute to the heart disease
    d. it may cause uremic poisoning

11. The following symptoms describe marasmus except for
    a. protein deficient
    b. edema
    c. calorie malnutrition
    d. emaciated appearance

12. Arrange the following foods into two lists, one with the best sources of complete proteins and one with the best sources of incomplete proteins.

Scrambled eggs	Refried beans
Tofu	
Chickpeas and rice	Fat-free milk
Turkey burger	Baked beans
Filet of sole	Grilled chicken
Peanuts	Swiss cheese

CASE IN POINT

ANNELIESE: HIGH-PROTEIN DIETS

Anneliese is a college exchange student from Germany. While attending college, she noticed she had gained some weight. She is 5-ft 6-in tall and is now 163 lb. Some of her friends were using the Atkins diet in an attempt to lose weight. They discussed how to follow the diet with her. She has been trying it out for the past two months and has seen some weight loss. However, she is finding it increasingly difficult to adhere to. She grew up in Germany eating many fruits and vegetables daily. She has been trying to find a new diet that will allow her to consume a larger variety of foods. In researching further, she discovers many diets that all promise the weight loss she desires. She decides a different diet might be the answer to her dilemma. She would definitely prefer one that incorporates more fruits and vegetables in with the high-protein foods. She believes this may help with the constipation she has been experiencing as well. One of her friends is studying nutrition and suggests Anneliese meet with a dietitian to help her choose a diet that is healthy. Anneliese hopes meeting with a dietitian will be the best way for her to lose weight, keep it off, and enjoy the foods she loves.

ASSESSMENT

1. What data do you have about Anneliese's eating habits?
2. What do you know about her ability to develop habits?
3. What is the cause of the current problem?

DIAGNOSIS

4. Complete the following diagnostic statement: Imbalanced nutrition, more than body requirements, as evidenced by _____.
5. Complete the following diagnostic statement: Deficient knowledge related to a lack of information about _____.

PLAN/GOAL

6. What are two possible measurable, reasonable goals for Anneliese?

IMPLEMENTATION

7. What foods need to be altered in Anneliese's diet?
8. What does Anneliese need to add to her diet?
9. Using preferences, suggest some alternative menus that would help Anneliese lose weight.

EVALUATION/OUTCOME CRITERIA

10. What criterion would a dietitian use to measure Anneliese's success?

11. What diseases would Anneliese avoid by reducing her high-fat protein intake?

THINKING FURTHER

12. Which protein sources are most economical and are low in calories?
13. How could this information be useful in other situations?

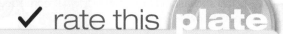

✔ rate this plate

Anneliese does not need a high amount of protein in order to lose weight. She only needs 5½ oz of protein per day. By lowering the amount of protein in the diet, calories will decrease and weight will be lost. Rate what she ate on the Atkins diet before seeing the dietitian.

7 oz deep-fried chicken breast

Spinach salad with tomatoes, onions, egg, dried cranberries, and croutons

Vinaigrette dressing

¾ cup of broccoli

What changes can be made to this plate to encourage healthy choices and continued weight loss without the Atkins diet plan?

CASE IN POINT

TALIL: PROTEIN ENERGY MALNUTRITION

Erin is a registered dietitian who is currently traveling with a medical missionary team of nurses and physicians throughout southern Asia. Their team's goal is to reach many of the people in that area who have never received any kind of medical attention. Talil lives in southern Asia with his family. Their primary source of food is the rice they grow and the fruits and berries they find on trees and bushes nearby. His mother is concerned about 2-year-old Talil. After giving birth to her second child eight months ago, she weaned Talil so she could feed the new baby. Since that time, Talil has become extremely thin, yet his belly is distended and his face is puffy. She doesn't understand why he is only gaining weight in his belly and his face. She has also noticed recently that some areas of his skin are lighter in pigment and others are more reddened and rashlike. He seems lethargic and irritable and has even had several bouts of diarrhea. His mother brings him to the clinic where the mission team is working. The doctor diagnoses Talil with kwashiorkor. He asks Erin to meet with Talil's mother and explain what kwashiorkor is and what needs to be done to improve Talil's health and well-being. Erin explains to Talil's mother that he is not getting adequate protein. She discusses the need for either meat or dairy sources in his diet. If meat and dairy are not available, then lentil beans need to be incorporated with the rice in his diet. She gives Talil's mom a case of lentils. The team brought several cases knowing the high incidence of kwashiorkor in this area of the world. She discusses with Talil's mom the importance of finding an additional source of protein for him before the lentils run out. Talil's mom asks Erin if consuming fish from the nearby lake would be a good protein source. Erin assures her that this would be an excellent way to start incorporating protein.

ASSESSMENT

1. What is deficient in Talil's diet?
2. What causes kwashiorkor?
3. What caused Talil to develop kwashiorkor?
4. If Talil's kwashiorkor continues, what consequence could follow as a result?

DIAGNOSIS

5. Write a nursing diagnosis for Talil.

PLAN/GOAL

6. What can Erin do as a dietitian to help Talil's mother correct his kwashiorkor?

IMPLEMENTATION

7. What could Talil's mom do to help prevent further kwashiorkor in her children or other children in their village?
8. Explain what happens in kwashiorkor that causes edema, skin lesions, and changes in pigment of the skin.

EVALUATION/OUTCOME CRITERIA

9. How will Talil's mom know that the strategies she has implemented have resolved the kwashiorkor?

THINKING FURTHER

10. Shown in Table 6-6, what are the key differences between kwashiorkor and marasmus?

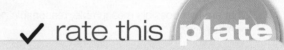
✔ rate this plate

Talil was diagnosed with kwashiorkor due to inadequate protein intake. His mother has asked the dietitian for good sources of protein and milk that she can find in her area. Talil's mother prepared the following meal. Rate this plate on protein content:

1 oz cooked fish

⅓ cup rice

¼ cup of vegetables

4 oz soy milk

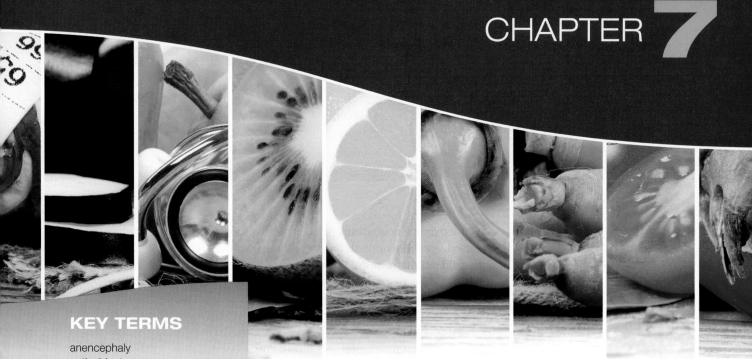

CHAPTER 7

KEY TERMS

anencephaly
antioxidant
ascorbic acid
avitaminosis
beriberi
biotin
carotenoids
coagulation
cobalamin
coenzymes
collagen
fat soluble
folate/folic acid
free radicals
heme iron
hemolysis
hemorrhage
hypervitaminosis
international units (IUs)
intrinsic factor
megadoses
megaloblastic anemia
myelin
neural tube defects (NTDs)
niacin
niacin equivalent (NE)
nonheme iron
pantothenic acid
pellagra
pernicious anemia
precursor
prohormone
provitamin
retinol
retinol equivalent (RE)
riboflavin
scurvy
spina bifida

VITAMINS

OBJECTIVES

After studying this chapter, you should be able to:

- State one or more functions of each of the 13 vitamins discussed
- Identify at least two food sources of each of the vitamins discussed
- Identify some symptoms of, or diseases caused by, deficiencies of the vitamins discussed

Vitamins are organic (carbon-containing) compounds that are essential in small amounts for body processes. Vitamins themselves do not provide energy. They enable the body to use the energy provided by carbohydrates, fats, and proteins. The name "vitamin" implies their importance, as in Latin *vita* means "life." They do not, however, represent a panacea (universal remedy) for physical or mental illness or a way to alleviate the stressors in life. They should not be overused—more is not necessarily better. In fact, **megadoses** can be toxic (poisonous). It was once believed that a healthy person eating a balanced diet would obtain all the nutrients—including vitamins—needed. That was in the past. Today's reality is such that with after-school sports, dance lessons, band practice or lessons, both parents working, and more, people are in a time and energy crunch. So in many homes, home-cooked family meals have been replaced by fast food, home delivery, carry-out, vending machines, and processed foods. Most of these choices are not found in the fruit and vegetable recommendation from MyPlate.

TABLE 7-1 Vitamins

FAT SOLUBLE (4)	WATER SOLUBLE (9)	
Vitamin A	Vitamin B complex	
Vitamin D	• Thiamine (B$_1$)	• Vitamin B$_{12}$ (cobalamin)
Vitamin E	• Riboflavin (B$_2$)	• Folate
Vitamin K	• Niacin	• Biotin
	• Vitamin B$_6$	• Pantothenic acid
	Vitamin C (ascorbic acid)	

The existence of vitamins has been known since early in the 20th century. It was discovered that animals fed diets of pure proteins, carbohydrates, fats, and minerals did not thrive as did those fed normal diets that included vitamins.

Vitamins were originally named by letter. Subsequent research has shown that many of the vitamins that were originally thought to be a single substance are actually groups of substances doing similar work in the body. Vitamin B proved to be more than one compound—B$_1$, B$_6$, B$_{12}$, and so on—and consequently is now known as B complex. Many of the 13 known vitamins are currently named according to their chemical composition or function in the body (Table 7-1).

Vitamins are found in minute amounts in foods. The specific amounts and types of vitamins in foods vary.

DIETARY REQUIREMENTS

Since 1997, the Food and Nutrition Board of the Institute of Medicine has been establishing Dietary Reference Intakes (DRIs) to replace the Recommended Dietary Allowances (RDAs) as outlined in Table 7-2. Tolerable upper limits (ULs) have also been set for some vitamins and minerals. The UL is the maximum level of daily intake unlikely to cause adverse effects and is not a recommended level of intake. Vitamin allowances are given by weight—milligrams (mg) or micrograms (µg or mcg).

TABLE 7-2 Adequate Intakes for Biotin and Pantothenic Acid

CATEGORY	AGE	BIOTIN (mg)	PANTOTHENIC ACID (mg)
Infants	0–6 mo	5	1.7
	7–12 mo	6	1.8
Children and	1–3 y	8	2
Adolescents	4–8 y	12	3
	9–13 y	20	4
	14–18 y	25	5
Adults	19–70 y	30	5
Pregnancy		30	6
Lactation		35	6

Source: Reprinted with permission from the National Academies Press, Copyright © 2006, National Academy of Sciences. *Dietary Reference Intakes: The Essential Guide to Nutrient Requirements.*

megadoses
extraordinarily large amounts

SPOTLIGHT *on Life Cycle*

Hypervitaminosis can be very dangerous. Several years ago, I received a letter from my sister informing me that she had been diagnosed with Alzheimer's disease and had approximately three years until she would no longer recognize me. I was devastated. My sister is a very intelligent person who keeps up with the latest nutrition information about diabetes (she has type 2), nutrition in general, and supplements. Over the years, we had many discussions about what supplements would be beneficial for her age, which is currently 84.

What I didn't know was that she and my brother-in-law, who live in Florida, had been going to a health food store and had been talked into taking a multitude, I mean handfuls, of vitamins, minerals, and herbal supplements. During my next visit, I discovered one entire dresser drawer full of bottles of vitamins, minerals, and herbal supplements that they had been taking for about two years. My brother, who visited my sister more often than I, knew that there had been a change in my sister's cognition. She would stop talking in midsentence, lose her train of thought, and even slur her speech. That explained why, when I would call, she would not want to talk for very long. My brother and I found it hard to believe she really had Alzheimer's, given her symptoms.

During my next visit, my brother and I got rid of all the supplements and helped my sister apply and thankfully be accepted into the assisted-living section of a retirement community. We did this so that my sister's medication and approved supplements would be given at designated times. Since then, two years have gone by, and my sister does not have Alzheimer's. Her cognition is fine she longer slurs her speech or has low blood pressure (caused by excessive potassium) and is just a little forgetful. I almost lost my sister because of overconsumption of vitamins, minerals, and herbal supplements, and now I have her back. I am so grateful!

Vitamin deficiencies can occur and can result in disease. Persons inclined to vitamin deficiencies because they do not eat balanced diets include alcoholics, the poor and incapacitated elderly, clients with serious diseases that affect appetite, intellectually disabled persons, and young children who receive inadequate care. Also, deficiencies of fat-soluble vitamins occur in clients with chronic malabsorption diseases such as cystic fibrosis, celiac disease, and Crohn's disease.

The term **avitaminosis** means "without vitamins," whereas **hypervitaminosis** is the excess of one or more vitamins. Either term followed by the name of a specific vitamin is used to indicate a serious lack thereof or excess of that particular vitamin. Either a lack or excess of vitamins can be detrimental to a person's health.

Vitamins taken in addition to those received in the diet are called **vitamin supplements**. One can acquire concentrated forms in tablets, capsules, and drops. Vitamin concentrates are sometimes termed *natural* or *synthetic* (manufactured). Some people believe that a meaningful difference exists between the two types and that the natural are far superior in quality to the synthetic. However, according to the U.S. Food and Drug Administration

avitaminosis
without vitamins

hypervitaminosis
condition caused by excessive ingestion of one or more vitamins

vitamin supplements
concentrated forms of vitamins; may be in tablet or liquid form

Exploring
THE WEB

Search the Web for vitamin supplements. Choose a supplement to report on. What claims are made by this product? What are they based on? Prepare a fact sheet that highlights the health benefits of this product and the adverse effects this product may have. What should consumers be aware of if they are taking this product?

(FDA), the body cannot distinguish between a vitamin of plant or animal origin and one manufactured in a laboratory because once they have been dismantled by the digestive system, the two types of the same vitamin are chemically identical.

Synthetic vitamins are frequently added to foods during processing. Such foods are described as enriched or fortified. Examples include enriched breads and cereals to which thiamine, niacin, riboflavin, folate, and the mineral iron have been added. Vitamins A and D are added to milk and fortified margarine.

Preserving Vitamin Content in Food

Occasionally, vitamins are lost during food processing. In most cases, food producers can replace these vitamins with synthetic vitamins, making the processed food nutritionally equal to the unprocessed food. Foods in which vitamins have been replaced are called enriched foods.

Because some vitamins are easily destroyed by light, air, heat, and water, it is important to know how to preserve the vitamin content of food during its preparation and cooking. Vitamin loss can be avoided by the following:

- Buying the freshest, unbruised vegetables and fruits locally and using them within a day's time

- Preparing fresh vegetables and fruits just before serving

- Heating canned vegetables quickly and in their own liquid

- Following package directions when using frozen vegetables or fruit

- Using as little water as possible when cooking and having it boil before adding vegetables, or preferably steaming them

- Covering the pan, cooking vegetables until bright in color and crisp tender

- Saving any cooking liquid for later use in soups, stews, and gravies

- Storing fresh vegetables and most fruits in a cool, dark place

- Microwaving fruits and vegetables in 1–2 tablespoons of water

- Cooking corn on the cob in a microwave by wrapping in a paper towel

- Roasting vegetables to retain nutrients rather than boiling them

CLASSIFICATION

fat soluble
can be dissolved in fat

water soluble
can be dissolved in water

coenzymes
active parts of an enzyme

precursor
something that comes before something else; in vitamins it is also called a provitamin, something from which the body can synthesize the specific vitamin

provitamin
a precursor of a vitamin

carotenoids
plant pigments, some of which yield vitamin A

Vitamins are commonly grouped according to solubility. Vitamins A, D, E, and K are **fat soluble**, and B complex and C are **water soluble** (Table 7-3). In addition, vitamin D is sometimes classified as a hormone, and the B-complex group may be classified as catalysts or **coenzymes**. When a vitamin has different chemical forms but serves the same purpose in the body it is sometimes called a vitamer. Vitamin E is an example. Sometimes a **precursor**, or **provitamin**, is found in foods. This is a substance from which the body can synthesize (manufacture) a specific vitamin. **Carotenoids** are examples of precursors of vitamin A and are referred to as provitamin A.

TABLE 7-3 Fat-Soluble and Water-Soluble Vitamins

NAME	FOOD SOURCES	FUNCTIONS	DEFICIENCY/TOXICITY
Fat-Soluble Vitamins			
Vitamin A (retinol)	Animal • Liver • Whole milk • Butter • Cream • Cod liver oil Plants • Dark-green leafy vegetables • Deep yellow or orange fruit • Fortified margarine	• Maintenance of vision in dim light • Maintenance of mucous membranes and healthy skin • Growth and development of bones • Reproduction • Healthy immune system • Antioxidant	Deficiency • Night blindness • Xerophthalmia • Respiratory infections • Bone growth ceases Toxicity • Birth defects • Bone pain • Anorexiant • Enlargement of liver
Vitamin D (calciferol)	Animal • Salmon and tuna • Fortified milk and yogurt • Fortified margarine • Fortified orange juice Plants • None Other sources • Sunlight	• Regulation of absorption of calcium and phosphorus • Building and maintenance of normal bones and teeth • Prevention of tetany • Immune and muscular function • Reduction of inflammation	Deficiency • Rickets • Osteomalacia • Osteoporosis • Poorly developed teeth and bones • Muscle spasms Toxicity • Kidney stones • Calcification of soft tissues
Vitamin E (tocopherol)	Animal • None Plants • Leafy green vegetables • Margarine • Salad dressing • Wheat germ • Vegetable oils • Nuts	• Antioxidant • Considered essential for protection of cell structure, especially of red blood cells	Deficiency • Destruction of red blood cells Toxicity • bleeding
Vitamin K	• Animal • Liver • Milk Plants • Leafy green vegetables • Cabbage, broccoli • Brussels sprouts	• Blood clotting	Deficiency • Prolonged blood clotting or hemorrhaging Toxicity • Hemolytic anemia • Interferes with anticlotting medications
Water-Soluble Vitamins			
Thiamine (vitamin B₁)	Animal • Lean pork • Beef • Liver • Eggs • Fish Plants • Whole and enriched grains • Legumes • Brewer's yeast	• Metabolism of carbohydrates and some amino acids • Maintains normal appetite and functioning of nervous system	Deficiency • Gastrointestinal tract, nervous system, and cardiovascular system problems • Beriberi Toxicity • None

(continues)

TABLE 7-3 *(continued)*

NAME	FOOD SOURCES	FUNCTIONS	DEFICIENCY/TOXICITY
Riboflavin (vitamin B$_2$)	Animal • Liver, kidney, heart • Milk • Cheese Plants • Leafy green vegetables • Cereals • Enriched bread	• Aids release of energy from food • Health of the mouth tissue • Healthy eyes	Deficiency • Cheilosis • Eye sensitivity • Dermatitis • Glossitis • Photophobia Toxicity • None
Niacin (nicotinic acid)	Animal • Milk • Eggs • Fish • Poultry Plants • Enriched breads and cereals	• Energy metabolism • Healthy skin and nervous and digestive systems	Deficiency • Pellagra—dermatitis, dementia, diarrhea Toxicity • Vasodilation of blood vessels
Pyridoxine (vitamin B$_6$)	Animal • Pork • Fish • Poultry • Liver, kidney • Milk • Eggs Plants • Whole-grain cereals • Legumes	• Conversion of tryptophan to niacin • Release of glucose from glycogen • Protein metabolism and synthesis of nonessential amino acids	Deficiency • Cheilosis • Glossitis • Dermatitis • Confusion • Depression • Irritability Toxicity • Depression • Nerve damage
Vitamin B$_{12}$ (cobalamin)	Animal • Seafood • Poultry • Liver, kidney • Muscle meats • Eggs • Milk • Cheese Plants • None	• Synthesis of red blood cells • Maintenance of myelin sheaths • Treatment of pernicious anemia • Folate metabolism	Deficiency • Degeneration of myelin sheaths • Pernicious anemia • Sore mouth and tongue • Anorexia • Neurological disorders Toxicity • None
Folate (folic acid)	Animal • Liver Plants • Leafy green vegetables • Spinach • Legumes • Seeds • Broccoli • Cereal and flour fortified with folate • Fruit	• Synthesis of RBCs • Synthesis of DNA	Deficiency • Anemia • Glossitis • Neural tube defects such as anencephaly and spina bifida Toxicity • Could mask a B$_{12}$ deficiency

(continues)

TABLE 7-3 *(continued)*

NAME	FOOD SOURCES	FUNCTIONS	DEFICIENCY/TOXICITY
Biotin	Animal • Milk • Liver and kidney • Egg yolks Plants • Legumes • Brewer's yeast • Soy flour • Cereals • Fruit	• Coenzyme in carbohydrate and amino acid metabolism • Niacin synthesis from tryptophan	Deficiency • Dermatitis • Nausea • Anorexia • Depression • Hair loss Toxicity • None
Pantothenic acid	Animal • Eggs • Liver • Salmon • Poultry Plants • Mushrooms • Cauliflower • Peanuts • Brewer's yeast	• Metabolism of carbohydrates, lipids, and proteins • Synthesis of fatty acids, cholesterol, steroid hormones	Deficiency • Rare: burning feet syndrome; vomiting; fatigue Toxicity • None
Vitamin C (ascorbic acid)	Animal • None Plants • All citrus fruits • Broccoli • Melons • Strawberries • Tomatoes • Brussels sprouts • Potatoes • Cabbage • Green peppers	• Prevention of scurvy • Formation of collagen • Healing of wounds • Release of stress hormones • Absorption of iron • Antioxidant • Resistance to infection	Deficiency • Scurvy • Muscle cramps • Ulcerated gums • Tendency to bruise easily Toxicity • Raised uric acid level • Hemolytic anemia • Kidney stones • Rebound scurvy

FAT-SOLUBLE VITAMINS

The fat-soluble vitamins A, D, E, and K are chemically similar. They are not lost easily in cooking but are lost when mineral oil is ingested. Mineral oil is not absorbed by humans. After absorption, fat-soluble vitamins are transported through the blood by lipoproteins because they are not soluble in water. Excess amounts can be stored in the liver. Therefore, deficiencies of fat-soluble vitamins are slower to appear than are those caused by a lack of water-soluble vitamins. Because of the body's ability to store them, megadoses of fat-soluble vitamins should be avoided, as they can reach toxic levels.

Vitamin A

Vitamin A consists of two basic dietary forms: preformed vitamin A, also called **retinol**, which is the active form of vitamin A; and carotenoids, the inactive form of vitamin A, which are found in plants.

retinol
the preformed vitamin A

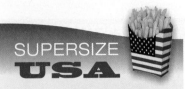

SUPERSIZE **USA**

A recent study conducted in China found that calcium intake plus vitamin D₃ supplementation facilitated fat loss in overweight and obese college students with low calcium consumption. Research has found that lower vitamin D levels are often found in overweight and obese adults. By increasing intakes of fatty fish, milk, fortified juices, and cereals as well as increasing exposure to sunshine, healthy vitamin D and calcium levels can be achieved. However, some resources indicate that just stepping outside and eating a calcium-rich diet may not be enough. Supplementing may be beneficial to ensure adequate vitamin D levels; however, further testing can be done to determine specific deficiencies.

Source: Wei, Z, et al. (2013). "Calcium Plus Vitamin D3 Supplementation Facilitated Fat Loss in Overweight and Obese College Students with Very Low Calcium Consumption: A Randomized Trial." *Nutrition Journal*, 12:43. http://www.ncbi.nlm.nih.gov/pubmed/23297844

antioxidant
a substance preventing damage from oxygen

free radicals
atoms or groups of atoms with an odd (unpaired) number of electrons that can be formed when oxygen interacts with certain molecules

retinol equivalent (RE)
the equivalent of 3.33 IUs of vitamin A

xerophthalmia
serious eye disease characterized by dry mucous membranes of the eye, caused by a deficiency of vitamin A

Functions

Vitamin A is a family of fat-soluble compounds that play an important role in vision, bone growth, reproduction, and cell division. It helps regulate the immune system, which helps fight infections. Vitamin A has been labeled as an **antioxidant** when, in fact, provitamin A (carotenoids) is the part of the family that functions as an antioxidant. Antioxidants protect cells from **free radicals**. Free radicals are atoms or groups of atoms with an odd (unpaired) number of electrons and can be formed when oxygen interacts with certain molecules. Once formed, these highly reactive radicals can start a chain reaction. When they react with important cellular components such as DNA or cell membranes, the most damage occurs. Antioxidants have the capability of safely interacting with free radicals and stopping the chain reaction before vital cells are damaged.

The first organic free radical was discovered in 1900 by Moses Gomberg. In the 1950s, Dr. Denman Harman was the first to propose the free radical theory of aging.

Sources

There are two forms of vitamin A: preformed vitamin A and provitamin A. Retinol is a preformed vitamin A and is one of the most active and usable forms of vitamin A. Retinol can be converted to retinal and retinoic acid, other active forms of vitamin A.

Provitamin A carotenoids can be converted to vitamin A from darkly colored pigments, both green and orange, in fruits and vegetables. Common carotenoids are beta-carotene, lutein, lycopene, and zeaxanthin. Beta-carotene is most efficiently converted to retinol. Eating "five-a-day" of fruits and vegetables is highly recommended. The best sources of beta-carotene are carrots, sweet potatoes, spinach, broccoli, pumpkin, squash (butternut), mango, and cantaloupe.

Research has shown that regular consumption of foods rich in carotenoids decreases the risk of some cancers because of its antioxidant effect. Taking a beta-carotene supplement has not shown the same results.

Preformed vitamin A (retinol) is found in fat-containing animal foods such as liver, butter, cream, whole milk, whole-milk cheeses, and egg yolk. It is also found in low-fat milk products and in cereals that have been fortified with vitamin A, but these are not the best sources.

Requirements

A well-balanced diet is the preferred way to obtain the required amounts of vitamin A. Vitamin A values are commonly listed as a **retinol equivalent (RE)**. A retinol equivalent is 1 mcg retinol or 6 mcg beta-carotene.

Hypervitaminosis

The use of a single vitamin supplement should be discouraged because an excess of vitamin A can have serious consequences. Signs of hypervitaminosis A may include birth defects, hair loss, dry skin, headaches, nausea, dryness of mucous membranes, liver damage, and bone and joint pain. In general, these symptoms tend to disappear when excessive intake is discontinued.

Deficiency

Signs of a deficiency of vitamin A include night blindness; dry, rough skin; and increased susceptibility to infections. Vitaminosis A can result in blindness or **xerophthalmia**, a condition characterized by dry, lusterless, mucous membranes of the eye. Lack of vitamin A is the leading cause of blindness in the world (discounting accidents).

Vitamin D

Vitamin D exists in two forms—D_2 (ergocalciferol) and D_3 (cholecalciferol). Each is formed from a provitamin when irradiated with (exposed to) ultraviolet light. Both forms are equally effective in human nutrition, but D_3 is the one that is formed in humans from cholesterol in the skin. D_2 is formed in plants. Vitamin D is considered a **prohormone** because it is converted to a hormone in the human body.

Vitamin D is heat-stable and not easily oxidized, so it is not harmed by storage, food processing, or cooking.

Functions

The major function of vitamin D is the promotion of calcium and phosphorus absorption in the body. By contributing to the absorption of these minerals, it helps to raise their concentration in the blood so that normal bone and tooth mineralization can occur and tetany (involuntary muscle movement) can be prevented. (Tetany can occur when there is too little calcium in the blood. This condition is called hypocalcemia.) Vitamin D has other roles in the body, involving cell growth, neuromuscular and immune function, and reduction of inflammation.

Vitamin D is absorbed in the intestines and is chemically changed in the liver and kidneys. Excess amounts of vitamin D are stored in the liver and in adipose tissue.

Sources

The best source of vitamin D is sunlight, which changes a provitamin to vitamin D_3 in humans. It is sometimes referred to as the sunshine vitamin. The amount of vitamin D that is formed depends on the individual's pigmentation (coloring matter in the skin) and the amount of sunlight available. The best food sources of vitamin D are oily fish, fortified milk, fish liver oils, egg yolk, butter, and fortified margarine. Because of the rather limited number of food sources of vitamin D and the unpredictability of sunshine, health authorities decided that the vitamin should be added to a common food. Since 1930, cow's milk has been fortified with 100 IU of vitamin D per cup.

Requirements

In late 2010, the Institute of Medicine (IOM) recommended an increase in vitamin D intake to 600 **international units (IUs)**—that is, 15 mcg for men and women aged 1–70 years old. To meet the vitamin D requirements through diet, one would have to consume 3 cups of milk, 1 egg, 6 oz of fortified yogurt, and 1 cup of fortified orange juice. Additional sources of vitamin D are listed in Table 7-4. Often it is difficult for consumers to fulfill their vitamin D requirement through diet; therefore, a vitamin D supplement may be necessary. Many general multivitamins contain 400 IUs of vitamin D_3. Calcium supplements contain varying amounts of vitamin D as well.

Vitamin D, or specifically cholecalciferol values, are given in micrograms on the DRI chart (Table 7-5); however, most supplements will state the amount in IUs.

Hypervitaminosis

Hypervitaminosis D must be avoided because it can cause deposits of calcium and phosphorus in soft tissues, kidney and heart damage, and bone fragility. Based on new research, the IOM has increased the tolerable upper limit that is safe to consume daily to 4,000 IUs for adults.

prohormone
substance that precedes the hormone and from which the body can synthesize the hormone

international units (IUs)
a unit of measurement of some vitamins; 5 mcg = 200 IUs

TABLE 7-4   Selected Food Sources of Vitamin D

Salmon (sockeye), cooked, 3 oz	447 IU
Tuna, water packed, drained, 3 oz	154 IU
Milk, fortified (nonfat, reduced fat, whole), 1 cup	115–124 IU
Yogurt, 6 oz fortified with 20% daily value of vitamin D	88 IU
Egg, 1 large	41 IU
Fortified margarine, 1 Tbsp	60 IU
Ready-to-eat cereal, fortified with 10% of daily value of vitamin D, ¾–1 cup	40 IU
Orange juice fortified with vitamin D, 1 cup	137 IU

Source: U.S. Department of Agriculture, Agricultural Research Service. 2011. *USDA National Nutrient Database for Standard Reference.*
Release 24. Nutrient Data Laboratory Home Page, http://www.ars.usda.gov/ba/bhnrc/ndl

TABLE 7-5   Recommended Dietary Allowances (RDAs) for Vitamin D

AGE	MALE	FEMALE	PREGNANCY	LACTATION
0–12 months*	400 IU (10 mcg)	400 IU (10 mcg)		
1–13 years	600 IU (15 mcg)	600 IU (15 mcg)		
14–18 years	600 IU (15 mcg)	600 IU (15 mcg)	600 IU (15 mcg)	600 IU (15 mcg)
19–50 years	600 IU (15 mcg)	600 IU (15 mcg)	600 IU (15 mcg)	600 IU (15 mcg)
51–70 years	600 IU (15 mcg)	600 IU (15 mcg)	600 IU (15 mcg)	600 IU (15 mcg)
>70 years	800 IU (20 mcg)	800 IU (20 mcg)		

*Adequate intake (AI).

Source: Reprinted with permission from the National Academies Press, Copyright © 2011, National Academy of Sciences. *Dietary Reference Intakes for Calcium and Vitamin D.*

Deficiency

The deficiency of vitamin D inhibits the absorption of calcium and phosphorus in the small intestine and results in poor bone and tooth formation. Vitamin D deficiency in children may lead to rickets, which causes malformed bones, pain, and poorly formed teeth (see Figure 7-1). Adults lacking sufficient vitamin D may develop osteomalacia, which is softening of the bones. Deficiency contributes to osteoporosis (brittle, porous bones).

People who are seldom outdoors, those who use sunscreens, and those who live in areas where there is little sunlight for three to four months a year should be especially careful that they attain the RDA for vitamin D. Other groups at risk for vitamin D deficiency include breast-fed infants, older adults, people with dark skin, those who have fat malabsorption, and those who are obese or who have undergone gastric bypass surgery. Vitamin D deficiency has been found to be widespread in the normal population, with some estimating deficiency as high as 40–75% of individuals. Recent research has shown that optimal blood levels are much higher than previously thought (>.30 ng/mL versus >.20 ng/mL). Emerging science is linking higher levels of vitamin D with reduced incidence of numerous diseases. Researchers document that vitamin D influences the expression of 229 genes in our bodies. If the current studies are confirmed, vitamin D status will play a central role in cancer protection, immunity, neuromuscular function, cardiovascular health, autoimmune disease protection, glucose tolerance, and diabetes.

tocopherols
vitamers of vitamin E

tocotrienols
a form of vitamin E

Vitamin E

Vitamin E consists of two groups of chemical compounds. They are the **tocopherols** and the **tocotrienols**. There are four types of tocopherols: alpha, beta, delta, and gamma. The most biologically active of these is alpha-tocopherol.

Rickets

Normal   Rickets

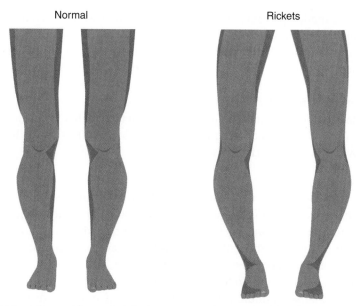

FIGURE 7-1 Bowed legs of rickets compared to normal leg formation.

Functions

Vitamin E is an antioxidant. It is aided in this process by vitamin C and the mineral selenium. It is carried in the blood by lipoproteins. When the amount of vitamin E in the blood is low, the red blood cells become vulnerable to a higher-than-normal rate of **hemolysis**. Vitamin E has been found helpful in the prevention of hemolytic anemia among premature infants. It may also enhance the immune system. Because of its antioxidant properties, it is commonly used in commercial food products to retard spoilage.

Sources

Vegetable oils made from corn, soybean, safflower, and cottonseed and products made from them, such as margarine, are the best sources of vitamin E. Wheat germ, nuts, leafy green vegetables, peanut butter, broccoli, and kiwi are also good sources. Animal foods, fruits, and most vegetables are poor sources.

Requirements

Research indicates that the vitamin E requirement increases if the amount of polyunsaturated fatty acids in the diet increases. In general, however, the U.S. diet is thought to contain sufficient vitamin E.

Hypervitaminosis

Although vitamin E appears to be relatively nontoxic, it is a fat-soluble vitamin, and the excess is stored in adipose tissue. Consequently, it would seem advisable to avoid long-term megadoses of vitamin E.

Deficiency

A deficiency of vitamin E has been detected in premature, low-birthweight infants and in clients who are unable to absorb fat normally. Malabsorption can cause serious neurological defects in children; in adults, it takes 5–10 years before deficiency symptoms occur.

hemolysis
the destruction of red blood cells

Vitamin K

Vitamin K is made up of several compounds that are essential to blood clotting. Vitamin K_1, commonly called phylloquinone, is found in dietary sources, especially leafy green vegetables such as spinach and in animal tissue. Vitamin K_2, called menaquinone, is synthesized in the intestine by bacteria and is also found in animal tissue. In addition, there is a synthetic vitamin K, called menadione. Vitamin K is destroyed by light and alkalies.

Vitamin K is absorbed like fats, mainly from the small intestine and slightly from the colon. Its absorption requires a normal flow of bile from the liver, and it is improved when there is fat in the diet.

Functions

Vitamin K is essential for the formation of prothrombin, which permits the proper clotting of the blood. It may be given to newborns immediately after birth because human milk contains little vitamin K and the intestines of newborns contain few bacteria. With insufficient vitamin K, newborns may be in danger of intracranial hemorrhage (bleeding within the head).

Vitamin K may be given to clients who suffer from faulty fat absorption; to clients after extensive antibiotic therapy (ingestion of antibiotic drugs to combat infection) because these drugs destroy the bacteria in the intestines; as an antidote for an overdose of anticoagulant (blood thinner such as warfarin—sometimes sold as Coumadin or warnerin); or to treat cases of **hemorrhage**.

Sources

The best dietary sources of vitamin K are leafy green vegetables such as broccoli, cabbage, spinach, and kale. Dairy products, eggs, meats, fruits, and cereals also contain some vitamin K. Cow's milk is a much better source of vitamin K than human milk. The synthesis of vitamin K by bacteria in the small intestine does not provide a sufficient supply by itself. It must be supplemented by dietary sources.

Requirements

Vitamin K is measured in micrograms. The AI for vitamin K is 120 mcg for men and 90 mcg for women. This is not increased during pregnancy or lactation. Infants up to 6 months should have 2.0 mcg a day. Those between 6 months and 1 year should receive 2.5 mcg a day. Vitamin K must be ingested daily. What is absorbed today will be utilized immediately with very little storage in the liver.

Hypervitaminosis

Ingestion of excessive amounts of synthetic vitamin K can be toxic and can cause a form of anemia.

Deficiency

The only major sign of a deficiency of vitamin K is defective blood **coagulation**. This increases clotting time, making the client more prone to hemorrhage. Human deficiency may be caused by faulty fat metabolism, antacids, antibiotic therapy, inadequate diet, or anticoagulants.

WATER-SOLUBLE VITAMINS

Water-soluble vitamins include B complex and C. These vitamins dissolve in water and are easily destroyed by air, light, and cooking. They are not stored in the body to the extent that fat-soluble vitamins are stored.

hemorrhage
unusually heavy bleeding

coagulation
thickening

Vitamin B Complex

Beriberi is a disease that affects the nervous, cardiovascular, and gastrointestinal systems. The legs feel heavy, the feet burn, and the muscles degenerate. The client is irritable and suffers from headaches, depression, anorexia, constipation, tachycardia (rapid heart rate), edema, and heart failure.

Toward the end of the 19th century, a doctor in Indonesia discovered that chickens that were fed table scraps of polished rice developed symptoms much like those of his clients suffering from beriberi. When these same chickens were later fed brown (unpolished) rice, they recovered.

Some years later, this mysterious component of unpolished rice was recognized as an essential food substance and was named vitamin B. Subsequently, it was named vitamin *B complex* because the vitamin was found to be composed of several compounds. The B-complex vitamins are listed in Table 7-1.

Thiamine

Thiamine, a coenzyme, was originally named vitamin B_1. It is partially destroyed by heat and alkalies and lost in cooking water.

Functions
Thiamine is essential for the metabolism of carbohydrates and some amino acids. It is also essential to nerve and muscle action. It is absorbed in the small intestine.

Sources
Thiamine is found in many foods, but generally in small quantities. Some of the best natural food sources of thiamine are unrefined and enriched cereals, whole grains, lean pork, liver, seeds, nuts, and legumes.

Requirements
Thiamine is measured in milligrams. The daily thiamine requirement for the average adult female is 1.1 mg a day, and for the average adult male it is 1.2 mg a day. The requirement is not thought to increase with age. In general, however, an increase in calories increases the need for thiamine.

Most breads and cereals in the United States are enriched with thiamine, so that the majority of people can and do easily fulfill their recommended intake.

Deficiency
Symptoms of thiamine deficiency include loss of appetite, fatigue, nervous irritability, and constipation. An extreme deficiency causes beriberi. Its deficiency is rare, however, occurring mainly among alcoholics whose diets include reduced amounts of thiamine while their requirements are increased and their absorption is decreased. Others at risk include renal clients undergoing long-term dialysis, clients undergoing bypass surgery for weight loss, and those who eat primarily rice.

Because some raw fish contain thiaminase, an enzyme that inhibits the normal action of thiamine, frequent consumption of large amounts of raw fish could cause thiamine deficiency. Eating raw fish is not recommended. Cooking inactivates this enzyme.

There are no known ill effects from excessive oral intake of thiamine, but it may be toxic if excessive amounts are given intravenously.

Riboflavin

Riboflavin is sometimes called B_2. It is destroyed by light and irradiation and is unstable in alkalies.

beriberi
deficiency disease caused by a lack of vitamin B_1 (thiamine)

thiamine
vitamin B_1

riboflavin
vitamin B_2

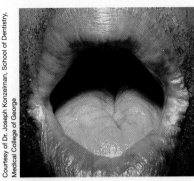

FIGURE 7-2 Cheilosis at the corners of the mouth is an indication of a riboflavin deficiency.

Functions

Riboflavin is essential for carbohydrate, fat, and protein metabolism. It is also necessary for tissue maintenance, especially the skin around the mouth, and for healthy eyes. Riboflavin is absorbed in the small intestine.

Sources

Riboflavin is widely distributed in animal and plant foods but in small amounts. Milk, meats, poultry, fish, and enriched breads and cereals are some of its richest sources. Some green vegetables such as broccoli, spinach, and asparagus are also good sources.

Requirement

Riboflavin is measured in milligrams. The average adult female daily requirement is thought to be 1.1 mg, and the adult male requirement is 1.3 mg. The riboflavin requirement appears to increase with increased energy expenditure. The requirement does not diminish with age.

Deficiency

Because of the small quantities of riboflavin in foods and its limited storage in the body, deficiencies of riboflavin can develop. The generous use of fat-free milk in the diet is a good way to prevent deficiency of this vitamin. It is important, however, that milk be stored in opaque containers because riboflavin can be destroyed by light. It appears that fiber laxatives can reduce riboflavin absorption, and their use over long periods should be discouraged.

A deficiency of riboflavin can result in cheilosis, a condition characterized by sores on the lips and cracks at the corners of the mouth (Figure 7-2), glossitis (inflammation of the tongue), dermatitis, and eye strain in the form of itching, burning, and eye fatigue. Its toxicity is unknown.

Niacin

Niacin is the generic name for nicotinic acid and nicotinamide. Niacin is fairly stable in foods. It can withstand reasonable amounts of heat and acid and is not destroyed during food storage.

Functions

Niacin serves as a coenzyme in energy metabolism and consequently is essential to every body cell. In addition, niacin is essential for the prevention of **pellagra**. Pellagra is a disease characterized by sores on the skin and by diarrhea, anxiety, confusion, irritability, poor memory, dizziness, and untimely death if left untreated. Niacin, when used as a cholesterol-lowering agent, must be closely supervised by a physician because of possible adverse side effects such as liver damage and peptic ulcers.

Sources

The best sources of niacin are meats, poultry, and fish. Peanuts and other legumes are also good sources. Enriched breads and cereals also contain some. Milk and eggs do not provide niacin per se, but they are good sources of its precursor, tryptophan (an amino acid). Vegetables and fruits contain little niacin.

Requirements

Niacin is measured as a **niacin equivalent (NE)**. One NE equals 1 mg of niacin or 60 mg of tryptophan. The general recommendation is a daily intake of 14 mg/NE for adult women and 16 mg/NE for adult men. Because excessive amounts of

niacin
B vitamin

pellagra
deficiency disease caused by a lack of niacin

niacin equivalent (NE)
unit of measuring niacin; 1 NE equals 1 mg niacin or 60 mg tryptophan

niacin have caused flushing due to vascular dilation (expansion of blood vessels), self-prescribed doses of niacin concentrate should be discouraged. Other symptoms include gastrointestinal problems and itching. If excessive amounts of niacin are ingested, liver damage may result.

Deficiency

A deficiency of niacin is apt to appear if there is a deficiency of riboflavin. Symptoms of niacin deficiency include weakness, anorexia, indigestion, anxiety, and irritability. In extreme cases, pellagra may occur.

Vitamin B$_6$

Vitamin B$_6$ is composed of three related forms: pyridoxine, pyridoxal, and pyridoxamine. It is stable to heat but sensitive to light and alkalies.

Functions

Vitamin B$_6$ is essential for protein metabolism and absorption, and it aids in the release of glucose from glycogen. With the help of vitamin B$_6$, amino acids present in excessive amounts can be converted to those in which the body is temporarily deficient. It also serves as a catalyst in the conversion of tryptophan to niacin, and it is helpful in the formation of other substances from amino acids. An example is the synthesis of neurotransmitters such as serotonin and dopamine.

Sources

Some of the nutrient-dense sources of vitamin B$_6$ are poultry, fish, liver, kidney, potatoes, bananas, and spinach. Whole grains, especially oats and wheat, are good sources of vitamin B$_6$, but because this vitamin is lost during milling and is not replaced during the enrichment process, refined grains are not a good source.

Requirements

Vitamin B$_6$ is measured in milligrams, and the need increases as the protein intake increases. For adult females, the daily requirement is 1.3–1.5 mg and for males, 1.3–1.7 mg. Vitamin B$_6$ is required for the body to manufacture the nonessential amino acids from the essential amino acids. Oral contraceptives interfere with the metabolism of vitamin B$_6$ and can result in a deficiency.

Deficiency

A deficiency of vitamin B$_6$ is usually found in combination with deficiencies of other B vitamins. Symptoms include irritability, depression, and dermatitis. In infants, its deficiency can cause various neurological symptoms and abdominal problems. Although its toxicity is rare, it can cause temporary neurological problems.

Vitamin B$_{12}$

Vitamin B$_{12}$ (**cobalamin**) is a compound that contains the mineral cobalt. It is slightly soluble in water and fairly stable to heat, but it is damaged by strong acids or alkalies and by light. It can be stored in the human body for three to five years.

Functions

Vitamin B$_{12}$ is involved in folate metabolism, maintenance of the **myelin** sheath, and healthy red blood cells. In order for vitamin B$_{12}$ to be absorbed, it must bind with a glycoprotein (**intrinsic factor**) present in gastric secretions in the stomach

cobalamin
organic compound known as vitamin B$_{12}$

myelin
lipoprotein essential for the protection of nerves

intrinsic factor
secretion of stomach mucosa essential for B$_{12}$ absorption

pernicious anemia
severe, chronic anemia caused by a deficiency of vitamin B_{12}; usually due to the body's inability to absorb B_{12}

folate/folic acid
a form of vitamin B, also called folacin; essential for metabolism

and travel to the small intestine, where it combines with pancreatic proteases, then travels to the ileum, where it attaches to special receptor cells to complete the absorption process. A client who has lost the ability to produce the gastric secretions, pancreatic proteases, intrinsic factor, or the special receptor cells because of disease or surgery will develop **pernicious anemia**.

Sources

The best food sources of B_{12} are animal foods, especially organ meats, lean meat, seafood, eggs, and dairy products.

Requirements

Vitamin B_{12} is measured in micrograms. The DRI for adults is 2–4 mcg a day, but it increases during pregnancy and lactation. The amount absorbed will depend on current needs.

Deficiency

Fortunately, a vitamin B_{12} deficiency is rare and is thought to be caused by congenital problems of absorption, which inhibit the body's ability to absorb or synthesize sufficient amounts of vitamin B_{12}. Vegan-vegetarians must choose their food wisely to avoid a B_{12} deficiency.

When the amount of B_{12} is insufficient, megaloblastic anemia may result. If the intrinsic factor is missing, pernicious anemia develops. Intrinsic factor could be missing because of surgical removal of the stomach, or a large portion of it, or because of disease or surgery affecting the ileum. Dietary treatment will be ineffective; the client must be given intramuscular injections of B_{12}, usually on a monthly basis.

Vitamin B_{12} deficiency may also result in inadequate myelin synthesis. This deficiency causes damage to the nervous system. Signs of vitamin B_{12} deficiency include anorexia, glossitis, sore mouth and tongue, pallor, neurological upsets such as depression and dizziness, and weight loss.

Folate

Folate, folacin, and **folic acid** are chemically similar compounds. Their names are often used interchangeably.

Functions

Folate is needed for DNA synthesis, protein metabolism, and the formation of hemoglobin. Researchers have concluded that folic acid helps to prevent colon, cervical, esophageal, stomach, and pancreatic cancers. Folic acid also increases homocysteine levels that help prevent strokes, blood vessel disease, macular degeneration, and Alzheimer's disease.

Sources

Folate is found in many foods, but the best sources are cereals fortified with folate, leafy green vegetables, legumes, sunflower seeds, and fruits such as orange juice and strawberries. Heat, oxidation, and ultraviolet light all destroy folate, and it is estimated that 50–90% of folate may be destroyed during food processing and preparation. Consequently, it is advisable that fruits and vegetables be eaten uncooked or lightly cooked when possible.

Requirements

Folate is measured in micrograms. The average daily requirement for all adults, both female and male, is 400 mcg. There is an increased need for folate during pregnancy and periods of growth because of the increased rate of cell division and the DNA synthesis in the body of the mother and of the fetus. Consequently, it is extremely important that women of child-bearing age maintain good folate intake. The recommended amount for a woman one month before conception and through the first six weeks of pregnancy is 600 mcg a day.

Deficiency

Folate deficiency has been linked to **neural tube defects (NTDs)** in the fetus, such as **spina bifida** (spinal cord or spinal fluid bulge through the back) (Figure 7-3) and **anencephaly** (absence of a brain). Other signs of deficiency are inflammation of the mouth and tongue, poor growth, depression and mental confusion, problems with nerve functions, and **megaloblastic anemia**, a condition in which red blood cells are large and immature and cannot carry oxygen properly.

Hypervitaminosis

The FDA limits the amount of folate in over-the-counter (OTC) supplements to 100 mcg for infants, 300 mcg for children, and 400 mcg for adults because consuming excessive amounts of folate can mask a vitamin B_{12} deficiency and inactivate phenytoin, an anticonvulsant drug used by epileptics.

Biotin

Biotin is a member of the B-complex group of vitamins and is also known as vitamin H.

Function and Sources

Biotin participates as a coenzyme in the synthesis of fatty acids and amino acids. Some of its best dietary sources are egg yolks, milk, poultry, fish, broccoli, spinach, and cauliflower. Biotin is also synthesized in the large intestine by microorganisms, but the amount that is available for absorption is unknown.

Requirements

Biotin is measured in micrograms. The Food and Nutrition Board of the Institute of Medicine has established an AI of 30 mcg for adults (see Table 7-2).

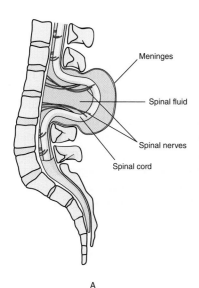

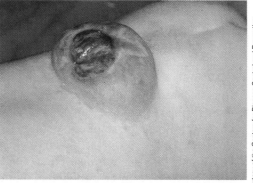

A   B

FIGURE 7-3 Infant with Spina Bifida.

neural tube defects (NTDs)
congenital malformation of brain and/or spinal column due to failure of neural tube to lose during embryonic development

spina bifida
spinal cord or spinal fluid bulge through the back

anencephaly
absence of brain

megaloblastic anemia
anemia in which the red blood cells are unusually large and are not completely mature

biotin
a B vitamin; necessary for metabolism

Courtesy of the Centers for Disease Control and Prevention.

Deficiency

Deficiency symptoms include nausea, anorexia, depression, pallor (paleness of complexion), dermatitis (inflammation of skin), and an increase in serum cholesterol. Toxicity from excessive intake is unknown.

Pantothenic Acid

Pantothenic acid is appropriately named because the Greek word *pantothen* means "from many places." It is fairly stable, but it can be damaged by acids and alkalies.

Functions

Pantothenic acid is involved in metabolism of carbohydrates, fats, and proteins. It is also essential for the synthesis of the neurotransmitter acetylcholine and of steroid hormones.

Sources

Pantothenic acid is found extensively in foods, especially animal foods such as meats, poultry, fish, and eggs. It is also found in whole-grain cereals and legumes. In addition, it is thought to be synthesized by the body.

Requirements

There is no DRI for pantothenic acid, but the Food and Nutrition Board has provided an estimated intake of 4–7 mg a day for normal adults (see Table 7-2).

Deficiency

Natural deficiencies are unknown. However, deficiencies have been produced experimentally. Signs include weakness, fatigue, and a burning sensation in the feet. Toxicity from excessive intake has not been confirmed.

Vitamin C

Vitamin C is also known as **ascorbic acid**. It has antioxidant properties and protects foods from oxidation, and it is required for all cell metabolism. It is readily destroyed by heat, air, and alkalies, and it is easily lost in cooking water.

Functions

Vitamin C is known to prevent **scurvy**. This is a disease characterized by gingivitis (soft, bleeding gums, and loose teeth); flesh that is easily bruised; tiny, pinpoint hemorrhages of the skin; poor wound healing; sore joints and muscles; and weight loss (Figure 7-4). In extreme cases, scurvy can result in death. Scurvy used to be common among sailors, who lived for months on bread, fish, and salted meat, with no fresh fruits or vegetables. During the mid-18th century, it was discovered that the addition of limes or lemons to their diets prevented this disease.

Vitamin C also has an important role in the formation of **collagen**, a protein substance that holds body cells together, making it necessary for wound healing. Therefore, the requirement for vitamin C is increased during trauma, fever, and periods of growth. Tiny, pinpoint hemorrhages are symptoms of the breakdown of collagen.

Vitamin C aids in the absorption of **nonheme iron** (from plant and animal sources and less easily absorbed than **heme iron**—see Chapter 8) in the small intestine when both nutrients are ingested at the same time. Because of this, it is called an iron enhancer.

pantothenic acid
a B vitamin

ascorbic acid
vitamin C

scurvy
a deficiency disease caused by a lack of vitamin C

collagen
protein substance that holds body cells together

nonheme iron
iron from animal foods that is not part of the hemoglobin molecule, and all iron from plant foods

heme iron
part of the hemoglobin molecule in animal foods

Vitamin C also appears to have several other functions in the human body that are not well understood. For example, it may be involved with the formation or functioning of norepinephrine (a neurotransmitter and vasoconstrictor that helps the body cope with stressful conditions), some amino acids, folate, leukocytes (white blood cells), the immune system, and allergic reactions.

It is believed to reduce the severity of colds because it is a natural antihistamine, and it can reduce cancer risk in some cases by reducing nitrites in foods. Vitamin C is absorbed in the small intestine.

Sources
The best sources of vitamin C are citrus fruits, melon, strawberries, tomatoes, potatoes, red and green peppers, cabbage, and broccoli (Figure 7-5).

Requirements
Vitamin C is measured in milligrams. Under normal circumstances, an average female adult in the United States requires 75 mg a day and an average male

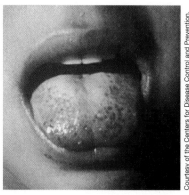

FIGURE 7-4 Scorbutic tongue related to scurvy.

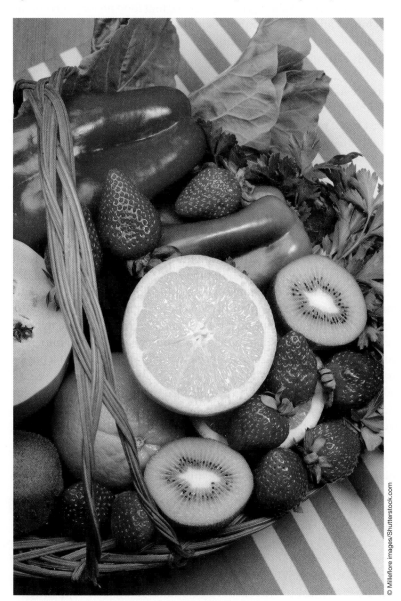

© Millefiore images/Shutterstock.com

FIGURE 7-5 Food sources of vitamin C.

90 mg. In times of stress, the need is increased. Regular cigarette smokers are advised to ingest 125 mg or more a day.

It is generally considered nontoxic, but this has not been confirmed. An excess can cause diarrhea, nausea, cramps, an excessive absorption of food iron, rebound scurvy (when megadoses are stopped abruptly), and possibly oxalate kidney stones.

Deficiency

Deficiencies of vitamin C are indicated by bleeding gums, loose teeth, tendency to bruise easily, poor wound healing, and, ultimately, scurvy.

SUPPLEMENTS

Healthy people who eat a variety of foods using the guidelines of MyPlate should be able to obtain all the vitamins needed to maintain good health. However, some people take supplements because they believe that food no longer contains the right nutrients in adequate quantities; supplements can "bulk up" muscles and enhance athletic performance; vitamins provide needed energy; and vitamins and minerals can cure anything, including heart trouble, the common cold, and cancer.

The facts are as follows: (1) A balanced diet would provide for the nutritional needs of healthy people, but many do not follow a healthy eating plan, they rely on fast food; processed foods; and heat, eat, and go foods. Therefore, the American Medical Association has recommended that everyone take one multivitamin a day. (2) No amount of vitamins will build muscles; only weight-lifting will do that. (3) Vitamins do not provide energy themselves. They help to release the energy within the carbohydrates, proteins, and fats that people ingest. (4) Only certain diseases caused by vitamin deficiencies (such as beriberi, scurvy, and rickets) can be cured with the help of vitamin supplements. Heart disease, cancer, and the common cold cannot.

Almost everyone can take a daily multivitamin and mineral supplement without fear of toxicity, but a megadose (10 times the RDA/DRI) to correct a deficiency or to help prevent disease should be prescribed by a physician. If a multivitamin-mineral is taken as a supplement, it is best not to exceed 100% of the RDA/DRI for each vitamin and mineral. An excess of one vitamin or one mineral can negatively affect the absorption or utilization of other vitamins and minerals. If vitamin supplements are thought to be necessary, it is best to consult a physician or registered dietitian.

Herbal products are also included under the heading "dietary supplements." Some people are interested in herbs because they believe certain ones can improve their health, they require no prescription, and they are often less expensive than prescription drugs.

The U.S. Food and Drug Administration (FDA) requires that manufacturers of prescription and over-the-counter drugs run, monitor, and report results of clinical trials of their products before selling them. Doses are established, and side effects and adverse reactions are reported in scientific journals. Also the FDA can inspect drug manufacturing facilities to confirm the purity of ingredients.

The Dietary Supplement Health and Education Act of 1994 however, exempts dietary supplements from FDA evaluation unless the FDA has evidence that a product is harmful. But before a suspect product can be removed from store shelves, the FDA must prove it is not safe. Manufacturers of supplements cannot claim their products can treat or prevent diseases, but they can make

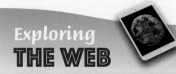

Exploring
THE WEB

Search the Web for information on vitamin deficiency disorders. Choose a disorder and research the signs and symptoms related to it. Prepare a diet for a client suffering from the disorder that would provide the vitamin content that is lacking in the client's current diet. What other factors do you need to consider in regard to planning a therapeutic diet?

"structure-function" claims. For example, they cannot say vitamin A prevents cancer, but they can say vitamin A has antioxidant properties and antioxidants have been linked to reduced rates of cancer.

Misinformation concerning supplements is widely available. Health care professionals must stay well informed concerning supplements, provide accurate information to their clients, and urge clients to consult with their physicians or registered dietitians before using any supplement. Some herbal products may indeed be helpful, but some may be harmful. Encourage clients to look for third-party certification for standardization of ingredients such as USP (United States Pharmacopia), NSF international, or Consumer Labs. There are many useful fact sheets available at the government's Office of Dietary Supplements.

HEALTH AND NUTRITION CONSIDERATIONS

Vitamins are a popular subject about which many people have strong beliefs. Some beliefs are based on fact; many are incorrect. Today's magazines, the Internet, and newspapers frequently contain articles about vitamins, but they are not always factual. Clients who have no other source of nutrition information tend to believe the statements in those articles. It is important that the client have correct information about vitamins (Figure 7-6). Continuation of a poor diet or continued abuse of vitamin supplements is potentially dangerous to the client.

Health care professionals will need a solid knowledge of vitamins, a convincing manner, and enormous patience to reeducate clients as may be needed. Some clients will believe that vitamin E will prevent heart attack, that the only source of vitamin C is orange juice, or that megadoses of vitamin A will prevent cancer. Others will confuse milligrams with grams.

Client education about vitamins may be difficult until the health care professional gains the confidence of the client. Simple and clear written materials to reinforce the information will be helpful to the client.

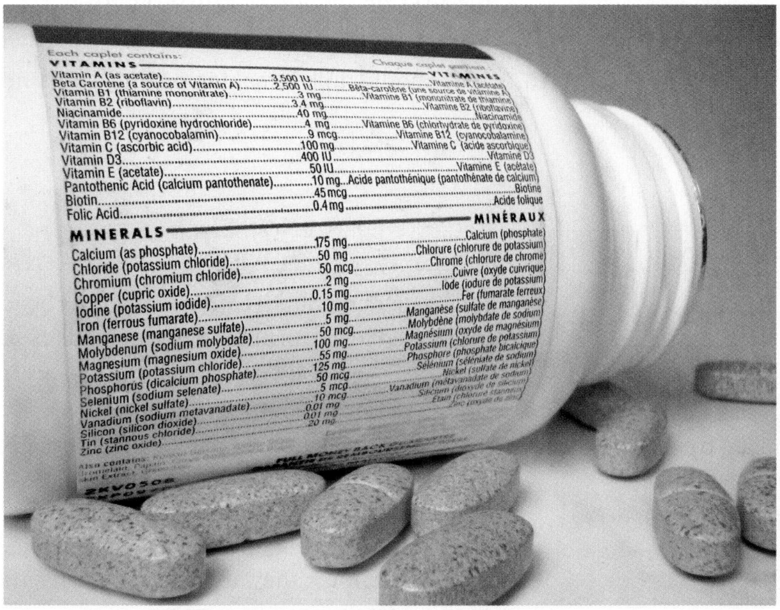

Exploring THE WEB

Search the Web for information on herbal dietary supplements. What claims are made by these products? Distinguish fact from fiction in the information that you uncover. Create a fact sheet for each of the herbal supplements you found and present the facts and the myths regarding use of the supplement. In addition, provide alternative food choices that would furnish the same benefits the supplement claims to make. What advice would you give a client inquiring about the use of these products?

FIGURE 7-6 Client education about vitamins is important.

SUMMARY

Vitamins are organic compounds that regulate body functions and promote growth. Each vitamin has a specific function or functions within the body. Food sources of vitamins vary, but generally a well-balanced diet provides sufficient vitamins to fulfill body requirements. Vitamin deficiencies can result from inadequate diets or from the body's inability to utilize vitamins. Vitamins are available in concentrated forms, but their use should be carefully monitored because overdoses can be detrimental to health. Vitamins A, D, E, and K are fat soluble. Vitamin B complex and vitamin C are water soluble. Water-soluble vitamins can be destroyed during food preparation. It is important that care is taken during the preparation of food to preserve its vitamin content.

DISCUSSION TOPICS

1. How do vitamins help to provide energy to the body?

2. Discuss possible times when avitaminosis of one or more vitamins may occur.

3. Discuss any vitamin deficiencies that class members have observed. What treatments were prescribed?

4. Discuss why it may be unwise for anyone but a physician or dietitian to prescribe vitamin supplements.

5. Discuss the terms *enriched* and *fortified*. What do they mean in relation to food products? Name foods that are enriched or fortified.

6. Discuss the proper storage and cooking of foods to retain their vitamin content.

7. If any member of the class has experienced night blindness, ask her or him to describe it. Discuss how this condition occurs and how it can be prevented.

8. Why is it advisable to use liquids left over from vegetable cooking? How might these be used?

9. Explain the role of vitamin C in collagen formation and wound healing.

10. If anyone in the class has taken concentrated vitamin C, ask why. If it was useful, ask how it helped.

11. Why are some vitamins called prohormones? Coenzymes? Give examples.

12. What is a precursor? Give an example.

13. Investigate why so many Americans have insufficient blood levels of vitamin D. If someone's blood level is low, what is the usual load dose to achieve normal levels? What other roles are they discovering vitamin D is involved with?

14. What is beriberi, and how can it be prevented?

15. Why should milk be sold in opaque containers?

SUGGESTED ACTIVITIES

1. Write a one-day that is especially rich in the B-complex vitamins. Underline the foods that are the best sources of these vitamins.

2. List the foods you have eaten in the past 24 hours. Write the names of the vitamins supplied by each food. What percentage of your day's food did *not* contain vitamins? Could this diet be nutritionally improved? How?

3. Plan a day's menu for a person who has been instructed to eat an abundance of foods rich in vitamin A.

4. Present a poster on the latest findings of vitamin D. Review how much sunshine is needed to form vitamin D and include food sources. Research supplementation and weigh in on whether the RDA is sufficient for most when so many are finding they are deficient or insufficient in this ultra-important nutrient.

REVIEW

Multiple choice. Select the *letter* that precedes the best answer.

1. The daily vitamin requirement is best supplied by
   a. eating a well-balanced diet
   b. eating one serving of citrus fruit for breakfast
   c. taking one of the many forms of vitamin supplements
   d. eating at least one serving of meat each day

2. All of the following measures preserve the vitamin content of food except
   a. using raw vegetables and fruits
   b. preparing fresh vegetables and fruits just before serving
   c. adding raw, fresh vegetables to a small amount of cold water and heating to boiling
   d. storing fresh vegetables in a cool place

3. Fat-soluble vitamins
   a. cannot be stored in the body
   b. are lost easily during cooking
   c. are dissolved by water
   d. are slower than water-soluble vitamins to exhibit deficiencies

4. Night blindness is caused by a deficiency of
   a. vitamin A
   b. thiamine
   c. niacin
   d. vitamin C

5. Good sources of thiamine include
   a. citrus fruits and tomatoes
   b. wheat germ and liver
   c. carotene and fish liver oils
   d. nuts and milk

6. Water-soluble vitamins include
   a. A, D, E, and K
   b. A, B_6, and C
   c. thiamine, niacin, and retinol
   d. thiamine, riboflavin, niacin, B_6, and B_{12}

7. Blindness can result from a severe lack of
   a. vitamin K
   b. vitamin A
   c. thiamine
   d. vitamin E

8. Organ meats are good sources of the vitamins
   a. thiamine, riboflavin, and B_{12}
   b. biotin and vitamin C
   c. vitamins E and K
   d. all of the above

9. Fortified milk is a good source of
   a. vitamin E
   b. vitamin D
   c. vitamin K
   d. vitamin C

10. Good sources of vitamin C are
    a. meats
    b. milk and milk products
    c. breads and cereals
    d. citrus fruits

11. The vitamin that aids in the prevention of rickets is
    a. vitamin A
    b. thiamine
    c. vitamin C
    d. vitamin D

12. The vitamin that is necessary for the proper clotting of the blood is
    a. vitamin A
    b. vitamin K
    c. vitamin D
    d. niacin

13. Vitamins commonly added to breads and cereals are
    a. vitamins A, D, and K
    b. thiamine, riboflavin, niacin, and folate
    c. vitamins E, B_6, and B_{12}
    d. ascorbic acid, pantothenic acid, and folate

14. The vitamin known to prevent scurvy is
    a. vitamin A
    b. vitamin B complex
    c. vitamin C
    d. vitamin D

15. The vitamin deficiency linked to neural tube defects such as spina bifida is
    a. vitamin K
    b. folate
    c. biotin
    d. vitamin E

16. Pernicious anemia is caused by a deficiency of
    a. vitamin B_6
    b. folate
    c. vitamin B_{12}
    d. vitamins A, C, and E

CASE IN POINT

KRYSTYNA: DEEP VEIN THROMBOSIS

Krystyna recently gave birth to her first child. She had lots of trouble with premature labor and had to be on bed rest during the last month of her pregnancy. She has been so relieved to be out of the house and enjoying her new baby and the sunshine. This morning she awoke and as she was getting out of bed she noticed quite a bit of pain in her left leg and calf. As she was getting dressed she noticed that her left leg was very swollen and even looked reddened. She was used to her legs being swollen during her pregnancy, but that had resolved since she gave birth. In addition, the leg swelling typically involved both legs, so Krystyna was concerned that it was just the left one.

She decided she was in enough pain that she would call the doctor. After examining Krystyna, the doctor told her that she had developed what is called a deep vein thrombosis. She told Krystyna that it was a blood clot that can sometimes occur after giving birth. Krystyna's doctor told her she needed to admit her to the hospital for treatment. She would run some additional tests and give Krystyna some blood thinning medications. In addition, she told Krystyna she would need to be cautious in consuming foods that had high levels of vitamin K in them, such as leafy green vegetables, among other things. The vitamin K in these foods could increase the chance of further clotting. Krystyna's doctor requested the hospital dietitian come and speak to her about these food sources.

ASSESSMENT

1. What data do you have about Krystyna?
2. What factors put Krystyna at risk for developing a deep vein thrombosis?
3. As the dietitian, what would you find helpful in Krystyna's history?

DIAGNOSIS

4. Write a nursing diagnosis for Krystyna.

PLAN/GOAL

5. What is a specific measurable goal for Krystyna in regard to her diet?

IMPLEMENTATION

6. What food sources are high in vitamin K and should be avoided by Krystyna?

EVALUATION/OUTCOME CRITERIA

7. What criteria should Krystyna use to evaluate the success of her actions?

THINKING FURTHER

8. Who else needs to be aware of Krystyna's vitamin K restriction?

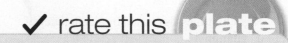

✔ rate this **plate**

The dietitian educated Krystyna on high vitamin K vegetables to avoid until her thrombosis had healed. Rate the plate that Krystyna ordered for lunch.

One 3 × 3 slice of spinach lasagna

1 garlic breadstick

½ cup steamed broccoli

⅙ slice of apple pie

12 oz iced tea

List the foods that are high in vitamin K and replace them with low sources of vitamin K.

CASE IN POINT
TINA: RECOVERING FROM ALCOHOLISM

Tina began drinking at a very young age. She can remember her parents drinking heavily at times as well. She was caught a few times in her early days, but Tina thought nothing of it. She had lots of friends who had experimented with alcohol. It was no big deal. When Tina went to college, she had a great time. There were bars and fraternities and all kinds of parties. Alcohol was everywhere. She would typically go out with a group of girls to the bar or a party, but often would find they were ready to go home long before she was. She would often tell her friends to go ahead and leave. She knew she could always find a ride home. One night, Tina's friends were really worried about her. By morning, she hadn't returned home and she hadn't called any of them. Finally, about noon she made it home. She had no shoes and her clothes were filthy with stains. She had walked home more than 2 miles from the party where they had been the night before. Tina assured her friends that she was fine. Over the course of time, this began happening again and

again. Tina would often arrive home in the morning with little memory of what had happened the night before. Finally, one night the police arrested Tina for public intoxication. Prior to transporting her to jail, she was taken to a local hospital for medical clearance. The emergency room doctor discovered that Tina had a blood alcohol level of 0.24. Tina's roommate arrived at the hospital and let the staff know that Tina had blacked out several times recently from alcohol abuse. She and her other friends were worried that Tina was an alcoholic. She would rarely eat, she had lost quite a bit of weight, and she could be found anytime day or night with a drink in hand.

At the hospital, Tina's doctor assesses her thiamine status. Knowing that many heavy abusers of alcohol are unable to absorb and utilize thiamine, this is one of the most common deficiencies among alcoholics. Indeed, Tina's thiamine levels are very low. He prescribes a thiamine replacement regimen and admits Tina to a rehabilitation facility.

ASSESSMENT

1. What are some of the red flags that may indicate that Tina is an alcoholic?
2. What are the consequences of Tina's body's inability to absorb thiamine as a result of excessive alcohol consumption?
3. Tina was arrested with a blood alcohol level of 0.24. How does her level compare to the legal blood alcohol limit in most states?

DIAGNOSIS

4. Write a nursing diagnosis for Tina related to her nutritional intake.
5. Write a nursing diagnosis for her alcohol abuse and rehabilitation.

PLAN/GOAL

6. Tina needs to begin reintroducing foods into her body. What would be the best way to go about this?

IMPLEMENTATION

7. What must Tina understand about her nutrition and her recovery?

EVALUATION/OUTCOME CRITERIA

8. What would you expect from Tina in six months if her recovery plan is successful?

THINKING FURTHER

9. Look at the web page for Alcoholics Anonymous. Read about this organization's programs and what it offers clients. Note the historical timeline of AA at http://www.aa.org/aatimeline/.

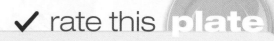
✔ rate this **plate**

Rate this plate that the dietitian at the rehabilitation facility ordered for Tina.

3 oz pulled pork on a whole-wheat bun

2 oz potato chips

1 medium orange

One 2 × 2 walnut brownie

8 oz milk

Did the dietitian do a good job at planning a meal rich in thiamine for Tina? Where could improvements be made in this meal?

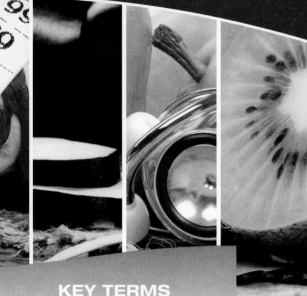

CHAPTER 8

KEY TERMS

acidosis
alkaline
alkalosis
cardiovascular
dehydration
demineralization
diuretics
edema
electrolytes
enriched foods
etiology
extracellular
hyperkalemia
hypertension
hypokalemia
intracellular
iodized salt
ions
iron deficiency anemia
Keshan disease
myoglobin
osmosis
tetany
toxicity

MINERALS

OBJECTIVES

After studying this chapter, you should be able to:

- List at least two food sources of given minerals
- List one or more functions of given minerals
- Describe the recommended method of avoiding mineral deficiencies

Chemical analysis shows that the human body is made up of specific chemical elements. Four of these elements—oxygen, carbon, hydrogen, and nitrogen—make up 96% of body mass. All the remaining elements are *minerals*, which represent only 4% of body weight. Nevertheless, these minerals are essential for good health.

A mineral is an inorganic (noncarbon-containing) element that is necessary for the body to build tissues, regulate body fluids, or assist in various body functions. Minerals are found in all body tissues. Any abnormal concentration of minerals in the blood can help diagnose different disorders. Minerals cannot provide energy by themselves, but in their role as body regulators, they contribute to the production of energy within the body.

Minerals are found in water and in natural (unprocessed) foods, together with proteins, carbohydrates, fats, and vitamins. Minerals in the soil are absorbed by growing plants. Humans obtain minerals by eating plants grown in mineral-rich soil or by eating animals that have eaten such plants. The specific

Exploring
THE WEB

Search the Web for information on sports drinks, drinks containing electrolytes, and energy drinks. What are the claims made by the makers of these drinks? What are the benefits, if any, that these drinks provide? Who is the target market for these drinks? What are some other dietary alternatives to these drinks? Are any warnings included for giving these drinks to babies?

mineral content of food is determined by burning the food and then chemically analyzing the remaining ash.

Highly processed or refined foods such as sugar and white flour contain almost no minerals. Iron, together with the vitamins thiamine, riboflavin, niacin, and folate, are commonly added to white flour and cereals, which are then labeled **enriched foods**.

Most minerals in food occur as salts, which are soluble in water. Therefore, the minerals leave the food and remain in the cooking water. Foods should be cooked in as little water as possible or, preferably, steamed, and any cooking liquid should be saved to be used in soups, gravies, and white sauces. Using this liquid improves the flavor as well as the nutrient content of foods to which it is added.

CLASSIFICATION

Minerals are divided into two groups. First are the major minerals, so named because each is required in amounts greater than 100 mg a day. Second, the trace minerals are needed in amounts smaller than 100 mg a day (Tables 8-1 and 8-2).

As mineral salts dissolve in water, they break into separate, electrically charged particles called **ions**. Ions, if positively charged, are called cations. When negatively charged, they are anions. The cations and anions must be balanced within the body fluids to maintain electroneutrality. For example, if body fluid contains 200 positive (+) charges, it must also contain 200 negative (−) charges. These ions are known as **electrolytes**.

Electrolytes are essential in maintaining the body's fluid balance, and they contribute to its electrical balance, assist in its transmission of nerve impulses and contraction of muscles, and help regulate its acid–base balance (see Chapter 9).

Normally, a balanced diet will maintain electrolyte balance. However, in cases of severe diarrhea, vomiting, high fever, or burns, electrolytes are lost, and the electrolyte balance can be upset. Medical intervention will be necessary to replace the lost electrolytes.

Scientists lack exact information on some of the trace elements, although they do know that trace elements are essential to good health. The study of these elements continues to reveal their specific relationships to human nutrition. A balanced diet is the only safe way of including minerals in the amounts necessary to maintain health.

The Food and Nutrition Board of the National Academy of Sciences, National Research Council (NRC) has recommended dietary allowances for minerals where research indicates knowledge is adequate to do so.

For those minerals where there remains some uncertainty as to amounts of specific human requirements, the NRC has provided a table of adequate intakes (AIs) of selected minerals (Table 8-3). The NRC recommends that the upper levels of listed amounts not be habitually exceeded. (Tables 8-1 and 8-2 list the best sources, functions, and deficiency symptoms of minerals.)

In addition, the Institute of Medicine has developed Daily Reference Intakes (DRIs) for calcium, fluoride, phosphorus, and magnesium. The DRI incorporates Estimated Average Requirements (EAR), the RDA, and Tolerable Upper Intake Levels.

enriched foods
foods to which nutrients, usually B vitamins and iron, have been added to improve their nutritional value

ions
electrically charged atoms resulting from chemical reactions

electrolytes
chemical compounds that dissolve in water break up into electrically charged atoms called ions

TABLE 8-1 Major Minerals

NAME	FOOD SOURCES	FUNCTIONS	DEFICIENCY/TOXICITY
Calcium (Ca^{++})	• Milk, cheese • Sardines • Salmon • Some dark-green leafy vegetables • Yogurt	• Development of bones and teeth • Transmission of nerve impulses • Blood clotting • Normal heart action • Normal muscle activity	Deficiency • Osteoporosis • Osteomalacia • Rickets • Tetany • Retarded growth • Poor teeth and bone formation
Phosphorus (P)	• Milk, cheese • Lean meat • Poultry • Fish • Whole-grain cereals • Legumes • Nuts	• Development of bones and teeth • Maintenance of normal acid–base balance of the blood • Constituent of all body cells • Necessary for effectiveness of some vitamins • Metabolism of carbohydrates, fats, and proteins	Deficiency • Poor teeth and bone formation • Weakness • Anorexia • General malaise
Potassium (K$^+$)	• Oranges, bananas • Dried fruits • Vegetables • Legumes • Milk • Cereals • Meat	• Contraction of muscles • Maintenance of fluid balance • Transmission of nerve impulses • Osmosis • Regular heart rhythm • Cell metabolism	Deficiency • Hypokalemia • Muscle weakness • Confusion • Abnormal heartbeat Toxicity • Hyperkalemia • Potentially life-threatening irregular heartbeats
Sodium (Na$^+$)	• Table salt • Beef, eggs • Poultry • Milk, cheese	• Maintenance of fluid balance • Transmission of nerve impulses • Osmosis • Acid–base balance • Regulation of muscle and nerve irritability	Deficiency • Nausea • Exhaustion • Muscle cramps Toxicity • Increase in blood pressure • Edema
Chloride (Cl$^-$)	• Table salt • Eggs • Seafood • Milk	• Gastric acidity • Regulation of osmotic pressure • Osmosis • Fluid balance • Acid–base balance • Formation of hydrochloric acid	Deficiency • Imbalance in gastric acidity • Imbalance in blood pH • Nausea • Exhaustion
Magnesium (Mg^{++})	• Leafy green vegetables • Whole grains • Avocados • Nuts • Milk • Legumes • Bananas	• Synthesis of ATP • Transmission of nerve impulses • Activation of metabolic enzymes • Constituent of bones, muscles, and red blood cells • Necessary for healthy muscles and nerves	Deficiency • Normally unknown • Mental, emotional, and muscle disorders
Sulfur (S)	• Eggs • Poultry • Fish	• Maintenance of protein structure • For building hair, nails, and all body tissues • Constituent of all body cells	Unknown

TABLE 8-2 Trace Minerals

NAME	FOOD SOURCES	FUNCTIONS	DEFICIENCY/TOXICITY
Iron (Fe⁺)	• Muscle meats • Poultry • Shellfish • Liver • Legumes • Dried fruits • Whole-grain or enriched breads and cereals • Dark green and leafy vegetables • Molasses	• Transports oxygen and carbon dioxide • Component of hemoglobin and myoglobin • Component of cellular enzymes essential for energy production	Deficiency • Iron deficiency anemia characterized by weakness, dizziness, loss of weight, and pallor Toxicity • Hemochromatosis (genetic) • Can be fatal to children • May contribute to heart disease • Injure liver
Iodine (I⁻)	• Iodized salt • Seafood	• Regulation of basal metabolic rate	Deficiency • Goiter • Cretinism • Myxedema
Zinc (Zn⁺)	• Seafood, especially oysters • Liver • Eggs • Milk • Wheat bran • Legumes	• Formation of collagen • Component of insulin • Component of many vital enzymes • Wound healing • Taste acuity • Essential for growth • Immune reactions	Deficiency • Dwarfism, hypogonadism, anemia • Loss of appetite • Skin changes • Impaired wound healing • Decreased taste acuity
Selenium (Se⁻)	• Seafood • Kidney • Liver • Muscle meats • Grains	• Constituent of most body tissue • Needed for fat metabolism • Antioxidant functions	Deficiency • Unclear, but related to Keshan disease • Muscle weakness Toxicity • Vomiting • Loss of hair and nails • Skin lesions
Copper (Cu⁺)	• Liver • Shellfish, oysters • Legumes • Nuts • Whole grains	• Essential for formation of hemoglobin and red blood cells • Component of enzymes • Wound healing • Needed metabolically for the release of energy	Deficiency • Anemia • Bone disease • Disturbed growth and metabolism Toxicity • Vomiting; diarrhea • Wilson's disease (genetic)
Manganese (Mn⁺)	• Whole grains • Nuts • Fruits • Tea	• Component of enzymes • Bone formation • Metabolic processes	Deficiency • Unknown Toxicity • Possible brain disease
Fluoride (F⁻)	• Fluoridated water • Seafood	• Increases resistance to tooth decay • Component of bones and teeth	Deficiency • Tooth decay • Possibly osteoporosis Toxicity • Discoloration of teeth (mottling)

(continues)

TABLE 8-2 *(continued)*

NAME	FOOD SOURCES	FUNCTIONS	DEFICIENCY/TOXICITY
Chromium (Cr)	• Meat • Vegetable oil • Whole-grain cereal and nuts • Yeast	• Associated with glucose and lipid metabolism	Deficiency • Possibly disturbances of glucose metabolism
Molybdenum (Mo)	• Dark-green leafy vegetables • Liver • Cereal • Legumes	• Enzyme functioning • Metabolism	Deficiency • Unknown Toxicity • Inhibition of copper absorption

TABLE 8-3 Recommended Dietary Allowances (RDA) and Adequate Intakes (AI) for Selected Trace Minerals

CATEGORY	AGE	COPPER (mcg)	MANGANESE (mg)	CHROMIUM (mcg)	MOLYBDENUM (mcg)
Infants	0–6 mo	200*	0.003*	0.2*	2*
	6–12 mo	220*	0.6*	5.5*	3*
Children and adolescents	1–3 y	340	1.2*	11*	17
	4–8 y	440	1.5*	15*	22
	9–13 y	700	1.9 males*	25 males*	34
	14–18 y	890	1.6 females*	21 females*	43
			2.2 males*	35 males*	
			1.6 females*	24 females*	
Adults	19–50 y	900	2.3 males*	35 males*	45
			1.8 females*	25 females*	
Adults	51–70		2.3 males*	30 males*	45
			1.8 females*	20 females*	
Pregnancy	14–18 y	1,000	2.0*	29*	50
	19–50	1,000	2.0*	30*	50
Lactation	14–18	1,300	2.6*	44*	50
	19–50	1,300	2.6*	45*	50

*Adequate intake (AI).

Reprinted with permission from the National Academies Press, Copyright © 2006, National Academy of Sciences. *Dietary Reference Intakes: The Essential Guide to Nutrient Requirements.*

TOXICITY

Because it is known that minerals are essential to good health, some would-be nutritionists will make claims that "more is better." Ironically, more can be hazardous to one's health when it comes to minerals. In a healthy individual who is eating a balanced diet, there will be some normal mineral loss through perspiration and saliva, and amounts in excess of body needs will be excreted in urine and feces. However, when concentrated forms of minerals are taken on a regular basis, over a period of time, accumulation of the mineral might occur, and toxicity develops. An excessive amount of one mineral can sometimes cause a deficiency of another mineral. In addition, excessive amounts of minerals can

toxicity
state of being poisonous

cause hair loss and changes in the blood, hormones, bones, muscles, blood vessels, and nearly all tissues. Concentrated forms of minerals should be used only on the advice of a physician.

MAJOR MINERALS

Calcium

The human body contains more calcium (Ca) than any other mineral. The body of a 154-lb person contains approximately 4 lb of calcium. Of that calcium, 99% is found in the skeleton and teeth. The remaining 1% is found in the blood.

Functions

Calcium, in combination with phosphorus, is a component of bones and teeth, giving them strength and hardness. Bones, in turn, provide storage for calcium. Calcium is needed for normal nerve and muscle action, blood clotting, heart function, and cell metabolism.

Regulation of Blood Calcium

Each cell requires calcium. It is carried throughout the body by the blood, and its delivery to the cells is regulated by the hormonal system. Normal blood calcium levels are maintained even if intake is poor.

When blood calcium levels are low, the parathyroid glands release a hormone that tells the kidneys to retrieve calcium before it is excreted. In addition, this hormone, working with calcitriol (the active hormone form of vitamin D), causes increased release of calcium from the bones by stimulating the activity of the osteoclasts (cells that break down bones). Both of these actions increase blood calcium levels. If calcium intake is low for a period of years, the amount withdrawn from the bones will cause them to become increasingly fragile. Osteoporosis may result.

If the blood calcium level is high, osteoblasts (cells that make bones) will increase bone mass. During growth, osteoblasts will make more bone mass than will be broken down. Bone mass is acquired until one is approximately 30 years old. With adequate consumption of calcium, phosphorus, and vitamin D, bone mass will remain stable in women until menopause. After menopause, bones will begin to weaken due to the lack of the hormone estrogen. A special x-ray, a DEXA scan, can be taken to determine bone density. If a person is at risk for injury due to decreased bone density, the physician will decide the best course of action. Drugs that help prevent further loss of bone mass are available.

Sources

The best sources of calcium are milk and milk products. They provide large quantities of calcium in small servings. For example, 1 cup of milk provides 300 mg of calcium (Figure 8-1). One ounce of cheddar cheese provides 250 mg of calcium.

Calcium is also found in some dark-green leafy vegetables. However, when the vegetable contains oxalic acid, as spinach and Swiss chard do, the calcium remains unavailable because the oxalic acid binds it and prevents it from being absorbed. When the intake of fiber exceeds 35 g a day, calcium will also bind with phytates (phosphorus compounds found in some high-fiber cereal), which also limits its absorption.

Factors that are believed to enhance the absorption of calcium include adequate vitamin D, a calcium-to-phosphorus ratio that includes no more

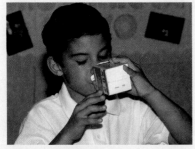

FIGURE 8-1 Milk is an important source of calcium and phosphorus. These minerals are essential for the normal growth and development of bones and teeth.

TABLE 8-4 Recommended Dietary Intakes for Calcium (mg/day)

0–6 mo*	200 mg
6–12 mo*	260 mg
1–3 y	700 mg
4–8 y	1,000 mg
9–18 y	1,300 mg
19–50 y	1,000 mg
51–70 y	1,000 mg males
	1,200 mg females
70+	1,200
Pregnant women, 14–18 y	1,300 mg
Pregnant women, 19–50 y	1,000 mg
Lactating women	Same as for nonlactating women of same age

*Adequate intake (AI).

Reprinted with permission from the National Academies Press, Copyright © 2011, National Academy of Sciences. *Dietary Reference Intakes: Calcium and Vitamin D.*

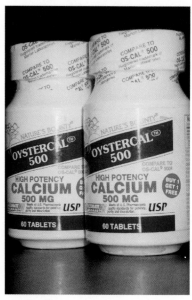

FIGURE 8-2 Always look for the USP seal of approval when purchasing supplements. NSF International or Consumer Labs also certify purity of supplements.

phosphorus than calcium, and the presence of lactose. A lack of weight-bearing exercise reduces the amount of calcium absorbed.

Requirements

The estimated requirement for calcium is now given as an AI level. Calcium is measured in milligrams (mg). The AIs for calcium at different ages and conditions are shown in Table 8-4. The recommendations were made to achieve optimal bone health and to reduce the probability of fractures in later life.

Calcium supplements are recommended for persons who are lactose intolerant, those who dislike milk, and those who are unable to consume enough dairy products to meet their needs. Calcium carbonate, the form found in calcium-based antacid tablets, has the highest concentration of bioavailable calcium. Calcium supplements appear to be absorbed most efficiently when consumed in doses of 500 mg.

When purchasing calcium supplements, check for the United States Pharmacopeia (USP) seal of approval on the product you select (Figure 8-2). USP-approved products are unlikely to contain lead or other toxins. Avoid bone meal products because they may contain lead.

Deficiency

Calcium deficiency may result in rickets. This is a disease that occurs in early childhood and results in poorly formed bone structure. It causes bowed legs, "pigeon chest," and enlarged wrists or ankles. Severe cases can result in stunted growth. Insufficient calcium can also cause "adult rickets" (osteomalacia), a condition in which bones become soft. And although the precise **etiology** of osteoporosis is unknown, it is thought that long-term calcium deficiency is a contributing factor. Other factors contributing to osteoporosis include deficiency of vitamin D and certain hormones. Further information on osteoporosis can be found in Chapter 13 under late adulthood section.

Insufficient calcium in the blood can cause a condition characterized by involuntary muscle movement, known as **tetany**. Excessive intake may cause constipation, or it may inhibit the absorption of iron and zinc.

etiology
cause

tetany
involuntary muscle movement

TABLE 8-5 Adequate Intakes and Recommended Dietary Allowances for Phosphorus

AI FOR PHOSPHORUS	
0–6 mo	100 mg*
7–12 mo	275 mg*
RDA FOR PHOSPHORUS	
1–3 y	460 mg
4–8 y	500 mg
9–18 y	1,250 mg
19–70 y	700 mg
Pregnant and lactating women	Same as for nonpregnant and nonlactating women of same age

*Adequate intake (AI).

Reprinted with permission from the National Academies Press, Copyright © 2006, National Academy of Sciences. Dietary Reference Intakes: *The Essential Guide to Nutrient Requirements.*

Phosphorus

Phosphorus (P), together with calcium, is necessary for the formation of strong, rigid bones and teeth. Phosphorus is also important in the metabolism of carbohydrates, fats, and proteins. Phosphorus is a constituent of all body cells. It is necessary for a proper acid–base balance of the blood and is essential for the effective action of several B vitamins. Like calcium, phosphorus is stored in bones, and its absorption is increased in the presence of vitamin D.

Sources

Although phosphorus is widely distributed in foods, its best sources are protein-rich foods such as milk, cheese, meats, poultry, and fish. Cereals, legumes, nuts, and soft drinks also contain substantial amounts of this mineral.

Requirements

The requirement for phosphorus is provided as AI for the first 12 months and as Estimated Average Requirements (EAR) after that (Table 8-5). Phosphorus is measured in milligrams.

Deficiency

Because phosphorus is found in so many foods, its deficiency is rare. Excessive use of antacids can cause it, because they affect its absorption. Symptoms of phosphorus deficiency include bone **demineralization** (loss of minerals), fatigue, and anorexia.

Potassium

demineralization
loss of mineral or minerals

intracellular
within the cell

osmosis
movement of a substance through a semipermeable membrane

Potassium (K) is an electrolyte found primarily in **intracellular** fluid. Like sodium, it is essential for fluid balance and osmosis. Potassium maintains the fluid level *within* the cell, and sodium maintains the fluid level *outside* the cell. **Osmosis** moves the fluid into and out of cells as needed to maintain electrolyte (and fluid) balance. There is normally more potassium than sodium inside the cell and more sodium than potassium outside the cell. If this balance is upset and the sodium inside the cell increases, the fluid within the cell also increases, swelling it and causing edema. If the sodium level outside the cell drops, fluid enters the cell to dilute the potassium level, thereby causing a reduction in **extracellular** fluid. With the loss of sodium and reduction of extracellular fluid, a decrease in blood pressure and dehydration can result.

Potassium is also necessary for transmission of nerve impulses and for muscle contractions.

Sources

Potassium is found in many foods. Fruits—especially melons, oranges, bananas, and peaches—and vegetables—notably mushrooms, Brussels sprouts, potatoes, tomatoes, winter squash, lima beans, and carrots—are particularly rich sources of it.

Deficiency or Excess

Potassium deficiency (**hypokalemia**) can be caused by diarrhea, vomiting, diabetic acidosis, severe malnutrition, or excessive use of laxatives or **diuretics**. Nausea, anorexia, fatigue, muscle weakness, and heart abnormalities (tachycardia) are symptoms of its deficiency. **Hyperkalemia** (high blood levels of potassium) can be caused by dehydration, renal failure, or excessive intake. Cardiac failure can result.

Sodium

Sodium (Na) is an electrolyte whose primary function is the control of fluid balance in the body. It controls the extracellular fluid and is essential for osmosis. Sodium is also necessary to maintain the acid–base balance in the body. In addition, it participates in the transmission of nerve impulses essential for normal muscle function.

Sources

The primary dietary source of sodium is table salt (sodium chloride), which is 40% sodium. One teaspoon of table salt contains 2,000 mg sodium. It is also naturally available in animal foods. Salt is typically added to commercially prepared foods because it enhances flavor and helps to preserve some foods by controlling growth of microorganisms. Note in Figure 8-3 that 77% of sodium in our diet comes from restaurant and processed foods. Fruits and vegetables contain little or no sodium. Drinking water contains sodium but in varying amounts. "Softened" water has a much higher sodium content than "hard," or unsoftened, water.

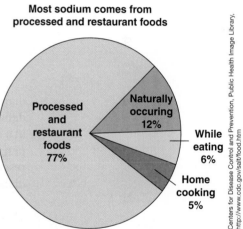

Most sodium comes from processed and restaurant foods

Processed and restaurant foods 77%

Naturally occuring 12%

While eating 6%

Home cooking 5%

Centers for Disease Control and Prevention, Public Health Image Library, http://www.cdc.gov/salt/food.htm

FIGURE 8-3 The majority of sodium in the diet comes from restaurant and processed foods.

Requirements

The DRI for sodium has been established at 1,500 mg for individuals 9 years of age through adulthood. This is considered an "adequate intake" (AI), as we all need a baseline amount of sodium for body processes. However, The Dietary Guidelines recommend to limit sodium to less than 2,300 mg (this is called the UL = upper limit) for individuals ages 14 years and older, as set by the Institutes of Medicine (IOM).

Deficiency or Excess

Either deficiency or excess of sodium can cause upsets in the body's fluid balance. Although rare, a deficiency of sodium can occur after severe vomiting,

extracellular
outside the cell

hypokalemia
low level of potassium in the blood

diuretics
substances used to increase the amount of urine excreted

hyperkalemia
excessive amounts of potassium in the blood

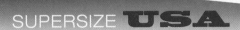
diarrhea, or heavy perspiration. In such cases, **dehydration** can result. A sodium deficiency also can upset the acid–base balance in the body. Cells function best in a neutral or slightly **alkaline** medium. If too much acid is lost (which can happen during severe vomiting), tetany due to **alkalosis** may develop. If the alkaline reserve is deficient as a result of starvation or faulty metabolism, as in the case of diabetes, **acidosis** (too much acid) may develop.

An excess of sodium is a more common problem and may cause **edema**. This edema adds pressure to artery walls that can cause **hypertension**. Thus, an excess of sodium is frequently associated with **cardiovascular** conditions such as hypertension and congestive heart failure. Certain groups have greater (or lesser) reduction in blood pressure in response to reduced sodium intake. Those with the greatest reductions in blood pressure have been termed *salt sensitive*, whereas those with little or no reduction in blood pressure have been termed *salt resistant*. Working with your cardiologist is the best way to determine which you are—sensitive or resistant. Depending on the diagnosis, the diet order may be either a 3–4 g (also called no-added salt or NAS) or a 1–2 g sodium-restricted diet. A physician rarely prescribes a diet of 1 g of sodium because compliance is difficult.

Chloride

Chloride (Cl) is an electrolyte that is essential for maintenance of fluid, electrolyte, and acid–base balance in the body. Like sodium, it is a constituent of extracellular fluid. It is also a component of gastric juices, where, in combination with hydrogen, it is found in hydrochloric acid, cerebrospinal fluid (of the brain and spinal cord), and muscle and nerve tissue. It helps the blood carry carbon dioxide to the lungs and is necessary during immune responses when white blood cells attack foreign cells.

dehydration
loss of water

alkaline
base; capable of neutralizing acids

alkalosis
condition in which excess base accumulates in, or acids are lost from, the body

acidosis
condition in which excess acids accumulate or there is a loss of base in the body

edema
abnormal retention of fluid by the body

hypertension
higher than normal blood pressure

cardiovascular
pertaining to the heart and entire circulatory system

SPOTLIGHT *on Life Cycle*

Older individuals, African Americans, and those with chronic diseases (including hypertension, diabetes, and kidney disease) are especially sensitive to the blood pressure–raising effects of salt and should follow their physician's or dietitian's advice on the amount of salt to consume daily. Their UL may be lower. These groups also experience an especially high incidence of high blood pressure related to cardiovascular disease. Orders may be either a 3–4 g (also called no added salt, or NAS) diet or a 1–2 g sodium-restricted diet. A physician rarely prescribes a diet of 1 g of sodium because compliance is difficult.

Sources

Chloride is found almost exclusively in table salt (sodium chloride) or in foods containing sodium chloride.

Requirements

The DRI for chloride for normal adults is 2,300 mg a day.

Deficiency

Because chloride is found in salt, deficiency is rare. It can occur, however, with severe vomiting, diarrhea, or excessive use of diuretics, and alkalosis can result. Also, it could occur in clients who follow long-term sodium-restricted diets. In such cases, clients can be provided with an alternative source of chloride.

Magnesium

Magnesium (Mg) is vital to both hard and soft body tissues. It is essential for metabolism and regulates nerve and muscle function, including the heart, and plays a role in the blood-clotting process.

Sources

Like phosphorus, magnesium is widely distributed in foods, but it is found primarily in plant foods. The nutrient-dense foods are leafy green vegetables, legumes, nuts, whole grains, and some fruits, such as avocados and bananas. Milk is also a good source if taken in sufficient quantity. For example, 2 cups of fat-free milk provide about 60 mg of magnesium.

Magnesium is lost during commercial food processing and in cooking water, so it is preferable to eat vegetables and fruits raw rather than cooked.

Requirements

The requirement for magnesium is provided as AIs (Table 8-6). Magnesium is measured in milligrams.

Deficiency

Because of the wide availability of magnesium, its deficiency among people on normal diets is unknown. When deficiency was experimentally induced, the symptoms included nausea and mental, emotional, and muscular disorders.

TABLE 8-6   Adequate Intakes (AIs) for Potassium, Sodium, Chloride, and Recommended Dietary Allowances for Magnesium

	POTASSIUM (g/d)	SODIUM (g/d)	CHLORIDE (g/d)	MAGNESIUM (mg/d)
LIFE STAGE GROUP				
Infants				
0–6 mo	0.4	0.12	0.18	30*
6–12 mo	0.7	0.37	0.57	75*
Children				
1–3 y	3.0	1.0	1.5	80
4–8 y	3.8	1.2	1.9	130
Males				
9–13 y	4.5	1.5	2.3	240
14–18 y	4.7	1.5	2.3	410
19–30 y	4.7	1.5	2.3	400
31–50 y	4.7	1.5	2.3	420
51–70 y	4.7	1.3	2.0	420
>70 y	4.7	1.2	1.8	420
Females				
9–13 y	4.5	1.5	2.3	240
14–18 y	4.7	1.5	2.3	360
19–30 y	4.7	1.5	2.3	310
31–50 y	4.7	1.5	2.3	320
51–70 y	4.7	1.3	2.0	320
>70 y	4.7	1.2	1.8	320
Pregnancy				
14–18 y	4.7	1.5	2.3	400
19–30 y	4.7	1.5	2.3	350
31–50 y	4.7	1.5	2.3	360
Lactation				
14–18 y	5.1	1.5	2.3	360
19–30 y	5.1	1.5	2.3	310
31–50 y	5.1	1.5	2.3	320

*Values are adequate intakes (AIs) for magnesium for infants.

Reprinted with permission from the National Academies Press, Copyright © 2006, National Academy of Sciences. *Dietary Reference Intakes: The Essential Guide to Nutrient Requirements.*

Sulfur

Sulfur (S) is necessary to all body tissues and is found in all body cells. It contributes to the characteristic odor of burning hair and tissue. It is necessary for metabolism.

Sources

Sulfur is a component of some amino acids and is consequently found in protein-rich foods.

Requirements or Deficiency

Neither the amount of sulfur required by the human body nor its deficiency is known.

TRACE MINERALS

Iron

The principal role of iron (Fe) is to deliver oxygen to body tissues. It is a component of hemoglobin, the coloring matter of red blood cells (erythrocytes). Hemoglobin allows red blood cells to combine with oxygen in the lungs and carry it to body tissues.

Iron is also a component of myoglobin, a protein compound in muscles that provides oxygen to cells, and it is a constituent of other body compounds involved in oxygen transport. Iron is utilized by enzymes that are involved in the making of amino acids, hormones, and neurotransmitters.

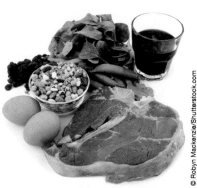

FIGURE 8-4 Food sources of iron, both heme and non-heme types.

Sources

Meat, poultry, and fish are the best sources of iron because only the flesh of animals contains heme iron. Heme iron is absorbed more than twice as efficiently as nonheme iron. Nonheme iron is found in whole-grain cereals, enriched grain products, vegetables, fruit, eggs, meat, fish, and poultry (see Figure 8-4). The rate of absorption of nonheme iron is strongly influenced by dietary factors and the body's iron stores. Factors affecting the absorption of both heme and nonheme iron are listed in Table 8-7.

For iron to be absorbed, it must be chemically changed from ferric to ferrous iron. This change is accomplished by the hydrochloric acid in the stomach. Absorption of nonheme iron can be enhanced by consuming a vitamin C–rich food and a nonheme iron–rich food at the same meal. Vitamin C holds onto and keeps the iron in its ferrous form, which facilitates absorption. Meat protein factor (MPF) is a substance in meat, poultry, and fish that aids in the absorption of nonheme iron.

Phytic acid and oxalic acid can bind iron and reduce the body's absorption of it. Polyphenols, such as tannins in tea and related substances in coffee, also reduce the absorption of iron. Antacids containing calcium and calcium supplements should be taken several hours before or after a meal high in iron because calcium also interferes with iron absorption.

Requirements

The NRC has determined that men lose approximately 1 mg of iron a day and that women lose 1.5 mg a day. On the assumption that only 10% of ingested iron is absorbed, the DRI for men has been set at 10 mg and for women from the age of 11 through the child-bearing years at 15 mg. This is doubled during pregnancy

TABLE 8-7 Factors That Affect Iron Absorption

INCREASE	DECREASE
Acid in the stomach	Phytic acid (in fiber)
Heme iron	Oxalic acid
High body demand for red blood cells (blood loss, pregnancy)	Polyphenols in tea and coffee
Low body stores of iron	Full body stores of iron
Meat protein factor (MPF)	Excess of other minerals (Zn, Mn, Ca) (especially when taken as supplements)
Vitamin C	Some antacids

myoglobin
protein compound in muscle that provides oxygen to cells

and is difficult to meet by diet alone. Consequently, an iron supplement is commonly prescribed during pregnancy. Women should make a special effort to include iron-rich foods in their diets at all times. The rapid growth periods of infancy and adolescence also produce a heavy need for iron.

Deficiency or Toxicity

Iron deficiency continues to be a problem, especially for women. Iron deficiency can be caused by insufficient intake, malabsorption, lack of sufficient stomach acid, or excessive blood loss, any or all of which can deplete iron stores in the body. Decreased stores of iron prevent hemoglobin synthesis. The result is an insufficient number of red blood cells to carry needed oxygen. What begins as iron deficiency can become iron deficiency anemia. Iron deficiency anemia takes a long time to develop, but it is the most common nutrient deficiency worldwide. Symptoms include fatigue, weakness, irritability, and shortness of breath. Clinical signs include pale skin and spoon-shaped fingernails.

Some people suffer from *hemochromatosis*. This is a condition due to an inborn error of metabolism and causes excessive absorption of iron. The onset of this disorder can happen at any age. Unless treated, this condition can damage the liver, spleen, and heart. To control the buildup of iron, the clients must have regularly scheduled sessions of phlebotomy. During each session, approximately a pint of blood is removed. However, this cannot be used for donation, since an excess of iron is in the blood.

Iodine

Iodine (I) is a component of the thyroid hormones, thyroxine (T_4) and triiodothyronine (T_3). It is necessary for the normal functioning of the thyroid gland, which determines the rate of metabolism.

Sources

The primary sources of iodine are iodized salt, seafood, and some plant foods grown in soil bordering the sea. Iodized salt is common table salt to which iodine has been added in an amount that, if used in normal cooking, provides sufficient iodine.

Requirements

The DRI for adults is 150 mg a day. Additional amounts are needed during pregnancy and lactation.

Deficiency

When the thyroid gland lacks sufficient iodine, the manufacture of thyroxine and triiodothyronine is retarded. In its attempt to take up more iodine, the gland grows, forming a lump on the neck called a goiter (Figure 8-5). Goiter appears to be more common among women than among men. A thyroid gland that doesn't function properly causes myxedema (hypothyroidism) in adults. The children of mothers lacking sufficient iodine may suffer from cretinism (retarded physical and mental development).

Zinc

Zinc (Zn) is a cofactor for more than 300 enzymes. Consequently, it affects many body tissues. It appears to be essential for growth, wound healing, taste acuity, glucose tolerance, and the mobilization of vitamin A within the body.

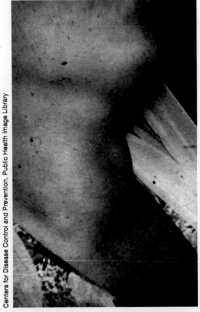

Centers for Disease Control and Prevention, Public Health Image Library

FIGURE 8-5 A goiter on the neck, which results primarily from iodine deficiency, is an enlargement of the thyroid gland.

iron deficiency anemia
condition resulting from inadequate amount of iron in the diet, reducing the amount of oxygen carried by the blood to the cells

iodized salt
salt that has the mineral iodine added for the prevention of goiter

Sources

The best sources of zinc are protein foods, especially meat, fish, eggs, dairy products, wheat germ, and legumes.

Requirements

The DRI for zinc is 11 mg in normal adult males and 8 mg in adult females, with increased requirements during pregnancy and further increases during lactation.

Deficiency

Decreased appetite and taste acuity, delayed growth, dwarfism, hypogonadism (subnormal development of male sex organs), poor wound healing, anemia, acne-like rash, and impaired immune response are all symptoms of zinc deficiency.

Selenium

Selenium (Se) is a constituent of most body tissues, but the heaviest concentration of the mineral is in the liver, kidneys, and heart.

Functions

Selenium is a component of an enzyme that acts as an antioxidant. In this way, it protects cells against oxidation and spares vitamin E.

Sources

The best sources of selenium are seafood, kidney, liver, and muscle meats.

Requirements

The DRI for selenium for an adult male and female is 70 mcg.

Deficiency or Toxicity

Symptoms of selenium deficiency are unclear, but selenium supplements appear to be effective in treating **Keshan disease**. High doses (1 mg or more daily) are toxic and can cause vomiting, loss of hair and nails, and skin lesions.

Copper

Copper (Cu) is found in all tissues, but its heaviest concentration is in the liver, kidneys, muscles, and brain. As an essential component of several enzymes, it helps in the formation of hemoglobin, aids in the transport of iron to bone marrow (soft tissue in bone center) for the formation of red blood cells, and participates in energy production.

Sources

Copper is available in many foods, but its best sources include organ meats, shellfish, legumes, nuts, cocoa, and whole-grain cereals. Human milk is a good source of copper, but cow's milk is not.

Requirements

The DRI for copper is 900 mg for adults.

Deficiency or Toxicity

Copper deficiency is extremely rare among adults, occurring only in people with malabsorption conditions and in cases of gross protein deficiency, such as kwashiorkor. It is apparent sometimes in premature infants and in people on long-term parenteral nutrition (feeding via a vein) programs lacking copper.

In The Media

Diet Supplement Dangers

The compound BMPEA, a chemical similar to the powerful stimulant amphetamine, has been found in numerous weight loss and work out supplements on sale across America. In late 2014, Canada pulled the supplement from its store shelves due to the potential serious health risk. But public health critics contend our FDA is reluctant to follow suit and pull the product as top agency regulators themselves come from the industry and have conflicts of interest. Regulation of the supplement industry has been an area of controversy. Under a 1994 law that was passed, supplements became exempt from more rigorous testing and oversight applied to prescription drugs. This means that supplements do not have to prove safety or effectiveness before they are sold to the public. In essence, the supplement industry is policing itself. Of course, proponents of the FDA feel it has an excellent safety record. It is worthwhile to note, however, that in 2013 and 2014, the National Products Association spent nearly $1.5 million on lobbying the FDA, Senate, and the FTC against a proposed Dietary Supplement Labeling Act, which would require labels to carry basic information about the product.

Source: O'Connor, Anahad. (2015, April 7). "Study Warns of Diet Supplement Dangers." New York Times blog. Accessed October 2015. http://well.blogs.nytimes.com/2015/04/07/study-warns-of-diet-supplement-dangers-kept-quiet-by-f-d-a/?_r=0

Keshan disease
condition causing abnormalities in the heart muscle

A copper deficiency can be caused by taking excess zinc supplements. Anemia, bone demineralization, and impaired growth may result.

Excess copper can be highly toxic. A single dose of 10–15 mg can cause vomiting. Wilson's disease is an inherited condition that results in accumulation of copper in the liver, brain, kidneys, and cornea. It can cause damage to liver cells and neurons. If the excess is detected early, copper-binding agents can be used to bind copper in the bloodstream and increase excretion.

Manganese

Manganese (Mn) is a constituent of several enzymes involved in metabolism. It is also important in bone formation.

Sources

The best sources of manganese are whole grains and tea. Vegetables and fruits also contain moderate amounts.

Requirements

The AI for adults is 2.3 mg for men and 1.8 mg for women.

Deficiency and Toxicity

Its deficiency has not been documented. Toxicity from excessive ingestion of manganese is unknown. However, people who have inhaled high concentrations of manganese dust have developed neurological problems.

Fluoride

Fluoride (F) increases one's resistance to dental caries. It appears to strengthen bones and teeth by making the bone mineral less soluble and thus less inclined to being reabsorbed.

Sources

The principal source of fluoride is fluoridated water (water to which fluoride has been added). In addition, fish and tea contain fluoride. Commercially prepared foods in which fluoridated water has been used during the preparation process also contain fluoride.

Requirements

The fluoride requirement AI is 4 mg for men and 3 mg for women.

Deficiency or Toxicity

The deficiency of fluoride can result in increased tooth decay. Excessive amounts of fluoride in drinking water have been known to cause permanent discoloration or mottling of children's teeth.

Chromium

Chromium (Cr) is associated with glucose and lipid metabolism. Chromium levels decrease with age except in the lungs, where chromium accumulates.

Sources

The best sources of chromium include meat, mushrooms, nuts, organ meats, and wheat germ.

Requirements

Although there is no DRI for chromium, there is AI for adults, which is 35 mg for men and 25 mg for women. There appears to be no difficulty fulfilling this requirement when one has a balanced diet.

Deficiency

Chromium deficiency appears to be related to disturbances in glucose metabolism.

Molybdenum

Molybdenum (Mo) is a constituent of enzymes and is thought to play a role in metabolism.

Sources

The best sources of molybdenum include milk, liver, legumes, and cereals.

Requirements

The estimated safe and adequate daily intake for adults is 45 mcg. This is normally fulfilled with a balanced diet.

Deficiency or Toxicity

No deficiencies have been noted in people who consume a normal diet. Excessive intake can inhibit copper absorption.

HEALTH AND NUTRITION CONSIDERATIONS

Second to vitamins, minerals are of great interest to the general public. They often are given mythic powers in current articles. It is imperative that the health care professional be aware of the dangers of even small doses of minerals and be able to transmit this information in a meaningful way to the clients.

Exploring THE WEB

Search the Web for information on mineral supplements. What claims are made regarding the use of these substances? Make a teaching checklist for a client outlining the health benefits and risks related to the use of these minerals. State other sources of attaining these minerals without the use of supplements.

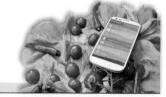

SUMMARY

Minerals are necessary to promote growth and regulate body processes. They originate in soil and water and are ingested via food and drink. Deficiencies can result in conditions such as anemia, rickets, and goiter. A well-balanced diet can prevent mineral deficiencies.

Concentrated forms of minerals should be taken only on the advice of a physician. Excessive amounts of minerals can be toxic, causing hair loss and changes in nearly all body tissues.

DISCUSSION TOPICS

1. Discuss the special importance of calcium and phosphorus to children and to pregnant women.

2. List ways of supplying an adequate amount of calcium in the diet of an adult who dislikes milk. Plan a day's menu for this adult.

3. Ask if any member of the class has suffered from anemia. If anyone has, ask the class member to describe the symptoms and treatment. What kind of anemia was it? If it's preventable, what measures are being taken to prevent a recurrence of the condition?

4. If a person is to decrease sodium in her or his diet, should animal foods be increased or decreased? Why?

5. Why does the FNB/NAS recommend that the upper limits of DRIs for minerals not be habitually exceeded?

6. If anyone in class knows someone with osteoporosis, ask for a description of the client, including sex, age, physical appearance, physical complaints, lifelong dietary habits, and medical treatment.

7. Explain the relationship of sodium and edema.

8. Why is it recommended that clients on sodium-restricted diets have the mineral content of their local water supply evaluated?

9. Explain the relationship of sodium and potassium.

10. Why would a doctor prescribe potassium at the same time a diuretic is prescribed?

11. Although rare, why does chloride deficiency sometimes occur in clients on long-term sodium-restricted diets?

12. Discuss the differences between heme and non-heme iron.

13. Why is iron commonly prescribed for pregnant women?

14. Why is selenium said to spare vitamin E?

SUGGESTED ACTIVITIES

1. Using outside sources, prepare a report on how sodium and potassium regulate the body's fluid balance.

2. Using other sources, write a report on at least one of the following:

    Rickets

    Goiter

    Hypothyroidism and hyperthyroidism

    Edema

    Osteoporosis

    Osteomalacia

3. Check four or five varieties of bread at the local supermarket. Using the labels on the breads, evaluate their mineral content.

4. List five good sources of heme iron and five sources of nonheme iron.

5. Spend 5–10 minutes observing customers at a drugstore display of various vitamin and mineral compounds. Write a short report on which minerals were most frequently purchased. Include your opinion about why this was the case.

6. Write a short essay on why iodized salt is a better choice than plain salt.

REVIEW

Multiple choice. Select the *letter* that precedes the best answer.

1. Minerals are inorganic elements that
   a. help to build and repair tissues
   b. are found only in bones
   c. provide energy when carbohydrates are lacking
   d. can substitute for proteins

2. The trace minerals in the human body are defined as
   a. those minerals that cannot be detected in laboratory tests
   b. those essential minerals found in very small amounts

   c. those minerals that are not essential to health
   d. only those minerals that are found in the blood

3. What mineral works with calcium to strengthen and maintain healthy bones and teeth?
   a. iron
   b. sulfur
   c. phosphorus
   d. molybdenum

4. Phosphorus is found in
   a. poultry
   b. common table salt
   c. vegetable oils
   d. leafy vegetables

5. The coloring matter of the blood is
   a. marrow
   b. lymph
   c. hemoglobin
   d. plasma

6. The main causes of iron deficiency are
   a. malabsorption
   b. lack of stomach acid
   c. insufficient intake
   d. all of the above

7. Some of the common signs of iron deficiency anemia are
   a. muscle spasms and pain in the liver
   b. bowed legs and an enlarged thyroid gland
   c. edema and loss of vision
   d. fatigue and weakness

8. Iodine is essential to health because it
   a. is necessary for red blood cells
   b. strengthens bones and teeth
   c. helps the blood to carry oxygen to the cells
   d. affects the rate of metabolism

9. Sodium is often restricted in cardiovascular conditions because it
   a. causes the heart to beat slowly
   b. encourages the growth of the heart
   c. contributes to edema
   d. raises the blood sugar

10. Iron is known to be a necessary component of
    a. adipose tissue
    b. hemoglobin
    c. thyroxine
    d. amino acids

11. Liquid from cooking vegetables should be used in preparing other dishes because
    a. mineral salts are soluble in water
    b. the hydrogen and oxygen in water aid the digestion of minerals
    c. the amino acids are soluble in water
    d. none of the above

12. Goiter can result from a deficiency of
    a. manganese
    b. magnesium
    c. copper
    d. iodine

13. A deficiency of calcium can cause
    a. lactose intolerance
    b. severe nausea
    c. tetany
    d. hypertension

14. Sodium is especially important in
    a. the blood-clotting process
    b. curing osteoporosis
    c. the prevention of osteomalacia
    d. osmosis

15. Sulfur
    a. is found only in bones and teeth
    b. is richly supplied in carbohydrates
    c. is found in all body cells
    d. deficiency is very common

16. Hypokalemia is
    a. caused by an abnormal heartbeat
    b. caused by potassium deficiency
    c. often a precursor of hyperkalemia
    d. a common result of chronic overeating

17. Delayed growth and hypogonadism are symptoms of what mineral deficiency?
    a. arsenic
    b. zinc
    c. selenium
    d. copper

18. What type of milk is a good source of copper?
    a. soy milk
    b. cow's milk
    c. goat's milk
    d. human milk

CASE IN POINT

LIAN: BALANCING EDEMA AND POTASSIUM LEVELS

Lian currently works as a secretary at a law firm. At work, she is primarily sitting at a desk during the day. She has never been particularly active, other than her household work and an occasional walk with her husband. She does try and take the stairs instead of the elevator while she is working to incorporate some activity throughout her day. Lian is 56 years old and is from China. She is small in stature at only 4-ft 10-in. She weighs 170 lb. She is currently 80 lb above her ideal body weight. She has noticed that she is increasingly out of breath when she does take the stairs. She rarely can climb more than one flight before needing to rest. Until recently, she has assumed that her shortness of breath was related to her inactivity. Lately though, she has noticed her ankles are swelling. She has been trying to keep her feet elevated after work to decrease the swelling. Finally, she decides that she needs to see her doctor. At her appointment, the nurse finds her blood pressure to be 192/98 and her heart rate is 96 bpm. Her doctor orders an EKG and the results are within normal limits. Lian's doctor suggests that she decrease the sodium in her diet to no more than 2,400 mg daily. He also tells Lian that she needs to work on losing weight and increasing her activity. The doctor explains that both of these will improve her stamina. In addition, her doctor prescribes a diuretic to help with both the swelling and the blood pressure. He explains that the diuretic could deplete her body of potassium so he also prescribes a potassium supplement. He asks her to return in three months for blood work. In an effort to cut back on her sodium intake, Lian begins replacing the salt in her diet with a salt substitute. She is unaware that the salt substitute contains potassium instead of sodium. When Lian returns in three months for her blood work, her doctor is really concerned. Her potassium level is very high. He explains that this can be a very dangerous problem and he will have to admit her to the hospital so she can be treated for hyperkalemia.

ASSESSMENT

1. How would you identify hidden sources of sodium in Lian's diet?
2. What contributing factors would cause her to have swelling?
3. What questions about thirst would be helpful to pinpoint?
4. What information from a 24-hour food diary could the doctor obtain?
5. What information about no added salt could be causing stress for Lian?
6. What information about Lian's lack of physical activity could benefit her in the future?

DIAGNOSIS

7. Write a nursing diagnosis for Lian.

PLAN/GOAL

8. What prepared foods can Lian have when starting to diet that would not interfere with her sodium restriction?
9. What foods are high in potassium that Lian may want to watch her consumption of?
10. What two goals would you set for Lian?

IMPLEMENTATION

11. What are the main topics you would have Lian understand about a no-added-salt, low-fat diet?
12. Explain the importance of drinking lots of water, even with edema.

EVALUATION/OUTCOME CRITERIA

13. How will Lian know if she is successful?

THINKING FURTHER

14. Look ahead to Chapter 18. What other factors could be influencing Lian's hypertension?
15. Why is it important for Lian to control her hypertension, and what are some of the consequences if she does not?

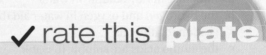 ✔ rate this **plate**

During her admission to the hospital, a registered dietitian educated Lian on a low-potassium, low-sodium diet. The dietitian regularly checked on the foods Lian ordered. Rate this plate.

Spaghetti and meatballs

1 breadstick

Side salad with Italian dressing

Are these food items permitted on a low-potassium, low-sodium diet? List some vegetables and fruits that are high in potassium.

CASE IN POINT

AISHA: IRON DEFICIENCY ANEMIA

Aisha first started her periods when she was 13 years old. She always had a great deal of difficulty with them each month. It was not uncommon for them to be seven to eight days in length, with five days of heavy bleeding. Her pediatrician told her that she would eventually outgrow this problem. Through the years, Aisha has learned to just live with her symptoms. She often had to stay home from school or work the first couple of days of her period. She usually was so fatigued she would have to nap throughout the day.

Aisha is now a 32-year-old woman. She is married and has a 2-year-old daughter. It took three years for her to conceive and give birth to her daughter. Since her daughter's birth, things have not improved for Aisha. She is increasingly more tired and short-tempered with her husband and family. She and her husband would like to have a second child, but Aisha feels too exhausted to even consider the idea. Aisha makes an appointment to see her OB/GYN. Results of her blood work reveal that Aisha has low iron stores and a low iron count. Her doctor diagnoses Aisha with iron deficiency anemia. He prescribes a medication to help regulate her periods. He also recommends an iron supplement as well as a stool softener. Her physician asks her to meet with a dietitian to help her better understand her nutritional needs. The dietitian discusses foods high in iron with Aisha. She also recommends Aisha take her iron tablet with vitamin C. She tells Aisha that this will help her body absorb the iron better.

ASSESSMENT

1. Would a 48-hour diet diary be helpful to you as a nurse?
2. What would you look for in the diet diary that would indicate a low iron store for Aisha?
3. What blood tests do you expect to see the doctor order for Aisha?
4. How much iron is lost by women, per day, according to the NRC?
5. What is the daily requirement for iron for women?

DIAGNOSIS

6. Complete the following diagnostic statement: Activity intolerance related to impaired oxygen transport secondary to diminished red blood cell count related to _____.
7. Complete the following diagnostic statement: Health-seeking behaviors related to lack of understanding of _____.

PLAN/GOAL

8. Name two reasonable goals for Aisha.

IMPLEMENTATION

9. Which food categories are priorities to include in Aisha's diet?
10. What can Aisha include as part of daily living to assist in absorption of iron?
11. Would Aisha benefit from taking an iron supplement?

EVALUATION/OUTCOME CRITERIA

12. In four months, when Aisha sees her doctor again, what could the doctor measure to evaluate the effectiveness of Aisha's compliance?

THINKING FURTHER

13. What changes could Aisha expect to see if she complies with her program?

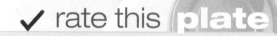

✔ rate this plate

No wonder Aisha is tired. She does not have enough iron to keep her going. The dietitian helped her realize that she could eventually keep her iron levels up by taking an iron supplement and eating a healthy diet. Rate this plate for iron intake.

5 oz sirloin steak

¾ cup rice pilaf

Vegetable medley with cauliflower and broccoli

Whole-wheat dinner roll with butter

Slice of chocolate cream pie

Lemonade

What on this plate is high in iron? If she wanted to limit red meat for health reasons, what other foods should she be including?

CHAPTER 9

KEY TERMS

acid–base balance
buffer systems
cellular edema
dehydrated
extracellular fluid (ECF)
homeostasis
hypothalamus
interstitial fluid
intracellular fluid (ICF)
milliequivalents
osmolality
pH
solute
solvent
vascular osmotic pressure

WATER

OBJECTIVES

After studying this chapter, you should be able to:

- Describe the functions of water in the body
- Explain fluid balance and its maintenance
- Name causes and consequences of water depletion
- Give causes and consequences of positive fluid balance
- Describe the acid–base balance of the human body

Although persons of average weight can live about 30–45 days without food, it is possible to live only 3–5 days without water. Water is a component of all body cells and constitutes 50–60% of normal adult body weight. The percentage is higher in males than females because men usually have more muscle tissue than women. The water content of muscle tissue is higher than that of fat tissue. The percentage of water content is highest in newborns (75%) and decreases with age.

Body water is divided into two basic compartments: intracellular and extracellular. **Intracellular fluid (ICF)** is water within the cells and accounts for about 65% of total body fluid (Figure 9-1). **Extracellular fluid (ECF)** is water outside the cells and accounts for about 35% of total body fluid. Extracellular fluid is made up of intravascular and **interstitial fluids**.

Although it is a component of all body tissues, water is the major component of blood plasma. It is a **solvent** for nutrients and waste products and helps

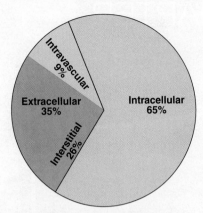

FIGURE 9-1 Body fluid compartments as percentage of total body fluid. All fluid in the body can be classified as either intracellular or extracellular.

TABLE 9-1 Functions of Water

- Component of all body tissues providing structure and form
- Solvent for nutrients and body wastes and chemical reactions
- Provides transport for nutrients and wastes via the blood and lymphatic system
- Essential for hydrolysis and thus metabolism
- Lubricant in joints and in digestion
- Helps regulate body temperature by evaporation of perspiration
- Serves as a shock absorber

transport both to and from body cells through blood. It is necessary for the hydrolysis of nutrients in the cells, making it essential for metabolism. It functions as a lubricant in joints and in digestion. In addition, it cools the body through perspiration and may, depending on its source, provide some mineral elements (Table 9-1).

The best source of water is drinking water. Table 9-2 lists the Dietary Reference Intake for water. One liter is equal to 33.8 ozs or 4.2 cups. Beverages of all types are the second-best source. A considerable amount is also found in foods, especially fruits, vegetables, soups, milk, and gelatin desserts. In addition, energy metabolism produces water. When carbohydrates, fats, and proteins are metabolized, their end products include carbon dioxide and water (Table 9-3).

TABLE 9-2 Dietary Reference Intake (Adequate Intake) for Water[1*]

LIFE STAGE GROUP	ADEQUATE INTAKE (L/DAY)
Infants	
0–6 mo	0.7
6–12 mo	0.8
Children	
1–3 y	1.3
4–8 y	1.7
Males	
9–13 y	2.4
14–18 y	3.3
19–30 y	3.7
31–50 y	3.7
51–70 y	3.7
>70 y	3.7
Females	
9–13 y	2.1
14–18 y	2.3
19–30 y	2.7
31–50 y	2.7
51–70 y	2.7
>70 y	2.7
Pregnancy	3.0
Lactation	3.8

*Total water includes all water contained in food, beverages, and drinking water.

Source: Reprinted with permission from the National Academies Press, Copyright © 2006, National Academy of Sciences. *Dietary Reference Intakes: The Essential Guide to Nutrient Requirements.*

intracellular fluid (ICF)
water within cells; approximately 65% of total body fluid

extracellular fluid (ECF)
water outside the cells; approximately 35% of total body fluid

interstitial fluid
fluid between cells

solvent
liquid part of a solution

TABLE 9-3 Estimated Daily Fluid Intake for an Adult

Ingested liquids	1,500 mL
Water in foods	700 mL
Water from oxidation	200 mL
Total	2,400 mL

FLUID AND ELECTROLYTE BALANCE

For optimum health, there must be homeostasis. For this to exist, the body must be in *fluid and electrolyte balance*. This means the water lost by healthy individuals through urination, feces, perspiration, and the respiratory tract must be replaced in terms of both volume and electrolyte content. Electrolytes are measured in milliequivalents/liter (mEq/L). An illness causing vomiting and diarrhea can result in large losses of water and electrolytes and must be addressed quickly. Water lost through urine is known as sensible (noticeable) water loss. Insensible (unnoticed) water loss is in feces, perspiration, and respiration. The body must excrete 500 mL of water as urine each day in order to get rid of the waste products of metabolism (Table 9-4).

homeostasis
state of physical balance; stable condition

milliequivalents
the concentrations of electrolytes in a solution

TABLE 9-4 Factors That Lead to Fluid Imbalances

FACTORS	FLUID DEFICIT	FLUID EXCESS
Environmental factors	• Exposure to sun or high atmospheric temperatures	
Personal behaviors	• Fasting • Fad diets • Exercise without adequate fluid replacement	• Excessive sodium or water intake • Venous compression due to pregnancy
Psychological influences	Decreased motivation to drink due to • Fatigue • Depression Excessive use of • Laxatives • Enemas • Alcohol • Caffeine	• Low protein intake due to anorexia
Consequences of diseases	Fluid losses due to • Fever • Wound drainage • Vomiting • Diarrhea • Heavy menstrual flow • Burns Difficulty swallowing due to • Oral pain • Fatigue • Neuromuscular weakness Excessive urinary output due to uncontrolled • Diabetes mellitus • Diabetes insipidus	Fluid retention due to • Renal failure • Cardiac conditions • Congestive heart failure • Valvular diseases • Left ventricular failure • Cirrhosis • Cancer • Impaired venous return

FIGURE 9-2 In osmosis, water passes through the selectively permeable cell membrane from an area of low-solute concentration to an area of high-solute concentration.

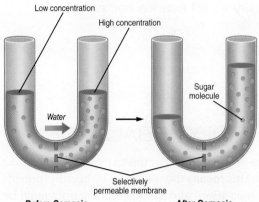

Low concentration

High concentration

Water

Sugar molecule

Selectively permeable membrane

Before Osmosis   **After Osmosis**

Water moves through cell walls by osmosis (Figure 9-2). Water flows from the side with the lesser amount of **solute** to the side with the greater solute concentration. The electrolytes sodium, chloride, and potassium are the solutes that maintain the balance between intracellular and extracellular fluids. Potassium is the principal electrolyte in intracellular fluid. Sodium is the principal electrolyte in extracellular fluid. **Osmolality** is the measure of particles in a solution.

When the electrolytes in the extracellular fluid are *increased*, ICF moves to the ECF in an attempt to equalize the concentration of electrolytes on both sides of the membrane. This movement reduces the amount of water in the cells. The cells of the **hypothalamus** (regulates appetite and thirst) then become **dehydrated**, as do those in the mouth and tongue, and the body experiences thirst. The hypothalamus stimulates the pituitary gland to excrete ADH (antidiuretic hormone) whenever the electrolytes become too concentrated in the blood or whenever blood volume or blood pressure is too low. This measurement is called **vascular osmotic pressure**. The ADH causes the kidneys to reabsorb water rather than excrete it. At such times, thirst causes the healthy person to drink fluids, which provide the water and electrolytes needed by the cells.

When the sodium in the ECF is reduced, water flows from the ECF into the cells, causing **cellular edema**. When this occurs, the adrenal glands secrete aldosterone, which triggers the kidneys to increase the amount of sodium reabsorbed. When the

solute
the substance dissolved in a solution

osmolality
number of particles per kilogram of solution; solutions with high osmolality exert more pressure than do those with fewer particles

hypothalamus
area at base of brain that regulates appetite and thirst

dehydrated
having lost large amounts of water

vascular osmotic pressure
high concentration of electrolytes in the blood; low blood volume or blood pressure

cellular edema
swelling of body cells caused by inadequate amount of sodium in extracellular fluid

In The Media

Coconut Water

We all know it is imperative to stay hydrated during exercise, but which type of beverage provides the most benefit? Coconut products have become the latest craze, with marketers claiming coconut water will hydrate better than water. Nutrition comparisons between sports drinks and coconut water show coconut water a lighter, more natural choice. One cup of pure coconut water contains about 45 calories, 11 g of carbohydrate, 70 mg of sodium, and 500 mg of potassium compared to a cup of sports drink containing 55 calories, 14 g of carbohydrate (all in the form of added sugar), 105 mg of sodium, and 30 mg of potassium. Few studies have been conducted between water, coconut water, and sports drinks and their hydrating properties with increased activity levels. For those who exercise 60 minutes or less under normal conditions, water remains the best option. When engaging in vigorous physical activity longer than 60 minutes, sipping on coconut water or a sports drink may be beneficial to enhance performance, exercise recovery, and fluid retention.

(Source: Adapted from Penner, Elle, MPH, RD. "Is Coconut Water More Hydrating" July 30, 2015. http://www.huffingtonpost.com/elle-penner/is-coconut-water-more-hydrating_b_7882330.html)

SPOTLIGHT *on Life Cycle*

Older adults often find liquids more acceptable in soups, fruit juices, milk products, soft drinks, tea, and coffee. If the client has difficulty swallowing thin liquids, especially water, foods with the consistency of gelatin, fruit ices, yogurt, custards, or puddings may be more desirable. Also, a powdered substance may be obtained to thicken thin liquids so that they can be more easily swallowed. Water is still the best choice if it can be swallowed easily without choking.

missing sodium is replaced in the ECF, the excess water that has been drawn from the ECF into the cells moves back to the ECF, and the edema is relieved.

The amount of water used and thus needed each day varies, depending on age, size, activity, environmental temperature, and physical condition. The average adult water requirement is 1 mL (milliliter) for every calorie in food consumed. For example, for every 1,800 kcal in food consumed, one needs to drink 7.5 glasses of fluid. The Institute of Medicine determined that the AI for men is roughly 3 L or about 13 cups of total fluid per day. The AI for women is 2.2 L or about 9 cups of total fluid per day. Youth, fever, diarrhea, unusual perspiration, and hyperthyroidism increase the requirement.

Dehydration

When the amount of water in the body is inadequate, dehydration can occur. It can be caused by inadequate intake or abnormal loss. Such loss can occur from severe diarrhea, vomiting, hemorrhage, burns, diabetes mellitus, excessive perspiration, excessive urination, or the use of certain medications such as diuretics. Signs and symptoms of dehydration include low blood pressure, thirst, dry skin, fever, and mental disorientation.

As water is lost, electrolytes are also lost. Thus, treatment includes replacement of electrolytes and fluids. Electrolyte content must be checked and corrections made if necessary. A loss of 10% of body water can cause serious problems. Blood volume and nutrient absorption are reduced, and kidney function is upset. A loss of 20% of body water can cause circulatory failure and death. Infants, for example, are at high risk of dehydration when fever, vomiting, and diarrhea occur. Intravenous fluids are often necessary if sufficient fluids cannot be consumed by mouth.

The thirst sensation often lags behind the body's need for water, especially in the elderly, children, athletes, and the ill. Feeling thirsty is not a reliable indicator of when the body needs water. Fluids should be drunk throughout the day to prevent dehydration (Figure 9-3 and Table 9-5).

Dehydration can occur in hot weather when one perspires excessively but fails to drink sufficient water to replace the amount lost through perspiration. Failure to

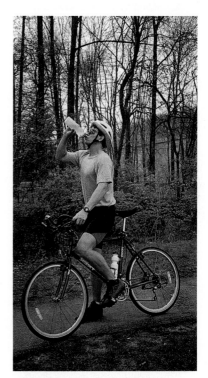

FIGURE 9-3 Preventing dehydration is an important element of proper nutrition.

TABLE 9-5 Signs of Dehydration

- Health history reveals inadequate intake of fluids.
- Decrease in urine output.
- Weight loss (% body weight): 3–5% for mild, 6–9% for moderate, and 10–15% for severe dehydration.
- Eyes appear sunken; tongue has increased furrows and fissures.
- Oral mucous membranes are dry.
- Decreased skin turgor (normal skin resiliency).
- Changes in neurological status may occur with moderate to severe dehydration.

replace water lost through perspiration could lead to progression through the four stages of heat illness: (1) *Heat fatigue* causes thirst, feelings of weakness, or fatigue. To combat this, one should go to a cool place, rest, and drink fluids. (2) *Heat cramp*, due to the loss of sodium and potassium, causes leg cramps and thirst. One should go to a cool place, rest, and drink fluids. (3) *Heat exhaustion* causes thirst, dizziness, nausea, headache, and profuse sweating. Treatment includes sponge baths with cool water, a two- to three-day rest, and the ingestion of a great deal of water. (4) *Heat stroke* involves fever and could produce brain and kidney damage. Emergency medical service (911) should be called, and the client should be put in chilled water and transported to the hospital. People can die from heat stroke. Those who are unable to perspire are at high risk for any of the stages of heat illness.

Fluid Balance During Exercise

Your average exerciser who works out for 30–60 minutes at moderate intensity three or four times a week can easily maintain water balance by eating and drinking normally. However, athletes who exercise hard day in and day out may become chronically dehydrated. Fluid needs vary greatly depending upon sport, body size, intensity of exercise, clothing worn, weather conditions, and how well trained you are. For many athletes, the thirst mechanism can be an unreliable signal to drink. This can also be problematic for child athletes and seniors as well.

Water is an excellent fluid for low-intensity or short-duration sports. However, professional trainers and sports nutritionists likely need to help more intense athletes with fluid balance by encouraging them to know their sweat rate. This can be discovered by weighing before and after training and competitions. In addition to fluid, sodium, potassium, and carbohydrate replacement needs should be addressed. The American College of Sports Medicine has a position statement on exercise and fluid replacement for further reference.

Excess Water Accumulation

Some situations cause an excessive accumulation of fluid in the body. This condition is called positive water balance. It occurs when more water is taken in than is used and excreted, and edema results. Hypothyroidism, congestive heart failure, hypoproteinemia (low amounts of protein), some infections, some cancers, and some renal conditions can cause such water retention because sodium is not being excreted normally. Fluids and sodium may then be restricted.

Water intoxication can occur and be life threatening when someone has overhydrated. This leads to hyponatremia. Under normal circumstances, accidently consuming too much water is a rare occurrence; however, it can occur in marathon runners when they consume too much fluid, or when persons are working in extreme heat or humidity for long periods and drink large amounts of water over short periods. Sometimes infants have issues if they take in more water relative to their body mass and sodium stores. There also is a psychiatric condition in which patients feel compelled to drink large quantities of water, putting them at risk for water intoxication.

ACID–BASE BALANCE

In addition to maintaining fluid and electrolyte balance, the body must also maintain **acid–base balance**. This is the regulation of hydrogen ions in body fluids (**pH** balance).

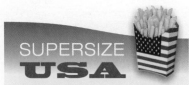

SUPERSIZE USA

According to a new study published in the Journal *Obesity*, drinking water before a meal can yield great weight loss results compared to not drinking water before meals. Participants in this 12-week study were randomized to either drinking 500 mL of water 30 minutes before their main meal, or to a control group where participants were asked to imagine their stomachs as full before meals. Those in the "pre-load" group lost 1.3 kg (2.87 lbs) more than the control group. Those who "pre-loaded" all three main meals of the day lost 4.3 kg (9.48 lbs) while those who only "pre-loaded" once or not at all lost only 0.8 kg (1.76 lbs). This simple strategy has the potential to make a big contribution to public health.

Source: "Efficacy of Water Preloading Before Main Meals as a Strategy for Weight Loss in Primary Care Patients with Obesity." *Obesity* (Silver Spring). 2015 Sep;23(9):1785–1791. Epub 2015 Aug 3. Accessed September 30, 2015. doi: 10.1002/oby.21167

acid–base balance
the regulation of hydrogen ions in body fluids

pH
symbol for the degree of acidity or alkalinity of a solution

In a water solution, an acid gives off hydrogen ions and a base picks them up. Hydrochloric acid is an example of an acid found in the body. It is secreted by the stomach and is necessary for the digestion of proteins. Ammonia is a base produced in the kidneys from amino acids.

Acidic substances run from pH 1 to 7, with the lowest numbers representing the most acidic (which contain the most hydrogen ions). Alkaline substances run from pH 7 to 14, with the alkalinity increasing with the number (as the number of hydrogen ions decreases). A pH of 7 is considered neutral. Blood plasma runs from pH 7.35 to 7.45. Intracellular fluid has a pH of 6.8. The kidneys play the primary role in maintaining the acid–base balance by selecting which ions to retain and which to excrete. For the most part, what a person eats affects the acidity not of the body but of the urine.

Buffer Systems

The body has **buffer systems** that regulate hydrogen ion content in body fluids. Such a system is a mixture of a weak acid and a strong base that reacts to protect the nature of the solution in which it exists. In a normal buffer system, the ratio of base to acid is 20:1. For example, when a strong acid is added to a buffered solution, the base takes up the hydrogen ions of the strong acid, thereby weakening it. When a strong base is added to a solution, the acid of the buffer system combines with this base and weakens it.

A mixture of carbonic acid and sodium bicarbonate forms the body's main buffer system. Carbonic acid moves easily to buffer a strong alkali, and sodium bicarbonate moves easily to buffer a strong acid. Amounts are easily adjusted by the lungs and kidneys to suit needs. For example, the end products of metabolism are carbon dioxide and water, and together they can form carbonic acid. The hemoglobin in the blood carries carbon dioxide to the lungs, where the excess is excreted. If the amount of carbon dioxide is more concentrated than it should be, the medulla oblongata in the brain causes the breathing rate to increase. This increase, in turn, increases the rate at which the body rids itself of carbon dioxide. Excess sodium bicarbonate is excreted via the kidneys. The kidneys can excrete urine from pH 4.5–8. The pH of average urine is 6.

Acidosis and Alkalosis

The healthy person eating a balanced diet does not normally have to think about acid–base balance. Upsets can occur in some disease conditions, however. Renal failure, uncontrolled diabetes mellitus, starvation, or severe diarrhea can cause acidosis. This is a condition in which the body is unable to balance the need for bases with the amount of acids it is retaining. Alkalosis can occur when the body has suffered a loss of hydrochloric acid from severe vomiting or has ingested too much alkali, such as too many antacid tablets.

HEALTH AND NUTRITION CONSIDERATIONS

Clients who are required to limit both their salt and liquid intake will probably be unhappy with their diets. In such cases, it is helpful when the dietitian can discuss realistic ways of planning menus for them and *with* them.

Exploring THE WEB

Search the Web for information related to the water needs of elderly and pediatric clients. How do the water needs differ in these two client populations? Why is there a difference? Why are these two populations at increased risk for dehydration? What tips can you provide to clients to maintain adequate water intake in these two client groups?

buffer systems
protective systems regulating amounts of hydrogen ions in body fluids

These menus should be based, of course, on good nutrition, but they also must be based on the client's normal habits and desires as much as possible. The client's former diet should be reviewed with the client. The high-salt and high-liquid foods should be pointed out and alternative foods presented in a positive manner.

SUMMARY

Water is a component of all tissues. It is a solvent for nutrients and body wastes and provides transport for both. It is essential for hydrolysis, lubrication, and maintenance of normal temperature. Its best sources are water, beverages, fruits, vegetables, soups, and water-based desserts.

Fluid balance and electrolyte balance are dependent upon one another. An upset in one can cause an upset in the other. An inadequate supply of water can result in dehydration, which can be caused by severe diarrhea, vomiting, hemorrhage, burns, or excessive perspiration or urination. Symptoms include thirst, dry skin, fever, lowered blood pressure, and mental disorientation. Dehydration can result in death. Positive water balance is an excess accumulation of water in the body. It causes edema.

Acid–base balance is the regulation of hydrogen ions in the body. Excessive acids or inadequate amounts of base can cause acidosis. Excessive base or inadequate amounts of acids can cause alkalosis.

Healthy people eating a balanced diet need not be concerned about fluid, electrolyte, or acid–base balance, as the body has intricate maintenance systems for all.

DISCUSSION TOPICS

1. Why can people live longer without food than without water?

2. Why does water constitute a larger proportion of a man's body weight than of a woman's?

3. Discuss the importance of proper fluid balance in those that exercise significantly. Address methods to hydrate correctly for best performance.

4. How do the lungs help to prevent excess acid from developing in the body?

5. What happens to the skin when it touches a red-hot pan? How might such developments on a large scale upset the body's fluid and electrolyte balance?

6. What is alkalosis? What causes it?

7. Explain how dehydration is dangerous in adults and in infants and children.

8. What does pH mean? How is it related to the homeostasis of the body?

SUGGESTED ACTIVITIES

1. Ask a nurse to describe what happens to body tissue when it is badly burned. Also ask about the treatment of burn clients, including diet.

2. Ask a nurse to describe a diabetic coma, explaining what causes it, why it can be life threatening, and how it can be treated.

REVIEW

Multiple choice. Select the *letter* that precedes the best answer.

1. Fluid within the cells is called
   a. interstitial fluid
   b. extracellular fluid
   c. intracellular fluid
   d. none of the above

2. Intravascular fluid contains
   a. interstitial fluid
   b. extracellular fluid
   c. intracellular fluid
   d. none of the above

3. In a mixture of sugar and water, water is the
   a. solute
   b. solvent
   c. solution
   d. none of the above

4. Water
   a. is essential for hydrolysis
   b. causes hydrogenation
   c. reduces hypoproteinemia
   d. is produced by hypothyroidism

5. Good sources of water include
   a. oranges and melon
   b. seafood and meats
   c. baked desserts and rice
   d. all of the above

6. The solute in the extracellular fluid principally responsible for maintaining fluid balance is
   a. potassium
   b. phosphorus
   c. calcium
   d. sodium

7. The solute in the intracellular fluid principally responsible for maintaining fluid balance is
   a. calcium
   b. phosphorus
   c. potassium
   d. sodium

8. ADH causes the kidneys to
   a. reabsorb water
   b. conserve fluid
   c. release additional sodium
   d. excrete increased amounts of urine

9. The amount of water needed by individuals
   a. varies from day to day
   b. is not affected by one's activities
   c. decreases with fever
   d. all of the above

10. Thirst is a symptom of
    a. osmosis
    b. hydrolysis
    c. cellular edema
    d. dehydration

11. What system in the body regulates acid–base balance?
    a. circulatory system
    b. buffer system
    c. respiratory system
    d. GI system

12. What are the three electrolytes that maintain the balance between intracellular and extracellular fluids?
    a. sodium, magnesium, and phosphorus
    b. sodium, chloride, and phosphorus
    c. sodium, chloride, and potassium
    d. sodium, potassium, and magnesium

CASE IN POINT

ESHE: COPING WITH DEHYDRATION

Eshe is a 52-year-old woman from South Africa. She has recently migrated to the United States. She is overwhelmed by the new lifestyle and culture that surrounds her. Eshe is very excited to have gotten a job working in a steel factory that makes parts for large machines. She was told when she was hired that the factory floor could often reach temperatures of 105°F. She was told that the shifts were 12 hours in length with periodic breaks in accordance with law. Her employer encouraged Eshe to take advantage of the breaks and to drink plenty of fluids. She is eager to please her boss and is a very hard worker.

Eshe had been working at the plant for two weeks. The factory is very warm and she finds herself sweating much more than she ever has. All aspects of her job are new to her so she has been working really hard to learn the tasks she is required to do. She has been taking her routine breaks, but has spent much of her break time asking questions and learning tips from other employees. She has not been able to drink as much water as she would like to at her breaks because of this. By the time she gets home she is so exhausted she will often go right to bed. The past two nights she was so tired after work, she even skipped dinner. Last night she was awakened with excruciating cramps in her calf and ankles.

ASSESSMENT

1. How can you explain to Eshe what is happening to her?
2. What data support your conclusion?
3. What does Eshe's increasing her physical exertion at work have to do with her condition?
4. What can be expected to occur if Eshe ignores the leg cramps?

DIAGNOSIS

5. Write a nursing diagnosis for Eshe.

PLAN/GOAL

6. What would be your immediate concern for Eshe?
7. What is your concern for her nursing shift?

IMPLEMENTATION

8. What fluid is most helpful to Eshe? Why?
9. How much fluid does she need to drink?
10. What else should Eshe's nurse be aware of during her nursing shift?

EVALUATION/OUTCOME CRITERIA

11. What should Eshe look for when her plan is effective?
12. Who else could benefit from this information?

THINKING FURTHER

13. At what point could Eshe have avoided her cramping problem?

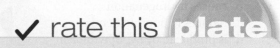
✔ rate this **plate**

Eshe is becoming dehydrated because she is not drinking enough fluids to replace the water lost through perspiration. How could Eshe's food intake improve her hydration status? Rate the plate.

Ham sandwich on whole-wheat bun

(the sandwich contains 3 oz lean ham, tomato, and lettuce)

2 oz corn chips

1 cup apple slices

8 oz milk

Use the Internet to look up the percentage of water in these foods. Which food ranked the highest in percent water and which one was the lowest? Would you change anything in this meal, and if so, what?

CASE IN POINT
BRANDON: CHRONIC RENAL FAILURE

Brandon is a 49-year-old African American male. He has a strong positive family history for hypertension. Brandon was diagnosed with hypertension in his early 20s. His doctor prescribed an antihypertensive medication, but Brandon felt fine and decided not to take it. He figured if there were truly something wrong with him he would have symptoms. Several years later he had a physical for work and was again told his blood pressure was elevated. The doctor again prescribed a medication to lower his blood pressure. Brandon did take the medication this time, but only for a while. His position was eliminated about a year later and Brandon lost his insurance. Frustrated, he quit taking the medication because now he was unable to afford it. In fact, he avoided seeing a doctor for several years so he didn't have to worry about his lack of insurance. Finally, after several months of not feeling well, he began to worry about his health. He was having difficulty breathing and his legs had been swollen for months. He often felt disoriented and confused. Finally, his symptoms are severe enough that Brandon decides to go to emergency room. Upon admission, Brandon's blood pressure is 232/108 with a heart rate of 112. The doctor orders several blood tests to further assess Brandon's problems. It is discovered that Brandon's BUN is 176 and his creatinine is 6.3. The doctor decides that Brandon needs immediate dialysis. A Quentin catheter is placed in Brandon's jugular vein as soon as possible and dialysis is initiated.

ASSESSMENT

1. What do you know about Brandon that puts him at risk for this problem?
2. How significant is his health problem?
3. How will dialysis alter his life?

DIAGNOSIS

4. Write a diagnostic statement about what Brandon needs to know about high blood pressure and renal failure.
5. Write a statement about the risk of excess fluid in the body.
6. Write a statement about the risk of noncompliance for renal clients.

PLAN/GOAL

7. Brandon's new renal diet is 3 g of sodium, 3 g of potassium, and 80 g of protein. How could you as a nurse help improve Brandon's knowledge of his new diet and encourage compliance?
8. What goals are important for Brandon?

IMPLEMENTATION

9. What major topics would be important for the dietitian to discuss with Brandon?
10. Create a day's menu for Brandon using the dietitian's new diet. Spread the protein intake throughout the day.
11. What teaching aids could the dietitian give Brandon to help him remember his new diet?
12. How could the website http://www.choosemyplate.gov help with meal planning?
13. What impact will his CRF have on his ability to be employed? What impact will it have on his physical and psychological status?

EVALUATION/OUTCOME CRITERIA

14. After discharge from the hospital, how will the physician know that Brandon has been compliant with his diet and medications?
15. During the dialysis treatment, what is important for Brandon to do in order to have the appropriate clearances of his blood and ultrafiltration of his fluids?

THINKING FURTHER

16. Why is it important for clients with hypertension to control it?
17. Why is it important for clients with diabetes to control it?

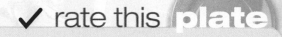 ✔ rate this **plate**

Now that Brandon is receiving dialysis, his protein, sodium, and potassium intake will have to be closely monitored. Before experiencing complications with his health, Brandon liked to prepare and eat the following meal. Rate the plate.

- **5 oz fried catfish filet**
- **1 cup sweet potato fries**
- **¾ cup collard greens made with fatback**
- **1 slice cornbread with butter**
- **½ cup watermelon and cantaloupe**
- **20 oz sweet iced tea**

In order to prevent further health complications, should Brandon continue to prepare this type of meal? How could this meal be changed to comply with his new meal plan?

SECTION 2

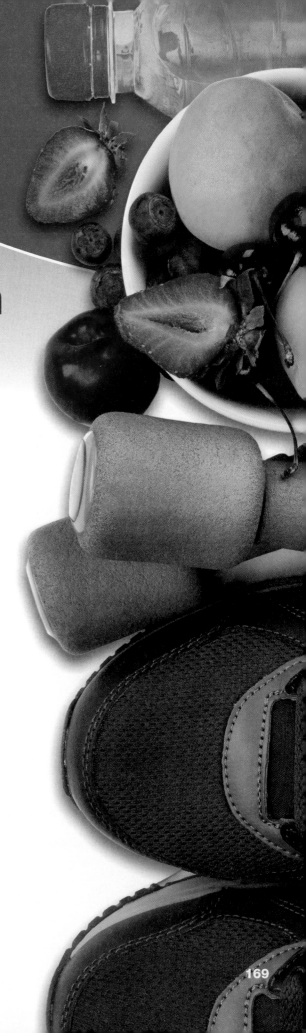

Nutrition through the Life Cycle

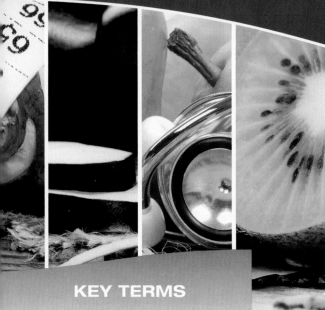

CHAPTER 10

KEY TERMS

amniotic fluid
anemia
eclamptic stage
fetal alcohol syndrome (FAS)
fetal malformations
fetus
gestational diabetes
hyperemesis gravidarum
lactation
lactation specialist
macrosomia
morning sickness
obstetricians
parenteral nutrition
pica
placenta
pregnancy-induced
  hypertension (PIH)
proteinuria
retardation
spontaneous abortion
trimester

NUTRITION DURING PREGNANCY AND LACTATION

OBJECTIVES

After studying this chapter, you should be able to:

- Identify nutritional needs during pregnancy and lactation
- Describe nutritional needs of pregnant adolescents
- Modify the normal diet to meet the needs of pregnant and lactating women

Good nutrition during the 38–40 weeks of a normal pregnancy is essential for both mother and child. In addition to her normal nutritional requirements, the pregnant woman must provide nutrients and calories for the **fetus**, the **amniotic fluid**, the **placenta**, and the increased blood volume and breast, uterine, and fat tissue.

In The Media

Fish Consumption During Pregnancy

One of the common myths with pregnancy is to avoid eating fish due to possible mercury exposure. High intakes of mercury while pregnant can lead to brain and neurological damage to the growing child. Research indicates, however, that consuming low-mercury fish can be beneficial to the growing baby and the mother. Fish contains many essential nutrients, such as protein, selenium, and vitamins E and D, among others. Those proven to have beneficial effects on brain development in particular are the polyunsaturated fatty acids DHA and EPA (omega 3). Consuming two to three servings of low-mercury seafood such as wild-caught salmon, tuna, shrimp, pollock, catfish, and cod each week can be beneficial. Seafood high in mercury that should be avoided includes swordfish, tilefish, shark, and king mackerel.

Source: Adapted from Radlicz, Christopher. (2015, October 8). "Fish Consumption During Pregnancy: Weighing the Risk-Benefit." The American Society for Nutrition.

fetus
infant in utero

amniotic fluid
surrounds fetus in the uterus

placenta
organ in the uterus that links blood supplies of mother and infant

retardation
delayed in mental development

trimester
three-month period; commonly used to denote periods of pregnancy

Studies have shown a relationship between the mother's diet and the health of the baby at birth. It is also thought that the woman who consumed a nutritious diet before pregnancy is more apt to bear a healthy infant than one who did not. Malnutrition of the mother is believed to cause decreased growth and mental **retardation** in the fetus. Low-birth-weight infants (less than 5.5 lb) have a higher mortality (death) rate than those of normal birth weight.

WEIGHT GAIN DURING PREGNANCY

Weight gain during pregnancy is natural and necessary for the infant to develop normally and the mother to retain her health. In addition to the developing infant, the mother's uterus, breasts, placenta, blood volume, body fluids, and fat must all increase to accommodate the infant's needs. The approximate total weight gain comes from the growing fetus (7.5 lb), the placenta (1 lb), the amniotic fluid and uterus (2 lb each), the breasts (1–3 lb), increased blood volume (4 lb), and maternal fat (4 lb plus).

The average weight gain during pregnancy is 25–35 lb. During the first **trimester** of pregnancy, there is an average weight gain of only 2–4 lb. Most of the weight gain occurs during the second and third trimesters of pregnancy, when it averages about 1 lb a week. This is because there is a substantial increase in maternal tissue during the second trimester, and the fetus grows a great deal during the third trimester.

Weight gain varies, of course. The Institute of Medicine updated guidelines in 2009 for weight gain in pregnancy. As noted in Table 10-1, the revised gestational weight gain guidelines are based on prepregnancy body mass index. Underweight women need to gain more than those who are overweight or obese. The Institute of Medicine also has guidelines, which can be referenced separately, for twin pregnancy.

No one should lose weight during pregnancy: this could cause nutrient deficiencies for both the mother and the infant. On average, a pregnant adult requires no additional calories during the first trimester of pregnancy, 340 additional calories during the second trimester, and 450 additional calories for the third trimester.

NUTRITIONAL NEEDS DURING PREPREGNANCY

Ideally when couples decide to have a child, they should make an appointment with their physician to discuss any health concerns or needed changes to the woman's diet. At that time, the physician needs to emphasize the importance of the woman taking a folic acid supplement at least one month prior to conception. During the 1990s, researchers established a correlation between taking folic acid before pregnancy and during the first trimester and having babies with brain and spinal cord defects. The results of this research led the U.S. government to require the addition of folic acid to grain products. The U.S. Public Health Service and the March of Dimes recommend that all women of child-bearing age take a multivitamin or 400 mcg of folic acid daily.

Lifestyle and habits also need to be taken into consideration before becoming pregnant. Certain medications, smoking, illegal drugs, and alcohol use by the mother can all be detrimental to the embryo. Related to the father's health,

TABLE 10-1 Institute of Medicine Weight Gain Recommendations for Pregnancy

PREPREGNANCY WEIGHT CATEGORY	BODY MASS INDEX	RECOMMENDED RANGE OF TOTAL WEIGHT (lb)	RECOMMENDED RATES OF WEIGHT GAIN IN THE 2ND AND 3RD TRIMESTERS (lb) (MEAN RANGE (lb/wk)
Underweight	Less than 18.5	28–40	1 (1–1.3)
Normal weight	18.5–24.9	25–35	1 (0.8–1)
Overweight	25–29.9	15–25	0.6 (0.5–0.7)
Obese (includes all classes)	30 and greater	11–20	0.5 (0.4–0.6)

Calculations assume a 1.1–4.4 weight gain in the first trimester. Modified from Institute of Medicine (US). *Weight Gain During Pregnancy: Reexamining the Guidelines.* Washington, DC: National Academies Press, 2009.

several studies have shown a slight connection between certain birth defects and birthweight with users of alcohol. Drug-dependent fathers usually have abnormalities in the sperm, which makes it impossible to fertilize the egg or results in a miscarriage within a few weeks. Nutrient deficiencies in the father's diet may increase the risk of birth defects and affects birth weight. Good nutrition and health habits for both parties are essential before becoming pregnant and during pregnancy.

NUTRITIONAL NEEDS DURING PREGNANCY

Some specific nutrient requirements are increased dramatically during pregnancy, as can be seen in Table 10-2. These figures are recommended for the general U.S. population; the physician may suggest alternative figures based on the client's nutritional status, age, and activities.

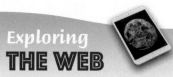

Exploring THE WEB

Search the website of the American College of Obstetricians and Gynecologists (http://www.acog.org) for information regarding pregnancy and nutrition. What information can you find related to nutritional needs before, during, and after pregnancy? How does lactation affect caloric needs?

TABLE 10-2 RDA and AI for Pregnancy and Lactation

				FAT-SOLUBLE VITAMINS				WATER-SOLUBLE VITAMINS		
Age	Weight (kg) (lb)	Height (cm) (in)	Protein (g/kg/day)	Vitamin A (µg RE)	Vitamin D (µg)	Vitamin E (mg α-TE)	Vitamin K (µg) (AI)	Vitamin C (mg)	Thiamine (mg)	Reboflavin (mg)
Pregnant			1.1	750; 700*	15	15	75; 90	80; 85	1.4	1.4
Lactating			1.3	1,200; 1,300*	15	19	75; 90	115; 2120	1.4	1.6

WATER-SOLUBLE VITAMINS				MINERALS							
Niacin (mg)	Vitamin B$_6$ (mg)	Folate (µg)	Vitamin B$_{12}$ (µg)	Calcium (mg)	Phosphorus (mg) (Ai)	Magnesium (mg)	Fluoride (mg) (Ai)	Iron (mg)	Zinc (mg)	Iodine (µg)	Selenium (µg)
18	1.9	600	2.6	1,300; 1,000	1,250; 700	360; 310	3	27	12; 11	220	60
17	2.0	500	2.8	1,300; 1,000	1,250; 700	360; 310	3	10	13; 12	290	70

*First value is for females 14–18 years old; second value is for females 19 years old and above.

Reprinted with permission from the National Academies Press, Copyright © 2006, National Academy of Sciences. *Dietary Reference Intakes: The Essential Guide to Nutrient Requirements* and the National Academies Press, Copyright © 2011, National Academy of Sciences. *Dietary Reference Intakes Calcium and Vitamin D.*

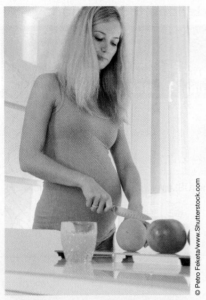

FIGURE 10-1 Healthy nutrition for a pregnant woman.

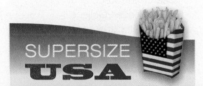

A common misconception during pregnancy is that the expecting mother should be "eating for two." In the first trimester, a woman needs no additional calories. Calorie needs increase by 340 calories a day in the second trimester and by 450 calories in the third. Incorporating healthy snacks such as cottage cheese and fruit, a whole-grain bagel with nut butter, hummus with veggies, or Greek yogurt with granola assist in meeting calorie goals during pregnancy. Choosing healthy, nutrient-dense snacks over junk food or calorie-dense foods is a better alternative for the mother and growing baby. Increasing whole-grain fiber, fruit, vegetable, and low-fat dairy intake will help provide the additional calories and nutrients needed during pregnancy.

obstetricians
doctors who care for mothers during pregnancy and delivery

The protein requirement is increased to 60 g of protein per day during pregnancy. Proteins are essential for tissue building, and protein-rich foods are excellent sources of many other essential nutrients, especially iron, copper, zinc, and the B vitamins.

Current research indicates there is no need for increased vitamin A during pregnancy. Excess vitamin A (more than 3,000 RE) has been known to cause birth defects such as hydrocephaly (enlargement of the fluid-filled spaces of the brain), microcephaly (small head), mental retardation, ear and eye abnormalities, cleft lip and palate, and heart defects. The required amount of vitamin D is 15 mcg or 600 IU. The requirement for vitamin E is 15 mg α-TE. The amount of vitamin K required is given as AI of 75–90 mcg, depending upon age. See Chapter 7 for specifics about the need for fat-soluble vitamins.

The requirements for all the water-soluble vitamins are increased during pregnancy. Additional vitamin C is needed to develop collagen and to increase the absorption of iron. The B vitamins are needed in greater amounts because of their roles in metabolism and the development of red blood cells.

The requirements for the minerals calcium, iron, zinc, iodine, and selenium are all increased during pregnancy. Calcium is, of course, essential for the development of the infant's bones and teeth as well as for blood clotting and muscle action. If the mother is not consuming adequate calcium in her diet, the baby will get its calcium from her bones.

The need for iron increases because of the increased blood volume during pregnancy. In addition, the fetus increases its hemoglobin level to 20–22 g per 100 mL of blood. This is nearly twice the normal human hemoglobin level of 13–14 mg per 100 mL of blood.

The infant's hemoglobin level is reduced to normal shortly after birth as the extra hemoglobin breaks down. The resulting iron is stored in the liver and is available when needed during the infant's first few months of life, when the diet is essentially breast milk or formula. Therefore, an iron supplement is commonly prescribed during pregnancy. However, if the pregnant woman's hemoglobin remains at an acceptable level without a supplement, the physician will not prescribe one.

FULFILLMENT OF NUTRITIONAL NEEDS DURING PREGNANCY

To meet the nutritional requirements of pregnancy, the woman should base her diet on MyPlate. Special care should be taken in the selection of food so that the necessary calories are provided by nutrient-dense foods (Figure 10-1).

One of the best ways to consume extra calories during pregnancy is by drinking an additional two servings of milk each day. The extra milk will provide protein, calcium, phosphorus, thiamine, riboflavin, and niacin. If whole milk is used, it will also contribute saturated fat and cholesterol and provide 150 calories per 8 oz of milk. Fat-free milk contributes no fat and provides 90 calories per 8 oz serving and thus is the better choice.

To be sure that the vitamin requirements of pregnancy are met, **obstetricians**, nurse midwives, and physician's assistants (PAs) may prescribe a prenatal vitamin supplement in addition to an iron supplement. However, it is *not* advisable for the mother to take any unprescribed nutrient supplement, as an excess of vitamins or minerals can be toxic to mother and infant.

The unusual cravings for certain foods during pregnancy do no harm unless eating them interferes with the normal balanced diet or causes excessive weight gain.

CONCERNS DURING PREGNANCY

Nausea

Sometimes nausea (the feeling of a need to vomit) occurs during the first trimester of pregnancy. This type of nausea is commonly known as **morning sickness**, but it can occur at any time. It typically passes as the pregnancy proceeds to the second trimester. The following suggestions can help relieve morning sickness:

- Eat dry crackers or dry toast before rising.
- Eat small, frequent meals.
- Avoid foods with offensive odors.
- Avoid liquids at mealtime.

In rare cases, the nausea persists and becomes so severe that it is life threatening. This condition is called **hyperemesis gravidarum**. The mother may be hospitalized and given **parenteral nutrition**, meaning she is given nutrients via a vein (see Chapter 21 for further discussion). Such cases are difficult, and these clients need emotional support and optimism from their caregivers.

Constipation

Constipation and hemorrhoids can be relieved by eating high-fiber foods, getting daily exercise, drinking at least eight glasses of liquid each day, and responding immediately to the urge to defecate.

Heartburn

Heartburn can result from relaxation of the cardiac sphincter and smooth muscles related to progesterone. Heartburn is a common complaint during pregnancy. As the fetus grows, it pushes on the mother's stomach, which may cause stomach acid to move into the lower esophagus and create a burning sensation there. Heartburn may be relieved by eating small, frequent meals; avoiding spicy or greasy foods; avoiding liquids with meals; waiting at least an hour after eating before lying down; and waiting at least two hours before exercising.

Excessive Weight Gain

If weight gain becomes excessive, the pregnant woman should reevaluate her diet and eliminate foods (except for the extra pint of milk) that do not fit within MyPlate. Examples include candy, cookies, rich desserts, chips, salad dressings (other than fat free), and sweetened beverages. In addition, she might drink fat-free milk, if not doing so, which would reduce her calories but not her intake of proteins, vitamins, and minerals. Except in cases in which the woman cannot tolerate lactose (the sugar in milk), it is not advisable to substitute calcium pills for milk because the substitution reduces the protein, vitamin, and mineral content of the diet.

A bowl of clean, crisp, raw vegetables such as broccoli or cauliflower, carrots, celery, cucumber, zucchini sticks, or radishes dipped in a low-fat salad dressing or salsa can provide interesting snacks that are nutritious, filling, satisfying, and low in calories. Fruits and custards made with fat-free milk make nutritious, satisfying desserts that are not high in calories. Broiling, baking, or boiling foods instead of frying can further reduce the caloric intake.

morning sickness
early morning nausea common to some pregnancies

hyperemesis gravidarum
nausea so severe as to be life threatening

parenteral nutrition
nutrition provided via a vein

Pregnancy-Induced Hypertension

Pregnancy-induced hypertension (PIH) was formerly called *toxemia* or *pre-eclampsia*. It is a condition that sometimes occurs during the third trimester, and is characterized by high blood pressure, the presence of albumin in the urine (**proteinuria**), and edema. The edema causes a somewhat sudden increase in weight. If the condition persists and reaches the **eclamptic** (convulsive) **stage**, convulsions, coma, and death of mother and child may occur. The cause of this condition is not known, but it occurs more frequently in first-time pregnancies, in multifetal pregnancies, in those women with morbid obesity, and among pregnant women on inadequate diets, especially protein-deficient diets. Pregnant adolescents have a higher rate of PIH than do pregnant adults.

Pica

Pica is the craving for nonfood substances such as starch, clay (soil), or ice. The reasons people get such a craving are not clear. Although both men and women are affected, pica is most common among pregnant women. Some believe it relieves nausea. Others think the practice is based on cultural heritage. The consumption of soil should be highly discouraged. Soil contains bacteria that would contaminate both mother and fetus. Ingesting soil can lead to an intestinal blockage, and substances in the soil would bind with minerals, preventing absorption by the body and thus leading to nutrient deficiencies. If any of the nonfood substances replaces nutrient-rich foods in the diet, this will result in multiple nutrient deficiencies. Eating laundry starch, in addition to a regular diet, will add unneeded calories and carbohydrates.

Anemia

Anemia is a condition caused by an insufficiency of red blood cells, hemoglobin, or blood volume. The patient suffering from it does not receive sufficient oxygen from the blood and consequently feels weak and tired, has a poor appetite, and appears pale. *Iron deficiency* is its most common form. During pregnancy, the increased volume of blood creates the need for additional iron. When this need is not met by the diet or by the iron stores in the mother's body, iron deficiency anemia develops. This may be treated with a daily iron supplement.

Folate deficiency can result in a form of megaloblastic anemia that can occur during pregnancy. It is characterized by too few red blood cells and by large immature red blood cells. The body's requirement for folic acid increases dramatically when new red blood cells are being formed. Consequently, the obstetrician might prescribe a folate supplement of 400–600 mcg a day during pregnancy.

Alcohol, Caffeine, Drugs, and Tobacco

Alcohol consumption is associated with subnormal physical and mental development of the fetus. This is called **fetal alcohol syndrome (FAS)**. Many infants with FAS are premature and have a low birth weight. Physical characteristics may include a small head, short eye slits that make eyes appear to be set far apart, a flat midface, and a thin upper lip. There is usually a growth deficiency (height, weight), placing the child in the lowest tenth of age norms. There is also evidence of central nervous system dysfunction, including hyperactivity, seizures, attention deficits, and microcephaly (small head) (Figure 10-2). Another condition caused by ingesting alcohol while pregnant is fetal alcohol effect (FAE). Children

pregnancy-induced hypertension (PIH)
typically occurs during late pregnancy; characterized by high blood pressure, albumin in the urine, and edema

proteinuria
protein in the urine

eclamptic stage
convulsive stage of toxemia

pica
abnormal craving for nonfood substance

anemia
condition caused by insufficient number of red blood cells, hemoglobin, or blood volume

fetal alcohol syndrome (FAS)
subnormal physical and mental development caused by mother's excessive use of alcohol during pregnancy

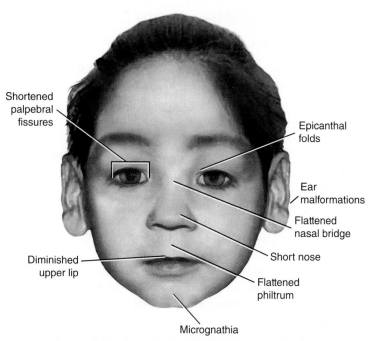

Shortened palpebral fissures

Epicanthal folds

Ear malformations

Flattened nasal bridge

Short nose

Flattened philtrum

Diminished upper lip

Micrognathia

FIGURE 10-2 Facial features in a child with fetal alcohol syndrome.

with FAE are born with less dramatic or no physical defects but with many of the behavioral and psychosocial problems associated with FAS. Those with FAE are not able to lead normal lives due to deficits in intelligence and behavioral and social abilities. When the mother drinks alcohol, it enters the fetal bloodstream in the same concentration as it does the mother's. Unfortunately, the fetus does not have the capacity to metabolize it as quickly as the mother, so it stays longer in the fetal blood than it does in the maternal blood. Abstinence is recommended.

Caffeine is known to cross the placenta, and it enters the fetal bloodstream. Birth defects in newborn rats whose mothers were fed very high doses of caffeine during pregnancy have been observed, but there are no data on humans showing that moderate amounts of caffeine are harmful. As a safety measure, however, it is suggested that pregnant women limit their caffeine intake to 2 cups of caffeine-containing beverages each day, or less than 300 mg/day.

Drugs vary in their effects, but self-prescribed drugs, including vitamins and mineral supplements and dangerous illegal drugs, can all damage the fetus. Drugs derived from vitamin A can cause **fetal malformations** and **spontaneous abortion**. Illegal drugs can cause the infant to be born addicted to whatever substance the mother used and, possibly, to be born with the human immunodeficiency virus (HIV). If a pregnant woman is known to be infected with HIV, her physician may prescribe AZT in an attempt to prevent the spread of the disease to the developing fetus.

Tobacco smoking by pregnant women has for some time been associated with babies of reduced birth weight. The more the mother smokes, the smaller her baby will be because smoking reduces the oxygen and nutrients carried by the blood. Other risks associated with smoking include sudden infant death syndrome (SIDS), fetal death, spontaneous abortion, and complications at birth. Smoking during pregnancy may also affect the intellectual and behavioral development of the baby as it grows up.

Because the substances discussed in this section may cause fetal problems, it is advisable that pregnant women avoid them.

fetal malformations
physical abnormalities of the fetus

spontaneous abortion
occurring naturally; miscarriage

DIET FOR THE PREGNANT WOMAN WITH DIABETES

Diabetes mellitus is a group of diseases in which one cannot use or store glucose normally because of inadequate production or use of insulin. This impaired metabolism causes glucose to accumulate in the blood, where it causes numerous problems if not controlled. (See Chapter 15 for additional information on diabetes mellitus.)

Some women have diabetes when they become pregnant. Others may develop **gestational diabetes** during pregnancy. In most cases, this latter type disappears after the infant is born; however, there is a 35–60% increased risk of developing type 2 diabetes later in life. Either type increases the risks of physical or mental defects in the infant, stillbirth, and **macrosomia** (birth weight over 9 lbs) unless blood glucose levels are carefully monitored and maintained within normal limits.

Every pregnant woman should be tested for diabetes between 24 and 28 weeks of gestation. Those found to have the disease must learn to monitor their diets to maintain normal blood glucose levels and to avoid both hypoglycemia and hyperglycemia.

In general, the nutrient requirements of the pregnant woman with diabetes are the same as for the normal pregnant woman. The diet should be planned with a registered dietitian or a certified diabetes educator because it will depend on the type of insulin and the time and number of injections. Patients with either gestational diabetes or preexisting diabetes who do not normally require insulin, may require insulin during their pregnancy to control blood glucose levels. A few of the oral hypoglycemic agents have also been approved for use during pregnancy. Between-meal feedings help maintain blood glucose at a steady level. Artificial sweeteners have been researched extensively and found to be safe for use during pregnancy.

Learning to eat healthy during pregnancy is important for any woman. Those with gestational diabetes not only need to learn the basics of healthy nutrition but must also learn how to plan their meals throughout the day. It may mean that the carbohydrate sources they typically consume must be distributed into smaller, more frequent amounts over the course of the day. Three meals and two to three snacks is typically the best way for the carbohydrates to be planned. These meals and snacks may be consumed two to three hours apart throughout the day. The breakfast meal is typically the most carbohydrate restrictive. Early morning rises in hormone levels make controlling the morning blood sugars more difficult. It is recommended that no more than 45 g of carbohydrate be consumed for breakfast and that simple carbohydrates, such as fruits or refined cereals, should be avoided until after lunch. It should be emphasized to these clients that healthy carbohydrates such as whole grains, fruits, and milk should not be eliminated. They are essential for fetal growth and brain formation. However, when reducing the amount of carbohydrates consumed during pregnancy, it is best to reduce the more highly processed and refined carbohydrates such as sweets and snack foods.

gestational diabetes
diabetes occurring during pregnancy; usually disappears after delivery of the infant

macrosomia
birth weight over 9 lbs

PREGNANCY DURING ADOLESCENCE

Teenage pregnancy is an increasing concern. The nutritional, physical, psychological, social, and economic demands on a pregnant adolescent are tremendous. With the birth of the infant, they increase. Young women who are themselves still in need of nurturing and financial support are suddenly responsible for a helpless newborn. If the mother does not have sufficient help, the total effect on her and the child can be devastating.

The young woman may need prenatal health care; infant care; and psychological, nutritional, and economic counseling as well as help in locating appropriate housing. And at this time, the young woman's family may or may not be supportive.

At such a time, nutritional habits can seem to some as being of slight importance. They are, however, of primary importance. An adolescent's eating habits may not be adequate to fulfill the nutritional needs of her own growing body. When the nutritional burden of a developing fetus is added, both are put at risk. Adolescents are particularly vulnerable to pregnancy-induced hypertension (PIH) and premature delivery. PIH can cause cardiovascular and kidney problems later. Premature delivery is a leading cause of death among newborns. Inadequate nutrition of the mother is related to both mental and physical birth defects.

These young women will need to know their own nutritional needs and the additional nutritional requirements of pregnancy (see Table 10-2). The government-funded Women, Infants, and Children (WIC) program can help with prenatal care, nutrition education, and adequate food for the best outcome possible. Pregnant teenagers will need much counseling and emotional support from caring, experienced people before nutritional improvements can be suggested.

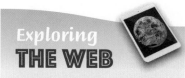

Exploring THE WEB

Search the Web for information on WIC programs. Become familiar with the services that are available to pregnant women. Research WIC services available in the area where you live.

LACTATION

A woman needs to decide whether to breastfeed before her infant is born. Almost all women can breastfeed; breast size is no barrier. Women who have chosen breast augmentation or reduction, however, are not able to breastfeed. Lactation, the production and secretion of breast milk for the purpose of nourishing an infant, is facilitated by an interplay of various hormones after delivery of the infant. Oxytocin and prolactin instigate the lactation process. Prolactin is responsible for milk production, and oxytocin is involved in milk ejection from the breast. The infant's sucking initiates the release of oxytocin, which causes the ejection of milk into the infant's mouth. This is called the let-down reflex. It is a supply-and-demand mechanism. The more an infant nurses, the more milk the mother produces.

It will take two to three weeks to fully establish a feeding routine; therefore, it is recommended that no supplemental feedings be given during this time. Human milk is formulated to meet the nutrient needs of infants for the first 6 months of life. Iron content in breast milk is very low, but it is very well absorbed; therefore, no iron supplement is needed for breastfed babies.

Lactation Specialist

A lactation specialist is an expert on breastfeeding and helps new mothers who may be having problems, such as the baby not latching on properly. This could cause the breast to become sore and could be discouraging to first-time mothers. Since the best first food for babies is breast milk, a lactation specialist can teach the proper techniques for successful breastfeeding. Lactation specialists are often part of general obstetric services of the hospital or may be employed by the physician practice or in their own private practice.

The Centers for Disease Control and Prevention in 2013 produced a helpful guide on strategies to support breastfeeding mothers and babies. In most

lactation
the period during which the mother is nursing the baby

lactation specialist
expert on breastfeeding

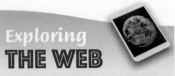

Exploring
THE WEB

Visit the website for the International Lactation Consultant Association (http://www.ilca.org). What information can you find on nutritional needs during lactation? Do these needs differ for older women and adolescents? Explore the benefits of breastfeeding. What are some of the common concerns that women have when making the decision to breastfeed? How would you respond to these concerns? Visit the International Breastfeeding Centre website (http://www.nbci.ca/) to watch videos and learn more about breastfeeding methods.

communities across America, resources exist to aid successful breastfeeding. This guide highlights the wealth of information that can be accessed, whether it be online education or printed materials, phone-in help from La Leche League International, or information on how to find professionally led or peer-led support groups.

Benefits of Breastfeeding

There are many positive reasons to breastfeed:

- Breast milk contains just the right mix of carbohydrate, protein, fat, vitamins, and minerals for brain development, growth, and digestion.
- Breastfeeding lowers the baby's risk of having asthma or allergies. Human milk contains at least 100 ingredients not found in formula.
- Breastfed babies have a lower incidence of ear infections, diarrhea, viruses, and hospital admissions. Breastfed babies receive immunities from their mothers for the diseases that the mother has had or has been exposed to. When a baby becomes ill, the bacteria causing the illness is transmitted to the mother while the baby is breastfeeding; the mother's immune system will start making antibodies for the baby.
- Sucking at the breast promotes good jaw development because it is harder work to get milk out of a breast than a bottle, and the exercise strengthens the jaws and encourages the growth of straight, healthy teeth.
- Breastfeeding facilitates bonding between mother and child. The skin-to-skin contact helps a baby feel safe, secure, and loved. Pediatricians encourage mothers of premature babies to hold their babies on their chests—skin to skin. This is called "kangaroo care," which has been shown to soothe and calm a baby and help maintain the baby's temperature. Fathers too can participate in kangaroo care by placing their infants against their bare chests.
- Benefits for mother include help in losing the pounds gained during pregnancy and stimulating the uterus to contract to its original size. Resting is important for a new mother, and breastfeeding gives her that opportunity. Breastfeeding is economical, always the right temperature, and readily available—especially in the middle of the night.

There is no need to stop breastfeeding when returning to work; a breast pump can be used to express milk for feedings when the mother is not available. Further, many companies provide areas for mothers to pump breast milk while they are at work. The CDC offers helpful information on proper handling and storage of expressed breast milk. In general, breast milk will keep:

- six to eight hours at room temperature (66–72°F)
- five days in the refrigerator
- three to six months in the refrigerator freezer
- six to twelve months in a deep freezer

Previously frozen milk must be used within 24 hours after defrosting in the refrigerator. Breast milk should not be heated in the microwave or directly on the stove. Those methods of heating breast milk will kill its immune-enhancing ability.

SPOTLIGHT *on Life Cycle*

Does breastfeeding lessen a baby's chances of developing obesity later in childhood? Several studies have indicated that breastfed infants have a lower risk of childhood obesity than formula-fed infants, while other studies have not reported a clear association. A large review study was undertaken in 2014 to provide a thorough look at the latest research. Twenty-five studies were reviewed from 1997 to 2014, with over 200,000 participants from 12 countries. This analysis revealed a dose-response effect between breastfeeding duration and reduced risk of childhood obesity and showed in particular that children breastfed for longer than seven months were significantly less likely to be obese in later childhood.

Source: Yan, et al. "The Association Between Breastfeeding and Childhood Obesity: A Meta-Analysis." *BMC Public Health* 2014, 14:1267. Accessed October 15, 2015

Calorie Requirements During Lactation

The mother's calorie requirement increases during lactation. The caloric requirement depends on the amount of milk produced. Approximately 85 calories are required to produce 100 mL (3.3 oz) of milk. During the first six months, average daily milk production is 750 mL (25 oz), and for this the mother requires approximately an extra 640 calories a day. During the second six months, when the baby begins to eat food in addition to breast milk, average daily milk production slows to 600 mL (20 oz), and the caloric requirement is reduced to approximately 510 extra calories a day.

The Institute of Medicine suggests an increase of 500 calories a day for the first six months of breastfeeding and 400 calories a day for seven to nine months. This is less than the actual need because it is assumed that some fat has been stored during pregnancy and can be used for milk production. The precise number of calories the mother needs depends on the size of the infant and its appetite and on the size and activities of the mother. Each ounce of human milk contains 20 calories.

If the mother's diet contains insufficient calories, the quantity of milk can be reduced, as seen in many Third World countries. Thus, lactation is not a good time to go on a strict weight loss diet. There will be some natural weight loss caused by the burning of the stored fat for milk production.

Nutrient Requirements During Lactation

In general, most nutrient requirements are increased during lactation. The amounts depend on the age of the mother (see Table 10-2). Protein is of particular importance because it is estimated that 10 g of protein are secreted in the milk each day.

MyPlate will be helpful in meal planning for the lactating mother. She should be sure to include sufficient fruits and vegetables, especially those rich in vitamin C. Extra fat-free milk will provide many of the additional nutrients and calories required during lactation. Chips, sodas, candies, and desserts provide little more than calories. Vegetarians will need to be especially careful to be sure they have sufficient calories, iron, zinc, copper, protein, calcium, and vitamin D. A vitamin B_{12} supplement can be prescribed for them.

It is important that the nursing mother have sufficient fluids to replace those lost in the infant's milk. Water and real fruit juice are the best choices.

The mother should be made aware that she must reduce her caloric intake at the end of the nursing period to avoid adding unwanted weight.

Medicines, Caffeine, Alcohol, and Tobacco

Most chemicals enter the mother's milk, so it is essential that the mother check with her obstetrician before using any medicines or nutritional supplements. Caffeine can cause the infant to be irritable. Alcohol in excess, tobacco, and illegal drugs can be very harmful. Illegal drugs, such as marijuana or cocaine, and prescription medication, such as methadone and oxycodone, can cause the baby to be excessively drowsy and to feed poorly. Stimulant drugs can cause the baby to be irritable. The biggest concern is addiction of the mother and baby.

HEALTH AND NUTRITION CONSIDERATIONS

Good nutrition during pregnancy can make the difference between a healthy, productive life and one shattered by health and economic problems—for both mother and child.

Most pregnant women will want the best nutrition for themselves and their children. They also will be concerned about their weight during and after pregnancy. It is essential that they receive advice from a properly trained health care professional. Articles in newspapers and magazines or in pamphlets from health food stores may or may not be correct and should not be taken at face value unless approved by a professional in the dietetic field.

Nutrition is currently a popular topic, and people are inclined to believe what is printed. It can be difficult to persuade people that the information they read is incorrect. As always, the health care professional must use great patience in reeducating those clients who may require it.

The pregnant teenager can present the greatest challenge. Her needs are vast, but her experience, and thus her perspective, is limited. Teaching pregnant adolescents about good nutrition may be difficult but, if successful, can help not only that particular client but also her child and her friends.

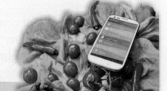

SUMMARY

A pregnant woman is most likely to remain healthy and bear a healthy infant if she follows a well-balanced diet. Research has shown that maternal nutrition can affect the subsequent mental and physical health of the child. Anemia and pregnancy-induced hypertension (PIH) are two conditions that can be caused by inadequate nutrition. Caloric and most nutrient requirements increase for pregnant women (especially adolescents) and women who are breastfeeding. The average weight gain during pregnancy is 25–35 lb.

DISCUSSION TOPICS

1. Discuss the statement, "A pregnant woman must eat for two."

2. Why is it especially important for a pregnant woman to have a highly nutritious diet?

3. Discuss weight gain during pregnancy from the first month through the ninth. Why is an excessive weight gain during pregnancy undesirable? Is pregnancy a good time to lose weight? Explain.

4. Why are protein-rich foods important during pregnancy?

5. It is common for an iron supplement to be prescribed during pregnancy. Why? What may

happen if the mother-to-be does not receive an adequate supply of iron? How might such a condition affect her baby? Discuss the advisability of the pregnant woman's taking a self-prescribed iron or vitamin supplement in addition to that prescribed by the obstetrician.

6. Discuss why the obstetrician regularly checks the pregnant woman's blood pressure, urine, and weight during pregnancy.

7. What is morning sickness, and how can it be helped? If any class member has been pregnant, ask her questions regarding morning sickness. Can this be a truly serious problem? Explain.

8. Why is it a good idea for a pregnant woman to include a citrus fruit or melon with every meal?

9. Why is the average weight gain 25–35 lb during pregnancy when the infant weighs approximately 7–8 lb?

10. Describe pica. Why is it undesirable?

11. Discuss the dangers to the fetus if the mother uses drugs.

12. How can the mother's diabetes affect the fetus?

SUGGESTED ACTIVITIES

1. Ask a dietitian to speak to the class on the importance of adequate nutrition before and during pregnancy. Ask the speaker questions regarding the effects of good and poor nutrition on the health of the mother, prenatal development, infant mortality, and the growth and development of the child. Ask the speaker's opinion regarding the use of alcohol, caffeine, and tobacco during pregnancy and during lactation.

2. Invite a nurse practitioner to speak to the class on the symptoms and dangers of PIH.

3. Invite a certified diabetes educator to speak to the class on the problems that can occur during the pregnancy of a diabetic mother.

4. Visit the International Breastfeeding Centre (http://www.nbci.com) and search for breastfeeding help videos to learn more about feeding techniques and benefits.

REVIEW

Multiple choice. Select the *letter* that precedes the best answer.

1. The infant developing in the mother's uterus is called the
   a. sperm   c. placenta
   b. fetus   d. ovary

2. A common form of anemia is caused by
   a. pica
   b. an excess of vitamin A
   c. a lack of iron
   d. a lack of B vitamins

3. High blood pressure, edema, and albumin in the urine are symptoms of
   a. calcium deficiency
   b. anemia
   c. not enough sodium
   d. pregnancy-induced hypertension

4. A common name given nausea in early pregnancy is
   a. morning sickness
   b. pica
   c. pregnancy-induced hypertension
   d. mortality

5. Folate and vitamin B_{12} requirements increase during pregnancy because of their roles in
   a. building strong bones and teeth
   b. fighting infections in the placenta
   c. building blood
   d. enzyme action

6. The additional daily energy requirement for the pregnant woman during the second trimester is
   a. 100 calories   c. 520 calories
   b. 340 calories   d. 1,000 calories

7. The additional calories required during pregnancy can be met by
   a. eating steak each day
   b. drinking a malted milk each day
   c. using an additional two servings of fat-free milk each day
   d. using an iron supplement

8. Craving nonfood substances during pregnancy is known as
   a. anemia
   b. megaloblastic anemia
   c. nausea
   d. pica

9. During pregnancy, the average weight gain preferred for a normal weight mother is
   a. 15–24 lb
   b. 25–35 lb
   c. 11–24 kg
   d. 15–24 kg

10. Which of the following is *not* a known benefit of breastfeeding?
    a. lower incidence of allergies or infections in the baby
    b. strengthens the bonding between mother and child
    c. fathers can't participate
    d. helps mother to lose weight

11. Some appropriate substitutes for milk include
    a. orange juice and tomato juice
    b. cheese and yogurt
    c. breads and cereals
    d. vegetables and fruit juices

12. The DRI for additional calories for a nursing mother during the first six months is
    a. 100
    b. 300
    c. 500
    d. 1,000

13. The daily diet during pregnancy and lactation should
    a. be based on MyPlate
    b. include at least 2 quarts of milk
    c. be limited to 1,900 calories
    d. all of the above

14. Appropriate snacks for pregnant and lactating women include
    a. fruits and raw vegetables
    b. potato chips and pretzels
    c. sodas
    d. hard candies

15. The duration of a normal pregnancy is
    a. 34–36 weeks
    b. 36–38 weeks
    c. 38–40 weeks
    d. 40–42 weeks

16. The fluid surrounding the fetus in the uterus is the
    a. parenteral fluid
    b. intracellular fluid
    c. amniotic fluid
    d. synovial fluid

17. During pregnancy, parenteral nutrition may be necessary for clients
    a. with excessive weight gain
    b. suffering from hyperemesis gravidarum
    c. who cannot tolerate milk
    d. who do not eat meat

18. Heartburn may be prevented by
    a. eating small, frequent meals
    b. lying down immediately after eating
    c. taking an aspirin
    d. increasing fluids at meals

19. Pregnancy-induced hypertension
    a. is relieved with salty food
    b. may occur when diets contain insufficient protein
    c. tends to be a precursor of iron deficiency
    d. causes megaloblastic anemia

20. Gestational diabetes
    a. tends to cause low-birth-weight babies
    b. always develops into type 1 insulin–dependent diabetes mellitus
    c. usually disappears after the baby is born
    d. presents no danger to mother or child

21. Maternal malnutrition
    a. has little effect on the fetus
    b. may cause an increase in the fetal hemoglobin level
    c. often causes macrosomia
    d. can lead to developmental or mental retardation

22. The need for iron increases during pregnancy because
    a. it prevents maternal goiter
    b. it is essential to bone development
    c. it is necessary to fetal metabolism
    d. of the increased blood volume

23. Nutrient-dense foods provide substantial amounts of
    a. vitamins, minerals, and proteins
    b. calories per gram of food
    c. carbohydrates, fats, and water
    d. sodium, chloride, and water

24. Excessive vitamin A should be avoided during pregnancy because it may
    a. cause birth defects
    b. cause gestational diabetes
    c. contribute to gallstones in the fetus
    d. reduce the mother's appetite

CASE IN POINT
JESSICA: TEENAGE PREGNANCY

Jessica always had a strong desire to fit in with her peers and often found herself doing things she didn't want to just to be accepted by her friends. Now that she is in high school it seems she is particularly concerned with fitting in. She is a good student, with a 3.8 GPA, but her biggest concern is gaining approval from her friends. Since her freshman year, Jessica has been a cheerleader and on the dance team. She is now a junior and has a boyfriend. She has been dating Ryan for most of her junior year. When Ryan asked her to prom, Jessica was very excited. She and Ryan attended prom and after-prom activities, then stayed over at another friend's house that night. Jessica felt she was in love with Ryan and was easily persuaded to do anything he requested to ensure he would not break up with her.

After her junior year, Jessica worked at a local coffee shop during the summer break. She often felt sick to her stomach when she arrived for her morning shift. She began noticing that many of the scents of the flavored coffees were making her feel nauseated. She was often invited to hang out with her friends after work, but rarely felt up for it. She often went home and slept. Finally, she confided in Ryan that she had missed two monthly periods and was concerned she could be pregnant. He insisted she take a pregnancy test to confirm her suspicions. Jessica indeed was pregnant. She and Ryan were both scared and decided to confide in Jessica's mother. Jessica's mother made an appointment for Jessica to see a doctor.

The doctor confirmed Jessica's pregnancy. Jessica was given prenatal vitamins. She expressed to the doctor that she did not want to become fat during her pregnancy. The doctor discussed with her the importance of weight gain and the appropriate amount for her size. Jessica was afraid if she gained weight, Ryan would break up with her. Jessica's mother was very concerned for her daughter. She tried to talk to her about her nutrition and eating habits, but Jessica would not listen. She was eating like a bird and gaining no weight. At her next appointment, Jessica's doctor notes she has lost 2 lb. After discussing this with Jessica and her mother, he decides she should see a dietitian to discuss appropriate foods for a healthy pregnancy. He also encourages Jessica to bring Ryan to the appointments so that he also understands what is happening to Jessica during the pregnancy.

ASSESSMENT

1. What objective data do you have about Jessica?
2. What caused Jessica to eat the way she did?
3. What was the cause of Jessica's noncompliance?
4. Which prenatal behaviors of Jessica were helpful? Which were not?

DIAGNOSIS

5. Complete the following diagnosis statement: Jessica's deficient knowledge about a healthy pregnancy and infant health is demonstrated by her lack of _____.
6. Write a nursing diagnosis for Jessica that would be appropriate for her situation.

PLAN/GOAL

7. What is your plan for Jessica's health after the birth?
8. What is your goal for the baby's health related to reducing the risk of SIDS and delayed development?

IMPLEMENTATION

9. What topics does Jessica need to be taught about her baby's health and development? What does she need to know about apnea and SIDS? What does she need to learn about normal infant growth and development?
10. Who else needs to be present for the teaching?
11. As a teenage mother, Jessica needs what type of medical and nursing follow-up? Would home health care nursing visits help?
12. What is your primary concern for the baby?

EVALUATION/OUTCOME CRITERIA

13. At the next visit, what criteria will the nurse practitioner be using to see if Jessica is eating healthy and caring for herself?

THINKING FURTHER

14. What other issues make this situation more difficult for a teen mother to be successful?
15. What other types of support may be helpful to a teenage mother?

✔ rate this **plate**

Jessica and Ryan met with a registered dietitian to learn about adequate nutrition during pregnancy and proper weight gain to support a healthy baby. The dietitian emphasized the importance of eating a nutrient-rich diet containing good sources of protein and iron. Rate the meal that Jessica purchased for her lunch while working at the coffee shop.

1 medium raisin bagel

2 Tbsp low-fat cream cheese

½ cup mixed fruit

10 oz regular coffee with cream and sugar

How many calories, grams of protein, and iron did Jessica consume in this meal? Is it enough for a pregnant teen? Why or why not?

CASE IN POINT

AH MAR MO: MANAGING GESTATIONAL DIABETES

Ah Mar Mo is currently 28 weeks pregnant with her first child. She has migrated to the United States from Myanmar and is just beginning English language lessons. During her pregnancy, she has been receiving prenatal care and a translator has attended her appointments with her. Ah Mar is 5-ft 3-in tall. Her weight prior to pregnancy was 149 lb. Her current weight is 174 lb. Today at her appointment, her doctor informed her that she has developed gestational diabetes. He tells her that her body is not processing the sugar in her food well enough and he wants her to meet with a certified diabetes educator to discuss some of the changes she will need to make in her diet.

The educator explains to Ah Mar Mo what is happening in her body and discusses possible complications both she and the baby could develop. She shows her how to monitor her blood sugar and instructs Ah Mar Mo on the types of foods that will raise her blood sugar. Rice and noodles are staples in Ah Mar Mo's meals and she rarely has a meal that does not contain one or the other. She also drinks large amounts of fruit juice with and between meals.

The educator discusses with Ah Mar Mo that she needs to have smaller, more frequent meals throughout the day and suggests three small meals and three snacks. She talks to Ah Mar Mo about replacing her consumption of juices with water and asks about her food preparation. Ah Mar Mo states that many of the foods she prepares are fried. Since the oils are very high in calories and eating fried foods could be contributing to her weight gain, they discuss alternative ways to prepare her foods. Ah Mar Mo also learns that she is eating much larger portions of rice and noodles than she should. The educator tells Ah Mar Mo that she was overweight prior to her pregnancy and is now at the high end of the weight gain recommendations for her prepregnancy weight. Ah Mar is not thrilled with changing her eating habits, but knows it is best for her and the baby.

ASSESSMENT

1. Why are elevated blood sugars during pregnancy a problem?
2. What are the consequences of high blood sugars for the baby during pregnancy?
3. What are the consequences of high blood sugars during pregnancy for the mom?
4. All pregnant women should be screened for gestational diabetes at what point during their pregnancy?

DIAGNOSIS

5. Write a nursing diagnosis for Ah Mar Mo related to her gestational diabetes.
6. Write a nursing diagnosis for Ah Mar Mo related to her nutrition.

PLAN/GOAL

7. Ah Mar Mo needs to be educated regarding her gestational diabetes. What would be the two most important things to instruct Ah Mar Mo about?
8. How often may the nurse practitioner or educator need to see Ah Mar Mo?

IMPLEMENTATION

9. What steps might the dietitian take to ensure that Ah Mar Mo is following the guidelines she was instructed on?

EVALUATION/OUTCOME CRITERIA

10. How could the physician, nurse practitioner, and dietitian be assured their goals were met?

THINKING FURTHER

11. What are some of the considerations necessary when using a translator to speak to a client?

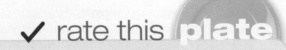

✔ rate this **plate**

Rate the plate that Ah Mar has chosen for lunch.

- **⅔ cup rice**
- **1 cup pork stir-fry made of bok choy, snow peas, and broccoli**
- **8 oz mango juice**
- **½ cup tapioca pudding with coconut**

Can you determine if her carbohydrates are correct for her meal? Yes or no, and why? What changes if any should be made to lower her caloric intake?

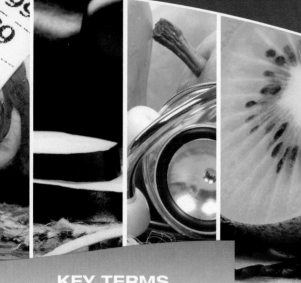

CHAPTER 11

KEY TERMS

amniocentesis
bonding
galactosemia
galactosuria
immunity
inborn errors of metabolism
isoleucine
leucine
Lofenalac
maple syrup urine disease
  (MSUD)
mutations
on demand
phenylalanine
phenylalanine hydroxylase
phenylketonuria (PKU)
psychosocial development
regurgitation
sterile
transferase
valine
weaning

NUTRITION DURING INFANCY

OBJECTIVES

After studying this chapter, you should be able to:

- State the effect inadequate nutrition has on an infant
- Discuss positive aspects of breastfeeding and bottle feeding
- Describe when and how foods are introduced into the baby's diet
- Describe inborn errors of metabolism and their dietary treatment

Food and its presentation are extremely important during the baby's first year. Physical and mental development are dependent on the food itself, and **psychosocial development** is affected by the time and manner in which the food is offered.

Infants react to their parents' emotions. If food is forced on a child, withheld until the child is uncomfortable, or if the food is presented in a tense manner the child reacts with tension and unhappiness. If the parent is relaxed, an infant's mealtime can be pleasurable for both parent and child (Figure 11-1).

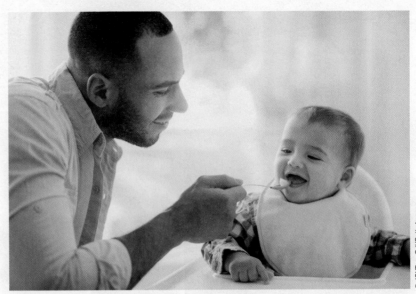

FIGURE 11-1 Food is better accepted and digested in a happy and relaxed atmosphere.

Although babies have been fed according to prescribed time schedules in the past, it is preferable to feed infants **on demand**. Feeding on demand prevents the frustrations that hunger can bring and helps the baby realize that his or her needs are being met. The newborn may require more frequent feedings, but normally the demand schedule averages approximately every four hours by the time the baby is 2 or 3 months old.

NUTRITIONAL REQUIREMENTS

The first year of life is a period of the most rapid growth in one's life. A baby doubles its birth weight by 6 months of age and triples it within the first year. This explains why the infant's energy, vitamin, mineral, and protein requirements are higher per unit of body weight than those of older children or adults. It is important to remember, however, that growth rates vary from child to child. Nutritional needs will depend largely on a child's growth rate.

During the first year, the normal child needs 98–108 calories per kilogram of body weight each day—approximately two to three times the adult requirement. Low-birth-weight infants and infants who have suffered from malnutrition or illness require more than the normal number of calories per kilogram of body weight. The nutritional status of infants is reflected by many of the same characteristics as those of adults.

The basis of the infant's diet is breast milk or formula. Either one is a highly nutritious, digestible food containing proteins, fats, carbohydrates, vitamins, minerals, and water.

It is recommended that infants up to 6 months of age have 2.2 g of protein per kilogram of weight each day, and from 6 to 12 months, 1.6 g of protein per kilogram of weight each day. This is satisfactorily supplied by human milk or by infant formulas (Figure 11-2).

Infants have more water per pound of body weight than adults. Thus, they usually need 1.5 mL of water per calorie. This is the same ratio of water to calories

psychosocial development
relating to both psychological and social development

on demand
feeding infants as they desire

as is found in human milk and in most infant formulas. Babies receive enough water in both breast milk and formula; additional water is not needed. Essential vitamins and minerals can be supplied in breast milk, formula, and food. Except for vitamin D, breast milk provides all the nutrients an infant needs for the first 4–6 months of life. An infant is born with a three- to six-month supply of iron. When the infant reaches 6 months of age, the pediatrician usually starts the infant on iron-fortified cereal.

Human milk usually supplies the infant with sufficient vitamin C. Iron-fortified formula is available, and its use is recommended by the American Academy of Pediatricians if the baby is not being breastfed. The pediatrician can prescribe a vitamin D supplement for infants who are nursed and who are not exposed to sunlight on a regular basis. Newborns lack intestinal bacteria to synthesize vitamin K, so they are routinely given a vitamin K supplement shortly after birth. In addition, some pediatricians prescribe fluoride for breastfed babies or for formula-fed babies living in areas where the water, such as well water, contains little fluoride.

Care must be taken that infants do not receive excessive amounts of either vitamin A or D because both can be toxic in excessive amounts. Vitamin A can damage the liver and cause bone abnormalities, and vitamin D can damage the cardiovascular system and kidneys.

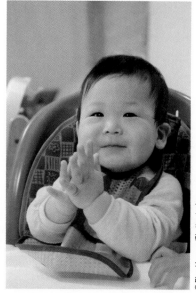

FIGURE 11-2 A happy, healthy, well-fed infant.

BREASTFEEDING

Although babies will thrive whether nursed or formula-fed, breastfeeding provides advantages that formulas cannot match. Breastfeeding is nature's way of providing a good diet for the baby. It is, in fact, used as the guide by which nutritional requirements of infants are measured (Figure 11-3).

Breast milk provides the infant with temporary **immunity** to many infectious diseases. It is economical, nutritionally perfect, and sanitary, and it saves time otherwise spent in shopping for or preparing formula. It is **sterile**, is easy to digest, and usually does not cause gastrointestinal disturbances or allergic reactions. Breastfed infants have fewer infections (especially ear infections) during the first few months of life than formula-fed babies, and because breast milk contains less protein and minerals than infant formula, it reduces the load on the infant's kidneys. Breastfeeding also promotes oral motor development in infants and decreases the infant's risk of obesity and diabetes.

Within the first several weeks of life, the infant will nurse approximately every two to four hours. As the infant grows and develops, a stronger sucking ability will allow more milk to be extracted at each feeding, and the frequency of nursing sessions will decrease. It is recommended that an infant nurse at each breast for approximately 5–10 minutes each session. Growth spurts occur at about 10 days, 2 weeks, 6 weeks, and 3 months of age. During this time, the infant will nurse more frequently to increase the supply of nutrients needed to support growth.

One can be quite confident the infant is getting sufficient nutrients and calories from breastfeeding if:

- there are six or more wet diapers a day
- there is normal growth
- there are one or two mustard-colored bowel movements a day
- the breast becomes less full during nursing

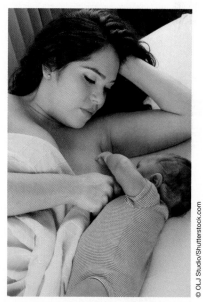

FIGURE 11-3 Breastfeeding offers many nutritional benefits to the newborn.

immunity
ability to resist certain diseases

sterile
free of infectious organisms

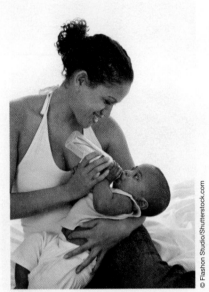

FIGURE 11-4 Feeding is a good time to provide the infant with love and attention.

From the mother's perspective at least, the **bonding** that occurs during breastfeeding is unmatched. In addition, breastfeeding helps the mother's uterus return to normal size after delivery, controls postpartum bleeding, and helps the mother more quickly return to her prepregnancy weight. Research has shown a correlation between breastfeeding and a decreased risk of breast cancer and osteoporosis in premenopausal women.

Breastfeeding rates continue to rise in the United States. In 2011, 79% of newborn infants started to breastfeed. Yet, breastfeeding is not continuing for as long as recommended. Of infants born in 2011, 49% were breastfeeding at 6 months and 27% at 12 months. *Healthy People 2020* has established goals for breastfeeding rates: 81.9% of newborns, 60.6% at 6 months, and 34.1% at 1 year. If the mother works and cannot be available for every feeding, breast milk can be expressed earlier, refrigerated or frozen, and used at the appropriate time, or a bottle of formula can be substituted. Never warm the breast milk in a microwave because the antibodies will be destroyed.

BOTTLE FEEDING

Some parents will choose to bottle-feed their babies. Some women fear they will be unable to produce enough breast milk. Some lack emotional support from their families, and some simply find breastfeeding foreign to their culture. Others who are employed or involved in many activities outside the home find bottle feeding more convenient. Either way of feeding is acceptable provided the infant is given love and attention during the feeding.

The infant should be cuddled and held in a semi-upright position during the feeding (Figure 11-4). It appears that babies fed this way are less inclined to develop middle ear infections than those fed lying down. It is believed that the upright position prevents fluid from pooling at the back of the throat and entering tubes from the middle ear. During and after the feeding, the infant should be burped to release gas in the stomach, just as the breastfed infant should be burped (Figure 11-5). Burping helps prevent **regurgitation**.

If the baby is to be bottle-fed, the pediatrician will provide information on commercial formulas and feeding instructions. Formulas are usually based on cow's milk because it is abundant and easily modified to resemble human milk.

bonding
emotional attachment

regurgitation
vomiting

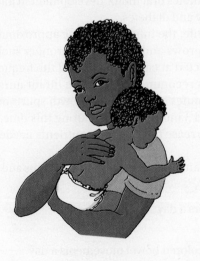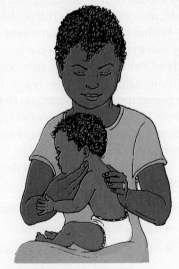

FIGURE 11-5 To burp a baby, hold in one of the two positions shown and gently stroke the back.

It must be modified because it has more protein and mineral salts and less milk sugar (lactose) than human milk. Formulas, such as soy formula, are developed so that they are similar to human milk in nutrient and caloric values.

When an infant is extremely sensitive or allergic to infant formulas, a synthetic formula may be given. Synthetic milk is commonly made from soybeans. Formulas with predigested proteins, commonly referred to as "hypoallergenic" formulas, are used for infants unable to tolerate all other types of formulas.

Formulas can be purchased in ready-to-feed, concentrated, or powdered forms. Sterile or boiled tap water must be mixed with the concentrated and powdered forms. The most convenient type is also the most expensive. The American Academy of Pediatrics' website, https://healthychildren.org, has information on how long formula can be stored as well as information to assess safety of water if it comes from a well. Formula remaining in a bottle that has been given to an infant must be discarded after one hour. Fresh formula that has been prepared for the infant is generally good for 24 hours. Ready-to-feed formula or formula made from concentrate is generally good for 48 hours.

If the type of formula purchased requires the addition of water, it is essential that the amount of water added be correctly measured. Too little water will create too heavy a protein and mineral load for the infant's kidneys. Too much water will dilute the nutrient and calorie value so that the infant will not thrive, and also it could lead to brain edema or seizures.

Infants under the age of 1 year should not be given regular cow's milk. Because its protein is more difficult and slower to digest than that of human milk, it can cause gastrointestinal blood loss. The kidneys are challenged by its high protein and mineral content, and dehydration and even damage to the central nervous system can result. In addition, the fat is less bioavailable, meaning it is not absorbed as efficiently as that in human milk.

Formula may be given cold, at room temperature, or warmed, but it should be given at the same temperature consistently. To warm the formula for feeding, place the bottle in a saucepan of warm water or a bottle warmer. The bottles should be shaken occasionally to warm the contents evenly. Warming the bottle in the microwave is not advisable because milk can heat unevenly and burn the infant's mouth. The temperature of the milk can be tested by shaking a few drops on one's wrist. The milk should feel lukewarm.

Infants should not be put to bed with a bottle. Saliva, which normally cleanses the teeth, diminishes as the infant falls asleep. The milk then bathes the upper front teeth, causing tooth decay. Also, the bottle can cause the upper jaw to protrude and the lower to recede. The result is known as the *baby bottle mouth* or *nursing bottle syndrome.* It is preferable to feed the infant the bedtime bottle, cleanse the teeth and gums with some water from another bottle or cup, and then put the infant to bed.

SUPPLEMENTARY FOODS

The age at which infants are introduced to solid and semisolid food has varied considerably over the years. At the beginning of the last century, doctors advocated that children be fed only breast milk during their first 12 months. By the 1950s, in response to parental demand, some pediatricians advised the introduction of solid food before the age of 1 year. Now, the general recommendation is that the infant's diet be limited to breast milk or formula until the age of 4–6 months and that breast milk or formula remain the major food source until the child is 1 year old. With the appropriate supplements of iron and vitamin D and possibly vitamin C and fluoride, breast milk or formula fulfills the nutritional requirements of most children until they reach the age of 6 months.

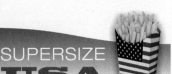

SUPERSIZE USA

Habits involving diet quality should begin in the first year of life, recent studies in the *Journal of Pediatrics* show. In the first study, infrequent intakes of fruits and vegetables during infancy continued as study participants reached age 6. A second study found that infants who were offered sugar-sweetened beverages were twice as likely to drink them daily at age 6. A third study found that participants who drank sugary beverages three times a week were twice as likely to be obese by the age of 6. Tips to help inspire healthy eating habits and decrease risks for obesity include:

- Breastfeeding your baby
- Having regular family meals
- Serving as a good role model for healthy eating
- Serving a variety of healthy food and snacks, especially fruits and vegetables
- Setting goals for activity and limiting screen time
- Involving kids in the meal-planning process
- Limiting or avoiding sugary beverages and high-fat foods/snacks
- Avoiding using food as a reward for young children

Source: Adapted from Saint Louis, Catherine. "Childhood Diet Habits Set in Infancy, Studies Suggest." *New York Times.* September 2, 2014. Accessed October 2015.

SPOTLIGHT *on Life Cycle*

The Women, Infants, and Children (WIC) program is federally funded and provides nutritious foods, nutrition education, and referrals to health and other social services to participants at no cost. Pregnant, postpartum, and breastfeeding women, infants, and children up to age 5 are eligible. Eligibility is based on income and nutritional risk, including conditions such as anemia, underweight or overweight, history of pregnancy complications, poor pregnancy outcomes, or dietary risks. Different food packages are offered, including infant cereal, iron-fortified adult cereal, vitamin C-rich fruit or vegetable juice, eggs, milk, cheese, peanut butter, dried and canned beans/peas, and canned fish. Vegetarian options are also available to accommodate the needs of the participants. Mothers can receive breastfeeding support and education as well as breast pumps to aide in the continuation of breastfeeding. During 2013, women, infants, and children who received benefits totaled 8.6 million participants per month.

Source: Adapted from "WIC Fact Sheet." Food and Nutrition Service, United States Department of Agriculture. April 2014. Accessed October 23, 2015 from http://www.fns.usda.gov

The introduction of solid foods before the age of 4–6 months is not recommended. The child's gastrointestinal tract and kidneys are not sufficiently developed to handle solid food before that age. Further, it is thought that the early introduction of solid foods may increase the likelihood of overfeeding and the development of food allergies, particularly in children whose parents suffer from allergies.

An infant's readiness for solid foods will be demonstrated by:

1. The physical ability to pull food into the mouth rather than always pushing the tongue and food out of the mouth (extrusion reflex disappears by 4–6 months)

2. A willingness to participate in the process (Figure 11-6)

3. The ability to sit up with support

4. Having head and neck control

5. The need for additional nutrients. If the infant is drinking more than 32 oz of formula or nursing 8–10 times in 24 hours and is at least 4 months old, then solid food should be started.

Solid foods must be introduced gradually and individually. One food is introduced and then no other new food in introduced for four or five days. If there is no allergic reaction, another food can be introduced, a waiting period allowed, then another, and so on. The typical order of introduction begins with a single grain cereal, usually iron-fortified oat, wheat, barley, or rice cereals, and then introduction of mixed cereals. In 2013, the FDA reported concerns in the amount of arsenic in rice cereals. This agency suggests rice cereal be used less often in the diet versus the other single grain options. Cooked and pureed vegetables follow, then cooked and pureed fruits, egg yolk, and, lastly, finely ground meats. A good rule of thumb for feeding during the first year of life is 2–4 tablespoons (1–2 oz) of each variety of food per meal. Between 6 and 12 months, toast, zwieback, teething biscuits, and Cheerios can be added in small amounts. Honey should never be given to an infant because it could be contaminated with *Clostridium botulinum* bacteria. After 6 months, sips of water can be given and no more than 4 oz of 100% juice. Breast milk and formula remain priority fluids.

Babies differ in the amount of food they eat from day to day. During that first important year of feeding, parents and their infants learn to read each other's verbal and non-verbal cues. It is important for the parent to learn how to be responsive with feeding by responding to the cues for hunger and fullness. In general, an infant will be fussy and cry when hungry (though sometimes they simply need a diaper change or some attention). Often parents get to know "types" of crying and eventually can discern the needs of the infant. Your infant may tell you she is hungry by sucking on her hands, moving her head toward the spoon, reaching for food, or using sounds or words to indicate hunger and cooing during feeding letting you know she wants to continue eating.

An infant will let you know when he or she is full in the following ways:

- Playing with the nipple on a bottle or a breast
- Looking around and no longer opening his or her mouth to solid food
- Pushing food away or clenching mouth
- Playing with food and shaking head to signal no

Parents usually are provided with guidelines on feeding from their physician. Table 11-1 shows appropriate foods and fluids needed daily for babies from 4 to 12 months.

By the age of 1 year, most babies are eating foods from all of the food groups and may have almost any food that is easily chewed and digested. However, precautions must be taken to avoid offering foods on which the child can choke. Examples include hot dogs, nuts, whole peas, grapes, popcorn, small candies, and small pieces of tough meat or raw vegetables. Foods should be selected according to the advice of the health care provider or pediatrician. It is not necessary to use the commercially prepared "third" foods. Table foods generally can be used, though they may need to first be mashed or run through a blender.

The USDA's Food and Nutrition information center has excellent resources for understanding infant food requirements. Its use will help guide the parent in supplying the appropriate foods and nutrients for their growing infant as well as help develop the correct feeding style to produce competent eaters. It is particularly important at this time to avoid excess sugar and salt in the infant's diet so that the child does not develop a taste for them and, consequently, overuse them throughout life.

Weaning actually begins when the infant is first given food from a spoon (Figure 11-7). It progresses as the child shows an interest in and an ability to drink from a cup. The child will ultimately discard the bottle or refuse the breast. If the child shows great reluctance to discard the bottle or still seeks the breast, then parents should discuss this with their health care provider.

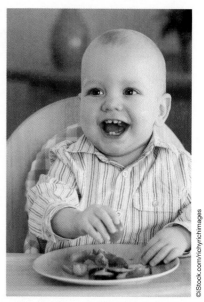

FIGURE 11-6 Infants sometimes find more pleasure in touching their food than tasting it.

©iStock.com/richyrichimages

ASSESSMENT OF GROWTH

In the clinical setting, health care professionals use standardized growth charts to assess growth of children, infants, and teens. The Centers for Disease Control and Prevention and the American Academy of Pediatrics recommend that health care providers in primary care settings in the United States use the WHO growth standard charts to monitor the growth of children aged birth to younger than 2 years regardless of type of feeding; and to use the 2000 CDC growth reference charts to monitor growth of children aged 2 until age 20 years. The CDC has a growth chart

weaning
training an infant to drink from the cup instead of the nipple

TABLE 11-1 Feeding Guidelines for Infants

FEEDING	4–6 MONTHS	6–8 MONTHS
Early morning	Breast milk or formula*	Breast milk or formula*
Breakfast	1–2 T infant cereal 1–2 T fruit or veggies	2–4 T infant cereal 2–3 T fruit or veggie 1 egg yolk mashed
Mid-morning	Breast milk or formula*	Breast milk or formula*
Lunch	Breast milk or formula*	1–4 T infant cereal 2–3 T fruit or veggies ½ c yogurt
Late afternoon	Breast milk or formula*	Breast milk formula*
Supper	Breast milk or formula* 1–2 T infant cereal or meat 1–2 T fruit or veggie	Breast milk formula*
		2–3 T meat or non-meat alternative Serving of grain (2 crackers or ½ slice bread 2–3 T veggies or fruit
Evening	Breast milk or formula*	Breast milk or formula* (optional)
Total breast milk/formula	4–6 feedings/day, 28–32 oz	3–5 feedings/day, 30–32 oz

Babies differ in the amounts of food they eat. Expect your baby's appetite to vary from day to day.

FEEDING	8–10 MONTHS	10–12 MONTHS
Morning	Breast milk or formula*	Breast milk or formula*
Breakfast	4–6 T infant cereal[†] 2–4 T fruit or veggie 1 egg yolk, mashed	5–8 T infant cereal[†] Well-cooked egg Soft chopped fruit
Mid-morning	Breast milk or formula*	½ c yogurt with cut-up fruit
Lunch	Breast milk or formula* 2–3 T meat or meat alternative 2–4 T veggies or fruit, chopped Serving of grain (4 T pasta)	Breast milk formula* 2–3 T meat or meat alternative 2–4 T veggies or fruit, chopped Serving of grain (¼–½)
Late afternoon	2–4 T fruit ½ c yogurt	Breast milk or formula* 2 T fruit, chopped ½ oz cheese
Supper	Breast milk or formula* 2–3 T meat or meat alternative 2–4 T vegetables Serving of grain	Breast milk or formula* 2–3 T meat or meat alternative 3–5 T vegetables 2–3 T fruit
Evening	Breast milk or formula* (optional)	Breast milk or formula* (optional)
Total breast milk/formula	3–5 feedings/day, 30–32 oz	3–4 feedings/day, 24–30 oz

*If baby is not breastfed, iron-fortified, commercial infant formula is recommended for the first 9–12 months.
[†]Iron-fortified infant cereal is recommended for babies during the first 2 years.

training website, which offers a set of self-directed, interactive training courses for health care professionals to accurately interpret growth status. There are low birth weight and very low birth weight charts used for premature infants. Additionally, there are growth charts developed for children with special health care situations such as cerebral palsy and Prader-Willi and Down's syndrome.

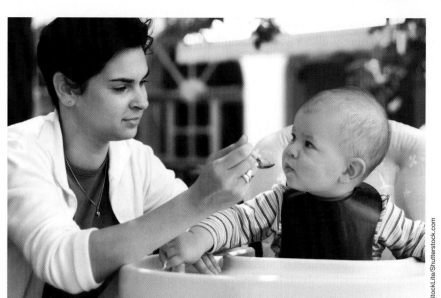

FIGURE 11-7 Solid foods are introduced at 4–6 months. Breast milk or formula continues to be the main source of calories at this age.

SPECIAL CONSIDERATIONS FOR INFANTS WITH ALTERED NUTRITIONAL NEEDS

Premature Infants

An infant born before 37 weeks' gestation is considered to be premature. These babies have special needs. The sucking reflex is not developed until 34 weeks of gestation, and infants born earlier must be fed by total parenteral nutrition, tube feedings, or bolus feedings (Figure 11-8). The best food for a premature infant is its mother's breast milk, which contains more protein, sodium, immunologic properties, and some other minerals than does the milk produced by mothers of full-term infants. Other concerns in preterm infants are low birth weight, underdeveloped lungs, immature GI tract, inadequate bone mineralization, and lack of fat reserves. Many specialized formulas are available for premature infants, but breast milk is best because its composition is made just for the baby, and it changes according to the baby's needs. Mothers of premature babies should be encouraged to pump their milk until the infant is able to nurse. Growth is assessed on the special growth charts for premature infants.

Infants with Cystic Fibrosis

Cystic fibrosis (CF) is an inherited disease that causes the body to produce abnormally thick, sticky secretions (mucus) within cells lining organs such as the lungs and pancreas. The thick mucus also obstructs the pancreas, preventing enzymes from reaching the intestines to help break down and digest food. Of those children with CF, 85% have exocrine pancreatic insufficiency (PI) and are at nutritional risk due to decreased production of digestive enzymes. Malabsorption of fat is also associated with CF; therefore, the recommendation is for 35–40% of total calorie intake to be fat. Digestive enzymes are taken in capsule form when

In The Media

Vegetarian and Vegan Diets for Infants and Toddlers

The Academy of Nutrition and Dietetics and the American Academy of Pediatrics both agree that vegetarian and vegan eating patterns are healthy for infants and children. Careful planning of meals and snacks can help ensure that young children are getting the nutrients they need to help them grow. When weaning a baby from breast milk, it is recommended to use an iron-fortified formula versus cow's milk, soy milk, rice milk, or homemade formulas until the first year of life. When introducing solid foods, meat can be replaced with pureed tofu, or beans and soy dairy products. Nutrients to pay close attention to include vitamin B12, vitamin D, calcium, iron, protein, and fiber. By including soy beverages, fortified cereals, beans, yogurt, eggs, grains, nut butters, and various fruit and vegetables, a well-rounded diet can be realized.

Source: Adapted from Hayes, Dayle. *Feeding Vegetarian and Vegan Infants and Toddlers.* May 4, 2015. Accessed October 2015. www. eatright.org.

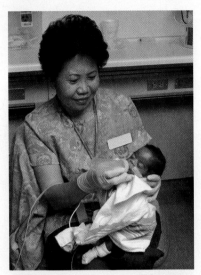

FIGURE 11-8 This premature infant receives a specially designed formula to meet his nutritional needs; note the placement of a nasogastric tube.

inborn errors of metabolism
congenital disabilities preventing normal metabolism

mutations
changes in the genes

food is eaten, and supplementation of fat-soluble vitamins should also be done at mealtime. There is also a water-miscible form of fat-soluble vitamins that can be administered if normal levels cannot be maintained with the use of only fat-soluble vitamins. It is not unusual for those having CF to be malnourished, even with supplementation, due to malabsorption of nutrients and increased needs. One possible solution would be nighttime tube feedings to supplement oral intake if adequate nutrition and weight cannot be maintained.

Infants with Failure to Thrive

Failure to thrive (FTT) can be determined by plotting the infant's growth on standardized growth charts (Figure 11-9); consideration must be made for genetic and ethnic variations. Weight for height is the first parameter affected when determining FTT. Later, height and head circumference are affected. Other signs might be slow development or lack of physical skills such as rolling over, sitting, standing, and walking. Mental and social skills will also be delayed. Babies grow the most in the first 6 months of life, and this is when their brain undergoes crucial development, which can affect the rest of their lives. Failure to thrive can have many causes, such as watered-down formula, congenital abnormalities, AIDS, lack of bonding, child abuse, or neglect.

Infants with Cleft Palate

Cleft lip and cleft palate are birth defects that occur when a baby's lip or roof of the mouth (palate) does not develop properly (Figure 11-10). A baby may have a cleft lip, cleft palate, or both malformations. Children with a cleft lip with or without a cleft palate, or a cleft palate alone, often have problems with feeding and speaking in a clear fashion. Surgery to repair the cleft is recommended before 12 months of life.

Because of the cleft, the baby cannot create the suction that is needed to efficiently pull milk from the bottle or breast. It is imperative to find the correct feeding modality for the cleft child, so that nutrition needs are met and growth advances. The mother can express breast milk and use one of the special cleft nursers or a Pigeon or Haberman special needs bottle. There are many accredited cleft palate multidisciplinary teams around the country that can assist the family. The Cleft Palate Foundation at www.cleftline.org has excellent resources for parents and clinicians to assist in feeding.

SPECIAL CONSIDERATIONS FOR INFANTS WITH METABOLIC DISORDERS

Some infants are born with the inability to metabolize specific nutrients. These congenital disabilities are called **inborn errors of metabolism**. They are caused by **mutations** in the genes. There is great variation in the seriousness of the conditions caused by these defects. Some cause death at an early age, and some can be minimized so that life can be supported by adjustments in the normal diet. Children born with these defects, however, face the common danger of damage to the central nervous system because of their abnormal body chemistry. This results in mental retardation and sometimes retarded growth. Early diagnosis of these inborn errors, combined with diet therapy, increases the chances of preventing retardation. Hospitals test newborns for some of these disorders as

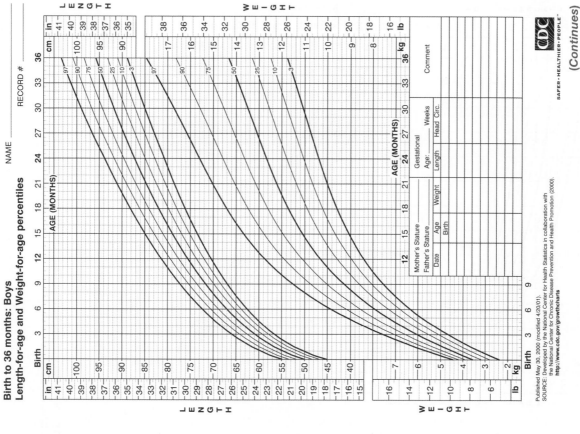

FIGURE 11-9 Physical growth charts.

Source: Centers for Disease Control and Prevention, National Center for Health Statistics in collaboration with the National Center for Chronic Disease Prevention and Health Promotion. 2000 CDC Growth Charts: United States. http://www.cdc.gov/growthcharts, updated April 20, 2001.

(Continues)

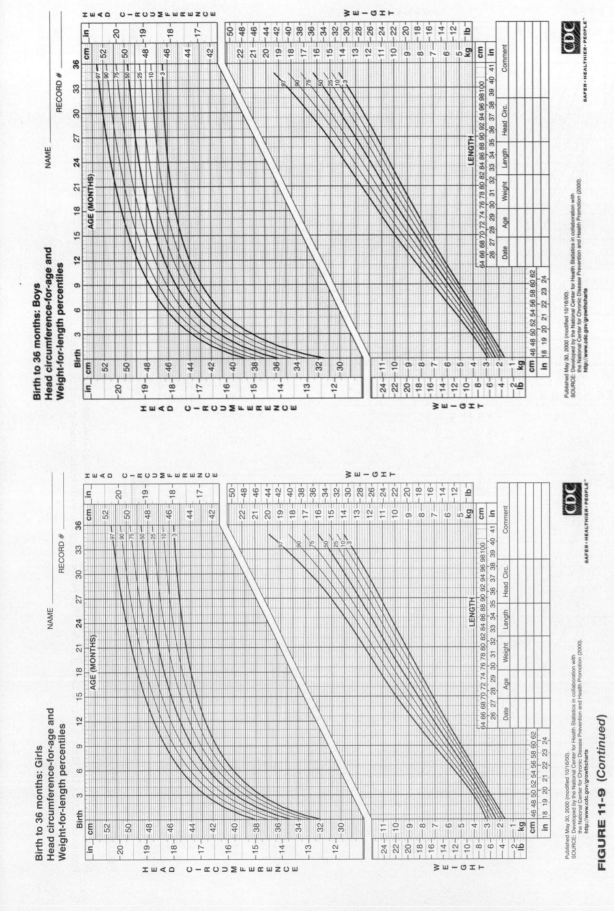

FIGURE 11-9 *(Continued)*

Source: Centers for Disease Control and Prevention, National Center for Health Statistics in collaboration with the National Center for Chronic Disease Prevention and Health Promotion. 2000 CDC Growth Charts: United States. http://www.cdc.gov/growthcharts, updated April 20, 2001.

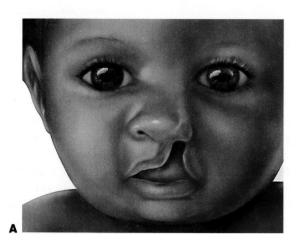
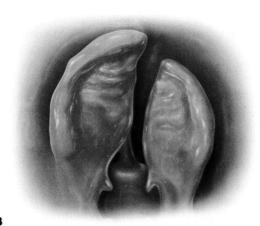

A   **B**

FIGURE 11-10 A. Cleft lip, B. Cleft palate.

a matter of course. If there is a family history of a certain genetic disorder, genetic screening can be done. In addition, some of these abnormalities can be discovered by **amniocentesis**.

Infants with Galactosemia

Galactosemia is a condition that affects 1 in 30,000 live births and is caused by the lack of the liver enzyme **transferase**. Transferase normally converts galactose to glucose. (Galactose is the simple sugar resulting from the digestion of lactose, the sugar found in milk; see Chapter 4.) When an infant who lacks transferase ingests anything containing galactose, the amount of galactose in the blood becomes excessive. As a result of this toxic level, the newborn suffers diarrhea, vomiting, edema, and abnormal liver function. Cataracts may develop, **galactosuria** occurs, and mental retardation ensues.

Diet Therapy

Diet therapy for galactosemia is the exclusion of anything containing milk from any mammal. During infancy, the treatment is relatively simple because parents can feed the baby lactose-free, commercially prepared formula and can provide supplemental minerals and vitamins. As the child grows and moves on to adult foods, parents must be extremely careful to avoid any food, beverage, or medicine that contains lactose. Nutritional supplements of calcium, vitamin D, and riboflavin must be given so that the diet is nutritionally adequate. This restricted diet may be necessary throughout life, but some physicians allow a somewhat liberalized diet as the child reaches school age. This may mean only small amounts of baked or processed foods that contain small amounts of milk. Even this restricted diet must be accompanied by careful and regular monitoring for galactosuria.

Infants with Phenylketonuria

In **phenylketonuria (PKU)**, infants lack the liver enzyme **phenylalanine hydroxylase**, which is necessary for the metabolism of the amino acid **phenylalanine**. Infants seem to be normal at birth, but if the disease is not treated, most of them become hyperactive, suffer seizures between 6 and 18 months of age, and become mentally retarded. Public health law requires

amniocentesis
a test to determine the status of the fetus in utero

galactosemia
inherited error in metabolism that prevents normal metabolism of galactose

transferase
liver enzyme that converts galactose to glucose

galactosuria
galactose in the urine

phenylketonuria (PKU)
condition caused by an inborn error of metabolism in which the infant lacks an enzyme necessary to metabolize the amino acid phenylalanine

phenylalanine hydroxylase
liver enzyme necessary to metabolize the amino acid phenylalanine

phenylalanine
amino acid

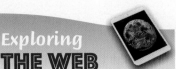

Exploring THE WEB

Visit the National PKU News website (http://www.pkunews.org). Read through the diet-related material and prepare a list of acceptable safe foods for clients with PKU. Read through some of the personal stories and be prepared to share some support group references with the parents of an infant with PKU.

most hospitals today to screen newborns for phenylketonuria. PKU babies typically have light-colored skin and hair. In the United States, PKU occurs in 1 out of every 10,000–15,000 births.

Diet Therapy

There is a special, nutritionally adequate, commercial infant formula available for PKU babies, called **Lofenalac**, with 95% of phenylalanine removed from its protein source. It provides just enough phenylalanine for basic needs, but no excess. The specific amount depends on the infant's size and growth rate. Regular blood tests determine the adequacy of the amounts. Diets are carefully monitored for calorie and nutrient content and are adjusted frequently as needs change. Except for fats and sugars, all foods contain some protein; and of that protein, some are phenylalanine, so diets for the growing child eating normal food must be carefully planned.

The two varieties of synthetic milk available for older children include *Phenyl-free* and *PKU-1*, *2*, or *3*. None of these contains any phenylalanine. They can be used as beverages or in puddings and baked products. The special formula and low-protein food product options do not yield a pleasurable and satisfying diet for most. Lifelong adherence to the diet is low; however, frequent monitoring by a metabolic medical team can help. It is important that diets be monitored throughout life to avoid mental retardation and to control hyperactivity and aggressive behavior.

Infants with Maple Syrup Urine Disease

Maple syrup urine disease (MSUD) is a congenital defect resulting in the inability to metabolize three amino acids: **leucine**, **isoleucine**, and **valine**. It is named for the odor of the urine of these infants and affects 1 in 100,000–300,000 live births. When the infant ingests food protein, there are increased blood levels of these amino acids, causing ketosis. Hypoglycemia, apathy, and convulsions occur very early. Depending on the extent of the disease, if not treated promptly, the child can die from acidosis. Mild forms of the disease, if left untreated, will cause mental retardation and bouts of acidosis.

Diet Therapy

The diet must provide sufficient calories and nutrients but with extremely restricted amounts of leucine, isoleucine, and valine. A special formula and low-protein foods are used. Diet therapy appears to be necessary throughout life.

HEALTH AND NUTRITION CONSIDERATIONS

Although the physical and mental development of infants depend on the nutrients and calories they receive, their psychosocial development depends on *how and when* these nutrients and calories are provided. Some new parents will have a solid knowledge of the nutrition information needed but lack a real understanding of the importance of how and when food should be presented to infants. They may hold the infant during feedings but focus instead on the television or newspaper.

Lofenalac
commercial infant formula with 95% of phenylalanine removed

maple syrup urine disease (MSUD)
disease caused by an inborn error of metabolism in which the body cannot metabolize certain amino acids

leucine
an amino acid

isoleucine
an amino acid

valine
an amino acid

Other parents may know instinctively how important cuddling and attention are to an infant, but they lack accurate knowledge of infant nutrition.

Parents from both groups are apt to have opinions that may or may not be correct. The health care professional will help these parents most by listening carefully to them. The parents are more inclined to listen to advice when a two-way discussion follows.

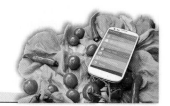

SUMMARY

It is particularly important that babies have adequate diets so that their physical and mental development are not impaired. Breastfeeding is nature's way of feeding an infant, although formula feeding is acceptable. Cow's milk is primarily used in formulas because it is most available and is easily modified to resemble human milk. Health care teams in pediatric offices will need to offer advice on growth and feeding. Infant feeding charts are useful when solid foods begin between 4 and 6 months. It is important that the parent be supportive, timely, and responsive with feeding.

Inborn errors of metabolism cause various problems, ranging from mental retardation to death, if not properly treated. In these conditions, diet therapy is the primary tool in maintaining the client's health.

Infants who are premature, have cystic fibrosis, or failure to thrive have special nutritional needs.

DISCUSSION TOPICS

1. Do any of the students know a woman who has breastfed her baby? If so, what were her reactions to the experience?

2. Why is breastfeeding not always possible?

3. Discuss the possible effects of regularly propping the baby's bottle instead of holding the baby during feeding.

4. Why is a rigid time schedule for feeding a baby not advisable? Explain why feeding infants on demand the first few months can lead to a regular feeding schedule.

5. How may weaning be accomplished?

6. What is meant by inborn errors of metabolism? What causes them? How might they affect infants?

7. Discuss PKU. Include its cause, symptoms, effects, and treatment.

8. Why should the mother give her baby special attention during feedings?

9. How is a bottle warmed? Is it always necessary to warm the bottle? Explain. Why is a microwave oven not recommended?

10. Why is it not advisable to give peanuts to an 8-month-old child?

SUGGESTED ACTIVITIES

1. Hold a panel discussion on the advantages and disadvantages of breastfeeding. Invite lactation specialists, doctors, and parents as panelists.

2. Observe a demonstration of the actual feeding and burping of a baby.

3. Visit a store that carries prepared infant formulas and compare their prices and nutritional values.

4. Invite a physician or nurse practitioner to give a talk on inborn errors of metabolism.

REVIEW

Multiple choice. Select the *letter* that precedes the best answer.

1. The most rapid growth in a child's life occurs during
    a. its first month
    b. the month following weaning
    c. the first 6 months
    d. its first year

2. The amount of protein needed by a child during its first year
    a. is greater during the first 6 months than during the second
    b. is greater during the second 6 months than during the first
    c. does not change over the course of the year
    d. increases on a weekly basis

3. After the initial supplement of vitamin K following birth, breast milk provides all the nutrients an infant needs during the first 4–6 months except for
    a. vitamin A
    b. vitamin B
    c. vitamin C
    d. vitamin D

4. The vitamin in question 3 might be provided
    a. by injection
    b. in diluted orange juice
    c. by regular walks in the sunshine
    d. in pasteurized apple juice

5. Breastfed babies are more resistant to infection than are bottle-fed babies because mother's milk provides
    a. sterile environment
    b. synthetic antibiotics
    c. leucine
    d. immunity

6. The development of emotional attachment to a child is called
    a. transferase
    b. bonding
    c. psychosocial development
    d. immunity

7. It is recommended that, at each feeding, a newborn nurse at each breast for approximately
    a. 3–5 minutes
    b. 5–10 minutes
    c. 10–15 minutes
    d. 20 minutes

8. It can be said that infant formulas
    a. are usually based on cow's milk
    b. have the same protein content as cow's milk
    c. contain fewer minerals than cow's milk
    d. contain no sugar

9. Infants with sensitivities to infant formulas may be given
    a. goat's milk
    b. synthetic milk, often made from soybeans
    c. formula with predigested carbohydrates
    d. any of the above

10. By the age of 6 months, a child
    a. may be introduced to a new formula
    b. is usually completely weaned
    c. is usually introduced to solid foods
    d. is no longer given milk

CASE IN POINT

DIEGO: OVERCOMING FAILURE TO THRIVE

Bonita's youngest child, Diego, was born four weeks ago at 7 lb 14 oz and 20-in long. Bonita was unable to take six weeks off work after Diego was born. Bonita is 34 years old. She and her husband are from Colombia and own a restaurant that serves authentic Colombian cuisine. Their head chef resigned shortly before Diego was born and Bonita was going to have to fill in as chef until a new one could be hired and trained. Diego was born during the height of the summer tourism season in their town and Bonita was desperately needed back at work. Bonita had hired the neighbor girl to care for Diego while she was working. The neighbor reported that Diego was often very cranky and would refuse his bottle. Bonita wasn't terribly concerned.

Her first child had been very colicky so it wouldn't surprise her that Diego was as well. Finally, Bonita and her husband were able to find a new chef for the restaurant and Bonita was able to take some much needed time off. By now, Diego was 4 months old. Bonita began realizing she never saw Diego smile like her other babies. He also seemed unable to track objects, such as toys, when she played with him. Bonita thought he seemed smaller than her other children at this age, but she wasn't sure how much smaller. At Diego's next well-baby check, his weight was 10 lb 14 oz and he only measured 21-in long. The doctor explained to Bonita that Diego was not growing adequately and diagnosed him with FTT.

ASSESSMENT

1. What data do you have about Bonita?
2. What data do you have about Diego?
3. What factors contributed to Diego's problem?
4. Using the growth charts in Figure 11-9, determine a baby's normal weight and height at 4 months. What should Diego weigh, and how long should he be?
5. What should Diego be doing developmentally at 4 months?
6. How severe is Diego's failure to thrive?

DIAGNOSIS

Complete the following nursing diagnoses:

7. Diego's failure to thrive is related to

   _____.

8. Diego's imbalanced nutrition, less than body requirements, is secondary to _____.
9. Bonita's ineffective feeding is a result of

   _____.

PLAN/GOAL

10. What is your immediate goal for Diego?
11. What is your long-term goal for Diego?
12. What is your short-term goal for Bonita?
13. What is your long-term goal for Bonita?

IMPLEMENTATION

14. What changes need to occur for Diego to thrive?
15. What does the NP need to teach Bonita?
16. How else can the NP help Bonita?
17. Who else needs to be involved in Diego's care?

EVALUATION/OUTCOME CRITERIA

18. After the plan has been in place for six weeks, what changes should Bonita see in Diego?
19. What will the NP measure and observe in Diego and Bonita if the plan is successful?

THINKING FURTHER

20. Why is it important for infants to have a good start in life? Why is their nutrition so critical? What future complications can be avoided as a result?

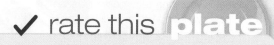 ✔ rate this **plate**

Diego is now 6 months old and Bonita will have to experiment with different foods to get him back on track. He has only been getting formula, but it's time to try solid foods. Rate this plate for lunch:

5 oz infant formula

2 Tbsp infant rice cereal

2 Tbsp pureed green beans

1 Tbsp pureed applesauce

Are the servings correct for a 6-month-old infant? If not, what corrections should be made to this meal?

CASE IN POINT

CADEN: INTRODUCING SOLID FOODS

Ann is a new mom. Her son Caden was born four months ago. Up until this time, she has been exclusively breast-feeding him. She is reading about introducing solid foods into his diet. As she begins to feed Caden cereal, she notices that he spits each bite back out of his mouth. She is concerned that he does not like the cereal. She is afraid he is a picky eater and will not continue to gain weight if he doesn't like cereal. Her mother suggests she try the cereal in a bottle for him, but she remembers the pediatrician saying that is not how cereal should be introduced. Caden has a well-baby exam this week, so she decides to wait and see what the doctor has to say. During the visit, Ann expresses her concerns about Caden's refusal of cereal. She tells him that Caden seems to spit back with his tongue every bite she feeds him. The doctor tells Ann that when Caden pushes the cereal out of his mouth with his tongue it is not because he doesn't care for the food. This is a reflex infants have called the *extrusion reflex*. It gradually disappears between 4 and 6 months of age. He assures her it is perfectly normal and even suggests she wait another month or two to try again. He graphs Caden's length of 25 in, and weight of 15 lb, on the age-appropriate chart. He reassures Ann that Caden is growing just fine. He suggests to Ann that she attend a class offered by the dietitians at a local hospital. The class is designed to educate new moms on how and when to introduce foods. Ann is very relieved that Caden is growing well. She makes plans to attend the next class offered by the dietitians.

ASSESSMENT

1. What are the benefits of breastfeeding?
2. Use Figure 11-9 to assess Caden's growth percentile for length and weight.
3. How many ounces of breast milk or formula would you expect a baby Caden's age to need? Use Table 11-1.
4. What would you expect Caden's calorie and protein needs to be at his age?

DIAGNOSIS

5. Write a nursing diagnosis for Caden.

PLAN/GOAL

6. What is the immediate goal for Caden?
7. What is your long-term goal for Caden?
8. What is your short-term goal for Ann?
9. What is your long-term goal for Ann?

IMPLEMENTATION

10. What does Ann need to learn from the dietitian's class?
11. Who else needs to be involved in Caden's care?

EVALUATION/OUTCOME CRITERIA

12. What might you expect of Caden by the time he is 1 year old?

THINKING FURTHER

13. The American Dietetic Association has a new web page for children. Check out http://www.eatright.org/kids and see the information offered. How would a website like this be helpful for Ann as Caden grows?

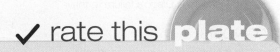
✔ rate this **plate**

Since Caden is not ready for solid foods, it would be recommended to wait and try again every week to see when his extrusion reflex disappears. At 10 months, Caden is now able to eat solid foods. Rate the meal that Ann has prepared for his lunch.

6 oz formula

4 Tbsp infant cereal

1 Tbsp baby chicken

3 Tbsp pureed sweet potatoes

4 Tbsp pureed pears

Does this meal meet the recommendations? If not, what can be changed?

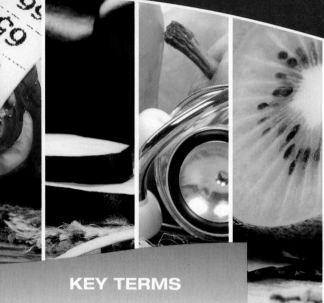

NUTRITION DURING CHILDHOOD AND ADOLESCENCE

OBJECTIVES

After studying this chapter, you should be able to:

- Identify nutritional needs of children ages 1–12 and of adolescents
- Describe attributes of a healthy feeding environment and style
- State the effects of inadequate nutrition during the growing years
- Describe eating disorders that can occur during adolescence
- Explain the growing concern over obesity, pre-diabetes, and type 2 diabetes in youth
- Discuss nutrition basics for the athlete

Although specific nutritional requirements change as children grow, nutrition always affects physical, mental, and emotional growth and development. Studies indicate that the mental ability and size of an individual are directly influenced by nutrition during the early years. Children who have an inadequate supply of nutrients—especially of protein—and calories during their early years may be shorter and less intellectually able than children who receive an adequate diet. Parents and caregivers have the all-important task of producing the blueprint for healthy eating. When a good foundation is laid, children will maximize their learning and growth potential.

CHILDREN AGED 1–12

A child's relationship to food and basic eating habits develops in early childhood. The caregiver's goal is to feed children age-appropriate food that meets nutrition needs and do this in a way that allows adequate support and encouragement. Micromanaging a child's eating or providing little support or chaotic feeding methods can increase emotional and physical problems such as irritability, fatigue, under or over nutrition, and possibly illness.

Because children learn partly by imitation, learning good eating habits is easier if parents role model those habits. Nutritious foods should be available at mealtime as well as snack time. Meals should include a wide variety of foods to ensure good nutrient intake. Families do best with structured meals and snacks, eaten at the kitchen table. When children are allowed constant food handouts and free rein of the kitchen, nutrition usually suffers and meal intake is suboptimal.

The most effective approach to feeding children is using an authoritative feeding style. This is characterized by responsiveness to the children, structure and boundaries around mealtime, and respect for the children's food choices in context of what the parent is serving at the meal or snack. The parent makes sure meals are served on time, responds to the child's hunger and fullness, allows reasonable choice around food, and lets the child regulate her own eating (deciding how much and which foods to eat from the foods presented at the mealtime). This type of feeding style is in stark contrast to the parent who tries to constantly control the child's intake (authoritarian) by insisting the child eat exactly the way the parent wants. And it differs from a permissive style of feeding in which there are few boundaries with eating, or from a neglectful style in which healthy family nutrition is barely a thought or a priority.

Eating together as a family should always be encouraged (Figure 12-1). Studies show that children who eat together with their family have healthier bodies, do better in school, have less risk-taking behaviors with drugs and alcohol, and have improved self-esteem. It is hard to dispute that it is one of the simplest and most effective ways for parents to be engaged in their children's lives.

Parents should be aware that it is not uncommon for children's appetites to vary. The rate of growth is not constant. As the child ages, the rate of growth actually slows. The approximate weight gain of a child during the second year of life

FIGURE 12-1 A family sitting down for a meal together.

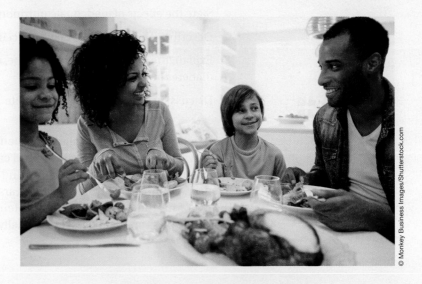

© Monkey Business Images/Shutterstock.com

is only 5 lb. In addition, children's attention is increasingly focused on their environment rather than their stomachs. Consequently, their appetites and interest in food commonly decrease during the early years. Children between the ages of 1 and 3 undergo vast changes. Their legs grow longer, they develop muscles, they lose their baby shape, they begin to walk and talk, and they learn to feed and generally assert themselves. A 2-year-old child's statement "No!" is his or her way of saying "Let me decide!"

As children continue to grow and develop, they are anxious to show their growing independence. Parents should respect this need within safe and loving limits. Children's likes and dislikes may change. New foods should be introduced gradually, in small amounts, and made attractive to the eye. Parents need to understand very young children are generally **neophobic** and that it can easily take up to 10 times of exposure before a new food is eaten. Allowing children to assist in purchasing and preparing a new food is often a good way of arousing interest in the food and a desire to eat it. Playing with pretend food not only helps children with fine motor skill development but can serve as a teachable "food" moment as they role model and have imaginary play (see Figure 12-2).

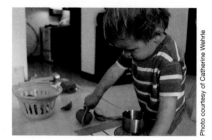

FIGURE 12-2 Learning about food and preparation can start with creative play.

Children should be offered nutrient-dense foods because the amount eaten often will be small. Fats should not be limited before the age of 2 years, but still avoid fat-laden meals and snacks. Whole milk is recommended until the age of 2 as extra fat is needed for brain development. Low-fat or fat-free milk should be served from age 2 and beyond. It is recommended that children not salt their food at the table or have foods prepared with a lot of salt. The same can be said for sugary foods or use of sugar at the table. Young children are especially sensitive to and reject hot (temperature) foods, but they will like crisp textures, mild flavors, and familiar foods. They may be wary of foods covered in sauce or gravy. Table 12-1 details serving sizes needed of the various food groups according to a child's age. Calorie needs will depend on rate of growth, activity level, body size, metabolism, and health.

Children can have food jags, such as eating only one or two foods, or rituals, such as not letting foods touch on the plate or using a different spoon for each food eaten. Choking is prevalent in young children. To prevent choking, do not give children under 4 years of age peanuts, grapes, hot dogs, raw carrots, hard candy, or thick peanut butter.

Often young children need a snack every two to three hours for continued energy. Children often prefer finger foods for snacks. Snacks should be nutrient dense and as nutritious as food served at mealtime. Fruit, a fiber-rich unsweetened cereal, and low-fat cheese make good snacks. Mealtime should be pleasant, and food should not be forced on the child. *The parents' primary responsibility is to provide nutritious*

neophobic
fear of anything new

TABLE 12-1 Food Plan for Preschool and School-Age Children Based on MyPlate

FOOD GROUP	APPROXIMATE SERVING SIZES PER DAY			
	AGES 1–2	**AGES 3–4**	**AGES 5–6**	**AGES 7–12**
Milk	1½–2 cups	2½ cups	3 cups	3 cups
Protein	1–2 oz	3–4 oz	5 oz	5–6 oz
Vegetable	½–1 cup	1½ cups	2 cups	2–3 cups
Fruit	½–1 cup	1½ cups	1½ cups	1½–2 cups
Grains	1½–3 oz	4–5 oz	5 oz	5–7 oz
Oils and fats are not represented as one of the major food groups, but you need some for good health. Appropriate ranges are provided here. Plant-based fats are recommended as the major fat source.				
Oils/Fat	3 tsp	4 tsp	4 tsp	5 tsp
Discretionary calorie allowance can range from 100–200 cal/day.				

Source: Adapted from United States Departments of Agriculture. *Daily Food Plans.* 2015. http://www.choosemyplate.gov

TABLE 12-2 Estimated Daily Calorie Needs for Children

CHILDREN	SEDENTARY TO ACTIVE (IN CALORIES)
2–3 yr	1,000–1,400
4–8 yr girl	1,200–1,800
4–8 yr boy	1,400–2,000
9–13 yr girl	1,600–2,200
9–13 yr boy	1,800–2,600

Source: U.S. Department of Agriculture and U.S. Department of Health and Human Services. *Dietary Guidelines for Americans, 2015* (8th ed.). Washington, DC: U.S. Government Printing Office. http://www.cnpp.usda.gov

food in a pleasant setting, and the child's responsibility is to decide how much food to eat or whether to eat, according to child expert Ellyn Satter (1995). When a child is hungry, he or she will eat. Forcing a child to eat can cause disordered eating and, ultimately, chronic overeating, **anorexia nervosa**, or **bulimia** (discussed later in this chapter).

Calorie and Nutrient Needs

The *rate* of growth diminishes from the age of 1 until about 10 years; thus, the caloric requirement per pound of body weight also diminishes during this period. For example, at 6 months, a girl needs about 54 calories per pound of body weight, but by the age of 10, she will require only 35 calories per pound of body weight. See Table 12-2 for estimated calorie needs of young children.

anorexia nervosa
psychologically induced lack of appetite

bulimia
condition in which client alternately binges and purges

My Daily Food Plan

Based on the information you provided, this is your daily recommended amount for each food group.

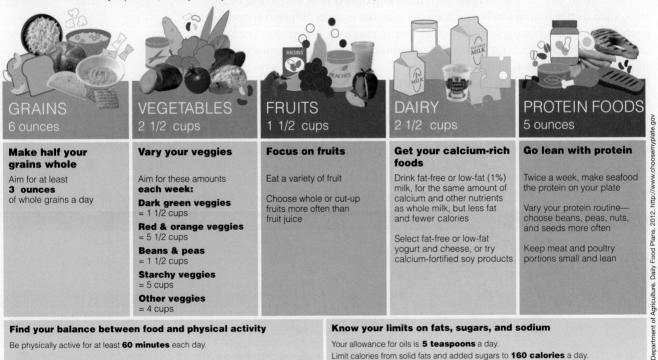

GRAINS 6 ounces	VEGETABLES 2 1/2 cups	FRUITS 1 1/2 cups	DAIRY 2 1/2 cups	PROTEIN FOODS 5 ounces
Make half your grains whole Aim for at least **3 ounces** of whole grains a day	**Vary your veggies** Aim for these amounts **each week:** **Dark green veggies** = 1 1/2 cups **Red & orange veggies** = 5 1/2 cups **Beans & peas** = 1 1/2 cups **Starchy veggies** = 5 cups **Other veggies** = 4 cups	**Focus on fruits** Eat a variety of fruit Choose whole or cut-up fruits more often than fruit juice	**Get your calcium-rich foods** Drink fat-free or low-fat (1%) milk, for the same amount of calcium and other nutrients as whole milk, but less fat and fewer calories Select fat-free or low-fat yogurt and cheese, or try calcium-fortified soy products	**Go lean with protein** Twice a week, make seafood the protein on your plate Vary your protein routine—choose beans, peas, nuts, and seeds more often Keep meat and poultry portions small and lean

Find your balance between food and physical activity
Be physically active for at least **60 minutes** each day.

Know your limits on fats, sugars, and sodium
Your allowance for oils is **5 teaspoons** a day.
Limit calories from solid fats and added sugars to **160 calories** a day.
Reduce sodium intake to less than **2,300 mg** a day.

Your results are based on a 1,800-calorie pattern.   Name: _____

This calorie level is only an estimate of your needs. Monitor your body weight to see if you need to adjust your calorie intake.

U.S. Department of Agriculture. Daily Food Plans. 2012. http://www.choosemyplate.gov

FIGURE 12-3 Use ChooseMyPlate to view a customized daily food plan.   *(Continued)*

My Daily Food Plan Worksheet

Check how you did today and set a goal to aim for tomorrow

Write in Your Food Choices for Today	Food Group	Tip	Based on a 1,800-calorie pattern. Your Goals Are:	Match Your Food Choices with Each Food Group	Estimate Your Total
_____ _____ _____ _____	GRAINS	Make at least half your grains whole grains	6 ounce equivalents (1 ounce equivalent is about 1 slice bread; 1 ounce ready-to-eat cereal; or ½ cup cooked rice, pasta, or cereal)	_____ _____ _____	ounce equivalents
_____ _____ _____ _____	VEGETABLES	Aim for variety every day; pick vegetables from several subgroups: Dark green, red & orange, beans & peas, starchy, and other veggies	2½ cups (1 cup is 1 cup raw or cooked vegetables, 2 cups leafy salad greens, or 1 cup100% vegetable juice)	_____ _____	cups
_____ _____ _____	FRUITS	Select fresh, frozen, canned, and dried fruit more often than juice	1½ cups (1 cup is 1 cup raw or cooked fruit, ½ cup dried fruit, or 1 cup 100% fruit juice)	_____ _____	cups
_____ _____ _____	DAIRY	Include fat-free and low-fat dairy foods every day	2½ cups (1 cup is 1 cup milk, yogurt, or fortified soy beverage; 1½ ounces natural cheese; or 2 ounces processed cheese)	_____ _____	cups
_____ _____ _____ _____	PROTEIN FOODS	Aim for variety—choose seafood, lean meat & poultry, beans, peas, nuts, and seeds each week	5 ounce equivalents (1 ounce equivalent is 1 ounce lean meat, poultry, or seafood; 1 egg; 1 Tbsp peanut butter; ¼ cup cooked beans or peas; or ½ ounce nuts or seeds)	_____ _____	ounce equivalents
_____ _____ _____	PHYSICAL ACTIVITY	Be active every day. Choose activities that you like and fit into your life.	Be physically active for at least 60 minutes each day.	Some foods and drinks, such as sodas, cakes, cookies, donuts, ice cream, and candy, are high in fats and sugars. Limit your intake of these.	minutes

How did you do today? ☐ Great   ☐ So-So   ☐ Not So Great

My food goal for tomorrow is: _____

My activity goal for tomorrow is: _____

FIGURE 12-3 *(Continued)*

Nutrient needs, however, do not diminish. From the age of 6 months to 10 years, nutrient needs actually *increase* because of the increase in body size. Therefore, it is especially important that young children are given nutritious foods *that they will eat.* The Dietary Reference Intake (DRI) tables show the amount of macronutrients (carbohydrates, protein, and fat) needed for children at different ages. The micronutrients (vitamins, minerals, and trace elements) are shown on the other DRI tables by life stage. The Choose MyPlate Daily Food Plans (Figure 12-3) serve as a good foundation for developing meal plans that, with adjustments, will suit all family members. These can be accessed on the Choosemyplate.gov site under "interactive tools."

The new *Dietary Guidelines* published in 2015 address eating changes for individuals starting at age 2. Americans are encouraged to consume more of certain foods and nutrients such as fruits, vegetables, whole grains, fat-free and low-fat dairy products, seafood, and alternative protein sources such as starchy beans, nuts, and seeds. We are cautioned to consume fewer foods with sodium (salt), saturated fats, trans fats, added sugars, refined grains, and animal-based foods such as red meat due to health and sustainability issues.

High-nutrition vegetables include choices in the broccoli family, orange vegetables, and leafy-green vegetables. High-nutrition fruits include citrus and berries. These have been coined the "powerhouse fruits and vegetables." Researchers believe that if Americans ate more of these nutrient-rich plant foods, a significant impact in public health would occur with disease prevention.

TABLE 12-3 Fiber Needs for Children

AGE	ADEQUATE INTAKE (AI) (IN GRAMS)
1–3 yr	19
4–8 yr	25
9–13 yr male	31
14–18 yr male	38
9–13 yr female	26
14–18 yr female	26

Reprinted with permission from the National Academies Press, Copyright © 2006, National Academy of Sciences. Dietary Reference Intakes: *The Essential Guide to Nutrient Requirements.*

Children also need water and fiber in their diet. Generally, fluid requirements are estimated at 1 mL of water for every calorie consumed: 1,200 calories intake = 1,200 mL or 5 cups. It should be noted, however, that many fruits and vegetables and milk will contribute to hydration and help fulfill fluid needs.

The Dietary Reference Intake charts list the requirement for fiber in children (Table 12-3). Fiber is often lacking in children's diets due to a marketplace that is flooded with refined, processed foods. Fiber is needed for bowel health and regularity as well as maintenance of healthy cholesterol levels. Fiber ideally needs to come in natural forms: beans, whole grains, fruits, and vegetables (Figure 12-4). These foods contain a mix of different fibers as well as key vitamins, minerals, and healthful plant chemicals, or phytochemicals. Some food products sold today have added fiber and may be useful in boosting fiber to the recommended intake level providing that individuals strive for the natural forms first.

The most recent Healthy Eating Index-2010 analysis from National Health and Examination Survey (NHANES) data underscores that the diet of children 2–17 years fell considerably short of recommendations. The data showed only 22% of children meeting whole grain requirements, and only 20% meeting requirement for dark greens and starchy bean intake. Whole fruit intake results show that 70% of our children are meeting recommendations.

As children get older, the following also occurs:

- Reduction in regular breakfast consumption
- Increase in foods prepared away from home
- Increase in snacking
- Increase in fried foods (especially French fries) and nutrient-poor food
- Increase in portion size
- Increase in sweetened beverages and sugar

Poor diet patterns and imbalances can set children up for health issues such as obesity, cardiovascular disease, high blood pressure, and pre-diabetes. Positive nutrition education and practices therefore need to happen broadly—in primary care settings, schools, and homes across the nation and start at a young age.

As kids desire sweets and prefer these to nutrient-rich foods, sugar-laden dessert and snack foods should be given sparingly. Sweetened drinks and fruit juices should be limited. The gold standard is for health practitioners to suggest limiting juice to only 4–6 oz per day for children aged 1–6, and ensure that it is 100% juice. The appropriate range of juice for older children is 8–12 oz per day. Frequent exposure of teeth to sugary foods, especially sticky sweet foods, increases the likelihood of dental caries.

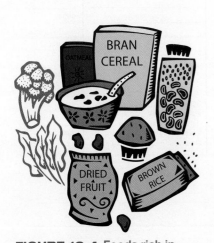

FIGURE 12-4 Foods rich in fiber.

In The Media

Food Insecurity and Children's Health

A new report from the American Academy of Pediatrics (AAP) stresses that pediatricians screen all children for food insecurity. It is known that more than 15 million U.S. children live in households struggling with hunger. These children suffer a myriad of consequences, such as getting sick more often, recovering more slowly from illness, poorer overall health, and more frequent hospitalizations. Children and adolescents affected by food insecurity are more likely to be iron deficient. They may also suffer from obesity and metabolic syndrome. Lack of food is tied to poorer ability to concentrate and perform in school and is linked to higher levels of behavioral and emotional problems. AAP recommends that doctors become familiar with community resources and advocate for policies that support adequate access to nutritious foods.

Source: Adapted from "Lack of Adequate Food Is Ongoing Health Risk to US Children." *Science Daily*. October 23, 2015. www.sciencedaily.com

Assessing Growth

Pediatric growth charts from the Centers for Disease Control and Prevention (CDC) have been used by pediatricians, dietitians, nurses, and parents to track the growth of infants, children, and adolescents in the United States since 1977 (Figure 12-5). It is recommended that health care providers use the following:

- World Health Organization (WHO) growth standards to monitor growth for infants and children 0–2 years of age in the United States
- CDC growth charts for children 2 years of age and older in the United States

The growth charts for youth 2–20 years of age measure stature-for-age, weight-for-age, and body mass index-for-age and consist of a series of percentile curves that illustrate the distribution of these measurements in children. As mentioned in the infancy chapter, the CDC has a self-directed interactive

Exploring THE WEB

Visit the Action for Healthy Kids website (www.actionforhealthykids.org) to learn what resources are available to help our youth stay well in the school setting. Learn about strategies that can help change school policy, environment, and systems and why school and family partnerships are so vital.

SUPERSIZE USA

Chronic sleep deprivation is linked to obesity in our youth. It is known that 68% of high schoolers do not get eight hours of sleep. Late bedtimes are to blame. For each hour of delaying sleep on weeknights, there was a more than two-point increase in body mass index (BMI). And the quality of sleep seems to be suffering as well. If there is increased phone use before bed, a negative impact is seen on alertness the next day. Nearly 62% of kids used their smartphone before bed, with nearly 57% texting, tweeting, or messaging in bed. Just over 20% of teens awoke to texts throughout the night. Excessive stimulation at night from the light of electronic devices can suppress melatonin, which helps to promote sleep. This poor-quality sleep may be linked to depression, anxiety, and ADHD. Parents should be encouraged to limit phone usage at night and to shuttle kids off to bed at a decent time for good health.

Adapted from Preidt, Robert. (2015, Oct 2). "For Teens, Late Bedtime May Lead to Weight Gain." *HealthDay*. U.S. National Library of Medicine. Accessed October 2015. Also adapted from Preidt, Robert. (2015, Oct 7). "Bedtime Texting May be Hazardous to Teen's Health." *HealthDay*. U.S. National Library of Medicine. Accessed October 2015.

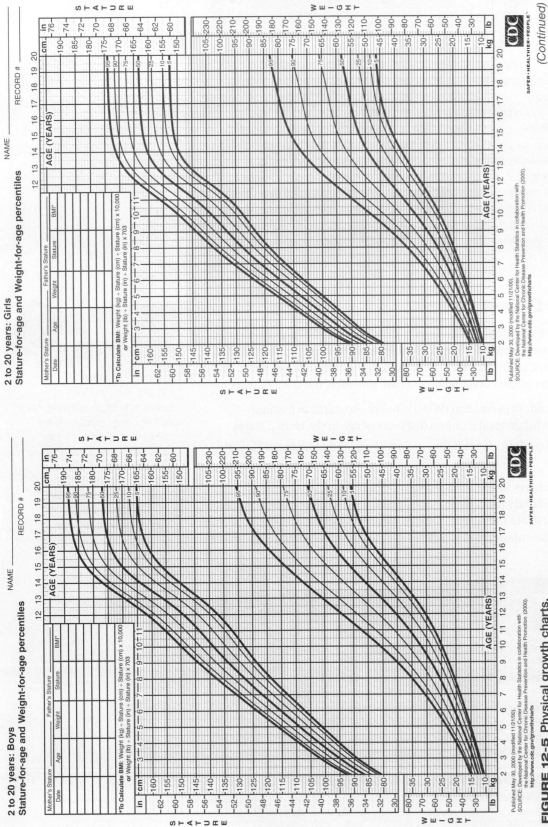

FIGURE 12-5 Physical growth charts.

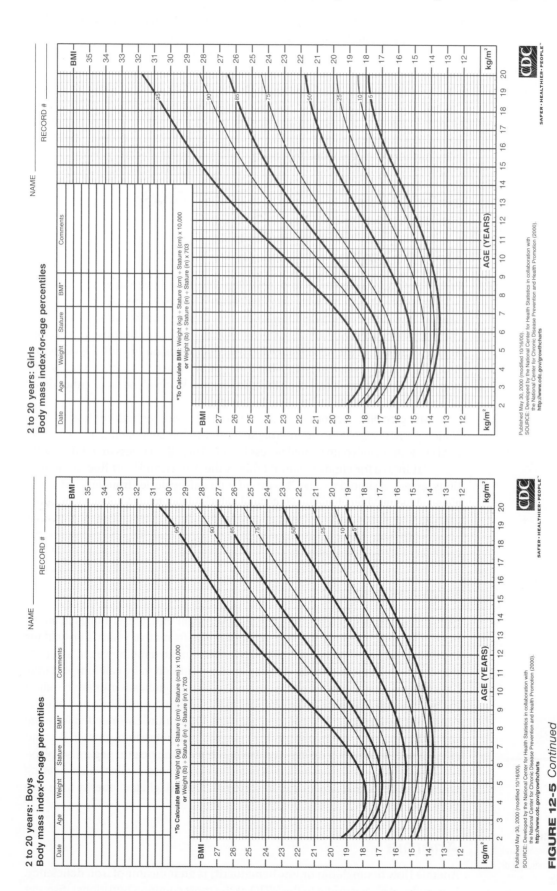

FIGURE 12-5 *Continued*

Centers for Disease Control and Prevention, National Center for Health Statistics in collaboration with the National Center for Chronic Disease Prevention and Health Promotion. 2000 CDC Growth Charts: United States. http://www.cdc.gov/growthcharts, retrieved October 2015. Additional clinical growth charts with the 3rd and 97th percentiles can be found on the CDC website.

training course for the growth charts on its website. **Body mass index (BMI)** is a number calculated from a person's weight and height and is a fairly reliable indicator of body fatness for most people. A BMI calculator is available on the MyPlate website (http://www.choosemyplate.gov), under the SuperTracker tab.

Growth charts are not intended to be used as the only diagnostic instrument but can contribute to forming an overall clinical impression for the child being measured. Clinicians find it useful to track children's growth over time to see if growth is happening in a predictable way. Changes in the growth chart alert practitioners to delve further into current health practices that have been affecting growth.

SPECIAL HEALTH CONCERNS DURING CHILDHOOD

Heart Health

Proper nutrition is vital to heart health. Recent studies have shown that children with one or both parents who have had heart disease before age 60 were more likely to have atherosclerosis themselves. Further, researchers know the risk of coronary artery disease increases progressively with age. Because it has been demonstrated that the atherosclerotic process can begin in youth, good nutrition, a physically active lifestyle, and absence of tobacco use are of utmost importance. These factors can contribute to lower risk prevalence and either delay or prevent the onset of cardiovascular disease.

Many health practitioners screen children at age 2 for high cholesterol. The National Cholesterol Education Program and AAP has suggested that acceptable total cholesterol for youth should be less than 170 mg/dl (LDL less than 110 mg/dl).

Fat intake for children should follow the American Heart Recommendations: ages 1–3 should receive 30–40% of total daily calories from fat, and youth ages 4–18 should receive 25–35% of total calories from fat. If aiming for no more than 30% total calories from fat, an ideal fat distribution would be saturated fat at no more than 7%, polyunsaturated fat at no more than 8%, and monounsaturated fat at 15% of total calories.

Bone Health

Optimizing bone health in youth results in stronger and denser bones in adulthood. Consumption of adequate calcium in the formative years is critical for the development of peak bone mass. Nutrient intake data, however, suggests that some children and teens do not consume enough daily calcium and may have less than ideal bone health. Vitamin D is also a significant nutrient required for bone health. As described elsewhere in this text, many children and adolescents may be lacking this important nutrient. Other nutrients needed for bone strengthening are protein, phosphorus, magnesium, potassium, vitamin B_{12}, and zinc. Genetics and physical activity also influence bone health. Regarding physical activity, lower levels of activity among our youth, especially weight-bearing types, have been linked to greater fracture risk. Overweight and obesity have also been linked to compromised bone health in children.

Anemia

Anemia (low hemoglobin or low hematocrit) is an indicator of iron deficiency. Iron deficiency, according to the WHO, is the most common nutritional disorder

body mass index (BMI)
a number calculated from a person's weight and height as a fairly reliable indicator of body fatness for most people

in the world. It is currently affecting millions of children in developing countries. Anemia is associated with developmental delays and behavior problems in children. The CDC reports that anemia occurs in 14% of U.S. toddlers (age 1–2 years). At this time of life, toddlers transition from their iron-rich infant foods to table food and cow's milk, which contains less iron.

The incidence of anemia is slightly higher in low-income children and varies by racial and ethnic groups, with the highest prevalence among African American children. The AAP recommends screening for anemia between the ages of 9 and 12 months with additional screening between the ages of 1 and 5 years for clients at risk. Red meat, poultry and seafood, egg yolk, and iron-fortified breads and cereals can help meet iron needs. Vegetables and fruits such as spinach and other greens, peas, broccoli, dried beans, and dried fruit (raisins, dates, apricots) are iron rich as well. Vitamin C–containing foods eaten along with iron-rich foods enhance absorption of the iron.

Medicines That Increase or Decrease Appetite

Certain medications (psychostimulants) used to treat attention deficit and hyperactivity disorder (ADHD) in children cause marked decrease in appetite. According to the CDC, in the United States, 9.5% or 5.9 million children aged 3–17 have an ADHD diagnosis, as of 2012. In practice, parents of the medicated ADHD child often see a compromised appetite especially at the lunch meal, when the medicine is most active.

If a child's appetite decreases after taking ADHD medicine, it is recommended to give the dose after breakfast so that he or she will eat better in the morning. A parent may then want to serve a large dinner in the evening, when the drug is beginning to wear off. Often the bedtime snack needs to turn into the "third meal." Parents will need to keep plenty of healthy snacks on hand; a balanced diet with nutritious, higher-calorie foods and drinks will help to offset any weight loss from the ADHD medication.

Some health care providers may see changes in the growth of a child on some of these stimulants. If the child's poor appetite lasts for a long period, the health care provider may reduce the dose or stop the drug on weekends or summer breaks to allow appetite to return to normal. The provider may reevaluate the medication chosen.

On the other end of the spectrum, children and adolescents who take some of the newer generation of antipsychotic medications for mood stabilization and behavior issues have increased appetite. Users of those medicines risk rapid weight gain and metabolic changes that could lead to diabetes, hypertension, and other illnesses. Some children on those medicines were recorded to have an average weight gain of 1–1.5 lb a week. Doctors believe, however, that these drugs still have their place in behavioral health, as they can spare children from psychological suffering. But practitioners are learning that they must be prescribed more cautiously and that the benefits must be weighed against the risks.

Food Allergies

Researchers are now estimating that as many as 1 out of 13 children under age 18 have allergies to at least one food. Preschoolers (age 3–5 years) have been shown to have the highest prevalence of allergies. Allergies to peanuts were the most commonly reported, affecting 2% of children. Milk and shellfish allergies ranked

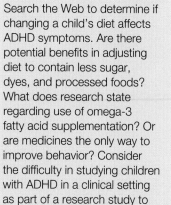

Exploring THE WEB

Search the Web to determine if changing a child's diet affects ADHD symptoms. Are there potential benefits in adjusting diet to contain less sugar, dyes, and processed foods? What does research state regarding use of omega-3 fatty acid supplementation? Or are medicines the only way to improve behavior? Consider the difficulty in studying children with ADHD in a clinical setting as part of a research study to determine diet effectiveness.

second and third. Tree nuts, egg, fish, strawberry, wheat, and soy rounded out the top nine food triggers. Some children with food allergies have mild cases and they outgrow them in time; however, researchers are discovering that 40% of children experience severe reactions, including wheezing and anaphylaxis. The Food Allergy Network (http://www.foodallergy.org) has useful information for families that are experiencing allergies. See Chapter 20 for further discussion on food allergies.

OBESITY AND RELATED HEALTH COMPLICATIONS

In America today, unprecedented numbers of our youth are being diagnosed with overweight and obesity. This is leading to a cascade of serious illnesses including pre-diabetes, diabetes, hypertension, and cardiovascular disease.

Obesity

Childhood overweight and obesity is a result of an imbalance between the energy taken in from food and beverages and the energy expended for normal growth and development as well as physical activity. No single factor causes obesity; rather, researchers believe it can stem from many factors, including genetic, behavioral, and environmental issues. Childhood obesity has more than doubled in children and quadrupled in adolescents in the past 30 years. The CDC estimates that approximately 17% (or 12.7 million) of children and adolescents aged 2–19 years are obese.

The obesity epidemic is disproportionally higher among children living in low-income, low-education, and higher-unemployment households, according to data from the National Survey of Children's Health. There are significant racial and ethnic disparities in obesity prevalence among U.S. children and adolescents. Hispanic youth and non-Hispanic black youth stand out as the groups experiencing higher rates of obesity. Further discussion on childhood obesity occurs in the weight management chapter (Chapter 14).

Pre-Diabetes and Diabetes

The prevalence of pre-diabetes and diabetes in youth has increased significantly. A study in the *Journal of Pediatrics* in 2012 reported that rates increased from 9% to 23% between the years 1999 and 2008. Pre-diabetes means that the blood sugar level is higher than normal, but not increased enough to be classified as type 2 diabetes. Pre-diabetes is defined as a fasting blood sugar between 100 and 126 mg/dl. Another name associated with pre-diabetes is *metabolic syndrome* or *insulin resistance*. Besides the elevated blood sugar, other factors may sometimes be present: high waist circumference, increasing blood pressure, and impaired lipids such as high triglycerides and low HDL (high-density lipoprotein). Exercise, diet, and weight changes are effective at turning around pre-diabetes. Specific to diet, research is beginning to show that fiber in addition to a high phytochemical intake from plant foods helps improve pre-diabetes.

Acanthosis nigricans is a hyper-pigmentation of the skin characterized by dark, thick, velvety skin in body folds and creases. Most practitioners see these skin changes around the neck during routine exams. This disorder is often associated with conditions that increase insulin level, such as type 2 diabetes or being overweight. If the insulin level is too high, the extra insulin may trigger activity in skin cells. This may cause the characteristic skin changes.

The increasing frequency of both type 1 and type 2 diabetes in youth has been one of the more troubling aspects of the diabetes epidemic. Type 1 diabetes (formerly called juvenile diabetes) is a chronic condition in which the pancreas produces little or no insulin. Nearly 167,000 U.S. youth younger than age 20 had type I diabetes in 2009. More than 18,000 new cases of type 1 are estimated to be diagnosed among U.S. youth each year. More information is available in Chapter 15.

Type 2 diabetes in children and adolescents already appears to be a significant and growing problem, with more than 5,000 new cases estimated to be diagnosed each year. Overall, diabetes is on the rise for all ages. In fact, the CDC states that one in three children born after the year 2000 will develop diabetes. Children and adolescents diagnosed with type 2 diabetes are generally between 10 and 19 years old, obese, have a strong family history for type 2 diabetes, and have insulin resistance. Diabetes screening is recommended for all children and adolescents at high risk, even if they have no signs or symptoms of the condition.

Those affected with type 2 diabetes belong to all ethnic groups, but it is more commonly seen in non-white groups. CDC data indicates American Indian youths have the highest prevalence of type 2 diabetes. Diabetics are at higher risk of heart disease, kidney disease, and neuropathy, among others. Children with type 2 diabetes should see a certified diabetes educator to learn what to eat to control their diabetes. This specialist will also prescribe daily exercise and attention to fiber intake, both of which help control blood glucose.

Hypertension

High blood pressure in children may be the result of an underlying disease process or the early onset of hypertension. Hypertension among overweight or obese youth worsens with time if left untreated. Diagnosing hypertension in children is done using the National Heart Lung and Blood Institute's blood pressure tables for children and adolescents, which look at age, gender, and height (http://www.nhlbi.nih.gov). Several blood pressure percentile readings over the 95th percentile suggest a diagnosis of hypertension. Regular aerobic activity, normalization of BMI, and watching sodium all improve blood pressure in youth.

Cardiovascular Disease

Children with the highest risks of developing cardiovascular disease are those who are sedentary and obese and may have diabetes or pre-diabetes. Youth who also have high blood pressure and high LDL cholesterol are at increased risk as well. Many children in late childhood or early adolescence already have fatty streaks in their coronary arteries. An overweight child who is sedentary, or one who consumes a diet high in saturated fat, should have routine cholesterol screenings throughout their youth.

A multipronged approach of sound health messaging will need to be communicated to youth. Parents hold the primary reigns for the change to begin. Health care providers, schools and daycares, government agencies and others will need to work in tandem to change the culture of health if we are to turn the tide in obesity, pre-diabetes and diabetes in our youth.

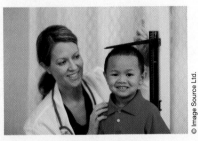

FIGURE 12-6 The doctor measures a child's height to record on the growth chart.

ADOLESCENTS

In general, a person between the ages of 13 and 20 is considered an adolescent. Adolescence is a period of rapid growth that causes major changes. It tends to begin between the ages of 10 and 13 in girls and between 13 and 16 in boys. A **growth spurt** may yield a height increase of 3 inches a year for girls and 4 inches a year for boys (Figure 12-6). Bones grow and gain density, muscle and fat tissue develop, and blood volume increases. Sexual maturity occurs: boys' voices change, girls experience the onset of **menses**, and both may experience acne. Note that acne is not caused by eating specific foods but by having overactive sebaceous glands of the skin.

These changes are obvious and have a tremendous effect on an adolescent's psychosocial development. No two individuals will develop in the same way. One girl may become heavier than she might like, another may be thin, a boy may not develop the muscle or the height he desires, and some may develop serious complexion problems. Many teens will accept their changes, while others may need psychological counseling.

Food Habits

Adolescents, especially boys, typically have enormous appetites. When good eating habits have been established during childhood and there is nutritious food available, the teenager's food habits should present no serious problem.

Adolescents are imitators, like children, but instead of imitating adults, adolescents prefer to imitate their **peers** and do what is popular. Unfortunately, foods that are popular such as potato chips, sodas, and candy, often have low nutrient density. These foods provide mainly carbohydrates and fats and very little protein, vitamins, and minerals, except for salt, which is usually provided in excess. According to the Center for Science in the Public Interest, on average, teens get 13% of their calories from carbonated and noncarbonated soft drinks. It provides the average 12–19-year-old boy with about 15 tsp of refined sugars a day and the average girl with about 10 tsp a day—an amount that has public health officials concerned (Figure 12-7).

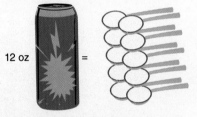

12 oz =

FIGURE 12-7 One 12 oz can of soda = 10 tsp of sugar.

The concern of soda is not simply all the sugary calories, but for what soda pushes out of the diet. Youth used to consume twice as much milk as soft drinks. On average at present, boys and girls consume twice as much soda pop as milk.

Adolescents' eating habits can be seriously affected by busy schedules, part-time jobs, athletics, social activities, and the lack of an available adult to prepare nutritious food when they are hungry or have time to eat. When adolescents' food habits need improvement, it is wise for adults to tactfully inform them of nutritional needs and of the poor nutrition quality of their food choices. The adolescent has a natural desire for independence and may resent being told what to do.

Before attempting to change food habits, carefully check an adolescent's food choices for nutrient content. It is too easily assumed that because the adolescent chooses the food, the food is automatically a poor choice in regard to nutrient content. It might be a good choice. An adolescent who has a problem maintaining an appropriate weight may need some advice regarding diet.

Calorie and Nutrient Needs

Because of adolescents' rapid growth, calorie requirements naturally increase. Boys' calorie requirements tend to be greater than girls' because boys are

growth spurt
significant rapid gain in size near the onset of adolescence

menses
another term for menstruation

peers
people who are approximately one's own age

generally bigger, tend to be more physically active, and have more lean muscle mass than girls.

The requirement for energy-containing nutrients, vitamins, and minerals all dramatically increase more during adolescence than at any other time of life except pregnancy and lactation. The DRI table provides such changes by life stage. Because of menstruation, girls have a greater need for iron than boys. Calcium requirements are high to support peak bone mass. Optimizing calcium intake for bone health is particularly important during adolescence, as peak use of calcium for bone mineralization occurs on average at 12.5 years in girls and 14.0 years in boys. In a three- to four-year period in adolescence, 40% of total adult bone mass is accumulated. It has been understood that low calcium intake in adolescence is problematic in America. It has been estimated that greater than 50% of our teens do not meet the requirement for calcium in their diets.

SPECIAL HEALTH CONCERNS DURING ADOLESCENCE

Adolescence is a stressful time for most young people. They are unexpectedly faced with numerous physical changes, an innate need for independence, increased work and extracurricular demands at school and jobs, and social and sexual pressures from their peers.

Anorexia Nervosa

While eating disorders may begin with an innocent attempt at dieting and losing weight, they are most often about much more than this. People with eating disorders often use food and the control of food in an attempt to compensate for difficult feelings and emotions that may seem overwhelming in their lives. Low self-esteem, troubled relationships, being teased about body issues, and stress are just some of the factors that play into the development of an eating disorder. Some may fear growing up. Many have overachieving personalities and are perfectionistic. Cultural factors also come into play, as many want to resemble the slim fashion models exhibited in the media (Figure 12-8). As many as 10 million females and 1 million males are fighting a battle with an eating disorder. Some individuals switch from one eating disorder pattern to another, or have a mixture of disordered eating traits.

Anorexia nervosa is a serious, potentially life-threatening eating disorder characterized by self-starvation and excessive weight loss. Anorexia nervosa has four primary symptoms:

1. Failure to maintain body weight at or above a minimally normal weight for age and height; usually 85% of expected weight
2. Intense fear of weight gain or being "fat," even though underweight
3. Disturbance with body weight or shape
4. Loss of menstrual periods in girls and women post-puberty

Anorexia, a psychological disorder, is more common in women than men. It can begin as early as late childhood, but usually begins during the teen years or early 20s. The dramatic reduction in calories causes altered metabolism, hair loss, low blood pressure, weakness, **amenorrhea**, brain damage, and even death.

Individuals with anorexia usually set a maximum weight for themselves and become an expert at "counting calories" to attain their chosen weight.

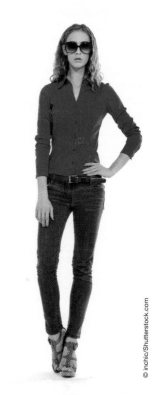

FIGURE 12-8 The average model is 5'10" and weighs 110 lb; however, an average 5'5" teen is 125–130 lb.

amenorrhea
the stoppage of the monthly menstrual flow

They also often exercise excessively to control or reduce their weight. Often once they achieve their weight goal, they are not satisfied and want to lose even more weight. If weight declines too far, organ failure will occur and the anorexic will ultimately die.

Treatment requires the following:

1. Development of a strong and trusting relationship between the client and the health care professionals involved in the case.

2. That the client learn and accept that weight gain and a change in body contours are normal during adolescence.

3. Nutritional therapy so the client will understand the need for both nutrients and calories and how best to obtain them.

4. Individual and family counseling by a licensed family therapist, ideally with a specialty in eating disorder counseling.

5. Medical monitoring by the doctor and full health care professional team.

6. Dedication to following up in an outpatient setting and progressing with goals, or movement to a partial hospitalization or full hospitalization program if further support is needed.

7. Time and patience from all involved. Often if someone has been hospitalized for an eating disorder, it can be difficult to return home with the influence of family and friends. Therapy usually addresses this important transition.

Bulimia

Bulimia is a syndrome in which an individual alternately binges on food then purges by inducing vomiting or using laxatives or diuretics, or overexercises, to compensate and "rid" oneself of ingested food. Bulimics are said to fear that they cannot stop eating. They tend to be high achievers who are perfectionistic, obsessive, and depressed. They generally lack a strong sense of self and have a need to seem special. They know their binge–purge syndrome is abnormal but also fear being overweight. This condition is more common among women than men and can begin any time from the late teens into the 30s.

A bulimic usually binges on high-calorie foods such as cookies, ice cream, pastries, and other "forbidden" foods. The binge can take only a few moments or can run several hours—until there is no space for more food. It occurs when the person is alone. Bulimia can follow a period of excessive dieting, and stress usually increases the frequency of binges. Bulimia is not usually life threatening, but it can irritate the esophagus and cause electrolyte imbalances, malnutrition, dehydration, and dental caries. Laxative abuse can cause disturbance in sodium, potassium, magnesium, and phosphorus levels. Disrupting these electrolytes and minerals can cause issues with the colon and heart. Laxative abuse can result in severe dehydration, and dependence on increasing doses of laxatives to move the bowels.

Treatment involves helping the person learn how to live at peace with oneself and the food environment. Therapists, doctors, social workers, and dietitians are also involved with the treatments of this eating disorder. Returning to scheduled eating times, doing appetite awareness training and journaling, and developing alternate coping skills to destress are usual tactics that clients use to overcome bulimia.

Binge Eating Disorder

Another recognized eating disorder is binge eating, also known as compulsive overeating. This disorder manifests itself by periods of uncontrolled or impulsive eating beyond normal fullness. Individuals suffering from this do not purge; however, the binge may be precipitated by a fast or strict diet measure. Once a binge has occurred, feelings of guilt and shame usually occur. Individuals that compulsively overeat often struggle with anxiety, depression, and loneliness. While many binge eaters are obese, some may be only moderately overweight or even normal weight. Experts believe the binge eating disorder can easily start in the childhood or teen years.

Signs may include:

- A large amount of food missing from the refrigerator or pantry
- Visibly seeing a child eating a lot of food quickly
- A pattern of eating in response to emotional stress, such as family conflict, peer rejection, or poor academic performance
- A child feeling ashamed or disgusted by the amount eaten
- Finding food containers or wrappers hidden in a child's room
- An increasingly irregular eating pattern, such as skipping meals, eating lots of junk food, and eating at unusual times (such as late at night)

A parent must be coached on addressing this issue in a very gentle and loving way, so the child feels safe talking about the issue. Blaming, scolding, or punishing the child will only backfire. Mental health professionals can help address the underlying issues.

More and more health practitioners are seeing what is described as the female athletic triad. The symptoms of this are disordered eating, amenorrhea, and osteoporosis. Female athletes who exercise and train intensely have lower levels of estrogen. This combined with not eating enough calories (and commonly restricting fat) leads to menstrual irregularities or absence of menses, stress fractures, and early osteoporosis.

Eating disorder awareness and prevention are key. Parents of youth must model healthy body image and healthy self-esteem if their children are to develop these important attributes. It is clear that children are watching their parents at all times and observing the way they talk about themselves and their body. Respect and appreciation for what our bodies do for us must be part of the discussion we have with our youth. It's important we value ourselves based on character, talent, and accomplishments, rather than what we look like or what we weigh.

Overweight and Obesity in Teens

Being overweight during adolescence is particularly unfortunate because it is apt to diminish an individual's **self-esteem** and, consequently, can exclude her or him from the normal social life of the teen years, further diminishing self-esteem. Also, it tends to make the individual prone to overweight as an adult.

Genetics may play a role in overweight, but it's the environment that triggers overweight or obesity. Overfeeding during infancy and childhood can be a contributing factor. Once someone is overweight, isolative behavior may ensue. For example, if a teenager becomes the center of his classmates' jokes, he or she may prefer to spend time alone, perhaps watching television and finding comfort in food. This behavior adds more calories, reduces activity, and thus worsens the condition. Overweight or obese youth are at more risk for depression. In fact, obese children who were surveyed about their quality of life rated it as being as

self-esteem
feelings of self-worth

low as children receiving chemotherapy for cancer treatment. The problem of being overweight during adolescence is especially difficult to solve until the individual involved makes the independent decision to change lifestyle habits. After making such a decision, the teenager should see a physician to ensure proper health. The health care provider can play an important role by offering guidance on changing eating habits, increasing exercise, and adopting a healthier lifestyle. This issue is further addressed in the weight management chapter (Chapter 14).

Fast Foods

Many Americans have become extremely fond of fast foods. Data from the mid-1990s has shown that one-third of young people eat fast food. Portion sizes offered by fast food restaurants also grew during this time period, with individual items from two to five times larger than they were when originally introduced (Figure 12-9).

FIGURE 12-9 Fast food portion sizes have grown greatly from prior decades.

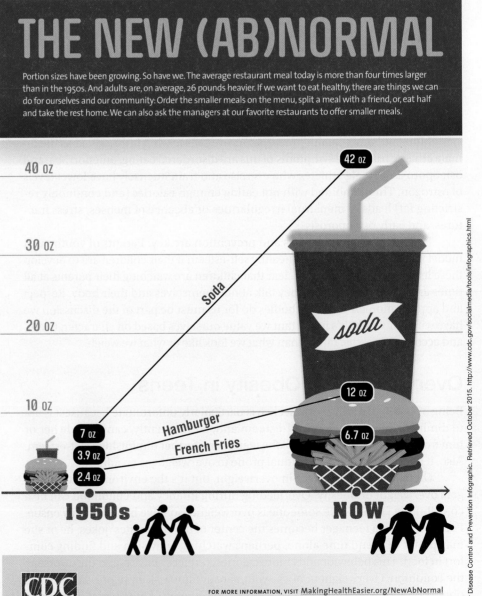

THE NEW (AB)NORMAL

Portion sizes have been growing. So have we. The average restaurant meal today is more than four times larger than in the 1950s. And adults are, on average, 26 pounds heavier. If we want to eat healthy, there are things we can do for ourselves and our community: Order the smaller meals on the menu, split a meal with a friend, or, eat half and take the rest home. We can also ask the managers at our favorite restaurants to offer smaller meals.

40 oz — 42 oz

30 oz

Soda

20 oz

10 oz — 12 oz

7 oz

Hamburger — 6.7 oz

French Fries

3.9 oz

2.4 oz

1950s — **NOW**

CDC

FOR MORE INFORMATION, VISIT <u>MakingHealthEasier.org/NewAbNormal</u>

Center for Disease Control and Prevention Infographic. Retrieved October 2015. http://www.cdc.gov/socialmedia/tools/infographics.html

Teenager favorites include hamburgers, cheeseburgers, French fries, milkshakes, pizza, sodas, tacos, fried chicken, and onion rings. These and other choices in fast food restaurants are high in fat, especially saturated fats, sodium, and sugar, and high in total calories. Generally speaking, many menu choices in a fast food restaurant are nutrient poor and energy dense. Vitamin, mineral, and fiber content are usually sorely lacking in these high-calorie foods.

Many fast food companies have the nutrient content of their products available to help the public make better choices. The Federal Drug Administration (FDA) now has a menu labeling compliance rule (effective December 2016) for establishments that have 20 or more locations. Most restaurants do offer some healthful and lower calorie choices on their menus, such as salads, grilled chicken, oatmeal, and fruit cups. Children can substitute apple or orange slices in place of French fries. These items are not big sellers, however, and unhealthy options are usually chosen.

The fast food industry spends more than $4 billion a year on media advertising to promote its products. Fast food has increasingly become inexpensive with the introduction of "dollar menu choices." Therefore, for a relatively small amount of money, we can become quite full. Health can suffer over the long term, however, with frequent fast food choices. Table 12-4 shows the nutrient content of a sample day of fast food eating for a teenage girl compared with the nutrients her body needs.

Alcohol

In a process called **fermentation**, sugars and starches can be changed to alcohol. Enzyme action causes this change. Alcohol is typically made from fruit, corn, rye, barley, rice, or potatoes. It provides 7 calories per gram but almost no nutrients.

Alcohol is a substance that can have serious side effects. Initially, it causes the drinker to feel "happy" because it lowers inhibitions. This feeling affects the drinker's judgment and can lead to accidents and crime. Ultimately, alcohol is a depressant; continued drinking leads to sleepiness, loss of consciousness, and, when too much is consumed in a short period, death.

Abuse (overuse) of alcohol is called **alcoholism**. Alcoholism can destroy the lives of families and devastate the drinker's nutritional status and thus health. It affects absorption and normal metabolism of glucose, fats, proteins, and vitamins. When thiamine and niacin cannot be absorbed, the cells cannot use glucose for energy. Blood cells, which depend on glucose for energy, are particularly affected. Alcohol causes kidneys to excrete larger-than-normal amounts of water, resulting in an increased loss of minerals. In a poor nutritional state, the body is less able to fight off disease.

In addition, excessive, long-term drinking can cause high blood pressure and can damage the heart muscle. It is associated with cancer of the throat and the esophagus and can damage the reproductive system.

The risks to the drinker are obvious. When a pregnant or lactating woman drinks, however, she puts the fetus or the nursing infant at risk as well. Alcohol can lower birth weight and cause fetal alcohol syndrome or fetal alcohol effect, with related developmental disorders (see Chapter 10).

Unfortunately, many teenagers ignore the dangers of alcohol and use it in an effort to appear adult. The 2013 Youth Risk Behavior Survey from the CDC found that among high school students, during the past 30 days: 34.9% drank some amount of alcohol and 20% binge drank. Alcohol use in teens has decreased since 1999. In addition to the damage to their own health, potential accidents, and the random acts of violence caused by their drinking, teenagers' behavior sets a poor example for younger children who emulate them.

fermentation
changing of sugars and starches to alcohol

alcoholism
chronic and excessive use of alcohol

TABLE 12-4 Calorie and Nutrient Content of a Fast Food Day of Eating Compared with Requirements for a Teenage Girl

SAMPLE DAY OF EATING FOR TEENAGE GIRL	AMOUNT	CALORIES	PROTEIN (g)	FAT (g)	CALCIUM (mg)	IRON (mg)	SODIUM (mg)	VITAMIN A (re)	VITAMIN C (mg)	FIBER (g)
Sausage muffin with egg	1	450	20	28	300	3	930	115	1	2
Hot chocolate	16 oz	100	0	0	0	0	85	0	0	0
Hamburger	1	292	15	11	84	3	555	3	0	2
French Fries, medium		389	5	21	16	2	235	0	3	4
Chocolate shake	10 oz	379	9	12	280	2	167	74	1	2
Pizza, pepperoni	¼ of 12"	500	22	20	282	4	1,144	127	0	3
Soda	16 oz	182	0	0	10	0	20	0	0	0
Daily Total		2,292	71	92	972	14	3,136	127	5	13
DRI/RDA for teenage girl		2,200	44	73	1,200	15	2,300	800	60	26

The health professional is in a good position to spread the message that alcohol is a substance that can cause severe economic and family problems, as well as addiction, disease, and death.

Marijuana

Approximately 23% of high school teens used marijuana one or more times within a 30-day period according to the latest Youth Risk Behavioral Surveillance System (2013). One marijuana cigarette is as harmful as four or five tobacco cigarettes, because the marijuana smoke is held in the lungs for a longer period of time. As a person smokes marijuana, the lungs absorb the fat-soluble active ingredient, delta-9-tetrahydrocannabinol (THC), and store it in the fat. Experts believe that the use of marijuana can lead to the use of other drugs, such as cocaine. Some common names for marijuana are *pot, grass, herb, weed, Mary Jane, reefer, dope, bud,* and *ganja.*

Cocaine

Cocaine is highly addictive and extremely harmful. It causes restlessness, heightened self-confidence, euphoria, irritability, insomnia, depression, confusion, hallucinations, loss of appetite, and a tendency to withdraw from normal activities. Cocaine can cause cardiac irregularities, heart attacks, and cardiac arrests, resulting in death. Weight loss is very common, mostly because it decreases appetite; addicts would give up food for the drug. The smokable form of cocaine is *crack,* which is more addictive than any other drug. It is estimated that half of all crimes against property committed in major cities are related to the use of crack cocaine and the addict's need for money to buy the drug.

Tobacco

Nicotine is dangerous for kids of any age. It is known that adolescence is a critical time for brain development and that the use of nicotine may cause lasting harm. It is highly addicting and can lead to sustained tobacco use. While cigarette smoking has declined from 2011 to 2014 per CDC data, the use of other tobacco products has increased. For all tobacco products, which include cigarettes, e-cigarettes, hookahs, and smokeless tobacco, 24.6% of high schoolers and 7.7% of middle schoolers used a tobacco product, or multiple products. Teenagers smoke to "be cool," to look older, to lose weight, or to impress peers. Smoking can influence appetite, nutrition status, and weight. Smokers need the DRI for vitamin C plus 35 mg, because smoking alters their metabolism. Low intakes of vitamin C, vitamin A, beta-carotene, folate, and fiber are common in smokers. Smoking increases the risk of lung cancer and heart disease.

Other Addictive Drugs

Methamphetamine, also known as crystal meth, is the most potent form of amphetamines. Amphetamines cause heart, breathing, and blood pressure rates to increase. The mouth is usually dry, and swallowing is difficult. Urination is also difficult. Appetite is depressed. The users' pupils become dilated, and reflexes speed up. As the drug wears off, users experience feelings of fatigue or depression. Street names include *crank, speed, crystal, meth, zip,* and *ice.* Ecstasy, a slang term for MDMA, is known as the "club drug." This drug is found in capsule or tablet form.

In The Media

E-Cigarettes

Electronic cigarettes are often advertised as a way to help smokers quit, but are they truly a better alternative? E-cigarettes are sold in many colors, shapes, sizes, and flavors and run on a battery vaporizer and cartridge that makes a mist that is inhaled. One e-cigarette can have as much nicotine as a whole pack of cigarettes, and e-cigarettes are not currently regulated by the FDA. E-cigarette use is increasing in our youth. As most e-cigarette cartridges have 20 mg of nicotine, health care professionals are growing increasingly alarmed, as a dose that is as little as 10 mg can be easily addictive and fatal to a child. Parents should be aware of the signs and symptoms of addiction and seek options approved by the FDA to assist their teen to quit smoking.

Source: Adapted from Korioth, Trisha. (2015, Aug 8). "E-Cigarettes: Dangerous, Available, and Addicting." American Academy of Pediatrics. http://www.healthychildren.org

Inhalants are chemicals whose fumes are inhaled into the body and produce mind-altering effects. Some inhalants are gasoline, lighter fluid, tool-cleaning solvents, model airplane glue, and permanent ink in felt-tip pens. Inhalants are both physically and psychologically addictive. Individuals who inhale may risk depression and apathy, nosebleeds, headaches, eye pain, chronic fatigue, heart failure, loss of muscle control, and death. Drugs can affect food intake, body weight, and taste preferences.

Energy Drinks

Energy drinks are sold legally and are advertised to boost energy. They contain stimulants, usually caffeine, as well as sugar. The AAP has stated that these energy drinks have no place in the diet of a child or adolescent; however, energy drinks are quite popular, especially in some athletic circles. The danger is that youth may view these as performance enhancers and consider them in the same category as fluid replacement drinks, which they are not. Further, energy drinks may interact with prescription medicines, especially ADHD medicine children or adolescents might be taking.

Many energy drinks contain about 80 mg of caffeine per 8 oz serving. Most energy drinks, however, are often packaged in 20–24 oz containers, which offer a dose of 200–240 mg of caffeine. Mix-your-own powders or concentrates are in the marketplace as well and in strengths researchers say ranges from 50 to 500 mg per serving.

The FDA limits the amount of caffeine a cola can have, but because energy drinks are marketed as a supplement, no such regulation on caffeine exists as yet. Energy drinks have been known to cause insomnia, nervousness, nausea, rapid heartbeat, and even more severe reactions, such as seizures, cardiac irregularities, and cardiac arrest.

Caffeine, regardless of its form, is a central nervous system stimulant and causes a transient rise in blood pressure. From a nutrition standpoint, caffeine may cause the body to lose small amounts of calcium and magnesium.

Nutrition for the Athlete

Good nutrition during the period of life when one is involved in athletics can prevent unnecessary wear and tear on the body as well as maintain the athlete in top physical form (Figure 12-10). The specific nutritional needs of the athlete are not numerous, but they are important. The athlete needs additional water, calories, thiamine, riboflavin, niacin, sodium, potassium, iron, and protein.

The body uses water to rid itself of excess heat through perspiration. This lost water must be regularly replaced during the activity to prevent dehydration. Athletes should be well hydrated before exercise and drink enough fluid during and after exercise to balance fluid levels. While plain water is the beverage of choice for light to moderate exercise lasting under one hour, other nutrition is needed when engaging in endurance activities lasting longer than that. To determine fluid needs to match heavier exercise, a sweat rate determination is needed. An athlete can weigh himself before and after an hour of exercise. For every pound of weight lost, he would need to drink about 80–100% (13–16 oz) of that loss while exercising to stay in optimal fluid balance. It is helpful to know from a practical level how many sips of water equates to 16 oz. By knowing sweat loss rate, you can stagger fluids during exercise to minimize sweat losses.

Sports beverages containing carbohydrates and electrolytes may be consumed before, during, and after exercise to help maintain blood glucose concentration, provide fuel for muscles, and decrease risk of dehydration and hyponatremia. Fruit, carbohydrate gels, and energy bars can help fuel these

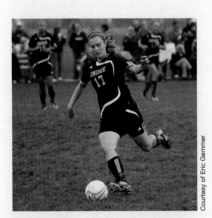

FIGURE 12-10 Participating in sports is great exercise for the mind and body.

Courtesy of Eric Gemmer

workouts. Interestingly, a recent study found that drinking 16 oz of fat-free chocolate milk with its mix of carbohydrates and protein (compared to mainstream sports drinks) led to greater concentration of glycogen in muscles at 30 and 60 minutes post-exercise.

The increase in calories depends on the activity and the length of time it is performed. The requirement could be double the normal, up to 6,000 calories per day. Because carbohydrates, not protein, are used for energy, the normal diet proportions of 50–55% carbohydrate, 30% fat, and 10–15% protein are advised during moderate physical activity.

There is an increased need for B vitamins because they are necessary for energy metabolism. They are provided in the breads, cereals, fruits, and vegetables needed to bring the calorie count to the total required. Some extra protein is used during training, when muscle mass and blood volume are increasing. Protein recommendations for endurance and strength-trained athletes range from 1.2 to 1.7 g/kg of body weight. These recommended protein intakes can generally be met through diet alone, without the use of protein or amino acid supplements. The minerals sodium and potassium are needed in larger amounts because of loss through perspiration. This amount of sodium can usually be replaced just by salting food to taste, and orange juice or bananas can provide the extra potassium. As stated, electrolyte replacement drinks may be needed for endurance activities lasting longer than one hour.

A sufficient supply of iron is important to the athlete, particularly to the female athlete. Iron-rich foods eaten with vitamin C–rich foods should provide sufficient iron. The onset of menstruation can be delayed by the heavy physical activity of the young female athlete, and amenorrhea may occur in those already menstruating.

When weight is a concern of the athlete, such as with wrestlers, care should be taken that the individual does not become dehydrated by refusing liquids in an effort to "make weight" for the class.

When weight must be added, the athlete will need an additional 3,500 calories to develop 1 lb. The additional foods eaten to reach this amount of calories should contain the normal proportion of nutrients. A high-fat diet should be avoided because it increases the potential for heart disease. Athletes should reduce calories when training ends.

In general, the athlete should select foods using MyPlate. The pregame meal should be eaten three hours before the event and should consist primarily of carbohydrates and small amounts of protein and fat. Concentrated sugar foods are not advisable because they may cause extra water to collect in the intestines, creating gas and possibly diarrhea.

Glycogen loading (carb-loading) is sometimes used for endurance activities. To increase muscle stores of glycogen, the athlete begins six days before the events. For three days, the athlete eats a diet consisting of only 10% carbohydrate and mostly protein and fat as she or he performs heavy exercise. This depletes the current store of glycogen. The next three days, the diet is 70% carbohydrate, and the exercise is very light so that the muscles become loaded with glycogen. Carbohydrate loading isn't right for every endurance athlete and may not be as effective in women as it is in men. A carbohydrate-loading diet can cause some discomfort or side effects, such as:

1. *Weight gain*. Much of this gain is extra water, but if it hampers performance, it's recommended to skip the extra carbohydrates.

2. *Digestive discomfort*. It may be important to avoid or limit some high-fiber foods (e.g., beans, bran, broccoli) for one to two days before the event, as these can cause gassy cramps, bloating, and loose stools.

glycogen-loading (carb-loading) process in which the muscle store of glycogen is maximized; also called carb-loading

3. *Blood sugar changes.* Carbohydrate loading can affect your blood sugar levels. Some athletes monitor their blood sugar during training or practices.

A qualified sports dietitian or U.S. board-certified specialist in sports dietetics can provide individualized nutrition direction as needed.

Creatine is currently the most widely used ergogenic aid among athletes wanting to build muscle and enhance recovery. Creatine has been shown to be effective in repeated short bursts of high-intensity activity in sports such as sprinting and weightlifting but not for endurance sports such as distance running. Ergogenic aids that are dangerous, banned, or illegal are anabolic or androgenic steroids, ephedra, and human growth hormone, among others. Steroid drugs can affect the fat content of the blood, damage the liver, change the reproductive system, and even alter facial appearance. Good diet, good health habits and practice, combined with innate talent, remain the essentials for athletic success.

HEALTH AND NUTRITION CONSIDERATIONS

The health care professional who works with young children may encounter poor appetites and eating habits in clients. Compounding this problem will be the anxiety of the clients' parents. They will understandably be concerned about their children's appetites and physical conditions. The health care professional can be most helpful to all concerned by exhibiting patience and understanding and by listening to parents and the client.

Adolescence is a rapid time of change. Sound nutrition is needed to optimize growth and health during these years, which may be tumultuous. As some teens are experiencing issues with overweight and obesity, a supportive health practitioner can serve as a gateway for positive nutrition and exercise messages. As many teens try to diet, some will be at risk for disordered eating. Screening tools will be valuable assets to determine if an eating disorder is developing or has developed. A team of professionals will need to be called upon to provide the best medical care.

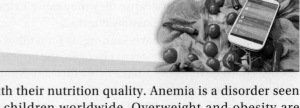

SUMMARY

Children's nutritional needs vary as they grow and develop. The rate of growth slows between the ages of 1 and 10, and the child's calorie requirement per pound of body weight slows accordingly. However, nutrient needs gradually increase during these years. During adolescence, growth is rapid, and nutritional and calorie requirements increase substantially. A positive feeding environment with sound, reliable nutrition will set the stage for optimum learning, growth, and development.

Unfortunately, health issues surface during childhood and adolescence. Many of our youth fall short with their nutrition quality. Anemia is a disorder seen in children worldwide. Overweight and obesity are on the rise. More of our youth experience pre-diabetes and type 2 diabetes, which were once considered adult-onset. Eating disorders experienced by youth are complex and underdiagnosed. Alcohol can be a serious problem for adolescents, and it is essential that they understand its potential dangers. The nutrition needs of athletes need to be carefully planned for maximum performance.

DISCUSSION TOPICS

1. Discuss how parents' anxieties about children's food habits may affect those habits.

2. In what ways does being overweight affect an adolescent's self-esteem?

3. Why can it be especially difficult for a parent to influence her or his adolescent's attitudes about food?

4. Discuss the nutrient content and food value of average fast food choices. Discuss healthier options available and go online to find a fast food restaurant's nutrition facts.

5. What could result if a 30-year-old lawyer continued to eat as he did as a 17-year-old football player?

6. Describe anorexia nervosa. Ask if anyone in the class knows of someone who has suffered from it. Ask that individual for descriptions of the person's attitude, physical condition, possible causes, and today's condition.

7. Discuss the use of growth charts in the primary care physician setting. What deviations in the growth chart of a child would raise cause for concern?

8. Why is it important to spot pre-diabetes in youth? What screening methods are used?

9. When do significant deposits in bone mass occur in youth? Discuss why this is especially critical and name the key nutrients involved.

SUGGESTED ACTIVITIES

1. List your favorite snack foods. Now list the most nutritious snack foods of your favorites. Check the calorie values of these foods and compare lists for nutrition and taste. Discuss possible improvements in your list of favorite snacks.

2. Plan a talk for fourth-grade students on the importance of good food habits. Research major nutrients, calories, fiber, and food needs to meet requirements of a 9-year-old boy and girl. Begin with an outline and develop it into a narrative that 9-year-old children will understand. If possible, ask permission of a fourth-grade teacher to deliver this talk to the class.

3. Role-play a situation in which your younger sister, who is somewhat overweight, has just asked you to help her get in shape. Ask her what food and lifestyle habits she believes have led to her feeling less healthy. Brainstorm three simple changes with her regarding food and exercise habits. Be positive and nonjudgmental; let her voice the realistic changes she wants to make, both short and long term.

4. Invite a registered dietitian to speak to the class on sports nutrition. Seek out a dietitian who has as a special interest or practice in this. Ideally, this person would be a certified sports nutrition professional. Often large universities or fitness centers know of these individuals. The Academy of Nutrition and Dietetics (http://www.eatright.org) may be able to put you in touch with a local dietetic association.

5. Invite a counselor who specializes in adolescent eating disorders to speak to the class.

6. Hold a panel discussion on alcohol and drugs. Assign the following topics to individual class members. They should prepare themselves by doing outside research before the panel discussion.

   What is alcohol?

   What are some commonly abused drugs?

   Why do people use alcohol or drugs?

   How do alcohol and drugs affect the human body?

   How can alcohol and drug abuse affect one's nutritional status?

   What are the dangers of drinking or using drugs during pregnancy?

REVIEW

Multiple choice. Select the *letter* that precedes the best answer.

1. Anorexia nervosa
   a. is characterized by binges and purges
   b. causes severe acne
   c. is a psychological disorder
   d. typically causes overweight

2. A child's eating habits
   a. can reflect his or her desire to assert self
   b. seldom change after the child reaches the age of 1 year
   c. usually improve when parents force the child to try new foods
   d. have no relation to the child's growth rate

3. Children's appetites
   a. vary
   b. are static
   c. are irrelevant to their nutritional status
   d. are entirely dependent on the size of the child

4. The Healthy Eating Index from NHANES data indicates that
   a. generally children are meeting nutrition needs, except for protein
   b. generally children are meeting nutrition needs, except for eating too many fried foods
   c. consumption of whole grains, greens, and legumes (starchy beans) is lacking
   d. consumption of adequate fiber is the only nutrient lacking

5. At what age should children be screened for high cholesterol, especially if there is a family history of heart disease?
   a. 5 years   c. 2 years
   b. 12 years   d. 16 years

6. Children's iron requirement is high because iron is needed for
   a. healthy bones and teeth
   b. fighting infections
   c. prevention of night blindness
   d. carrying oxygen

7. As a child grows, his or her calorie requirement per pound of body weight
   a. remains unchanged
   b. increases
   c. becomes less
   d. doubles each year

8. What age group has the highest prevalence of food allergies?
   a. toddlers
   b. preteens
   c. preschoolers
   d. midteens

9. A teenager who consumes frequent fast food
   a. is at risk for becoming overweight
   b. likely has a diet high in salt and fat, which could contribute to disease later in life
   c. is influenced to some degree by fast food marketers when making food choices
   d. experiences all of the above

10. Although adolescent boys usually need more calories than adolescent girls, the girls usually need more
    a. protein
    b. vitamin C
    c. iron
    d. vitamin D

CASE IN POINT

ELIZABETH: IDENTIFYING ANOREXIA NERVOSA

Elizabeth loves hanging out with her friends. She also loves to read. In addition to books, she loves to read magazines. She loves to look at the latest fashion trends in hair, makeup, and clothing. She would like to be a fashion designer when she is older. She is currently 5-ft 2-in. tall and weighs 80 lb. She has gotten taller over the past year, but her waist and hip measurements have changed only slightly.

Elizabeth and her family rarely have a night where they are all home together for supper. Elizabeth's dad works second shift and is always gone in the evenings. Now that Elizabeth is 14 years old, her mother has decided to pick up a second job as a waitress a few nights a week to help make ends meet. Elizabeth is in charge of her younger sister on the evenings when her parents are both gone. Elizabeth's mom would typically have something easy for the girls to fix for supper while she was working. Elizabeth's sister, Hannah, is

12 years old. She has started noticing that Elizabeth is no longer eating supper with her. At first, she thought Elizabeth was taking food to her room because she just wanted to be alone. But now, she is realizing that Elizabeth isn't eating much, if at all. Lately, Elizabeth has complained about being tired and told Hannah to eat supper without her. She often naps on the weekend and after school instead of playing with her friends. Her afterschool snacks have gone from choices such as cheese and crackers or granola bars, to no more than a small piece of fruit.

One night Hannah confronted Elizabeth and asked why she wasn't eating. Elizabeth admitted to Hannah that she was hungry, but wasn't going to eat because she did not want to gain weight. Her sister immediately informed her parents of this, and her parents are now watching her eating habits and behaviors more closely.

ASSESSMENT

1. What objective information do you have about Elizabeth?
2. What subjective information do you have about Elizabeth?
3. Which psychological issues are having an effect on Elizabeth's understanding of proper nutrition?
4. What are the psychological needs of preteens?
5. What would lead you to believe that Elizabeth may be having appearance issues?

DIAGNOSIS

6. Complete the following statement: Elizabeth's imbalanced nutrition is secondary to _____.
7. What signs of anorexia nervosa does Elizabeth exhibit?

PLAN/GOAL

8. What is the major nutritional goal for Elizabeth?
9. What is the priority for Elizabeth's physical development?

IMPLEMENTATION

10. What should Elizabeth and her mother be taught about good nutrition?
11. What needs to be taught about anorexia nervosa? Who else needs this information?
12. Would a counselor be of assistance to Elizabeth and her mother?
13. What can be done to prevent anorexia nervosa in her sister? Does anorexia nervosa have an age limit?

EVALUATION/OUTCOME CRITERIA

14. What criteria could be used to demonstrate that her anorexia nervosa was under control?
15. Can anorexia nervosa be cured?

THINKING FURTHER

16. How can parents, teachers, and coaches help preteens who have eating disorders?
17. Will Elizabeth's younger sister be at risk for anorexia nervosa?

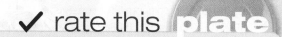

✔ rate this **plate**

Elizabeth may be feeling pressured to look a certain way and be a particular weight by the magazines she reads. As she continues to grow throughout her teen years, her calorie and nutrient needs will increase. Elizabeth needs nutrient-dense foods. Rate the plate she ate for dinner:

2 chicken nuggets

¼ cup instant mashed potatoes

½ cup diced pineapple

8 oz fruit punch drink

Are any of these foods nutrient dense? Are any of these foods calorie dense? If so, which one(s)? How could this meal be improved to provide Elizabeth with adequate calories and nutrients to support growth throughout her teenage years?

CASE IN POINT

JORDAN: CHILDHOOD OBESITY

Jordan's parents divorced two years ago, when she was 4 years old. She spends the majority of her time at her mother's house. Her father sees her every other weekend and on Wednesday nights for supper. Her mother used to stay home with her but was forced to go back to work full time after the divorce. Jordan is often shuffled between different babysitters when her parents are working. Her parents are so busy that many of the meals they provide for Jordan have become fast food or convenience foods. Every Wednesday night, Jordan and her Dad go to a fast food restaurant for supper. Jordan loves that she gets a new toy each week!

Jordan used to take dance lessons and play soccer, but she has had to give both activities up because her parents simply can't afford them since the divorce. Jordan started kindergarten this fall and her mother is hoping that will fill the void of friendship she lost since discontinuing her activities. Jordan is a very smart girl, but she tells her mom she hates school. She cries each morning when she gets up and complains that she does not want to go. Finally, she reveals to

her mother that the other kids are making fun of her. She says that they tell her she is fat. Jordan's mom is heartbroken. She knows Jordan has gained a lot of weight, but she had no idea it was affecting her at school. Jordan's mom makes an appointment for Jordan with her pediatrician. She asks Jordan's dad to attend the appointment as well. At the doctor's office, Jordan measures 45-in tall and weighs 61 lb. The doctor informs her parents that he is concerned about her weight and would like them to meet with a registered dietitian to discuss a plan for Jordan and to set some goals for her weight. Despite their differences, Jordan's parents are both concerned about Jordan's weight. Both Jordan's parents have struggled with their own weight through the years and have made numerous attempts to lose weight. They are concerned that Jordan is headed down the same path. They both agree to meet with the dietitian and work on this together for Jordan. They have also discussed ways to encourage Jordan to increase her activity and decrease the amount of less nutritious foods and snacks she consumes.

ASSESSMENT

1. What objective data do you have about Jordan?
2. Using Figure 12-5, what percentile weight and height is Jordan in for a 6-year-old girl?
3. How do diet, activity, heredity, and family lifestyle impact her current weight?
4. How significant is this problem?

DIAGNOSIS

Complete the following diagnostic statements:
5. Imbalanced nutrition; more than body requirements related to _____.
6. Deficient knowledge related to _____.

PLAN/GOAL

7. State two reasonable and measurable goals for Jordan.
8. At Jordan's checkup, the doctor agreed with her mom and referred them to a dietitian. As a dietitian, what personal goals are appropriate for Jordan and her parents, including their activities and foods?

IMPLEMENTATION

9. What information does the dietitian need to know to help Jordan?
10. Who needs to be involved in the plan for it to be successful?
11. What are the two big changes that need to occur to help Jordan stop gaining weight?
12. What strategies could you suggest so Jordan would be successful but have fun in the process?
13. How can playing outdoors with friends be helpful?
14. How can her family help?

EVALUATION/OUTCOME CRITERIA

15. How often should Jordan be weighed?
16. What outcome is reasonable in three months? In six months?

THINKING FURTHER

17. Why is it important to intervene with Jordan's weight now? What are the future consequences of a lifetime of being overweight? Why is this a community health issue in America now?
18. What would the Internet be able to provide?
19. In March 2012, the National Nutrition Standards for school lunches were revised. You can read the current guidelines by visiting http://www.fns.usda.gov/cnd/governance/regulations.htm.

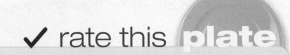

✔ rate this plate

Jordan still enjoys the occasional treats from a fast food restaurant when she visits her father on Wednesday nights. Rate the meal that her father ordered for her.

- **1 kid-size cheeseburger**
- **1 small order French fries**
- **4 oz vanilla yogurt**
- **½ cup apple slices**
- **12 oz orange juice drink**

Check a fast food menu online to determine total calories. Is this too much food? If so, where can calories be decreased in this meal?

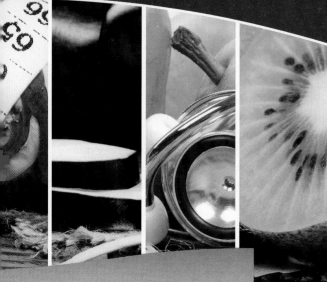

NUTRITION DURING ADULTHOOD

OBJECTIVES

After studying this chapter, you should be able to:

- Identify the nutritional needs of young, middle, and late-age adults

- Discuss diet-related diseases that may present themselves in adulthood and tactics that may prevent or manage them

- Explain sensible, long-range weight control for this age group, including exercise

- Identify physiological, economic, and psychosocial problems that can affect an older adult's nutrition

YOUNG AND MIDDLE ADULTHOOD

Young adulthood is a time of excitement and self-exploration. The age range spans 18–40 years of age. Individuals are alive with plans, desires, and energy as they begin searching for and finding their place in the mainstream of adult life. They appear to have boundless energy for both social and professional activities. They are often interested in exercise for its own sake and may participate in athletic events as well.

The middle period spans 40–65 years of age. This is a time when the physical activities of young adulthood typically begin to decrease, resulting in lowered caloric requirement for most individuals. Table 13-1 shows equations that Registered Dietitians use in assessing energy (calorie) requirements. For a person who simply wants an estimate of one's calorie intake, he or she can assess information from www.choosemyplate.gov. During these years, people seldom have young children to supervise, and the strenuous physical labor of some occupations may be delegated to younger people. Middle-agers may tire more easily than they did when they were younger. Therefore, they may not get as much exercise as they did in earlier years. Because appetite and food intake may not decrease, there is a common tendency toward weight gain during this period.

During young to middle adulthood, the beginnings of osteoporosis may also be evident. A diet rich in calcium, vitamin D, magnesium, and fluoride is thought to help prevent osteoporosis.

TABLE 13-1 Equations to Estimate Energy Requirements for Adults

IRETON-JONES

For calculation of resting energy expenditure (REE) or resting metabolic rate (RMR), where weight (W) in kilograms (kg), height (H) in centimeters, and age (A) in years use these equations.

- Spontaneously breathing: $629 - 11(A) + 25(W) - 609(O)$
- Ventilator-dependent (original, 1992): $1925 - 10(A) + 5(W) + 281(S) + 292(T) + 851(B)$
- Ventilator-dependent (revised, 2002): $1784 - 11(A) + 5(W) + 244(S) + 239(T) + 804(B)$
- B = Diagnosis of burn (present = 1, absent = 0)
- O = Obesity, body mass index (BMI) >.27 kg/m² (present = 1, absent = 0)
- S = Sex (male = 1, female = 0)
- T = Diagnosis of trauma (present = 1, absent = 0)

MIFFLIN–ST JEOR

According to the American Academy of Nutrition and Dietetics, if it is not possible to measure RMR, then the Mifflin–St Jeor equation using actual weight is the most accurate for estimating RMR for overweight and obese individuals.

- Men: $(9.99 \times W) + (6.25 \times H) - (4.92 \times A) + 5$
- Women: $(9.99 \times W) + (6.25 \times H) - (4.92 \times A) - 161$

HARRIS–BENEDICT EQUATION

- Men: RMR = $66.47 + (13.75 \times W) + (5 \times H) - (6.75 \times A)$
- Women: RMR = $655.09 + (9.56 \times W) + (1.84 \times H) - (4.67 \times A)$

Total energy requirements (TEE) = REE × (activity factor) × (injury factor) ± 500 calories (for desired weight loss or weight gain, if applicable) + fever factor

ACTIVITY FACTORS	INJURY FACTORS
• Comatose: 1.1	• Surgery
• Confined to bed: 1.2	○ Minor: 1.0–1.2
• Confined to chair: 1.25	○ Major: 1.1–1.3
• Out of bed: 1.3	• Skeletal trauma: 1.1–1.6
• Normal activities of daily living (ADLs): 1.5	• Head trauma: 1.6–1.8

FEVER FACTOR	INJURY FACTORS		
Fahrenheit scale: add 7% of REE for every 1° over normal	• Pressure ulcers	• Infection	• Burns (% body surface area)
Centigrade scale: add 13% of REE for every 1° over normal	○ Stage I: 1.0–1.1	○ Mild: 1.0–1.2	○ < 20% BSA: 1.2–1.5
	○ Stage II: 1.2	○ Moderate: 1.2–1.4	○ 20%–40% BSA: 1.5–1.8
	○ Stage III: 1.3–1.4	○ Severe: 1.4–1.8	○ >40% BSA: 1.8–2.0
	○ Stage IV: 1.5–1.6		

Source: Adapted from Jeor, M.S. *Energy Requirements for Adults*. Accessed October 2015. http://www.nutrition411.com

SPOTLIGHT *on Life Cycle*

Whether we like it or not, our body shape will change naturally as we age. Our lifestyle choices will affect how fast or slow the change takes place. After age 30, we tend to lose muscle (lean tissue). The amount of body fat likewise increases. Older individuals may have almost one-third more fat compared to their youth. Fat builds up around the internal organs and near the center of the body. Related to height, people also lose one-half in. every 10 years after age 40. Height loss occurs even more quickly once you hit 70. Overall, it is not uncommon for someone to lose 1–3 in. of height. Men often gain weight until middle age, around age 55; however, they then begin to lose weight later in life. Women usually gain weight until age 65, but then begin to lose weight.

Source: Adapted from "Aging Changes in Body Shape." *MedlinePlus.* NIH, U.S. National Library of Medicine. Accessed October 2015.

The onset of rheumatoid arthritis (RA), an **autoimmune disease**, usually occurs between the ages of 30 and 50 and will affect approximately 1.3 million Americans, of which about 70% are women. RA affects the wrists, joints of the fingers other than those closest to the fingernail, hips, knees, ankles, elbows, shoulders, feet, and neck. Although there is no specific diet for sufferers of rheumatoid arthritis, an eating style similar to the Mediterranean may help symptoms and progression of disease. Rheumatoid arthritis is less severe in some Mediterranean countries such as Greece and Italy due in part to the anti-inflammatory nature of the diet. Best foods to choose include fatty fish such as salmon and tuna, soy foods, extra virgin olive oil, cherries and berries, green tea, citrus, whole grains, and nuts. A multiple vitamin containing vitamin D and a calcium supplement should be taken daily. Pro-inflammatory foods such as sugar, saturated and trans fat, and refined carbohydrates should be limited.

Nutritional Requirements for Young and Middle Adulthood

Growth is usually complete by age 25 years. Consequently, except during pregnancy and lactation, the essential nutrients are needed only to maintain and repair body tissue and to produce energy. During these years, the **nutrient requirements** of healthy adults change very little.

The iron requirement for women throughout the child-bearing years remains higher than that for men. Extra iron is needed to replace blood loss during menstruation and to help build both the infant's and the mother's extra maternal blood needed during pregnancy. After menopause, this requirement for women matches that of men.

Protein needs for healthy adults are thought to be 0.8 g per kilogram of body weight. To determine the specific amount, one must divide the weight in pounds by 2.2 to obtain the weight in kilograms and then multiply the weight in kilograms by 0.8.

The current requirement for calcium for adults age 19–50 is 1,000 mg, and for vitamin D, 15 μg per day (or 600 IUs). Both calcium and vitamin D are essential for strong bones, and both are found in milk. Bone loss begins slowly, at about age 35–40, and can later lead to osteoporosis. Therefore, it is wise for

autoimmune disease
an illness that occurs when the body tissues are attacked by its own immune system

nutrient requirements
amounts of specific nutrient needed by the body

young people, especially women, to consume foods that provide more than the requirements for these two nutrients. Three glasses of milk a day nearly fulfill the requirement for calcium; however, the level of vitamin D in three glasses of milk still falls short of the newer recommended allowance. Most people will need to include other vitamin D sources, or more likely add a supplement of vitamin D. Increasing this amount could prevent osteoporosis. Fat-free milk or foods made from fat-free milk should be consumed to limit the amount of fat in the diet.

Calorie Requirements for Young and Middle Adulthood

Calorie requirements begin to diminish after age 25, as basal metabolism rates decrease. After age 25, a person will gain weight if the total calories are not reduced according to actual need, which will be determined by activity, BMI (REE), and amount of lean body mass. Those who are more active will require more calories than those who are less active.

Special Considerations Related to Nutrition Concerns for Young and Middle Adulthood

It is especially important to maintain good eating habits during young and middle adulthood. Those who may be concerned about weight, cost of food, or time can easily develop nutrient deficiencies. For example, a woman who settles for a piece of pie at lunchtime while her husband eats a hamburger and salad is not obtaining adequate nutrients. If she continues to eat like this, she will jeopardize her health.

A hamburger can have 250–400 calories. The salad will contain less than 50 calories without dressing, and the dressing could be limited to 1 Tbsp, or approximately 100 calories, for a total intake of 400–550 calories. Pies average 100 calories per 1-in slice. Most slices are about 3.5 in. A scoop of ice cream on the pie would bring the total to at least another 100 calories.

Although the calorie intakes of the husband and wife would be comparable, the nutrient intakes would differ. The wife's would be inadequate. If the woman is of child-bearing age and plans to have children, she or her children could suffer from such habits. It would have been better to have ordered a grilled chicken sandwich instead of a hamburger along with a side salad. Replacing the hamburger and pie choices with healthier, more nutrient-dense items such as mixed fruit or a side salad with assorted vegetables will result in lower calorie intake and higher nutrient intake.

In general, people today are concerned about nutrition and want to limit fats, cholesterol, sugar, salt, and calories and increase fiber. Many know the sources of these items; others do not. Unfortunately, both groups tend to select their food because of cost, convenience, and flavor rather than nutritional content. It is easier to drive through a fast food restaurant or heat a prepared frozen dinner than it is to shop for individual food items, cook them, and clean up after the meal. Consequently, many people ingest more fats, sugar, salt, and high-calorie foods and less fiber and other nutrients than they should.

Many physical changes also take place during middle adulthood. For women, **menopause** is a time where it is important to incorporate healthy lifestyle choices such as reducing calories and increasing physical activity to make the transition into middle adulthood easier. On average, women meet menopause at age 51. As a woman ages, the two main hormones essential in reproduction, called estrogen

calorie requirements
number of calories required daily to meet energy needs

menopause
the end of menstruation

and progesterone, begin to decrease. As hormone levels decrease, menstrual periods become shorter and eventually cease. Due to the lessening of hormone levels, weight maintenance during the 40s and 50s may be a challenge. Research shows that to maintain weight in the mid to late 40s, women need about 200 fewer calories per day. Eating smaller meals throughout the day along with participating in physical activity will maintain metabolism and prevent significant weight gain. For the adult male, a diet that supports reducing the risk for heart disease is especially important because males develop heart disease at a younger age than women. Both regular exercise and weight-bearing exercise are important to promote bone health.

Adults will not outgrow their need for essential vitamins and minerals as they age. Although calcium is necessary for growing bones, it's also needed to help keep bones strong throughout adulthood. Three servings of dairy foods per day provide adequate calcium for adults. Fiber is also an essential nutrient for overall health. Fiber is known best for maintaining bowel regularity and preventing intestinal conditions such as diverticular disease; however, research has also proven that fiber can lower risks of heart disease, high blood pressure, cancer, and type 2 diabetes. Fiber can also help lower cholesterol levels by absorbing fat and cholesterol from the blood. Fiber is also relatively low in calories and increases satiety, therefore controlling weight. Whole-grain products as well as beans, fruits, and vegetables are rich sources of fiber. Women of child-bearing age need adequate intake of folic acid and iron in order to prevent birth defects and iron-deficiency anemia during pregnancy. Food sources of folate include lentils, spinach, broccoli, and other leafy green vegetables. Other vitamins and minerals of concern during adulthood include magnesium, potassium, and vitamins E, A, D, and C. Magnesium contributes to bone strength, immunity, and numerous body functions. Potassium plays a critical role in muscle contractions, nerve impulses, and maintaining fluid balance in the body. Eating a variety of green vegetables, beans, and dairy products will provide potassium. Vitamins A, E, and C contain powerful antioxidant properties that offer a variety of health benefits including maintaining eye health and vision, combating free radicals, and repelling germs to achieve a healthy immune system. Consuming a diet balanced with fruits, vegetables, whole grains, lean protein, and dairy will provide essential nutrients needed through young and middle adulthood.

Weight Control for Young and Middle Adulthood

Weight control is one of the top concerns of U.S. adults. Whether for reasons of vanity, health, or both, most people are interested in controlling their weight. It is advisable because overweight can introduce health problems. Cases of diabetes mellitus, metabolic syndrome, hypertension, and other diseases are more numerous among the overweight than among those of normal weight. Overweight individuals are poor risks for surgery, and their lives are generally shorter than others who are not overweight. They are prone to social and emotional problems because overweight and obesity can reduce self-esteem.

The causes of overweight are not always known, but the most common cause appears to be **energy imbalance**. In other words, if one is overweight, chances are that more calories have been taken in than were needed for energy.

An intake of 3,500 calories more than the body needs for maintenance and activities will result in a weight gain of 1 lb. An individual who overeats by only 200 calories a day can gain 20 lb in one year. Obviously, when nutrient requirements remain static but calorie requirements decrease, people must select their foods carefully to fulfill their nutrient requirements.

Exploring THE WEB

Search the "Nutrition source" section of the Harvard University School of Public Health website. Focus on the section on disease prevention in particular for information related to diet and disease and disorders. What conditions are directly affected by diet? Can these conditions be prevented by changing one's nutritional status? How can this be done? What resources are available for individuals experiencing a nutrition-related disorder?

SUPERSIZE USA

Making healthy choices while traveling can be a challenge. When eating fast food, seek out restaurants that have healthy options such as Panera, Subway, and Atlanta Bread. Avoid fried foods, choose whole-grain breads, avoid adding cheese to sandwiches or burgers, and choose lean protein sources such as grilled options instead of fried. You may think salads would be a healthier meal alternative, but many entrée salads have a lot of calories, especially if you add full-fat dressing or breaded chicken. Chili is a better side option compared to other choices. When choosing a beverage, opt for water or unsweetened tea or coffee instead of regular or diet soda.

Source: Health, United States, 2014. National Center for Health Statistics, CDC. Accessed October 2015.

energy imbalance
eating either too much or too little for the amount of energy expended

In The Media

HDL Cholesterol and Menopause

New research suggests that having higher levels of HDL cholesterol (commonly known as the "good" cholesterol), can be harmful to women going through menopause in that it may increase plaque buildup in the arteries. Results were independent of other factors such as body weight and levels of bad cholesterol. For the study, 225 women in their middle to late 40s were followed for up to 9 years. All participants were free of heart disease prior to the study. Results indicated that as women aged and went through menopause, increasing levels of good cholesterol were linked with greater plaque buildup. Researchers speculate that the increase in fat to the abdomen and around the heart can cause inflammation and change HDL levels. More research is needed to truly understand the process.

Source: Adapted from Reinberg, Steven. 2015, October 16). "During Menopause, 'Good' Cholesterol May Lose Protective Effect on Heart." *HealthDay.* www.consumer.healthday.com

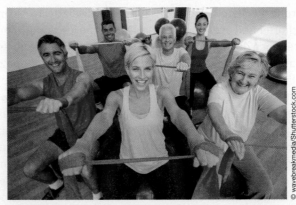

FIGURE 13-1 The need for exercise continues throughout life, no matter your age.

Individuals who are overweight simply because of energy imbalance can solve the problem by eating less and increasing physical exercise. Exercise will increase the number of calories burned (Figure 13-1). However, unless the exercise is sufficient to burn more calories than the ingested food contains, exercise alone will not solve the problem. By far the most effective method of weight loss is increased exercise combined with reduced calories. This will help tone the muscles as excess fat is lost. Exercise may also increase lean body mass in such a way that weight loss will not be necessarily significant; in this case, a decrease in clothing size may be a better indicator of fat loss.

When weight reduction is necessary, clients should confirm with their physician that they are in good health. It is important for clients to be coached on cooking more meals at home, eating mindfully away from distractions and media, slowing down and savoring food, and reducing screen time and "sitting" throughout their day. There are many online resource and support groups available. With the help of a registered dietitian, individuals can develop a healthy eating plan to fit their lifestyle. A healthy eating plan is easiest to follow when it is based on MyPlate (Table 13-2). This plan will aid dieters in obtaining needed nutrients, will help change previously unsatisfactory eating habits, and will allow them to adapt and thus enjoy meals anywhere—at home, parties, or in restaurants. For additional information about weight loss diets, see Chapter 14.

Health and Nutrition Considerations for Young and Middle Adulthood

The young and middle years of life are busy. Most people feel they have too many things to do and too little time to accomplish them. Most have families, jobs, and social obligations and, thus, more responsibilities. In their fast-paced world, drive-thru meals become common place. This can lead to obesity not only in young and middle aged adults but in their children as well.

LATE ADULTHOOD

Currently, the fastest-growing age group in the United States is that of people age 85 and older. The average life expectancy in this country is now 81 years for women and 76 years for men (National Center for Health Statistics, 2014). In the

TABLE 13-2 1,600-Calorie Daily Menu

BREAKFAST	LUNCH
• 1¼ cup oatmeal cooked in 8 oz skim milk • 2 tbsp raisins • 2 tbsp chopped pecans • 1 hard-boiled egg **Beverage:** coffee	**Tuna salad** • 5 oz water pack tuna • 2 tbsp onion • 1 tbsp light mayonnaise and 1 tbsp. chopped celery • 4 whole-wheat crackers • 1 cup chopped Romaine lettuce and 3 slices tomato • 1 medium orange **Beverage:** water or tea
DINNER	**SNACKS**
Roasted chicken • 3 oz cooked chicken breast • 1 large sweet potato, roasted • 1 cup steamed broccoli • 2 tsp tub margarine • 1 cup berries **Beverage: 1 cup skim milk**	• 6 baby carrots • 2 tbsp hummus

Source: Adapted from www.nutrition411.com. October 2015.

year 2014, people 65 and older represented 14.5% of the population. This percentage is expected to grow to 21.7% of the population by the year 2040. Consequently, **gerontology**, the study of aging, is of increasing importance.

The rate of aging varies. Each person is affected by heredity, emotional and physical stress, and nutrition. Research continues to reveal more about the causes of aging and the role of nutrition in the aging process.

The Effects of Aging

As people age, **physiological**, psychosocial, and economic changes occur that affect nutrition.

Physiological Changes

The body's functions slow with age, and the ability of the body to replace worn cells is reduced. The metabolic rate slows; bones become less dense; lean muscle mass is reduced; eyes do not focus on nearby objects as they once did, and some grow cloudy from cataracts; poor **dentition** is common; the heart and kidneys become less efficient; and hearing, taste, and smell are less acute. If poor nutrition has been chronic, the immune system may be compromised.

Osteoarthritis and its debilitating effects are of great concern to the elderly. Arthritis can limit the ability to perform activities of daily living (ADLs). The role that diet plays in arthritis has been of increasing interest to researchers. Excessive weight, certain vitamin deficiencies, and the type of diet being followed may influence some types of arthritis. Eating a healthy, well-balanced diet that includes an abundance of fruits and vegetables, along with whole grain products, lean poultry, oily fish, nuts, seeds and beans, along with adequate calcium

gerontology
the study of aging

physiological
relating to bodily functions

dentition
arrangement, type, and number of teeth

and vitamin D is likely very beneficial for arthritis sufferers. As mentioned earlier in the text, limiting pro-inflammatory foods such as sugar, refined grains, and unhealthy fats help as well. Your physician or dietitian may also recommend taking a multiple vitamin daily. In addition, exercise helps most sufferers of osteoarthritis.

Digestion is affected because the secretion of hydrochloric acid and enzymes is diminished. This in turn decreases the intrinsic factor synthesis, which leads to a deficiency of vitamin B_{12}. The tone of the intestines is reduced, and the result may be constipation or, in some cases, diarrhea.

Psychosocial Changes

Feelings do not decrease with age. In fact, psychosocial problems can increase as one grows older. Age does not diminish the desire to feel useful, appreciated, and loved by family and friends. Retirement years may not be "golden" if one suffers a loss of self-esteem from feelings of uselessness. Grief over the loss of a spouse or close friend, combined with the resulting loneliness, can be devastating. Physical disabilities that develop in the senior years and prevent one from going out independently can destroy a social life. Becoming a fifth wheel in a grown child's home or a resident of a nursing home can lead to severe depression. Problems such as these can diminish a person's appetite and ability to shop and cook.

Economic Changes

Retirement typically results in decreased income. Unless one has carefully prepared for it, this can affect one's quality of life by reducing social activities, adding worry about meeting bills, and causing one to select a less than healthy diet by choosing foods on the basis of cost rather than nutrient content.

Sidestepping Potential Problems

Healthy eating habits throughout life, an exercise program suited to one's age, and enjoyable social activities can prevent or delay physical deterioration and psychological depression during the senior years. The benefits can be said to be circular. The first two contribute largely to one's physical condition, and social activities can prevent or diminish depression. Healthy eating habits and a suited exercise program give purpose to the day, happiness to life, and zest to the appetite. Whenever an elderly person is depressed, his or her nutrition and lifestyle should be carefully reviewed.

Food–drug interactions must be monitored closely in the elderly. Frequently, specific foods will prevent, decrease, or enhance the absorption of a particular drug. Dairy products should not be consumed within two hours of taking the antibiotic tetracycline, or it will not be absorbed. A person taking a blood clot–reducing drug such as coumadin or warfarin (often called an anticoagulant) needs to consume vitamin K– rich food in moderation, as it counteracts blood thinners. Even vitamin supplements can cause interactions. The antioxidant vitamins are not to be taken with blood clot–reducing medications because they also have a tendency to thin the blood.

Drug–drug interactions as well as food–drug interactions can contribute to decreased nutritional status. These interactions could affect appetite as well as absorption of nutrients from the food eaten. Careful monitoring is recommended (see Appendix D).

Nutritional Requirements for Late Adulthood

Although the nutritional needs of growth disappear with age, the normal nutritional needs for maintaining a constant state of good health remain throughout

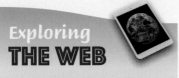

Exploring
THE WEB

Visit the National Institute on Aging (http://www.nia.nih.gov) for guidelines on good nutrition throughout life. What are some of the challenges and concerns facing older adults in relation to healthy eating?

life. Good nutrition can speed recovery from illness, surgery, or broken bones and generally can improve the spirits and quality, and even the length, of life.

Despite the physical changes that the body undergoes beyond age 50, only a few of the DRIs and AIs in this age category are less than those for younger people.

The protein requirement remains at the average 50 g per day for women and 63 g for men. This is based on the estimated need of 0.8 g per kilogram of body weight. However, newer research is pointing to the fact that after age 65, it may be advisable to increase one's daily protein intake to 1.0 g per kilogram of body weight in order to preserve muscle mass. In general, vitamin requirements do not change after the age of 51, except for a slight decrease in the DRIs for thiamine, riboflavin, and niacin. The need for these three vitamins depends largely on the calorie intake, and calorie requirement is reduced after the age of 51. The need for iron is decreased after age 51 in women because of menopause.

The calorie requirement decreases approximately 2% per decade after age 20, because metabolism slows and activity is reduced. If the calorie intake is not reduced, weight will increase. This additional weight would increase the work of the heart and put increased stress on the skeletal system. It is important that the calorie requirement not be exceeded and just as important that the nutrient requirements be fulfilled to maintain good nutritional status. An exercise plan appropriate for one's age and health can be helpful in burning excess calories and toning and strengthening the muscles.

Food Habits for Late Adulthood

A lifetime of poor food habits are more likely to continue as one ages. These habits will not be easy to change. Poor food habits that begin during old age can also present problems. Decreased income during retirement, lack of transportation, physical disability, and inadequate cooking facilities may cause difficulties in food selection and preparation. Anorexia caused by grief, loneliness, boredom, depression, or difficulty in chewing can decrease food consumption. Dementia and Alzheimer's disease may cause the elderly to think they have eaten when in fact they have not.

Studies indicate that many senior citizens consume diets deficient in protein; vitamins C, D, B_6, B_{12}, and folate; and the minerals calcium, zinc, iron, and sometimes fiber and calories.

skeletal system
body's bone structure

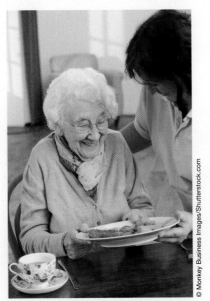

FIGURE 13-2 A volunteer delivers a warm meal to an elderly woman.

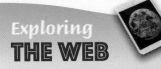

Exploring

THE WEB

Search the Web for information on food fads. What makes the elderly vulnerable to food fads? Are these types of diets and fads geared toward the elderly population? Why? What advice would you provide to an elderly client inquiring about one of these fads?

food faddists
people who have certain beliefs about particular foods or diets

An elderly client's diet plan should be based on MyPlate and the nutrients should be checked against the DRIs and AIs. Older persons' needs can vary considerably, depending on their conditions, so each person should be examined by a physician to determine specific requirements. A general multivitamin-mineral supplement is recommended likely with additional vitamin D.

Variety and nutrient-dense foods should be encouraged, as should water. Water is important to help prevent constipation, to maintain urinary volume, to prevent dehydration, and to prevent urinary tract infections (UTIs). When there is serious protein energy malnutrition (PEM), the reason may be economic or psychosocial. Elderly people who have long hospital stays can develop PEM in the hospital. They may dislike the food, drugs may dull the appetite, and they may be lonely and depressed. Sometimes poor or missing teeth can make eating protein foods difficult. In such cases, protein-rich supplements can be used.

If overweight is a problem, it may be caused by overeating, lack of exercise, drugs, or alcohol.

Any adjustment in food habits will require thorough explanation, and plans for changes must be based on the individual's total situation.

Food Fads for Late Adulthood

Some older people are consciously or unconsciously searching for eternal life, if not youth. Consequently, they are frequently susceptible to the claims of **food faddists** who seek to profit from their ignorance. Senior citizens spend money on unnecessary vitamins, minerals, and special honey, molasses, bread, milk, and other foods that may be guaranteed by the salesperson to prevent or cure various diseases. This money could be much more effectively used on ordinary foods from MyPlate that would cost considerably less. It would be better to spend money on foods that represent MyPlate than on food supplements.

Appropriate Diets for Late Adulthood

The diets of older adults should be planned around MyPlate. When special health problems exist, the normal diet should be adapted to meet individual needs (see Section 3, Medical Nutrition Therapy).

The federal government provides the states with funds to serve hot meals at noon in senior centers across the country. These senior centers become social clubs and are immensely beneficial to the elderly. They provide companionship in addition to nutritious food. Frequently, the noon meal at "the center" becomes the focal point of an older person's day (Figure 13-2).

The federal government also provides transportation for those who are otherwise unable to reach the senior center for the meal. When individuals are completely homebound, arrangements can be made for the meals to be delivered to their homes. Some communities have Meals-on-Wheels projects. Participating people pay according to ability. In addition, food stamps are available and can sometimes be used for the Meals-on-Wheels programs.

Special Considerations for the Chronically Ill Older Adult

The CDC reports that approximately 80% of older adults have one chronic condition and 50% have at least two. Examples include osteoporosis, arthritis, cataracts, cancer, diabetes mellitus, hypertension, heart disease, and periodontal disease. The branch of medicine that is involved with diseases of older adults is called **geriatrics**.

Osteoporosis

Osteoporosis is a condition in which the amount of calcium in bones is reduced, making them porous. The International Osteoporosis Foundation estimates that osteoporosis and low bone mass are currently a major public health threat for almost 54 million U.S. women and men aged 50 and older. Those at higher risk for osteoporosis are small-boned women, Caucasian, smokers, those who drink more than moderately, and those who do little or no exercise. Men are also at risk due to the same factors as women. A bone density scan (DEXA scan) can be done with a special x-ray to diagnose osteoporosis. It is typically unnoticed at its onset, which occurs at approximately age 45, and it may not be noticed at all until a fracture occurs. One of its symptoms is a gradual reduction in height.

Doctors are not certain of its cause. It is thought that years of a sedentary life coupled with a diet deficient in calcium, vitamin D, and fluoride contribute to it, as does **estrogen** loss, which occurs after menopause. Some physicians are still recommending estrogen replacement therapy (ERT) to help prevent osteoporosis. Some doctors are also advising clients to consume 1,500 mg of calcium, which would require the daily consumption of over 1 qt of milk or its equivalent. Calcium tablets, preferably calcium citrate, could be used instead, but the client would also require supplementary vitamin D. A diet with sufficient calcium and vitamin D plus an appropriate exercise program begun early in the adult years is thought to help prevent this disease. Because many individuals are deficient in vitamin D, it is recommended they get their blood levels tested to determine their status.

New research is also leaning toward the importance of eating a diet abundant in fruits and vegetables, especially for osteoporosis. Not only is the potassium and other nutrients they provide important for bone health, but eating more fruits and vegetables tends to yield an alkaline environment, which may produce less leaching of calcium from bone on a daily basis. Eating meat and grains produces more of an acidic environment, which may result in leaching of calcium from bone to keep blood pH normal. Ensuring that protein needs are met from alternative protein sources such as soy, beans, nuts, and seeds is advantageous. Slowing down on salty foods, reducing or eliminating alcohol, and not smoking are other tactics that can affect bone health.

Another possible cause of osteoporosis may be a diet containing excessive amounts of phosphorus, which can speed bone loss. It is known that Americans are ingesting increasing amounts of phosphorus. Sodas and processed foods contain phosphorus, and their consumption is increasing as milk consumption is decreasing in the United States. Soda intake is linked to osteoporosis in so far as it is replacing milk consumption. Some believe that **periodontal disease** may be linked to osteoporosis. Periodontal disease is characterized by bone loss in the jaw, which can lead to loosened teeth and infection in the gums.

Arthritis

Arthritis is a disease that causes the joints to become painful and stiff. It results in structural changes in the cartilage of the joints. A client with arthritis should be especially careful to avoid overweight because the extra weight adds stress to joints that are already painful. If the client is overweight, a weight reduction program should be instituted.

The regular use of aspirin by these clients may cause slight bleeding in the stomach lining and subsequent anemia, so their diets may require additional iron. Arthritis can greatly complicate one's life because it may partially or

geriatrics
the branch of medicine involved with diseases of the elderly

estrogen
hormone secreted by the ovaries

periodontal disease
disease of the mouth and gums

arthritis
chronic disease involving the joints

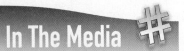

Can a Certain Diet Cut the Risk for Alzheimer's?

Researchers have tested a unique diet that appears to reduce the risk for developing Alzheimer's disease. The study, conducted by researchers at Rush University Medical Center in Chicago, designed the MIND diet, which is similar to the heart-healthy Mediterranean diet and DASH diet. The MIND diet, however, differs as it places particular emphasis on eating "brain health" foods such as berries, leafy green vegetables and other vegetables, starchy beans, whole grains, fish, poultry, olive oil, and wine. Participants, with a median age of 81, were followed on average for 4.5 years. Subjects whose diet choices adhered closely to the MIND diet had a 53% reduced risk for developing Alzheimer's.

Source: Adapted from Reddy, Sumathi. "A Diet Might Cut the Risk of Developing Alzheimer's." *The Wall Street Journal.* April 20, 2015. Accessed October 2015.

Exploring THE WEB

Search the Web for information on exercises that are appropriate for the elderly. What information can you find? Cite references of safe and effective exercises for the elderly. What benefits can these exercises bring to the elderly client? If an elderly client is active, how does that affect his or her nutritional needs?

occlusions
blockages

completely immobilize one so much that shopping, moving around, and cooking become difficult.

Aspirin and other anti-inflammatory drugs do help relieve the pain of arthritis, but there is as yet no cure. Clients should be well informed of this to prevent them from wasting their money on so-called miracle cures recommended by health food faddists or quacks.

Cancer

Research about the role of nutrition in cancer development continues. The American Cancer Society that it is important to stay at a healthy weight, increase physical activity, and eat a diet full of plant foods, while avoiding processed meats (see Chapter 19).

Diabetes Mellitus

Diabetes mellitus is a chronic disease. It develops when the body does not produce sufficient amounts of insulin or does not use it effectively for normal carbohydrate metabolism. Diet is very important in the treatment of diabetes. Chapter 15 discusses this treatment in detail.

Hypertension

Hypertension, or high blood pressure, can lead to strokes. It is associated with diets high in salt or possibly low in calcium. Most Americans ingest from two to six times the amount of salt needed each day. It is thought that the earlier a person reduces salt intake, the better that person's chances of avoiding hypertension, particularly if there is a family history of it. Hypertension is discussed in detail in Chapter 16.

Heart Disease

Heart attack and stroke are the major causes of death in the United States. They occur when arteries become blocked (occluded), preventing the normal passage of blood. These **occlusions** (blockages) are caused by blood clots that form and are unable to pass through an unnaturally narrowed artery. Arteries are narrowed by plaque, a fatty substance containing cholesterol that accumulates in the walls of the artery. This condition is called atherosclerosis. It is believed that excessive saturated fats in the diet and an intake high in sugars and refined carbohydrates (promoting obesity and inflammation) over many years contribute to this condition. The therapeutic diet appropriate for atherosclerosis is discussed in Chapter 16.

Effects of Nutrition

Current research about the role of nutrition in preventing or relieving these chronic diseases continues. The effects of nutrition are cumulative over many years. The effects of a lifetime of poor eating habits cannot be cured overnight. When diets have been poor for a long time, prevention of these chronic diseases may not be possible. It may be possible, however, to use nutrition to help stabilize the condition of such a client. The prevention of many of the diseases of the elderly should begin in one's youth (Figure 13-3).

Health and Nutrition Considerations for Late Adulthood

It is essential that the health care professional remember that each client is an individual with unique needs. It is easy for someone working exclusively with geriatric clients to group them together, but doing so diminishes the quality of the care they receive and adds to their unhappiness. The 80-year-old client is just as pleased to see a smile on the face of a nurse as is an 18-year-old client.

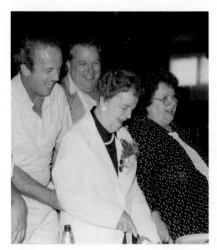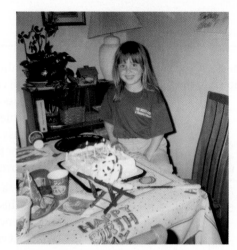

FIGURE 13-3 Celebrating an 80th birthday is as much fun as turning 8—when health is good, of course.

The 70-year-old overweight arthritic client deserves as much help with a weight loss program as the 45-year-old client. The 85-year-old client suffering from senility still enjoys a bright hello and a gentle pat on the back. People's feelings must never be forgotten. The incapacitation that can accompany old age is a terrible indignity, and these clients deserve special care.

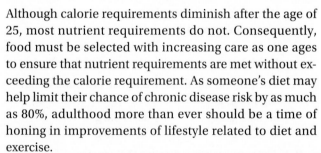

SUMMARY

Although calorie requirements diminish after the age of 25, most nutrient requirements do not. Consequently, food must be selected with increasing care as one ages to ensure that nutrient requirements are met without exceeding the calorie requirement. As someone's diet may help limit their chance of chronic disease risk by as much as 80%, adulthood more than ever should be a time of honing in improvements of lifestyle related to diet and exercise.

Overweight can cause health problems. If it is caused by energy imbalance, a program of weight loss, which includes exercise, should be undertaken. The diet should be based on MyPlate, and eating habits should be taught so that the lost weight will not be regained later.

The elderly are becoming an increasingly large segment of the U.S. population, and their nutritional needs are of growing concern. If a chronic disease is being experienced, often a modification in diet can help manage the disease. Most nutrient requirements do not decrease with age, but calorie requirements do. When food habits of senior citizens must be changed, adjustments require great tact and patience on the part of the dietitian. Older people are easily attracted to food fads that promise good health and prolonged life.

DISCUSSION TOPICS

1. Why do calorie requirements tend to diminish after the age of 25? Why do nutrient requirements not diminish at the same time?

2. Why does a 40-year-old road constructor require more calories than a 40-year-old administrative assistant?

3. Why are middle-age adults more inclined to be overweight than young adults?

4. Why does the iron requirement usually diminish for women after the age of 50?

5. In what ways can emotional stress affect eating habits? What kinds of emotional stress do the elderly sometimes suffer?

6. What is osteoporosis? Name the risk factors involved. Which risk factors do you or a close relative have for osteoporosis?

SUGGESTED ACTIVITIES

1. Keep a food diary for a day. Check off each food under MyPlate headings, as shown in the form provided.

	Fat/ Sweet	Dairy	Meats	Veg.	Fruit	Bread/ Grain
Recommended servings/day	Use sparingly	2–3	2–3	3–5	2–4	6–8
Breakfast						
Lunch						
Dinner						
Total						

a. Total the entries in the vertical columns. Which columns have the highest totals?
b. Discuss the shortages or excesses and the possible dangers of each.
c. Discuss realistic ways of improving your diet.
d. Repeat this exercise in a week. Evaluate for improvements.

2. Interview a relative or neighbor with osteoporosis. What is this person doing to prevent future pain and degeneration associated with the disease? What diet changes has this person undergone?

3. Research various autoimmune diseases. Is there any nutrition component that may help in these conditions?

4. If possible, visit a nursing home at mealtime. Write your evaluation of the food and a description of resident's reactions to it and to you, the visitor.

5. Research current food fads and pick one to discuss with the class, stating whether this product would help or hinder nutritional health.

REVIEW

Multiple choice. Select the *letter* that precedes the best answer.

1. Overweight during middle age is often due to
   a. obesity
   b. hypertension
   c. adipose tissue
   d. energy imbalance

2. The measure of energy in foods eaten is one's
   a. calorie requirement
   b. calorie intake
   c. nutrient requirement
   d. energy imbalance

3. Because of menstruation and pregnancy during the young and middle years, women have a greater need than men for
   a. proteins
   b. B vitamins
   c. iodine
   d. iron

4. Calorie requirements
   a. increase with age
   b. decrease with age
   c. remain unchanged throughout adult life
   d. none of the above

5. Nutrient requirements during adult life generally
   a. increase with age
   b. decrease with age
   c. change very little
   d. none of the above

6. Women's calorie requirements as compared with men's are generally
   a. lower
   b. higher
   c. the same
   d. none of the above

7. The protein needs for a 35-year-old male weighing 192 lb is
   a. 60.2 g
   b. 72.4 g
   c. 69.8 g
   d. 87.3 g

8. Osteoporosis is a disease that causes
   a. poor appetite
   b. a reduction in the number of red blood cells
   c. joints to become painful and stiff
   d. bones to become porous

9. Hypertension is related to diets high in
   a. cholesterol
   b. vitamin D
   c. calcium
   d. salt

10. Which of the following may cause depression in the elderly?
    a. loss of a family member
    b. lack of social ability
    c. physical disability
    d. all of the above

CASE IN POINT

MARY: DISCOVERING OSTEOPOROSIS

Fred and Mary have been married for 52 years. Throughout the years, they have been a very active and healthy couple. They have always tried to eat healthy, exercise, and see their doctor routinely. After Fred retired, he and Mary began playing tennis with a group at their local country club. They particularly enjoyed the doubles tennis and even participated in some senior tournaments. In one particularly exciting match, Mary fell and injured her wrist. She wasn't in too much pain at the time, but by the next morning her wrist was swollen, bruised, and painful to move. She decided to see a doctor to have it x-rayed. The x-ray revealed that her wrist had a small fracture. The doctor also noted that her bones didn't look quite as dense as they should on the x-ray film. The doctor explained to Mary that it is possible she had developed osteoporosis. Mary never liked to take pills and so she did not take an estrogen replacement therapy after menopause. In addition, she was now 2 inches shorter than she was in her younger days. Her doctor informed her that these were both risk factors for developing osteoporosis. The doctor asked Mary to have a bone density scan done as well. The doctor wanted further assessment of Mary's situation in hopes to prevent future fractures.

ASSESSMENT

1. What do you know about Mary's health?
2. What did the doctor suspect about Mary?
3. How significant is this problem?
4. How common is this problem in the elderly?

DIAGNOSIS

5. Write a diagnosis for Mary's alteration in health maintenance and its cause.
6. Write a diagnosis for Mary's deficient knowledge and the type of education she needs.

PLAN/GOAL

7. What must change in Mary's diet?

IMPLEMENTATION

8. What additions or alterations in Mary's diet would prevent further osteoporosis? What are the best sources of calcium? What about vitamin D?
9. What information does Mary need to make this change?
10. Who can help her learn?
11. How can regular exercise help?
12. How could information from the National Osteoporosis Foundation (http://www.nof .org) help Mary?

EVALUATION/OUTCOME CRITERIA

13. At her next office visit with the doctor, what will Mary report?
14. How long will it take before the doctor can measure an improvement in a DEXA scan?

THINKING FURTHER

15. From your review of the National Osteoporosis Foundation website (http://www.nof.org), what kind of information is available there?
16. Aside from calcium and vitamin D, how could other medications for osteoporosis help?
17. Why is it important to intervene with a person at any age who suffers from osteoporosis?
18. How can you use this lesson in other situations?

✔ rate this plate

Mary's problem was first noticed when she injured her wrist on the tennis court. She will need further testing to properly diagnose osteoporosis. Even though Mary has tried to eat healthy and live an active life, she may not have eaten adequate calcium and vitamin D to develop dense bones. Rate this plate on calcium content:

1 cup clam chowder

6 whole-wheat crackers

1 medium peach

½ cup tapioca pudding

Water with lemon

Will this meal give Mary a serving of calcium? How many milligrams of calcium is considered a serving? List foods that are good sources of calcium.

CASE IN POINT

MAX: DECREASING APPETITE

Max is a 95-year-old man. His wife of 64 years, Sophia, died after suffered a stroke 12 years ago. Max misses Sophia dearly, but tries to remain active and busy to keep his mind off of the sadness that he now has in his life. Max had been a salesman for many years and had a love for people and a gift for conversation. After Sophia's death, he decided to volunteer at the local hospital. For several years, he helped transport clients at discharge, offered books and magazines to clients, and delivered flowers and mail. About a year ago, the volunteer work began to be too much for him physically, so he decided to stop.

Max's daughter, Avery, and her children live nearby. Avery often stops to visit with her dad in the evenings, and cook meals and bring food to him on a regular basis. Max isn't much of a cook. Since Sophia's death, he has depended on Avery or restaurants for any hot meals. Recently, Avery has noticed that her Dad is eating less of the food she puts in his refrigerator. Max says that he doesn't have much of an appetite. Avery has also noticed that her father's hygiene practices are in decline, as he is not the neatly dressed, clean-shaven man she knows, but is bearded and usually dressed in pajamas. Avery is concerned because her father looks very pale and thin. Max has also reported feeling weak and dizzy. Avery decides it's time to take her father to the doctor.

ASSESSMENT

1. What do you know about Max and his health?
2. What do you know is a barrier in Max's life to maintaining health?
3. What nutrients are missing from Max's diet, and why?
4. How significant is the problem? What are the long-term consequences of the problem?

DIAGNOSIS

5. Complete the following statement: Imbalanced nutrition; less than body requirements related to _____.
6. What nutrition education does Avery need to help Max?

PLAN/GOAL

7. What are your goals for Max's diet?

IMPLEMENTATION

8. Identify how each of the following resources can help Max solve this problem and prevent further problems: his daughter, Avery; his grandchildren; his church; and local agencies.

EVALUATION/OUTCOME CRITERIA

9. At Max's next Nurse Practitioner (NP) appointment, what changes would the NP expect to note? What would the NP expect Avery to report?

THINKING FURTHER

10. Why it is so important in older persons to ensure that there is a balance between nutrition, medication, and chronic illness?
11. What would be the benefits of an assisted living setting for Max?
12. How can you use this lesson in other situations?

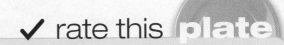

✔ rate this **plate**

Max's lack of energy and weakness could be directly related to his poor appetite. Avery brought Max a warm meal to encourage her father to eat, which included:

4 oz meatloaf

1 small baked potato with butter and sour cream

½ cup of green beans and corn

1 dinner roll

½ cup custard

Coffee

Are these choices good, or does any food need to be changed or added? Will this meal provide enough calories and nutrients for Max?

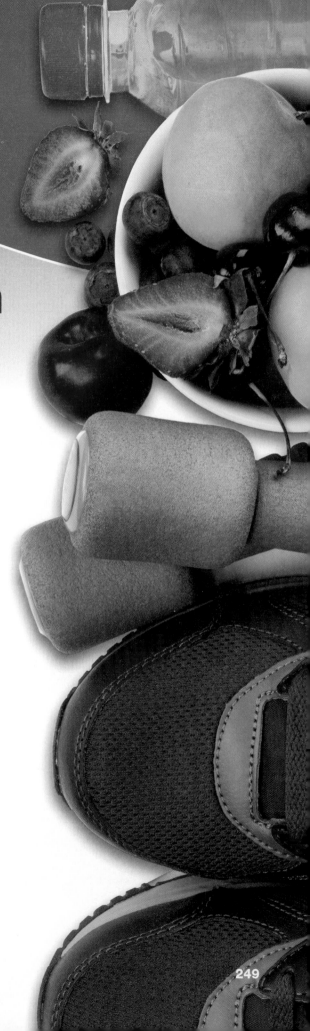

SECTION 3

Medical Nutrition Therapy

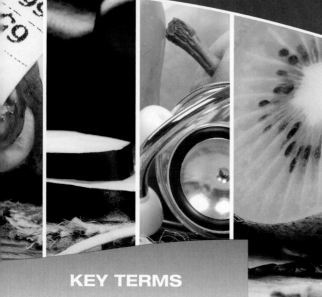

CHAPTER 14

KEY TERMS

built environment
ghrelin
Hamwi method
hyperthyroidism
hypothyroidism
leptin
motivational interviewing
plateau period
subcutaneous fat
visceral fat
yo-yo effect

WEIGHT MANAGEMENT ACROSS THE LIFE CYCLE

OBJECTIVES

After studying this chapter, you should be able to:

- Describe factors that contribute to energy balance and weight

- Describe changes in environment that have influenced obesity rates

- Understand medical complications of obesity for children and adults

- Explain treatment methods for overweight and obese children and adults, and where to find resources

- Discuss prevention strategies and national efforts to rein in the obesity epidemic

FIGURE 14-1 The places where you store your body fat affect your health. "Pear" shapes tend to store fat in the hips and buttocks. "Apple" shapes store fat around the waist, which may be associated with more health issues.

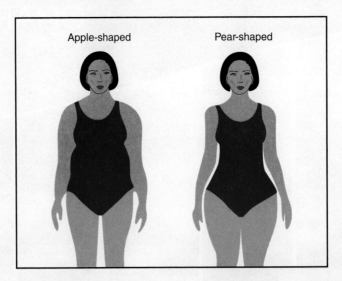

We are all born with the innate ability to regulate our eating so that we grow and develop properly and meet our energy needs over the life cycle. Our body's appetite regulation system is designed to guide us on the proper amount of food to consume, which in turn regulates our weight. But weight regulation is complex and influenced by many factors. Our genetics and physiology play key roles in how our body turns out—its shape, size, and weight distribution as well as susceptibility to disease (Figure 14-1). Our environment and lifestyle choices also exert considerable influence on our weight and health as well.

The very young are excellent food regulators; however, research shows that children near school age respond more to external influences and learn to bypass internal fullness cues. Eating in response to boredom or stress is a learned behavior that may surface between ages 5 and 9.

TRIGGERS FOR OVEREATING

If more food is set before us, overconsumption happens. If we smell or see appetizing food, we may eat it whether we are hungry or not. Boredom or stress are other external factors that can trigger eating. For many of us, we are not conscious of these effects. These habits can become ingrained and continue habitually throughout life. Pair these factors with a world of rich, plentiful, and highly marketed food, then sprinkle in liberal amounts of media time and low physical activity, and here lies the recipe for emerging obesity.

Parents can disrupt the natural flow of feeding by putting pressure on children to either eat more or eat less at meals, therefore pulling them away from natural feeding cues. Underweight children who are coerced to eat tend to back away from food. Children who are restricted in their diets, to lose weight, are prone to overeat in the absence of hunger. Some end up managing their eating well; others become distressed eaters, which then can follow into adulthood.

Many individuals struggle with balancing their weight in a healthy fashion. Obesity is commonplace in today's society. Some feel obesity is a result of the "thrifty" gene. The genes that helped our ancestors survive occasional shortages of food may now be working against us in a supply that is abundantly plentiful year round. Some researchers believe that genes may have a role in those who suffer from poor appetite regulation and those who have an easily stimulated capacity to store body fat. Likely, it is not one gene that predisposes a person to obesity, but a cluster of genes; and many researchers today believe obesity has strong ties to insulin resistance.

While genetics predisposes a person to obesity, it's really the environment and lifestyle factors that tip the scale in its favor. Our modern world has efficiently engineered the art of movement out of the culture: sedentary desk jobs, remote controls, elevators, cars, escalators, and more. Time- and energy-saving gadgets abound. Food is available 24 hours a day, around every corner, at every venue imaginable. The shifts are dramatic; higher fast food and soft drink consumption, reduced frequency of family meals, and increased portion sizes. Children and adults gravitate to television, video games, computers, and smartphones and, consequently, engage in little physical activity.

EATING REGULATION AND ENERGY BALANCE

Regulation of eating occurs primarily in the brain. In the hypothalamus, hunger and satiety chemicals work to regulate eating. The hormone **leptin** receives signals from fat and the intestine to make you feel full so eating will stop. The hormone **ghrelin** is released from the stomach and signals the hypothalamus that it's time to eat. Other key hormones and neurotransmitters are involved as well in food regulation.

The body needs a certain amount of energy (calories) from food to sustain basic life functions and, in children, growth. Body weight is maintained when calories eaten equal the number of calories the body expends, or "burns" (Figure 14-2). When more calories are consumed than burned, energy balance is tipped toward weight gain, overweight, and obesity.

As referenced in Chapter 3, the components of our energy "out" are basal metabolic rate (BMR), physical activity, and the thermic effect of food. Figure 14-3 breaks down these components into percentages. Activity level and basal metabolic rate can vary greatly. Factors that affect BMR include age, height, growth cycle, and body composition. Other factors that affect BMR are temperature (body temperature as well as climate temperature) and fasting, or undereating. If an individual is underproducing thyroid hormone, BMR can decrease. This condition is called **hypothyroidism**.

Regarding physical activity, only 31% of U.S. adults report that they engage in regular leisure-time physical activity (150 minutes per week of light to moderate

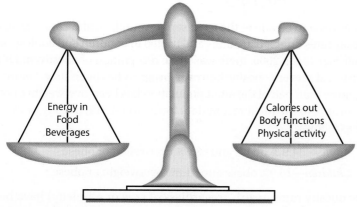

FIGURE 14-2 Balancing "energy in" and "energy out" will maintain weight.

leptin
an appetite-suppressing hormone involved in maintenance of body composition

ghrelin
a hormone from the stomach that signals the brain that it's time to eat

hypothyroidism
a condition in which the thyroid gland secretes too little thyroxine and T3, resulting in a lower basal metabolic rate

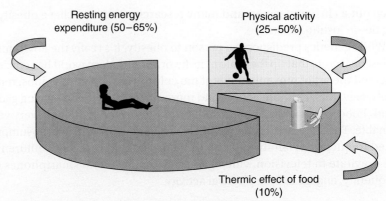

Resting energy
expenditure (50–65%)

Physical activity
(25–50%)

Thermic effect of food
(10%)

FIGURE 14-3 Components of basal metabolic rate.

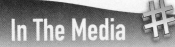

In The Media

Affordable Care Act to Cover Weight Loss Services

The Affordable Care Act (ACA), which was signed into law by President Obama in 2010, will now cover weight loss programs that involve professional weight loss doctors, nurses, and registered dietitians. According to a report published in the *New York Times*, "currently 23 states cover bariatric or gastric bypass surgery and 16 states now include some coverage for dietary and nutritional screening, counseling, and weight loss programs." Some weight loss aides, such as supplements, pills, and shakes are not covered under the current plan. While the ACA creates opportunities for practitioners to assist in weight loss promotion, it can also create an opportunity for some unproven weight loss methods. The public is cautioned on any diets that offer "quick fixes" for speedy weight loss.

Source: Adapted from "Affordable Care Act Will Cover Weight Loss Medical Services" (2015, July 9). ABC News. Accessed October 19, 2015. www.abcnews.go.com

physical activity or 60 minutes of vigorous activity per week). About 40% of adults report no leisure-time physical activity. Interestingly, when physical activity is measured by a device that detects movement, only about 3–5% of adults obtain 30 minutes of moderate or greater intensity physical activity on at least 5 days per week.

Without a doubt, many Americans are having a hard time balancing the "energy in" part of the equation. It appears that there has been a steady increase in calorie intake over the last 40 years. Adults on average are consuming approximately 450 more calories a day as of 2010 than they did in 1970. And a higher proportion of the calories we do take in comes from added sugars. Even though soda sales have leveled off and even decreased, our high sugar intake is coming in other forms, such as energy drinks and designer coffees.

It has also been documented that Americans have a greater consumption of low-nutrition, energy-dense foods. Cost seems to be a factor in driving that change. Adjusted for inflation, prices for low-nutrient, energy-dense foods and beverages, such as soda and fast food, have declined sharply, which makes them appealing for consumers with smaller food budgets. Unfortunately, on the flipside, research has documented a dramatic rise in the price of more nutritious foods, such as fruits, vegetables, lean meats, and low-fat dairy products.

About three-fourths of the population has an eating pattern that is low in vegetables and fruits. Most Americans exceed the recommendations for added sugars, saturated fats, and sodium.

OBESITY TRENDS

Obesity has risen to be one of the most serious public health concerns of our nation. Obesity rates doubled in adults and tripled in children and adolescents from 1980–2000. Starting in 2000, there was more recognition of obesity and intervention to treat and prevent obesity; however, progress has been slow. For more than 25 years, more than half of the adult population has been overweight or obese.

According to the most recent data from 2011–2012, obesity or overweight rates are as follows:

- *Adults*—34.9 % obese and 68.6% overweight or obese
- *Children*—16.9% obese and 31.8% overweight or obese

The obesity rates in girls (regardless of race or ethnicity) have been stable; however, the rate in men, boys, and African American and Hispanic women has increased. Obesity is more prevalent in families in poverty. Figure 14-4

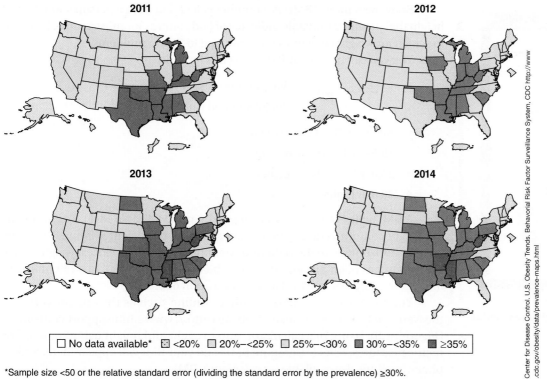

2011   2012

2013   2014

☐ No data available*   ▨ <20%   ☐ 20%–<25%   ☐ 25%–<30%   ■ 30%–<35%   ■ ≥35%

Center for Disease Control. U.S. Obesity Trends. Behavorial Risk Factor Surveillance System, CDC http://www .cdc.gov/obesity/data/prevalence-maps.html

*Sample size <50 or the relative standard error (dividing the standard error by the prevalence) ≥30%.

FIGURE 14-4 Prevalence of self-reported obesity among U.S. adults by state and territory, 2011–2014.

illustrates the increase in obesity by state in just the past several years in the adult population.

Defining Obesity

On a basic level, obesity can be defined as excess fat accumulation under the skin and around the organs in the body. Fat accumulated in the lower body (the pear shape) is **subcutaneous fat** (Figure 14-5). Fat in the abdominal area (the apple shape) is mostly **visceral fat**. Abdominal fat correlates more with health risks such as cardiovascular disease and type 2 diabetes. In women, it also correlates with breast cancer risk and gallbladder disease. Where we deposit fat is influenced by hormones and heredity.

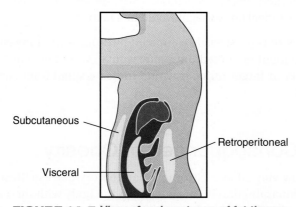

Subcutaneous

Retroperitoneal

Visceral

FIGURE 14-5 View of various types of fat tissue.

subcutaneous fat
fat stored directly under the skin

visceral fat
fat stored within the abdominal cavity

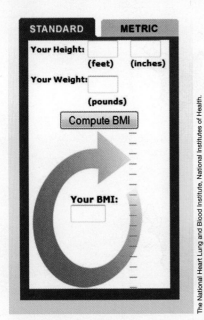

FIGURE 14-6 **Body mass index calculator.**

Body mass index (BMI) is a number calculated from a person's weight and height that provides a reliable indicator of body fatness for most people. It is used to screen for weight categories that may lead to health problems.

You can calculate your BMI using this formula:

$$\text{BMI} = \frac{\text{Weight (pounds)} \times 703}{\text{Height squared (inches}^2)}$$

- Below 18.5 = Underweight
- 18.5–24.9 = Healthy weight
- 25.0–29.9 = Overweight
- 30.0 or higher = Obese

A BMI table is a useful tool to approximate BMI (Table 14-1). To use, follow the height column vertically on the left side until the height is found. Trace the column horizontally to the right until you find your client's closest weight. Once the weight has been pinpointed, trace the column upward in a straight line to find out the approximate BMI and classification of BMI.

You may also use a BMI calculator online such as the one provided on the National Institutes of Health website (http://www.nhlbisupport.com/bmi/) (Figure 14-6). Using this calculator, enter weight and height using standard or metric measures. Select "Compute BMI" and your BMI will appear there. Smartphone apps are also available for calculating BMIs.

Although BMI can be used for most men and women, it does have some limits:

- It may overestimate body fat in athletes and others who have a muscular build.
- It may underestimate body fat in older persons and others who have lost muscle.

A way to quickly assess ideal body weight is to use the **Hamwi method**, which considers height, frame size, and gender. The Hamwi formula uses ideal body weight goals as follows:

- Men: 5-ft man at 106 lb. Add or subtract 6 lb for every inch above or below 5 ft. This is for a medium frame man. For small frame, deduct 10%, and for a large frame, add 10% to calculation. A 6-ft man with a medium frame therefore would have an ideal body weight of 178 lb.
- Women: 5-ft woman at 100 lb. Add or subtract 5 lb for every inch above or below 5 ft. For small frame, deduct 10%, and for a large frame, add 10% to calculation. A 5-ft 3-in woman of medium frame's ideal body weight would be 115 lb.

(Frame size is most easily estimated by doing a wrist measurement. The wrist measurement for a medium frame woman would be 6 in. and for a man 7 in. A smaller or larger number would indicate small frame or large frame, respectively.)

Health Consequences of Obesity

Hamwi method
a formula for estimating ideal body weight based on gender, height, and frame size

Obesity is now viewed as a chronic inflammatory disease. Researchers now believe that inflammation is "turned on" in the body with increasing visceral or abdominal fat. This in turn sets the stage for a cascade of chronic disease

TABLE 14-1 BMI Table

BMI	NORMAL						OVERWEIGHT					OBESE										EXTREME OBESITY		
	19	20	21	22	23	24	25	26	27	28	29	30	31	32	33	34	35	36	37	38	39	40	41	42
Height (Feet-Inches)	Weight (Pounds)																							
4' 10"	91	96	100	105	110	115	119	124	129	134	138	143	148	153	158	162	167	172	177	181	186	191	196	201
4' 11"	94	99	104	109	114	119	124	128	133	138	143	148	153	158	163	168	173	178	183	188	193	198	203	208
5' 00"	97	102	107	112	118	123	128	133	138	143	148	153	158	163	168	174	179	184	189	194	199	204	209	215
5' 01"	100	106	111	116	122	127	132	137	143	148	153	158	164	169	174	180	185	190	195	201	206	211	217	222
5' 02"	104	109	115	120	126	131	136	142	147	153	158	164	169	175	180	186	191	196	202	207	213	218	224	229
5' 03"	107	112	118	124	130	135	141	146	152	158	163	169	175	180	186	191	197	203	208	214	220	225	231	237
5' 04"	110	116	122	128	134	140	145	151	157	163	169	174	180	186	192	197	204	209	215	221	227	232	238	244
5' 05"	114	120	126	132	138	144	150	156	162	168	174	180	186	192	198	204	210	216	222	228	234	240	246	252
5' 06"	118	124	130	136	142	148	155	161	167	173	179	186	192	198	204	210	216	223	229	235	241	247	253	260
5' 07"	121	127	134	140	146	153	159	166	172	178	185	191	198	204	211	217	223	230	236	242	249	255	261	268
5' 08"	125	131	138	144	151	158	164	171	177	184	190	197	203	210	216	223	230	236	243	249	256	262	269	276
5' 09"	128	135	142	149	155	162	169	176	182	189	196	203	209	216	223	230	236	243	250	257	263	270	277	284
5' 10"	132	139	146	153	160	167	174	181	188	195	202	209	216	222	229	236	243	250	257	264	271	278	285	292
5' 11"	136	143	150	157	165	172	179	186	193	200	208	215	222	229	236	243	250	257	265	272	279	286	293	301
6' 00"	140	147	154	162	169	177	184	191	199	206	213	221	228	235	242	250	258	265	272	279	287	294	302	309
6' 01"	144	151	159	166	174	182	189	197	204	212	219	227	235	242	250	257	265	272	280	288	295	302	310	318
6' 02"	148	155	163	171	179	186	194	202	210	218	225	233	241	249	256	264	272	280	287	295	303	311	119	326
6' 03"	152	160	168	176	184	192	200	208	216	224	232	240	248	256	264	272	279	287	295	303	311	319	327	335
6' 04"	156	164	172	180	189	197	205	213	221	230	238	246	254	263	271	279	287	295	304	312	320	32a	336	344

Adapted from: George Bray, Pennington Biomedical Research Center, *Clinical Guidelines on the Identification, Evaluation, and Treatment of Overweight and Obesity in Adults: The Evidence Report*, National Institutes of Health, National Heart, Lung, and Blood Institute, September 1998.

Source: National Institute of Diabetes and Digestive and Kidney Diseases. Weight Control Information Network. (November 2008). *Understanding Adult Obesity*. Accessed January 2016. http://win.niddk.nih.gov

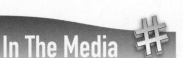

In The Media

Sitting Is a Negative Even If You Work Out

According to the World Health Organization, physical inactivity has been identified as the fourth-leading risk factor for death. Sedentary behavior can lead to cardiovascular disease, cancer, and diabetes. Researchers from Toronto analyzed 47 studies of sedentary behavior. Data was adjusted to incorporate the amount someone exercises in a day; however, researchers still found that the amount of sedentary time engaged in outweighed the benefit from exercise. Tactics to help you sit less include taking frequent breaks during the work day to stretch and walk, and decreasing TV time or taking time to stand up during commercial breaks.

Adapted from Christensen, Jn. "Sitting Will Kill You, Even if You Exercise." CNN News. www .cnn.com

possibilities. As weight increases to reach the levels referred to as "overweight" and "obese," the risks increase for:

- Coronary heart disease
- Insulin resistance and type 2 diabetes
- Cancers (endometrial, breast, and colon)
- Hypertension (high blood pressure)
- Dyslipidemia (e.g., high total cholesterol or high levels of triglycerides)
- Stroke
- Liver and gallbladder disease
- Sleep apnea and respiratory problems
- Osteoarthritis (a degeneration of cartilage and its underlying bone within a joint)
- Gynecological problems (abnormal menses, infertility)

Besides the physical consequences of obesity and overweight, emotional and social health is affected. Some overweight or obese individuals suffer from low self-esteem and negative body image. Often, those who suffer from weight issues can be depressed and feel that they are the object of discrimination.

Financial issues are a concern as well. On average, people who are considered obese pay 42% more in health care costs than normal-weight individuals. Our nation as a whole is seeing the staggering economic effect. The cost of overweight and obesity in the United States is estimated at $270 billion per year. This cost is related to the increased need for medical care and the loss of productivity from disability and death.

Waist Circumference

Because of the science behind the health risk of visceral fat, it is useful to measure waist circumference, along with BMI, and correlate this to disease risk. Note that in Table 14-2, you can see that the disease risk increases as waist circumference and BMI increase.

One important note is that BMI does not show the difference between fat and muscle. It does not always accurately predict when weight could lead to health problems. For example, when someone with a lot of muscle (such as a bodybuilder

TABLE 14-2 Classification of Overweight and Obesity by BMI, Waist Circumference, and Associated Disease Risks

	BMI (kg/m²)	OBESITY CLASS	DISEASE RISK* RELATIVE TO NORMAL WEIGHT AND WAIST CIRCUMFERENCE	
			MEN (40 in.) OR LESS WOMEN (35 in.) OR LESS	MEN >40 in. WOMEN >35 in.
Underweight	<18.5		—	—
Normal	18.5–24.9		—	—
Overweight	25.0–29.9		Increased	High
Obesity	30.0–34.9	I	High	Very high
	35.0–39.9	II	Very high	Very high
Extreme Obesity	40.0+	III	Extremely high	Extremely high

*Disease risk for type 2 diabetes, hypertension, and CVD. +Increased waist circumference also can be a marker for increased risk, even in persons of normal weight.

Source: The National Heart Lung and Blood Institute, National Institutes of Health. *Obesity and Physical Activity Information. Classification of Overweight and Obesity by BMI, Waist Circumference, and Associated Disease Risks*. Accessed January 2016. www.nhlbi.nih.gov

or football player) has a higher BMI, they may still be healthy and have little risk of developing secondary complications from overweight or obesity. Studies do show it's the level of fitness that correlates to long-term survival better than one's level of obesity. Simply put, research tends to show overweight people who are fit have a lower risk of death than normal-weight individuals who are sedentary.

Body fat assessment is much more specific to your actual fat content and thus provides a more accurate picture. The two most common methods used are skinfold measurement and bioelectrical impedance analysis (BIA) machines or scales. In skinfold measurement, a trained specialist uses calipers to measure specific spots on the body. These measurements are compared to a chart that estimates fat percentage. However, the accuracy of this method varies greatly based on the user's abilities.

Bioelectrical impedance analysis is the technology behind the many fat percentage machines in use at fitness centers and in scales sold for home use. However, the error rates for these can be as high as 8%. Body fat measures that are more accurate are x-ray analysis (DEXA scan) and water displacement methods, which are largely used in research institutions.

According to the American Council on Exercise, acceptable body fat percentages for women are between 25% and 31%, and for men between 18% and 24%. To be considered in the "fitness" body fat percentage range, women should be between 21% and 24%, and men between 14% and 17%. Despite the multiple factors that influence weight, altered food intake and decreased physical activity play into the equation in a significant way.

STRATEGIES FOR WEIGHT LOSS

When an individual begins the journey of weight loss, the road can begin to look very bumpy. There are numerous diet and self-help books available to the public. In fact, according to data from 2014, the diet industry overall adds up to nearly $60 billion.

Among America's 75 million dieters, 80% are trying to do it on their own. But the big questions remain: What works, and is it safe? Safe weight loss has been described in the medical literature for decades at 1–2 lb per week, in order to preserve lean body mass. That equates to roughly decreasing your intake between 500 and 1,000 calories a day. For very obese individuals, some references state that they can safely lose 1% of their body weight per week (325-lb man = 3.25 lb/week acceptable weight loss). Research has documented many benefits for persons losing as moderately as 5–10% of their body weight.

There are many eating styles that are healthy and safe and will yield weight loss. The Therapeutic Lifestyle Change (TLC) diet from the National Institute of Health is an all-around healthy plan aimed at improving heart health and lowering cholesterol. The same can be said of the Ornish diet and the Mediterranean diet. The DASH diet (Dietary Approaches to Stop Hypertension), also from the National Institutes of Health, works to improve hypertension and heart health. Common threads in these eating plans are consuming highly nutritious fruits; vegetables; high-fiber grains; and heart-healthy protein foods such as seafood, beans, very lean poultry, low-fat dairy, nuts, seeds, and small amounts of oil (Figure 14-7).

A way to assemble your plate that naturally trims calories would be to estimate portions using hand size:

- Cup your hands—very lean protein would fit in one palm; a higher fiber grain or healthy starchy vegetable/starchy bean dish would fit in the other palm.

- Fill in the rest of your plate with non-starchy vegetables in the form of salads, soups, and steamed or lightly sautéed vegetables. Besides

Exploring THE WEB

How have portion sizes changed in restaurants over the past 20 years? Research what the calorie content was of a fast food meal back in the 1970s. Compare that with a fast food meal of today. The term *portion distortion* describes the phenomenon that is happening. Check out the National Heart, Lung, and Blood Institute's slide set on portion distortion by going to http://www.nhlbi.nih.gov and typing "Portion Distortion Slide show" into the search bar.

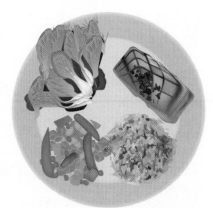

FIGURE 14-7 Healthy eating for weight management.

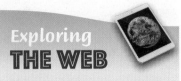

high nutrient value, they will add fullness and bulk to your eating
and help keep your calories in check for weight loss. Examples of nonstarchy vegetables include broccoli; spinach; tomatoes; green beans;
cucumbers; mushrooms; carrots; cabbage; peppers; summer squash,
such as zucchini, lettuce; and onion.

- Provide yourself with a serving of fruit, skim milk, and a small allowance
of healthy fat for optimal intake.

Mindful eating concepts have been incorporated into many weight management programs over the last few years. Mindful eating is eating with attention
and intention. It revolves around eating slowly at the table without distraction
and judgment, savoring the food you have, and allowing yourself to eat until you
are pleasantly satisfied. A recent systematic review found significant weight loss
documented in 13 out of 19 studies.

As discussed elsewhere in this text, Choose MyPlate (http://www.choose-
myplate.gov) offers mainstream advice to the public about healthy eating plans.
The website includes information for "dieters" and offers ways to track food intake using the SuperTracker. Other popular plans with focused weight loss goals
include the Mayo Clinic diet, the volumetric diet, Weight Watchers, and the *Biggest Loser* diet. Some individuals desiring weight loss swear by simply counting
calories or fat grams. Others learn to weigh and measure their food and follow an
exchange-type meal plan. Table 14-3 shows "less conventional" approaches to
weight loss and their advantages and disadvantages.

TABLE 14-3 Less Conventional Approaches to Weight Loss

DIET METHOD	PRO	CON
Low carbohydrate (<100 g/day) (Atkins, South Beach, Protein Power)	Rapid initial weight loss; low circulating glucose; may see drop in lipids	Much of initial weight loss is water; could cause poor stamina and ketosis; Atkins high in unhealthy fat; high protein taxes kidney; no higher weight loss shown with this eating vs. low-fat eating after 1 yr; artificial sweetener use touted; hard to follow long term
Extremely low fat (<20% calories from fat) (T-Factor, Pritikin, Ornish)	Wide variety of wholesome foods allowed at normal portions; reduces risk of heart disease and cancer	Satiety and palatability may be a concern for some; decreased absorption of fat-soluble vitamins and minerals
Novel diets promoting certain nutrients, foods, or combinations	May promote rapid weight loss	Nutritionally inadequate; doesn't promote permanent change in food habits or body weight
Paleo—hunter, gatherer diet	Makes you feel full, good weight loss, and control of blood sugar and blood pressure	Low in calcium, vitamin D, B-vitamins, and possibly folate; may be expensive due to high meat, poultry and seafood intake; nutritious food off limits such as legumes, whole grains, and dairy
Fit for Life	Encourages vegetables	Teaches food combining and diet is low in calcium, zinc, iron, and vitamins B_{12} and D
Enter the Zone	Six small eating sessions offer steady supply of energy	Low in fiber and marginal in some nutrients; portrays some high-glycemic foods as dangerous, even though they may have merit nutritionally
Very low calorie (<800 cal/day) or formula (Optifast, Medifast, Cambridge)	Quick weight loss Eliminates behavior cues and food decisions	Low-calorie diets can be dangerous if not monitored by a doctor; does not foster long-term behavior change
Premeasured (Jenny Craig, Nutrisystem)	Generally safe and effective Eliminates decision making from eating	Expensive, clients may have trouble transitioning to their own home-cooked meals

Sources: Adapted from Zonya Health International. *Zonya's Diet Comparison Chart.* 2003, 2006. www.zonya.com; Bastin, Sandra. *Fad Diets.*
UK Cooperative Extension Service. www.ca.uky.edu

Going on a rigid diet low in calories may result in an initial rapid weight loss. However, a higher portion of the weight loss may be lean body mass versus body fat. Sudden weight loss of this type lowers metabolic rate. Often individuals reach a **plateau period** as well in which weight does not decrease further. Due to the depriving nature of strict dieting, individuals are at risk for binge eating. Some may categorize food into "good" and "bad" categories, and if something forbidden is eaten, they feel guilty. Swings in eating then can lead to weight gain, until another diet method is tried. This can have a **yo-yo effect** on weight and impact health.

Behavior Change Methods

Regardless of which type of eating pattern is chosen for weight loss, true behavior change is a must. A skilled clinician must assess whether the patient is indeed, ready to change. More and more clinicians are being trained on the technique of **motivational interviewing**, which is an evidence-based conversational counseling style designed to help people plan for and begin the process of change. In this technique, clinicians help clients explore and resolve ambivalence and begin the "change talk."

Four core principles of motivational interviewing involve:

- *Expressing Empathy*—Use reflective listening to convey understanding of client's message.
- *Rolling with Resistance*—Meet the client's resistance with reflection rather than confrontation.
- *Developing Discrepancy*—Help client understand how deeply held values are different than current behavior.
- *Supporting Self-Efficacy*—Build confidence that change is possible.

Nurses, doctors, mental health professionals, dietitians, health coaches, and others are being trained to use this method to effectively facilitate behavior change in individuals.

There are a multitude of behavior patterns that influence energy balance and contribute to obesity. Skipping breakfast, eating in front of the television, late-night snacking, lack of adequate sleep, being too rushed to exercise, or eating to help manage stress or difficult emotions are just some of the patterns we engage in. What drives our behavior patterns, however, are often not evident but need to be brought to the surface before permanent change can be made. Clients need to evaluate their habits around food and exercise and find the source of the obstacle. We must trace and address underlying issues. Behavior change requires coming to a stage of readiness and being open to readily accept it.

Here are behavioral strategies for weight loss clients:

- Set specific, realistic goals to address changes in eating and exercise and begin to establish new routines.
- Keep a record of food intake and amount of physical activity. Many individuals today track their exercise and even their food intake, on some type of digital fitness tracker (Figure 14-8). Sometimes, clients will have startling self-discovery and eat differently once they know they will be recording it. Individuals may think they exercise more than they really do, but their log may tell them a different story. Reflecting on a personal log can inspire clients as they learn new habits. Wellness habits increase over the long term as clients develop higher self-esteem and better health.

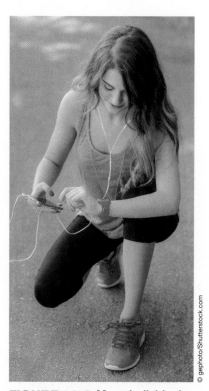

FIGURE 14-8 Many individuals today monitor their health using fitness devices.

© gephoto/Shutterstock.com

plateau period
period in which there is no change in weight

yo-yo effect
when a dieter's weight goes up and down over short periods due to swings in eating (from strict dieting to overconsumption)

motivational interviewing
an evidence-based counseling approach designed to facilitate behavior change by exploring and resolving ambivalence

- On their food record, clients may want to include emotions surrounding their eating patterns, and assess their level of hunger and satiety when finished eating. Sometimes eating happens in the absence of hunger (external drivers), and clients may eat until the stuffed or too full stage. Sensing normal hunger and fullness cues is important, as are triggers for eating.

- Encourage clients to change their surroundings to avoid overeating. For example, they can avoid eating in front of the television. Instruct to keep a pantry full of healthy food, not tempting snack foods and sweets, and to take balanced portions of food to work for lunch and snacks.

- Clients should reward their success in a non-food way. Once they've met a goal, treating oneself to a movie, music CD, an afternoon off from work, a massage, or personal time is gratifying.

- Clients need support from a health care provider, friend, or spouse. A call, e-mail, or even a text can boost support. Perhaps they should join a local support group for accountability.

- Instruct clients to weigh in only once a week for self-monitoring. Clients who are fearful of the scale may only want to measure themselves with a tape measure.

Physical Activity

Staying physically active to build and preserve muscle, in tandem with a healthier diet, are the ingredients for weight loss and healthy weight maintenance. The research on physical activity is compelling. Exercise provides these benefits:

- Lowers the risk of chronic disease (e.g., heart disease, diabetes, cancers) and can help improve blood pressure

- Strengthens lungs and helps them to work more efficiently

- Builds and strengthens muscles and keeps joints in good condition

- May slow bone loss

- Increases energy levels and builds self-confidence

- Helps in relaxation and coping skills by reducing stress and possibly lessening depression

- Helps provide solid sleep habits

- Boosts immunity

How much activity is needed?

- For good health and to reduce risk of disease, aim for at least 30 minutes of moderate physical activity most days of the week.

- To help manage body weight and prevent gradual weight gain, aim for 60 minutes of moderate-to-vigorous physical activity most days of the week.

- To maintain weight loss, aim for at least 60–90 minutes of daily moderate physical activity.

Breaking up exercise into 15-minute increments is useful for some people. If clients have been inactive for some time, they should start slowly and gradually increase their activity. For example, start walking for 10–15 minutes three times a week, then gradually build up to the recommended amount with brisk walking.

Some overweight individuals do not have success "going it alone" and may require formal instruction from a registered dietitian. A dietitian can meet with clients one-on-one for weight management counseling, or in a group setting. Group classes can offer participants moral support, enhanced learning, and significant accountability. Behavior therapy expertise as well as instruction from an exercise scientist forms the basis for comprehensive programming for weight management. Oversight and medical monitoring from a physician is also an important variable.

With new health care reform, the primary care physician's office is now referred to as the "medical home." Primary care doctors are the gatekeepers and serve to organize overall care. Many overweight and obese individuals do receive initial coaching on health habits to help lower their weight in this setting. Since late 2011, many individuals on Medicare with a BMI of 30 or more can receive weekly in-person weight management counseling visits for 1 month, followed by visits every 2 weeks for an additional 5 months. These are fully paid by Medicare with no co-pay.

Exploring THE WEB

Go to the Mayo Clinic website (http://www.mayoclinic.com) for a critique of popular over-the-counter weight loss pills. Review the different products and consider their claims, effectiveness, and safety.

Weight Loss Drugs

Some clients ask their physicians about prescription weight loss drugs. According to the 2015 Endocrine Society Practice Guidelines for Pharmacologic Management of Obesity, if a person has been unsuccessful with losing and maintaining weight loss, he may be a candidate for pharmacotherapy, provided he meets the guidelines on the drug label.

Prescription weight loss drugs are approved only for those clients with a BMI above 30, or a BMI of 27 and above with associated diseases such as hypertension, type 2 diabetes, or dyslipidemia. Appetite suppressants, approved by the FDA, are meant only to be used short term. Efficacy and safety of this therapy should be addressed monthly for the first three months, then at least every three months thereafter.

The top five most prescribed weight loss medicines are as follows:

- *Orlistat*—sold under the brand name Xenical (prescription) and Alli (over the counter). The drug is a lipase inhibitor that prevents absorption of fat from the food into the body. Side effects are gassiness, oily bowel movements and other bowel-related changes, and possible liver malfunction, signs and symptoms of which include yellow skin or eyes, itching, and loss of appetite. Weight loss studies show modest results.

- *Lorcaserin*—sold under the brand name Belviq. This drug acts on receptors in the brain to promote feelings of fullness, thus encouraging users to eat less. This drug, approved in 2012, cannot be used with other selective serotonin reuptake inhibitors (SSRIs). Side effects may include drowsiness, headache, and constipation. When combined with diet and exercise, users lost 3–3.7% more than with a placebo.

- *Phentermine + Topiramate*—sold under the brand name Qsymia. Phentermine is a stimulant that decreases appetite whereas Topiramate is an anti-seizure and migraine drug that also decreases appetite and causes a feeling of early satiety. Women of child-bearing age must use birth control due to the issues with possible birth defects. When combined with diet and exercise, users lost an average of 9% of their body weight compared with 1.5% of patients who took a placebo.

- *Bupropion + Naltrexone*—sold under the brand name Contrave. This drug targets the brain's hypothalamus, which controls hunger and the brain circuitry involving reward activity, including eating. This drug was initially rejected by the FDA due to concerns about long-term effects on the heart and cardiovascular system. It has a black box warning, as Bupropion is associated with increased risk of suicidal thoughts. In one study, 42% of patients lost at least 5% of their body weight taking this drug along with diet and exercise.

- *Liraglutide*—sold under the brand name Saxenda. This drug has a black box warning as animal studies showed it caused thyroid tumors. In studies, 62% of users lost 5% or more of their body weight compared to 34% who took a placebo.

Patients who do not lose at least 5% of their body weight after three months of use should discontinue the drug. The cost benefit should be weighed carefully in patients who are being considered for weight loss pharmacotherapy.

There are numerous over-the-counter weight loss pills and supplements promoting "fat burning." Most products have not been proven effective and some may be dangerous. Supplements and weight loss aids are not subject to the same rigid standards as prescription drugs, although the FDA does monitor their safety and can recall or ban a product if deemed necessary.

Weight Loss Surgery

When sustainable weight loss efforts have failed, some obese individuals opt to have bariatric surgery. The four types of operations common in the United States are as follows (Figure 14-9):

- *Adjustable gastric band (AGB).* A small bracelet-like band is placed around the top of the stomach to restrict the size of the opening from the throat to the stomach, thereby reducing food intake. The size of the opening can be controlled via a balloon inside the band.

- *Roux-en-Y gastric bypass (RYGB).* Food intake is limited as surgeons create a small pouch for the stomach. This pouch is then connected to a different part of the intestine (bypassing the stomach and duodenum), thereby changing the way food is absorbed. The pouch is only about the size of a walnut.

- *Vertical sleeve gastrectomy (VSG).* This newer procedure involves removing much of the stomach in a vertical fashion, allowing only a

FIGURE 14-9 Four types of bariatric surgery.

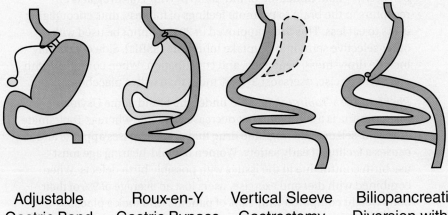

Adjustable Gastric Band (AGB)

Roux-en-Y Gastric Bypass (RYGB)

Vertical Sleeve Gastrectomy (VSG)

Biliopancreatic Diversion with a Duodenal Switch (BPD-DS)

tubular sleeve-shaped stomach, which empties into the duodenum. Because so much stomach is removed, there is less ghrelin, which reduces hunger more than banded gastroplasty.

- *Biliopancreatic diversion with duodenal switch (BPD-DS).* Sometimes this surgery is done 6–18 months after a sleeve surgery, as a "staged approach" to weight loss surgery. It involves rerouting the sleeve from much of the small intestine and diverting bile and gastric juices to change digestion and absorption.

Bariatric surgery may be an option for adults with a BMI ≥40, or a BMI ≥35 with a serious health problem linked to obesity (e.g., type 2 diabetes, heart disease, or severe sleep apnea). The FDA recently approved the use of the adjustable gastric band for patients with BMI ≥30 who also have at least one condition linked to obesity, such as heart disease or diabetes.

Before surgery is approved, clients must show proof they have tried traditional methods of weight loss and not found success. Often a psychological evaluation is done to determine if the client is a proper candidate and can respond well to the weight loss and change in body image. Surgeons require clients to demonstrate their full understanding of the undertaking and their motivation to follow extensive food, exercise, and medical guidance the rest of their lives. A surgeon, primary care doctor, psychologist, and dietitian are key people on the treatment team.

Side effects may include bleeding, infection, leaks from the site where the intestines are sewn together, diarrhea, and blood clots in the legs that can move to the lungs and heart. Side effects that may occur later include some nutrient deficiencies, especially in clients who do not take their prescribed vitamins and minerals. Vitamin B_{12}, iron, vitamin D, and folate are of special concern. Usually an individual is given 200% of the Daily Value of nutrients in a multi-vitamin along with sufficient calcium and vitamin D. Vitamin B_{12} is given sublingually. Dumping syndrome may occur, in which clients may experience cramping upon eating higher-fat, higher-sugar foods. Lactose intolerance, hair loss, and taste changes are also common effects after bariatric surgery. Complication rates among clients initially hospitalized for bariatric surgery is now 15%, which is lower than previous estimates. Many surgeries are now done laparoscopically.

After surgery, bariatric patients end up with a 1-oz size stomach pouch that takes six to eight weeks to heal. They begin a high-protein liquid diet for two to three weeks, then transition to soft-solid proteins for another four to six weeks. After this, they begin soft, moist whole foods. They must consume fluids separately from meals, and take 30–60 minutes to eat.

Once healing is complete during that six- to eight-week period, a bariatric patient's daily diet guidelines are as follows:

- 64 oz fluid
- Protein at 60–80 g via soft, chopped or ground meat, fish, or poultry or other protein source. Some may be intolerant to red meat.
- Three servings of fruits and vegetables. Some may have difficulty with raw forms.
- Three servings of whole grains (serving is ½ c). Some may have difficulty with rice, pasta, or doughy breads.
- Overall focus is on lower-fat, lower-sugar, high-protein eating

Weight loss surgery is considered successful when 50% of excess weight is lost and the loss is sustained up to 5 years. Bariatric surgeries may cost $20,000–$25,000, and insurance coverage varies by state and insurance plan.

A less invasive procedure is now approved by the FDA, which is a temporary implanted balloon device. Endoscopically, two connected balloons are inserted into the stomach and are filled with saline. This causes a full sensation when only a small amount of food is eaten, therefore prompting weight loss. This device is allowed to stay in the stomach for six months, at which time it is removed. There is an alternate product that mimics the same effect. This is a balloon in a pill with a tiny catheter attached, which is swallowed and through which saline is pumped through to fill the balloon. It operates from the same principle—the balloon creates a full sensation in the stomach. This balloon, however, naturally passes through the GI tract after a period of time.

Many individuals struggle with being successful at weight loss. Some attempt weight loss multiple times. There is a lot of talk that 95% of diets fail; however, if individuals are ready to change their thinking, habits, and environment, a healthy weight can be within their grasp. Research has shown that approximately 20% of overweight individuals are successful at long-term weight loss when defined as losing at least 10% of initial body weight and maintaining the loss for at least one year. Newer research has shown 29.7% of obese individuals being successful at one-year weight loss maintenance.

The National Weight Control Registry, established in 1994, serves as the largest prospective investigation of long-term successful weight loss maintainers. This registry, from Brown University School of Medicine, tracks over 10,000 people who have lost significant amounts of weight and kept it off for long periods of time.

Solid habits reported common among the participants include maintaining a low-calorie, low-fat diet and doing high levels of activity.

- 78% eat breakfast every day.
- 75% weigh themselves at least once a week.
- 62% watch less than 10 hours of television per week.
- 90% exercise, on average, about one hour per day.

CHILDHOOD WEIGHT ISSUES

As was discussed earlier in this chapter, a public health emergency has surfaced surrounding childhood obesity. Over the past three decades, childhood obesity rates in America have tripled. Today, nearly one in three children in America are overweight or obese. Unfortunately, childhood weight issues follow into adulthood—overweight adolescents have a 70% chance of becoming overweight or obese adults. This increases to 80% if at least one parent is overweight or obese.

In African American and Hispanic communities, nearly 40% of the children are overweight or obese. Nine of the ten states with the highest rates of obese children are in the South, which also correlates to poverty rates.

Because of the rising obesity rates, researchers speculate this may be the first generation of children who live shorter lives than their parents. Current research has found that obesity, glucose intolerance, and elevated blood pressure during childhood and adolescence are associated with increased rates of early death.

Risk factors for heart disease, such as high cholesterol and high blood pressure, occur with increased frequency in overweight children and adolescents compared to children with a healthy weight. Also, type 2 diabetes, previously considered an adult disease, has increased dramatically in children and adolescents. As discussed in Chapter 12, overweight and obesity are closely linked to type 2 diabetes and its precursor, insulin resistance. Asthma, hepatic steatosis (fatty liver), and sleep apnea are other disorders sometimes associated with overweight youth. Polycystic ovarian syndrome (PCOS), a hormonal imbalance that may be associated with insulin resistance, is sometimes seen in overweight teen girls.

The most immediate consequence of overweight as perceived by the children themselves is social discrimination. Overweight children may feel they are viewed as lazy or lacking discipline. Many overweight children are teased or bullied, which is associated with poor self-esteem and depression. Low self-esteem, in turn, can hinder academic and social functioning, and persist into adulthood (Figure 14-10).

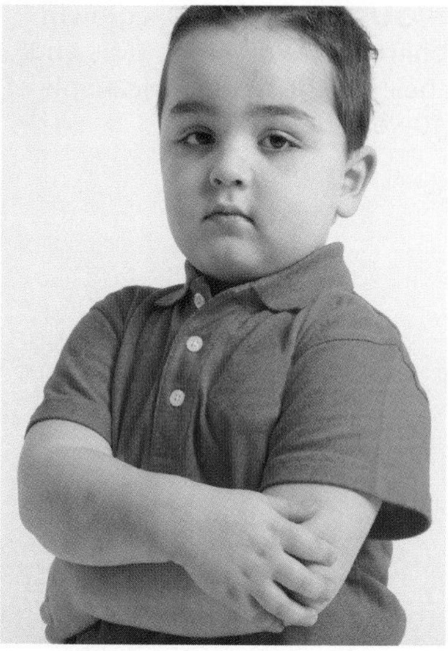

Children today lead different lives from their parents and grandparents, who as children played outdoors most of the time. Now neighborhoods may be less safe and outside play is limited. The walks to school have been replaced by car or bus rides. Gym class and after-school sports activities have been subject to program cuts. Researchers know that only 42% of children aged 6–11 obtain the recommended 60 minutes per day of physical activity and only 8% of adolescents achieve this goal.

FIGURE 14-10 Overweight children may suffer low self-esteem and feel isolated.

Afternoons and evenings are filled with "screen" time—television, video games, online computing, and texting. The average media time per U.S. child is 7.5 hours/day. Today's families share fewer home-cooked meals. Snacking between meals is rampant, as pantries are "fair game," and children can obtain out-of-control portion sizes any time of the day. It's no wonder researchers have used the term *toxic* to describe the food environment in America. Table 14-4 outlines key behaviors that contribute to childhood overweight and obesity.

The CDC and the American Academy of Pediatrics (AAP) recommend the use of BMI to screen for overweight and obesity in children beginning at age 2 years. BMI can be calculated for children and teens and the resulting number plotted on the CDC's "BMI-for-age" growth charts. These percentiles help practitioners assess growth relative to the averages set for children of the same sex and age. A BMI between the 85th and 95th percentile is considered overweight; one that falls above the 95th percentile is considered obese (Figure 14-11).

An important perspective for overweight and obese children and teens is to consider lifestyle changes that slow the rate of weight gain while allowing normal growth and development. If a child can simply slow or halt weight gain during the active growth years and allow their "height" to catch up, BMI can lower and normalize. However, if a child is experiencing other health complications such as high cholesterol, high blood pressure, high blood sugar, and is also overweight

TABLE 14-4 Contributors to Overweight and Obesity

- Skipping breakfast
- Low fruit and vegetable intake
- Sweetened beverage intake
- Excessive media time (especially TV in bedroom)
- Low physical activity level (sedentary behavior)
- Not eating meals together as a family
- Parental restriction of palatable foods

Source: Intermountain Health Care. Primary Care Guide to Weight Management in Children and Adolescents. 2007 (updated 2010). www.intermountainhealthcare.org.

FIGURE 14-11 CDC's growth chart shows different BMIs and their weight status in a sample of 10-year-old males.

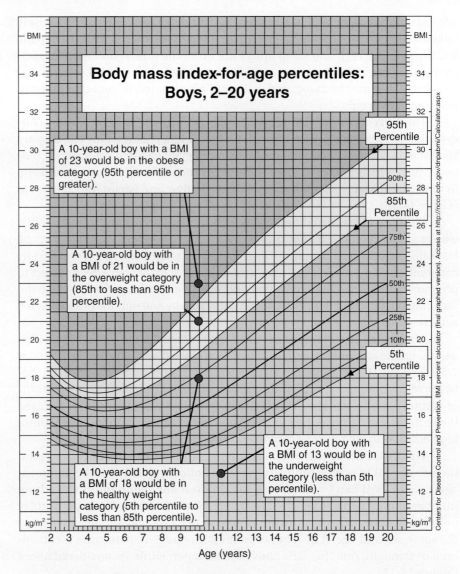

Body mass index-for-age percentiles: Boys, 2–20 years

A 10-year-old boy with a BMI of 23 would be in the obese category (95th percentile or greater).

A 10-year-old boy with a BMI of 21 would be in the overweight category (85th to less than 95th percentile).

A 10-year-old boy with a BMI of 18 would be in the healthy weight category (5th percentile to less than 85th percentile).

A 10-year-old boy with a BMI of 13 would be in the underweight category (less than 5th percentile).

95th Percentile
85th Percentile
5th Percentile

Age (years)

Centers for Disease Control and Prevention. BMI percent calculator (final graphed version). Access at http://nccd.cdc.gov/dnpabmi/Calculator.aspx

or obese, some weight loss is indicated. Table 14-5 shows weight management or loss guidelines for kids.

Strategies for Childhood Weight Loss

Treatment of the overweight or obese child or teen can happen with success. Parents can improve the food environment and keep their kids physically fit, especially if they serve as the role model. Measures are successful when surrounded with positive support and consistency. Important tactics would be to:

- Provide reliable meals and snacks at the table, with no food handouts at other times
- Model slow, mindful eating, with children being allowed to "trust" themselves to eat until satisfied
- Prepare fresh and balanced meals, but include small amounts of "treat" foods several times a week (cookies, chips) to prevent feeling deprived (and so these foods are not viewed as "forbidden")
- Consider that fiber and nutrient density are especially important for kids experiencing insulin resistance

TABLE 14-5 Weight Guidelines for Overweight or Obese Children

AGE RANGE	HEALTH	OVERWEIGHT (85TH–95TH PERCENTILE)	OBESE (>95TH PERCENTILE)
Age 2–7	Otherwise healthy	Maintenance	Maintenance
	Secondary complication*	Maintenance	Very slow weight loss (no more than 1 lb/mo)
Ages 7 and above	Otherwise healthy	Maintenance	Weight loss (2–4 lb/mo)
	Secondary complication*	Weight loss (2–4 lb/mo)	Weight loss (1–2 lb/week)

*Secondary complication could include high cholesterol, high blood pressure, insulin resistance, sleep apnea, fatty liver, joint problems, PCOS, or depression/anxiety.

Source: Intermountain Health Care. Primary Care Guide to Weight Management in Children and Adolescents. 2007 (updated 2010). www.intermountainhealthcare.org.

- Plan fun, home-based activity options, and encourage participation in sporting activities
- Understand a need for parental limits on media time that will naturally facilitate more activity
- Understand that healthy habit changes are a family affair—not just a measure you are undertaking for the overweight child

When families of overweight children need additional support, the answer may lie within family-based treatment programs in a hospital, clinic, recreation center, or school. Those that are most successful are behavioral-based healthy eating and exercise programs. Popular programs that can improve fitness and health while halting weight gain or promoting weight loss, among others, are the CATCH program (Child and Adolescent Trial for Cardiovascular Health), LEAP (Lifestyle Education for Activity Program), Project SPARK (Sports, Play, and Active Recreation for Kids), and youth programming at the local YMCAs.

Bariatric surgery is sometimes used to treat very obese youth. Teens can lose weight after bariatric surgery; however, many questions exist about the long-term effects on their developing bodies and minds. Doctors suggest that, as with adults, families consider surgery for their teens only after they have tried for six months to lose weight and were unsuccessful. Candidates must meet three criteria: have extreme obesity with a BMI >40; have reached their adult height (age 13 or older for girls and age 15 or older for boys); and have serious health problems linked to weight (type 2 diabetes or sleep apnea, for example). Doctors also need to assess the candidate's emotional stability and his or her willingness to follow through with lifestyle changes. Gastric bypass surgery is the main operation used. Adjusted gastric banding has not been approved in those under age 18 in the United States.

To reverse nationwide obesity will require a long-term effort where many entities work together for the greater good. Individuals, families, communities, schools, businesses, government, and other groups will be needed to turn the tide. How we handle this health crisis will be this generation's defining moment. The stakes are high, as this epidemic will affect the health of generations to come. Policy change is needed to strengthen the ability to make healthy decisions and remove obstacles for change, especially for those whose options have been limited.

The momentum is spreading to prevent and reduce obesity for the sake of America's health. Carrying this forward will be the challenge, as it will require increased and sustained efforts nationwide. In addition to government health entities, the Robert Wood Johnson Foundation has formulated one of its goals as reversing childhood obesity. Through their vision and influence on both private and public sectors, they are leading efforts to:

- Ensure that all food and beverages served in school meet or exceed the Dietary Guidelines for Americans
- Increase access to high-quality and affordable food through new or improved grocery stores and healthier corner stores
- Increase the time, intensity, and duration of physical activity during the school day and in after-school programs
- Increase physical activity by improving the **built environment** in communities
- Using pricing strategies (incentives and disincentives) to promote the purchase of healthier food
- Reduce youth's exposure to the marketing of unhealthy foods through regulation policy and effective industry self-regulation

There are a multitude of health resources for clients who want to journey toward health and a better weight. Websites such as the Weight Information Network, the CDC, the National Institutes for Health, and the American Heart Association provide easily accessible information and resources. Tips on prevention of childhood overweight can be found at most of these websites as well. The government's Let's Move program, in addition to the Action for Healthy Kids and the Alliance for a Healthy Generation, are other large platforms for excellent guidance and resources for childhood overweight. Healthy eating tips and recipes and physical fitness information abound in our culture via TV shows and media, magazines, books, the Internet, and medical literature, among others. There are online calorie and exercise calculators and counters, smartphone apps, and computerized fitness gear that can assist anyone's health pursuits.

UNDERWEIGHT

Although staying lean may be advantageous, being truly underweight could have its risks as well. Underweight status may be the result of a medical condition and/or compromised nutrition intake. Underweight is seen in anorexia, depression, and in those with cancer and a variety of other conditions. It can be the result of tissue wasting, poor absorption of nutrients, infection, excessive activity, or **hyperthyroidism**. Those who are underweight may have weaker immune systems. They may have lower muscle mass, compromised bone status, and substandard nutrition stores.

Adults with a BMI of ≤18.5 are considered underweight. Children who are at or below the 5th percentile on the BMI chart are considered underweight. In children, the inability to gain weight may be a condition called failure to thrive, which is referenced in Chapter 12. This may be caused by an illness, or issues related to swallowing and digestion, lack of feeding support, or an imbalanced diet. Genetics can play a factor in underweight, but so can the environment.

Underweight is treated by a high-calorie diet. If the goal is to gain 1 lb per week, then 500 extra calories a day must be eaten. Often those who need to gain weight must begin slowly, and eat a bit more with every meal and snack. Some clients need an extra vitamin or mineral supplement if they are not absorbing their food well, or if they have food intolerances.

The foods not recommended on a high-calorie diet would be ones that add too much bulk, fiber, or water content to the diet, thereby filling up the individual without providing a high amount of energy. Items to limit when desiring a high-calorie diet would be salads, broth-based soups, raw vegetables,

built environment
man-made resources and infrastructure designed to support health and activity (e.g., parks, walking and bike paths, access to healthy foods)

hyperthyroidism
condition in which the thyroid gland secretes too much thyroxine and T3 resulting in an unusually high metabolism

ultra-high-fiber cereals, and light or diet products made with artificial sweeteners. A high consumption of water would also be filling, especially just prior to a meal.

Tips that help with underweight include:

- Eat frequently (five or six small meals per day) to avoid feeling full.
- Eat foods that are dense in nutrients and calories (e.g., nuts, seeds, dried fruit, egg, avocado, yogurt). Limit heavy amounts of sugar or unhealthy fats.
- Add healthy fat to food in cooking such as olive or canola oil or mayonnaise. Butter, whole milk, and cheese have higher amounts of saturated fats and may need to be used with a little more discretion in those with cholesterol concerns.
- Pack foods to eat when away from home so there are no gaps in eating if a restaurant is not convenient.
- Check out high-calorie snack recipes to make at home, such as milk shakes and puddings, and dense foods, such as a homemade peanut butter granola bar.
- Consider supplement drinks to boost calories as needed.
- Encourage parents of underweight children to provide support, but not threaten, bribe, or force-feed their child, as their child will engage in the opposite behavior and back away from the food.
- Fully investigate the root cause of the underweight status.
- Consult a doctor or dietitian for a full evaluation and treatment plan.

HEALTH AND NUTRITION CONSIDERATIONS

Weight regulation is complex and governed by many factors. Often multiple attempts at weight loss occur before success happens. What works for one individual may not work for another. A permanent lifestyle change is required whereby clients change their mindset about healthy eating and movement throughout their environment. If a lapse occurs, individuals need to learn how to spot it and set in motion new behaviors to get back on track. A state of readiness needs to be present for clients to begin to change. Positive weight management resources, based on current science and "best practices," need to be available to clients. The health care provider can support clients to help them voice realistic changes, to attain better health and weight. As a health care provider, support and encouragement can help pave the way for change.

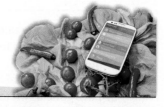

SUMMARY

Genetics, the environment, and lifestyle factors all affect weight. We are all engineered to be good food regulators, but some respond more to external influences and begin to overeat. Nationally, we have an obesity crisis on our hands and it is causing serious health consequences. Children who are overweight tend to become overweight adults. Altered food intake and decreased physical activity are to blame among other factors. Americans go on and off various diets at an alarming rate to reduce, when a long-term view of health is what contributes to a normal weight. Realistic and dedicated changes in eating and exercise can be the winning ticket with weight control. Our nation is pulling together to start policy change that will affect adults and children in a positive way. Community groups, health care providers, schools, among others are forming the web of change to get adults and children in our nation healthy again. Health care providers play key roles in helping individuals of every shape and size to lead healthier lives.

DISCUSSION TOPICS

1. Discuss ways to determine body mass index. Note BMI ranges for underweight, overweight, and obesity, including the stages of obesity, in adults. How would you assess BMI in children and determine if they are underweight, overweight, or obese?

2. What is the value in knowing waist circumference and how is it related to disease risk? Discuss the health consequences of obesity.

3. Discuss criteria used for assessing whether children need weight maintenance or weight loss.

4. How might an overweight athlete be in better shape and healthier than a sedentary person at normal weight?

5. Describe a balanced eating approach for weight loss and compare this to a fad diet. Which is sustainable? What might be the consequences of a fad diet?

6. Name three food changes and three behavior changes an individual could make to help begin weight loss. Why is it important to have a long-term view of healthful weight maintenance?

7. Describe at least three positive benefits of physical activity. Why is it important to record exercise in a log? What might be some types of exercise suited for persons with mobility problems? Who would they go to for guidance and advice?

8. Why might individuals be underweight? Name ways they could change their diet to gain weight.

SUGGESTED ACTIVITIES

1. Do a three-day food record on yourself, making sure one of the day's intake is on a weekend. Use the SuperTracker (http://www.choosemyplate. gov) to analyze your intake. Critique your eating based on MyPlate. If you needed to trim your eating for weight loss, what would you change?

2. The doctor you work for wants you to suggest to a client a weight management class taught by the office dietitian. Role-play this discussion with a fellow student. Begin with an assessment of the client's feelings, such as "How do you feel about your health and weight?" Be positive and supportive as you describe the weight management class and the referral. What happens if you hear resistance?

REVIEW

1. The complication rates for bariatric surgery
   a. have gone down from 40% to 30%
   b. are unchanged
   c. are less than 3%
   d. have gone down to 15%

2. If one or both parents are overweight or obese, an overweight child has a ___ chance that this will follow him or her into adulthood.
   a. 50%
   b. 25%
   c. 80%
   d. 70%

3. In studies, contributors to overweight and obesity in children include
   a. eating an evening snack
   b. not making the sports team at school
   c. skipping breakfast, drinking pop, and overdoing media time
   d. underperforming in school

4. A 13-year-old obese child with high blood pressure should
   a. maintain current weight and not gain any more
   b. lose 1–2 lb per week
   c. lose 2–4 lb per month
   d. engage in very slow weight loss of 1 lb per month

5. If a man has a waist circumference of 42 in and he has stage II obesity, what is he at increased risk of having, and what is his risk level?
    a. high level of risk for diabetes only
    b. increased risk for cardiovascular disease, hypertension, and/or diabetes
    c. high level of risk for reflux
    d. very high risk for cardiovascular disease, hypertension, and/or diabetes

6. A newer weight loss drug that is sometimes used short term when obese clients are at increased medical risk is
    a. phentermine and topiramate
    b. fenfluramine and dexfenfluramine
    c. sibutramine (Meridia)
    d. none of the above, as all amphetamines are good to use

7. Policy changes than can reduce obesity would be
    a. scheduling an exercise session with a fitness trainer
    b. calculating the calories daily from the foods eaten
    c. requiring local governments to plan neighborhoods with walking and bike paths and easy accessibility to healthy grocery stores and farmers' markets
    d. shopping the perimeter of the grocery store

8. If an underweight child's goal is to gain 1.5 lb per week, how many extra calories would he need to consume daily?
    a. 500   c. 250
    b. 750   d. 1,000

9. What is an external factor that can trigger eating?
    a. packing lunch for work every day
    b. walking by the donut shop and you see and smell the aroma of donuts
    c. feeling weak and light-headed when your stomach is growling
    d. consuming caffeine

10. According to the latest data, obesity continues to climb
    a. only in Hispanic women
    b. in the Mid-Atlantic and states of the West
    c. in those that have more education
    d. in African American and Hispanic women and men and boys

11. Factors that could affect BMR, include
    a. quantity of vitamin C containing foods eaten daily
    b. your age, size, and body composition
    c. whether there is a diagnosis of hypertension
    d. distance to the nearest gym

12. When an individual wants to find reliable resources to help with weight loss, she should
    a. talk to a local health food store representative
    b. talk to a health care provider and check out literature from the Weight Control Information Network and Choose MyPlate
    c. talk to a friend who lost 100 lb on a liquid diet
    d. decrease her calories to no more than 1,000 per day

CASE IN POINT

RIDA: GAINING WEIGHT IN RETIREMENT

Rida had been a fifth-grade teacher for 38 years and just retired this past school year. She and her husband have two daughters who are grown and married, so it is just the two of them at home. Rida had always packed her lunch through the years when she was working. She usually spent many of her evenings grading papers and preparing lesson plans. She and her husband would usually eat a light supper in the evening so she wouldn't have to spend a lot of time cooking. Now at age 63, Rida is enjoying her new lifestyle and less-stressful routine. She finally has time for some hobbies and crafts. She has always loved to cook and bake, but never had quite enough time to enjoy that, either. Since her retirement, Rida has been trying many new recipes. She enjoys cooking "fancier" meals for her husband now, including rich desserts.

In addition, Rida has been catching up with old friends. Many of the teachers she worked with through the years are also retired. Twice a week they meet for lunch to catch up and enjoy each other's company. Although she's enjoying her retirement, Rida gained 7 lb almost immediately. However, she felt the weight gain was worth it and was no cause for worry. But after 4 months, Rida's weight was up 16 lb. Then she decided it was time to make some changes.

ASSESSMENT

1. What information do you have about Rida's activity and eating habits before her retirement?
2. How did Rida's habits change after she retired?
3. How has the change affected her?
4. How long should Rida expect to take to lose the 16 lb she gained?

DIAGNOSIS

5. Write a diagnosis for Rida's alteration in nutrition.
6. Write a diagnosis for Rida's activity level change.

PLAN/GOAL

7. What is a reasonable, measurable goal for Rida's weight loss?

IMPLEMENTATION

8. List some strategies that match Rida's new priorities.
9. What can her husband and friends do to help her lose weight?
10. How can she enjoy her new routine without gaining weight?

EVALUATION/OUTCOME CRITERIA

11. What criteria would Rida use to determine the success of the plan?

THINKING FURTHER

12. How can she maintain weight control for the rest of her life?
13. How can websites such as SparkPeople.com be helpful to Rida?

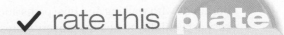

✔ rate this plate

Rida has been enjoying retirement by visiting with friends over lunch a few times a week. Since her recent weight gain, Rida has decided to pay closer attention to the meals she orders while out with her friends. Rate this plate:

2 cups orange chicken stir-fry with broccoli, snow peas, and carrots

1 cup steamed white rice

1 garlic breadstick

12 oz sweet iced tea

What questions could Rida ask the server before ordering the meal? What decisions could Rida make to improve the nutritional quality of her meal? What suggestions would you give Rida when choosing to eat out with friends?

CASE IN POINT

BELLA: STAYING HEALTHY FOLLOWING GASTRIC BYPASS SURGERY

Bella has been overweight most of her life. She never thought much about it because her parents were both overweight as well. She is currently 5-ft 3-in tall, 287 lb, and 58 years old. Most of her life her weight has fluctuated between 200 and 220 lb, but she began gaining more weight after menopause. Bella's family immigrated from Italy, and she has always maintained a taste for the authentic Italian foods she grew up eating. She remembers her mother saying on more than one occasion, "When there is a problem, a great Italian meal is the answer!" Bella's diet has always included many varieties of pasta. Her favorite recipes are prepared with creamy alfredo or wine and butter sauce. She loved the richness of her mother's soups when she prepared them with cream as well. Bella enjoys vegetables, but prefers them in a cheese sauce. To truly complete an Italian meal, says her mother, you always need a good decadent dessert. Ice cream and sorbets have been Bella's favorites since childhood. Bella has tried different diets through the years in an attempt to lose weight, but unsuccessfully. She seems to regain the weight she lost and a little extra as soon as she stops dieting.

Bella has noticed recently some swelling in her legs. She also seems to be having headaches on a regular basis. Her physician requests she have some blood work completed before seeing him. At her appointment, her doctor informs her that her blood pressure is 212/102. Her total cholesterol is 347 with an LDL of 200 and HDL of 26. Her fasting glucose level is 114 mg/dl. Her doctor is very concerned. He prescribes both blood pressure and cholesterol reduction medications. In addition, he informs her that her blood sugar level is considered to be in the range of pre-diabetes. He states that she must lose weight to improve all of her conditions. Bella asks her doctor about gastric bypass surgery. He emphasizes the changes she would need to make to even be a candidate for the surgery.

Bella underwent gastric bypass surgery 6 months later. Bella has been under the supervision of her physician, surgeon, and dietitian during this time. Only after Bella met the presurgical requirements and was deemed safe for the surgery, could it be performed. Bella's daughter was her health coach postoperatively. She assisted Bella throughout the presurgical time as well. Bella and her daughter attended classes on eating healthy, weight loss, exercise, and behavior modification. Bella felt confident her surgery would improve her health and the quality of her life.

ASSESSMENT

1. What do you know about Bella?
2. What was her new priority?
3. What is her ideal weight?
4. How many pounds does she need to lose to be at the high end of her ideal body weight?
5. How long should it take to be done safely without the assistance of gastric bypass?
6. What is her current BMI and what are her risks for health problems on the basis of her BMI?
7. What are her known health problems?
8. At what weight will her health risk be reasonable?
9. How long will it take to reach that reasonable health-risk weight?

DIAGNOSIS

10. Write a complete nursing diagnostic statement for Bella's nutrition problem.
11. Write a diagnosis for her activity intolerance.

PLAN/GOAL

12. Write at least three goals for Bella that are reasonable and measurable.

IMPLEMENTATION

13. What class of obesity was Bella in when she weighed 287 lb?
14. How much weight would Bella need to lose to move from category III obesity to the overweight category?
15. What topics are essential in Bella's nutrition classes?
16. Use the food items Bella liked to eat and list low-calorie, low-fat alternatives.
17. What are some behavior modification hints or tips related to where and when she eats that would help her?
18. Bella was instructed to turn in her home scale to the doctor's office and to see him every Friday morning to weigh in and have her blood pressure checked. What is the rationale for these directions?

(continued)

(continued)

19. How would the obesity information on the National Heart, Lung, and Blood Institute's website (http://www.nhlbi.nih.gov) be helpful to Bella?

EVALUATION/OUTCOME CRITERIA

20. What changes should the doctor see, hear, and be able to measure that are indicative of success?

THINKING FURTHER

21. Why is it important for Bella to persevere at weight reduction?
22. What are some of the serious potential complications of this surgery?

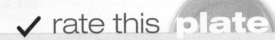
✔ rate this plate

After surgery, Bella allowed her stomach to start to heal by only consuming liquids and semisolid foods. She transitioned from semisolids to soft-solid foods after a few weeks and by eight weeks was ready to try solid foods. Four months after gastric bypass surgery, Bella has returned to a normal, healthy diet following the advice of her health care team. She continues to meet with a registered dietitian to assist in planning her meals. Rate this plate:

2 oz pork tenderloin

¼ cup sweet potatoes

¼ cup pears

¼ cup cottage cheese

6 oz water

Does this meal meet the recommendations for diet after gastric bypass surgery? If not, what can be improved?

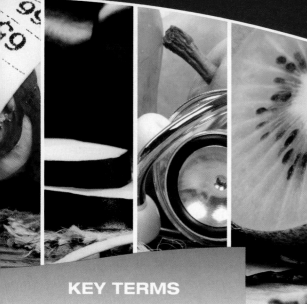

CHAPTER 15

KEY TERMS

A1C
acanthosis nigricans
coma
diabetes mellitus
dyslipidemia
endogenous insulin
exchange lists
exogenous insulin
glycosuria
insulin reaction
ketoacidosis
ketonemia
ketonuria
metabolic syndrome
nephropathy
neuropathy
oral diabetes medication
pre-diabetes
polydipsia
polyphagia
polyuria
renal threshold
retinopathy
type 1 diabetes
type 2 diabetes
vascular system

DIET, PRE-DIABETES, AND DIABETES

OBJECTIVES

After studying this chapter, you should be able to:

- Describe pre-diabetes and types of diabetes
- Describe the signs and symptoms of pre-diabetes and diabetes
- Explain the relationship of insulin to diabetes mellitus
- Discuss appropriate nutritional management of pre-diabetes and diabetes

Diabetes mellitus is the name for a group of serious and chronic (long-standing) disorders affecting the metabolism of carbohydrates. Due to the absence or misuse of insulin, these disorders are characterized by hyperglycemia (abnormally large amounts of glucose in the blood). A precursor to one of the types of diabetes (type 2) may occur, which is called **pre-diabetes**. This is a condition in which blood glucose levels are higher than normal, but not high enough for the diagnosis of diabetes. Pre-diabetes, also known as impaired glucose tolerance, can be realized when there is growing insulin resistance in which the body begins to not respond to and use the insulin it produces.

Sometimes insulin resistance is referenced when clinicians describe **metabolic syndrome**. Metabolic syndrome (or dysmetabolic syndrome) is a constellation of conditions that pose significant risk of developing heart disease, stroke, and diabetes. Metabolic syndrome individuals have abnormal cholesterol, excess body fat around the waist, and increased blood pressure and blood sugar.

Diabetes insipidus is a different disorder. It also generates large amounts of urine, but it is "insipid," not sweet. This is a rare condition, caused by a damaged pituitary gland. It is not discussed in this chapter.

According to the American Diabetes Association (ADA), 29.1 million people in the United States have diabetes (9.3% of U.S. population). An estimated 18.8 million people have been diagnosed with the disease, with 8.1 million more going undiagnosed. There are approximately 86 million people with pre-diabetes, and 1.7 million new cases of diabetes in people aged 20 years and older diagnosed in 2010. It is a major cause of blindness; heart and kidney disease; amputations of toes, feet, and legs; infections; and death.

Hundreds of years ago, a Greek physician named the condition *diabetes*, which means "to flow through," because of the large amounts of urine generated by clients. Later, the Latin word *mellitus*, which means "honey," was added because of the amount of glucose in the urine.

The body needs a constant supply of energy, and glucose is its primary source. Carbohydrates provide most of the glucose, but about 10% of fats and up to nearly 60% of proteins can be converted to glucose if necessary.

The distribution of glucose must be carefully managed for the maintenance of good health. Glucose is transported by the blood, and its entry into the cells is controlled by hormones. The primary hormone is insulin.

Insulin is secreted by the beta cells of the islets of Langerhans in the pancreas. When there is inadequate production of insulin or the body is unable to use the insulin it produces, glucose cannot enter the cells and it accumulates in the blood, creating hyperglycemia. This condition can cause serious complications.

Another hormone, glucagon, which is secreted by the alpha cells of the islets of Langerhans, helps release energy when needed by converting glycogen to glucose. Somatostatin is a hormone produced by the delta cells of the islets of Langerhans and the hypothalamus. All actions of this hormone are inhibitory. It inhibits the release of insulin and glucagons.

The amount of glucose in the blood normally rises after a meal. The pancreas reacts by providing insulin. As the insulin circulates in the blood, it binds to special insulin receptors on cell surfaces. This binding causes the cells to accept the glucose. The resulting reduced amount of glucose in the blood in turn signals the pancreas to stop sending insulin.

ETIOLOGY

The etiology (cause) of diabetes is not confirmed. Although it appears that diabetes may be genetic, environmental factors also may contribute to its occurrence. For example, viruses or obesity may precipitate the disease in people who have a genetic predisposition.

The World Health Organization indicates that the prevalence of the disease is increasing worldwide, especially in areas showing improvement in living standards.

SYMPTOMS

The abnormal concentration of glucose in the blood of clients with diabetes draws water from the cells to the blood. When hyperglycemia exceeds the **renal threshold**, the glucose is excreted in the urine, a process known as **glycosuria**.

diabetes mellitus
chronic disease in which the body lacks the normal ability to metabolize glucose

pre-diabetes
a condition in which blood glucose in higher than normal but not high enough for a diabetes diagnosis

metabolic syndrome
a cluster of conditions that contribute to increased risk of heart disease, stroke, and diabetes

renal threshold
kidneys' capacity

glycosuria
excess sugar in the urine

With the loss of the cellular fluid, the client experiences polyuria (excessive urination), and polydipsia (excessive thirst) typically results.

The inability to metabolize glucose causes the body to break down its own tissue for protein and fat. This response causes polyphagia (excessive appetite), but at the same time, a loss of weight, weakness, and fatigue occur. The body's use of protein from its own tissue causes it to excrete nitrogen.

The untreated client with diabetes cannot use carbohydrates for energy so, therefore, excessive amounts of fats are broken down, and consequently the liver produces ketones from the fatty acids. In healthy people, ketones are subsequently broken down to carbon dioxide and water, yielding energy. In clients with diabetes, fats break down faster than the body can handle. Ketone collection in the blood is known as ketonemia. Excretion of ketones in the urine, a necessary process, is known as ketonuria. Ketones are acids that lower blood pH, causing acidosis. Acidosis, caused by ketones, is known as ketoacidosis. Ketoacidosis can lead to loss of consciousness, which can result in death if the client is not treated quickly with fluids and insulin.

In addition to the symptoms previously mentioned, clients with diabetes are more likely to suffer from diseases of the vascular system, such as hypertension and atherosclerosis. Atherosclerosis is a condition in which there is a buildup of fatty substances inside artery walls. This can reduce blood flow and is a major cause of death among clients with diabetes. Neuropathy, damage to the nervous system, occurs in 60–70% of clients with diabetes. Damage to the small blood vessels in the eye is known as retinopathy. Retinopathy is the leading cause of blindness in the United States. Nephropathy, damage to the kidneys, is also a complication of diabetes. Nephropathy is the number one cause of the need for kidney dialysis. It is also common for clients with diabetes to suffer from frequent infections such as urinary tract infections.

Individuals with pre-diabetes may have no symptoms, or have mild symptoms of pre-diabetes. In summary, according to the American Diabetes Association, the symptoms of diabetes are:

- Urinating often
- Feeling very thirsty
- Feeling very hungry even though you have been eating
- Extreme fatigue
- Blurry vision
- Cuts or bruises that are slow to heal
- Weight loss—even though you are eating more (Type 1)
- Tingling pain or numbness in the hands or feed (Type 2)

CLASSIFICATION AND CRITERIA FOR TESTING AND DIAGNOSIS

Classification of this group of disorders can be made by the following:

- Pre-diabetes
- Type 1 diabetes
- Type 2 diabetes
- Gestational diabetes
- Types of diabetes due to other causes, such as drug or chemical-induced diabetes, among others.

polyuria
excessive urination

polydipsia
abnormal thirst

polyphagia
excess hunger

ketonemia
ketones collected in the blood

ketonuria
ketone bodies in the urine

ketoacidosis
unconsciousness caused by a state of acidosis due to too much sugar or too little insulin

vascular system
circulatory system

neuropathy
nerve damage

retinopathy
damage to small blood vessels in the eyes

nephropathy
damage to the kidneys

Pre-Diabetes

More than one out of three adults has pre-diabetes. Further troubling is that 9 out of 10 Americans do not know they have it. Pre-diabetes is usually spotted when someone is undergoing screening for diabetes.

Results indicating pre-diabetes include:

- A fasting glucose of 100 and 125 mg/dl
- An **A1C** of 5.7–6.4%
- An OGTT (oral glucose tolerance test) 2-hour blood glucose of 140–199 mg/dl

Pre-diabetes or diabetes testing in asymptomatic adults should be considered in all adults who are overweight (BMI >25) and ones that have additional risk factors. These risk factors would be physical inactivity; first-degree relative with diabetes; member of a high-risk race or ethnicity, such as African American, Latino, Native or Asian American, or Pacific Islander; women who delivered babies > 9 lb or had gestational diabetes; hypertension; abnormal lipids often called **dyslipidemia** (low HDL, high triglycerides); women with polycystic ovary syndrome; elevated labs as above; or other clinical conditions associated with insulin resistance (severe obesity, **acanthosis nigricans**) and history of cardiovascular disease.

For all patients, testing is recommended beginning at age 45 years. If results are normal, testing should be repeated at a minimum of three-year intervals.

Type 1 Diabetes

Type 1 diabetes, previously known as juvenile diabetes, develops when the body's immune system destroys the pancreatic beta cells. These are the only cells in the body that make the hormone insulin that regulates blood glucose. Type 1 diabetes is usually diagnosed in children and young adults. It accounts for 5% of all diagnosed cases of diabetes.

According to the 2016 guidelines of the American Diabetes Association's Standards of Medical Care in Diabetes, blood glucose rather than A1C should be used to diagnose acute onset of type 1 diabetes in individuals with symptoms of hyperglycemia. A fasting blood sugar of 126 mg/dl or above is the criteria for diagnosis.

Some risk factors include genetics, autoimmune status, and environmental factors. Clients with type 1 diabetes must use exogenous insulin to survive. Most people with type 1 diabetes should be treated with multiple dose insulin injections or continuous subcutaneous insulin infusions. There are a variety of insulins that can be used to maintain control of blood sugars. Insulins vary in their actions. They differ in onset, peak, and duration of their effectiveness. Table 15-1 identifies the different insulins and their actions.

Type 2 Diabetes

Type 2 diabetes was previously called adult-onset diabetes because it usually occurred in adults over the age of 40. But as obesity has become an epidemic, this has drastically increased the incidence of type 2 diabetes among adolescents and young adults. Besides obesity, type 2 is associated with a cluster of other risk factors mentioned previously.

A1C
a blood test to determine how well blood glucose has been controlled for the last three months

dyslipidemia
increased lipid in the blood

acanthosis nigricans
dark velvety discoloration in body folds and creases often found in people with obesity related insulin resistance

type 1 diabetes
diabetes occurring suddenly between the ages of 1 and 40; clients secrete little, if any, insulin and require insulin injections and a carefully controlled diet

type 2 diabetes
diabetes occurring usually after age 40; onset is gradual and production of insulin gradually diminishes; can usually be controlled by diet and exercise

TABLE 15-1 Insulin Actions

INSULIN TYPE	ONSET	PEAK	DURATION
Rapid acting			
Lispro (Humalog®)	10–15 minutes	30–90 minutes	2–4 hours
Aspart (Novolog®)	10–15 minutes	30–90 minutes	2–4 hours
Glulisine (Apidra®)	10–15 minutes	30–90 minutes	3–5 hours
Short acting			
Regular (Humulin® R, Novolin® R)	30 minutes	2–4 hours	6–8 hours
Intermediate acting			
NPH (Humulin® N, Novolin® N)	1–2 hours	6–12 hours	16–24 hours
Long acting			
Detemir (Levemir®)	1–2 hours	Minimal	24 hours
Glargine (Lantus®, Basaglar®, Toujeo®)	1–2 hours	Minimal	24 hours
Inhaled			
Afrezza®			
Premixed			
Humulin or Novolin 70/30: follows the actions of both regular and NPH insulins			
Novolog 70/30: follows the actions of both Novolog and NPH			
Humalog 75/25: follows the actions of both Humalog and NPH			
Humulin 50/50: follows the actions of both regular and NPH			

A diagnosis of type 2 diabetes is made with:

- A fasting blood glucose of 126 mg/dl (fasting must occur with no calorie intake for at least 8 hours)
- A 2-hour glucose of ≥ 200 mg/dl during an OGTT
- An A1C of ≥ 6.5%

Type 2 diabetes can usually be controlled by diet and exercise, or by diet, exercise, and an **oral diabetes medication**. However, insulin may also be necessary in type 2 diabetes as well. Table 15-2 shows types of oral glucose-lowering medications. Metformin, if not contraindicated, is the preferred initial pharmacological agent for type 2 diabetes. The goals of medical nutrition therapy for clients with type 2 diabetes include maintaining healthy glucose, blood pressure, and lipid levels. Also, because approximately 85% of type 2 clients are overweight, these clients may be placed on weight reduction diets to help achieve blood glucose levels that are within acceptable range. Thus, monitoring their weight loss also becomes part of their therapy.

The criteria for testing for type 2 diabetes or pre-diabetes in asymptomatic children include:

- Overweight (BMI > 85th percentile)
- Plus any two of the following: Family history of type 2 in first or second degree relative; race/ethnicity that are at risk as described above; and signs of insulin resistance or conditions associated with insulin resistance as described above, which also includes small-for-gestational age birth weight
- Age of initiation: age 10 years or at onset of puberty, if puberty occurs at a younger age

Frequency of testing is recommended every 3 years.

oral diabetes medication
oral hypoglycemic agent; medication that may be given to type 2 diabetes to lower blood glucose

TABLE 15-2 Types of Oral Diabetes (Glucose-Lowering) Medications

Meglitinide	• Repaglinide (Prandin®)
D-Phenylalanines	• Nateglinide (Starlix®)
Thiazolidinedione	• Pioglitazone (Actos®) • Rosiglitazone (Avandia®)
Nonsulfonylurea	• Metformin (Glucophage®) • Metformin and a time-released controlling polymer (Glucophage XR®)
Alpha-glucosidase inhibitor	• Acarbose (Precose®) • Miglitol (Glycet®)
Second-generation sulfonylureas	• Glyburide (DiaBeta®, Micronase, Glynase Prestabs) • Glipizide (Glucotrol®, Glucotrol XL®) • Glimepride (Amaryl®)
Class-bile acid sequestrants (primarily used to decrease cholesterol but also improves blood sugar control)	• Colesevelam (Welchol®)
DPP-4 inhibitors	• Sitagliptin (Januvia®) • Saxagliptin (Onglyza™) • Linagliptin (Tradjenta®) • Alogliptin (Nesina®)
SGLTZ inhibitors	• Canagliflozin (Invokana™) • Dapagliflozin (Farxiga™) • Empagliflozin (Jardiance®)
Dopamine receptor agonist	• Bromocriptine Mesylate (Cycloset®)
Combination drugs (in the interest of space, only brand names listed)	• Glucovance®, Avandamet®, Metaglip® • ACTOplus Met™, Avandaryl™, Duetact™, Janumet™, Kombiglyze™ XR, Kazano, Oseni, Juvisync™, Jentadueto™, Invokamet™, Xigduo™XT, Glyxambi®

Noninsulin Injectable Medications

There is a newer class of injectable medications used to improve blood sugar control, called incretin mimetics. The incretin mimetics on the market are Byetta®, Victoza®, Bydureon™, Tanzeum®, and Trulicity™. Incretin mimetics are injected the same as insulin, but they are not insulins. Another noninsulin injectable antihyperglycemic medication is pramlintide (Symlin®). It is used in clients with type 1 diabetes. It works to lower blood sugars by assisting insulin injected at meals to lower postmeal blood sugar levels. It also suppresses postmeal glucagon release, slows gastric emptying, and decreases appetite.

When food is eaten, incretin hormones are released from cells located in the small intestine. In the pancreas, incretins will act on the beta cells to increase glucose-dependent insulin secretions to ensure an appropriate insulin response after a meal. This medication can be used in conjunction with oral medications to help clients lower their A1C to less than 7%. The American Diabetes Association prefers the outcome to be less than 7% for a client with diabetes. The American College of Endocrinology has a target of less than 6.5% for clients with diabetes.

In The Media

Promising Research

Individuals with type I diabetes may soon be free from insulin injections because of a new diabetes treatment that will turn skin cells into healthy pancreatic cells. This new-found research has already proved successful in mice. Scientists at the University of California have found that a small amount of skin cells can be transferred into the patient's pancreas, where trillions of healthy cells can be made to assist in the production of insulin. Although this treatment is aimed toward those with type 1 diabetes, researchers also believe it could be used as a treatment option for type 2 diabetes. Although the research appears promising, scientists say the current process will not terminate the use of insulin shots yet. However, continued research and current success indicate that insulin shots may one day be obsolete.

Source: Adapted from West, Tara (2016, January 8). "Diabetics Soon to Be Free from Insulin Injections Thanks to Scientific Breakthrough Using Patient's Own Skin Cells." *Inquisitr.* Accessed January 9, 2016. http://www.inquisitr.com/2691961/diabetics-soon-to-be-free-from-insulin-injections-thanks-to-scientific-breakthrough-using-patients-own-skin-cells/

SPOTLIGHT *on Life Cycle*

Diabetes affects older Americans disproportionately. While just over 9% of U.S. citizens have diabetes, 25% of older Americans (60 years and above) have the disease. Researchers know that the aging of the U.S. population is one of the drivers of the diabetes epidemic. This manifests itself in many ways when it comes to longevity, functional status, and an increased risk for hospitalization and long-term care. To address this issue, the American Diabetes Association has developed a "Senior Signature Series" to offer diabetes resources and education for older adults. There are many Web-based resources to read and half-day educational events aimed to reach this audience and their caregivers (www.diabetes.org).

Adapted from www.diabetes.org

Exploring THE WEB

Search the Web for additional information on gestational diabetes. What are the presenting signs and symptoms of gestational diabetes? What are the dangers of gestational diabetes to the mother and to the fetus if left untreated? Are there factors that put certain women at a higher risk for developing gestational diabetes? If yes, what are these risks?

Gestational Diabetes

Gestational diabetes can occur in pregnancy between weeks 16 and 28. It is diagnosed with an OGTT. If it is not responsive to diet, exercise, or oral medications, insulin injection therapy will be used (Figure 15-1). It is recommended that a dietitian or a diabetic educator be consulted to plan an adequate diet that will control blood sugar for mother and baby.

Concentrated sugars should be avoided. Weight gain should continue, but not in excessive amounts. Usually, gestational diabetes disappears after the infant is born. Women who have gestational diabetes have a 35–60% chance of developing type 2 diabetes in the next 10–20 years.

Secondary diabetes occurs infrequently and is caused by certain drugs or by a disease of the pancreas. For example, steroid medications can increase blood sugars and a client can develop steroid-induced diabetes.

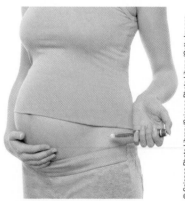

FIGURE 15-1 A pregnant woman can develop diabetes during her pregnancy that may need to be managed by insulin injections.

TREATMENT

Patients with pre-diabetes can prevent or delay progression to type 2 diabetes if they are committed to changing their lifestyle. Patients should be referred to an intensive diet and physical activity behavioral counseling program adhering to the tenets of the Diabetes Prevention Program (DPP), targeting a loss of 7% of body weight. They should increase their moderate-intensity physical activity (such as brisk walking) to at least 150 minutes a week. Technology-assisted resources, which include Web-based social networks, distance learning, mobile applications, and so forth, can be useful elements of effective lifestyle modification to prevent diabetes.

The treatment of diabetes is intended to do the following:

1. Control blood glucose levels
2. Provide optimal nourishment for the client
3. Prevent symptoms and thus delay the complications of the disease

Treatment is typically begun when blood tests indicate hyperglycemia, impaired glucose tolerance, or when other previously discussed symptoms occur. Normal blood glucose levels (called fasting blood sugar, or FBS) range from 70 to 100 mg/dl.

Treatment can be by diet alone or by a diet combined with insulin or an oral glucose-lowering medication plus regulated exercise and the regular monitoring of the client's blood glucose levels.

The physician and dietitian can provide essential information and counseling and can help the client prevent complications. The ultimate responsibility, however, rests with the client. When a person with diabetes uses nicotine, eats carelessly, forgets insulin, ignores symptoms, and neglects appropriate blood tests, he or she increases the risk of developing permanent complications.

NUTRITIONAL MANAGEMENT

According to the latest recommendations from the American Diabetes Associations 2016 Standards of Medical Care, diabetes nutrition therapy, preferably provided by a registered dietitian, can result in cost savings and improved outcomes. The dietitian will need to know the client's diet history, food likes and dislikes, and lifestyle at the onset. The client's calorie needs will depend on age, activities, lean muscle mass, size, and resting energy expenditure. Some clients will need to be taught a simplistic, yet effective approach emphasizing healthy food choices and portion control.

In the newest recommendation, there is no ideal macronutrient distribution of carbohydrate, protein, and fat; rather, distribution should be individualized while keeping total calorie and metabolic goals in mind. Carbohydrate intake from whole grains, vegetables, fruits, legumes, and dairy products with an emphasis on foods higher in fiber and lower in glycemic load should be advised over other sources, especially those containing sugars. Individuals with diabetes and those at risk should avoid sugary drinks and minimize the consumption of sucrose-containing foods that have the capacity to displace other healthier, more nutrient-dense food choices. The data on dietary fat amounts, according to research is still inconclusive; however, the Mediterranean style diet rich in monounsaturated fats can be an effective alternative to a diet low in total fat but relatively high in carbohydrate. Protein should be

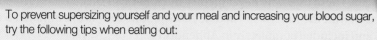

SUPERSIZE USA

To prevent supersizing yourself and your meal and increasing your blood sugar, try the following tips when eating out:

- Ask, ask, ask. Ask your waitress for the serving size of the entrée and how it is prepared. Special requests and substitutions to the menu can be made.
- Split a meal with a companion and order extra vegetables or salad. If dining alone, ask for a take-home container to save part of the meal for later.
- Eat slowly and pay attention to what you are eating and savor the flavor.
- Ask for sauces, gravies, and dressings on the side and avoid breaded and fried foods.
- Select items that are steamed in their own juice, broiled, baked, roasted, poached, and only lightly salted.
- Ask for fresh fruit instead of dessert.
- Limit alcohol consumption since it provides no nutrients, only additional calories.

as lean as possible and sodium should be limited to <2,300 mg a day, and for some, even lower.

Regardless of the percentages of energy nutrients prescribed, the foods ultimately eaten should provide sufficient vitamins and minerals as well as energy nutrients.

The client with type 1 diabetes needs a nutritional plan that balances calories and nutrient needs with insulin therapy and exercise. It is important that meals and snacks be composed of similar nutrients and calories and eaten at regular times each day. Small meals plus two or three snacks may be more helpful in maintaining steady blood glucose levels for these clients than three large meals each day. Medications and insulin dosing can help determine the number and timing of meals.

The client with type 1 diabetes should anticipate the possibility of missing meals occasionally and carry a few crackers and some cheese or peanut butter to prevent hypoglycemia, which can occur in such a circumstance.

The client with type 2 diabetes may be overweight. The nutritional goal for this client is not only to keep blood glucose levels in the normal range but also to lose weight. Exercise can help attain both goals.

Carbohydrate Counting

Carbohydrate counting is the newer method for teaching a client with diabetes how to control blood sugar with food. The starch and bread category, milk, and fruits have all been put under the heading of "carbohydrates." This means that these three carbohydrate-containing food groups can be interchanged within one meal. For example, a person is to have four carbohydrates for breakfast (two breads or starches, one fruit, and one milk). If there is no milk available, a bread or starch serving or fruit must be eaten in place of the milk. The exchange lists are utilized in carbohydrate counting as well as in traditional meal planning. Protein, approximately 3–4 oz, is eaten for lunch and dinner. No more than one or two fat exchanges are recommended for each meal. Two carbohydrates and 1 oz of protein should be eaten for an evening snack. These are only beginning guidelines. A dietitian or diabetic educator can help tailor this to the individual client.

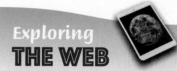

Exploring THE WEB

Today, cell phones are not just used to make phone calls or send messages. Smartphones are becoming more popular and there are numerous applications at our fingertips. Search the Web for nutrition, weight management, and meal tracker applications. What applications are available to assist clients with diabetes? How can these applications assist in diabetes management?

Diets Based on Exchange Lists

The method of diet therapy most commonly used for diabetic clients is based on **exchange lists**. These lists were developed by the American Diabetes Association in conjunction with the American Dietetic Association. They are summarized in Table 15-3 and included completely in Appendix E.

Under this plan, foods are categorized by type. The foods within each list contain approximately equal amounts of calories, carbohydrates, protein, and fats. This means that any one food on a particular list can be substituted for any other food on that *particular list* and still provide the client with the prescribed types and amounts of nutrients and calories.

The amounts of nutrients and calories on one list are not the same as those on any other list. Each list includes serving size by volume or weight and the calorie value of each food item, in addition to the grams of carbohydrates, and, when appropriate, proteins and fats. The number of calories a person needs will determine the number of items prescribed from any particular list. These lists also can be used to control calorie content of diets and are thus appropriate for low-calorie diets.

The total energy requirements for adult diabetic clients who are not overweight will be the same as for nondiabetic individuals. When clients are overweight, a reduction in calories will be built into the diet plans, typically allowing for a weight loss of 1 lb a week.

exchange lists
lists of foods with interchangeable nutrient and calorie contents; used in specific forms of diet therapy

TABLE 15-3 Summary of Exchange Lists

THE FOOD LISTS

The following chart shows the amount of nutrients in one serving from each list.

FOOD LIST	CARBOHYDRATE (g)	PROTEIN (g)	FAT (g)	CALORIES
Carbohydrates				
Starch: breads, cereals, and grains, starchy vegetables, crackers, snacks, and starchy beans	15	0–3	0–1	80
Fruits	15	—	—	60
Milk				
Fat free, low-fat, 1%	12	8	0–3	100
Reduced fat, 2%	12	8	5	120
Whole	12	8	8	160
Sweets	15	varies	varies	varies
Nonstarchy vegetables	5	2	—	25
Meat and Meat Substitutes				
Lean	—	7	0–3	45
Medium fat	—	7	4–7	75
High fat	—	7	8+	100
Plant-based proteins	varies	7	varies	varies
Fats	—	—	5	45
Alcohol	varies	—	—	100

Source: Reproduction of the Exchange Lists in whole or part, without permission of the American Dietetic Association or the American Diabetes Association, Inc., is a violation of federal law. This material has been modified from *Choose Your Foods: Exchange Lists for Diabetes*, which is the basis of a meal planning system designed by a committee of the American Diabetes Association and the American Dietetic Association. While designed primarily for people with diabetes and others who must follow special diets, the Exchange Lists are based on principles of good nutrition that apply to everyone. Copyright © 2008 by the American Diabetes Association and the American Dietetic Association. Academy of Nutrition and Dietetics (formerly the American Dietetic Association). Reproduced with permission.

The diet is given in terms of exchanges rather than as particular foods. For example, the menu pattern for breakfast may include one fruit exchange, one meat exchange, two bread or starch exchanges, and two fat exchanges. The client may choose the desired foods from the exchange lists for each meal but must adhere to the specific exchange lists named and the specific number of exchanges on each list. Vegetables (nonstarchy) are relatively free and can be eaten in amounts up to 1½ cups cooked or 3 cups raw. If more than this amount is eaten at one meal, count the additional amount as one more carbohydrate. Snacks are built into the plan. In this way, the client has variety in a simple yet controlled way.

When there are changes in one's physical condition, such as pregnancy or lactation, or in one's lifestyle, the diet will need to be modified. A change in job or in working hours can affect nutrient and calorie requirements. When such changes occur, the client should be advised to consult a physician or dietitian so that calorie and insulin needs can be promptly adjusted.

SPECIAL CONSIDERATIONS FOR THE CLIENT WITH DIABETES

Fiber

The therapeutic value of fiber in the diabetic diet has become increasingly evident. High-fiber intake appears to reduce the amount of insulin needed because it lowers blood glucose. It also appears to lower the blood cholesterol and triglyceride levels. "High fiber" may mean 25–35 g of dietary fiber a day. Such high amounts can be difficult to include. High-fiber foods should be increased very gradually, as an abrupt increase can create intestinal gas and discomfort. When increasing fiber in the diet, one must also increase water intake. An increased fiber intake can affect mineral absorption. For clients dosing insulin based on the grams of carbohydrate they are consuming, a portion of fiber may be subtracted. When reading food labels, if the fiber content is greater than 5 g, half the grams of fiber may be subtracted from the total carbohydrates for which the client is dosing.

Alternative Sweeteners

There are a variety of artificial sweeteners available in the market place. Some of the sweeteners have safety controversies, as some have not been studied as extensively as they should have been. The common artificial sweeteners in the marketplace are:

- Sucralose (brand name Splenda) is made from a sugar molecule that has been altered in such a way that the body will not absorb it. It is 600 times sweeter than sugar. Some believe this should be used with caution because of a 2012 independent study, not yet published, which linked it to increased leukemia in mice in utero.

- Aspartame (brand name Equal, Nutrasweet) is the generic name for a sweetener composed of two amino acids: phenylalanine and aspartic acid. It is 200 times sweeter than sugar. Consumer groups believe this tops the list of least desirable sweeteners to use (even avoid), because of independent studies showing cancer in rats in mice.

- Saccharin (brand name Sweet'N Low) is 350 times sweeter than sugar. Consumer safety groups believe this is to be avoided as studies on rodents showed saccharin caused bladder cancer, among other cancers.

- Acesulfame-Potassium (brand name Equal Original or Equal Spoonful) is 200 times sweeter than sugar and is generally used with sucralose or aspartame to cut bitterness. Many believe this sweetener should be avoided, as tests done 40 years ago were questionable in quality, with two of them showing risk for cancer in rats.
- Advantame is 20,000 times sweeter than sugar and was approved by the FDA in 2014. It is viewed as safe, especially due to the fact that such small amounts are used in foods.
- Neotame (brand name Newtame) is 8,000 times sweeter than sugar. There are no safety concerns; however, this sweetener is rarely used.
- Stevia Leaf Extract (Pure Via, Sweet Leaf, Truvia), which is highly purified, is viewed as safe; however, whole-leaf stevia or crude stevia is not allowed to be in foods.

Dietetic Foods

The use of diabetic or dietetic foods is generally a waste of money and can be misleading to the client. Often, the containers of foods will contain the same ingredients as containers of foods prepared for the general public, but the cost is typically higher for the dietetic foods. There is potential danger for diabetic clients who use these foods if they do not read the labels on the food containers and assume that because they are labeled "dietetic," they can be used in larger quantities. In reality, their use should be in specified amounts only, as these foods will contain carbohydrates, fats, and proteins that must be calculated in the total day's diet.

It is advisable for the client with diabetes to use foods prepared for the general public, but pay close attention to portion sizes. The important thing is for the diabetic client to *read the label* on all food containers purchased.

Alcohol

Although alcohol is not recommended for diabetic clients, its limited use is sometimes allowed if approved by the physician. However, some clients with diabetes who use hypoglycemic agents cannot tolerate alcohol. Clients must be very careful to only consume alcohol while eating. If alcohol is consumed on an empty stomach, the person may experience hypoglycemia. When used, alcohol must be included in the diet plan to account for the calories consumed.

Exercise

Exercise helps the body use glucose by increasing insulin receptor sites and stimulating the creation of glucagon. It lowers cholesterol and blood pressure and reduces stress and body fat as it tones the muscles. For clients with type 2 diabetes, exercise helps improve weight control, glucose levels, and the cardiovascular system.

However, for clients with type 1 diabetes, exercise can complicate glucose control. As it lowers glucose levels, hypoglycemia can develop. Exercise must be carefully discussed with a physician. If done, it should be on a regular basis, and it must be considered carefully as the meal plans are developed so that sufficient calories and insulin are prescribed. Clients should be educated on hypoglycemia signs and symptoms and its treatment. Clients need to have access to a meter and glucose tablets during exercise.

Insulin Therapy

Clients with type 1 diabetes must have injections of insulin every day to control their blood glucose levels (Figure 15-2). This insulin is called **exogenous insulin** because it is produced outside the body. **Endogenous insulin** is produced by the body.

Exogenous insulin is a protein. It must be injected because, if swallowed, it would be digested and would not reach the bloodstream as a complete hormone. For type 1 diabetes, after insulin treatment is begun, it is usually necessary for the client to continue it throughout life. With type 2 diabetes, patients may come off insulin if lifestyle changes and weight loss are significant.

Human insulin is the most common insulin given to clients. This insulin does not come from humans but is made synthetically by a chemical process in a laboratory. Human insulin is preferred because it is very similar to insulin made by the pancreas. Animal insulin comes from cows or pigs and is called beef or pork insulin. These insulins are rarely used because they contain antibodies that make them less pure than human insulin.

Various types of insulin are available. They differ in the time it takes for them to peak (if at all) and in the duration they continue to act. This latter category is called insulin action. Consequently, this insulin is classified as very rapid, rapid, intermediate, and long acting. Those insulins most commonly used are the very rapid acting, dosed just before meals, and the long acting, which provide the background insulin (i.e., the amount needed regardless of meals). For type 1 diabetes, insulin is often given in two or more injections daily and may contain more than one type of insulin. Injections are given at prescribed times.

More clients with insulin-dependent diabetes, both type 1 and type 2, are using insulin-pump therapy for better blood glucose control. Pumps deliver insulin in two ways: the basal rate and a pre-meal bolus. The basal rate is a small amount of very-rapid-acting insulin delivered continuously throughout the day. This insulin keeps blood glucose in check between meals and during the night. A pre-meal bolus of very-rapid-acting insulin is designed to cover the food eaten during a meal. This allows more flexibility as to when meals are eaten. Insulin pumps are not for everyone. An endocrinologist and diabetes educator can determine the best candidates for pump therapy.

Insulin Reactions

When clients do not eat the prescribed diet but continue to take the prescribed insulin, hypoglycemia can result. This is called an **insulin reaction**, or *hypoglycemic episode*, and may lead to **coma** and death. Symptoms include sweating, shaking, light-headedness, headache, blurred vision, confusion, poor coordination, and eventual unconsciousness. Insulin reaction is dangerous because if frequent or prolonged, brain damage can occur. The brain must have sufficient amounts of glucose in order to function. The physician should be consulted if an insulin reaction occurs or seems imminent.

Conscious clients may be treated by giving them glucose tablets or a beverage containing about 15–20 g of sugar. If in 15 minutes the individual is still hypoglycemic, the procedure is repeated. Once blood sugar returns to normal, a meal or snack should be given. If the client is unconscious, glucagon can be injected or an intravenous treatment of dextrose and water is given. It is advisable for the clients with diabetes to carry identification explaining the condition so that people do not think they are drunk when, in reality, they are experiencing an insulin reaction.

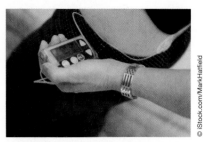

FIGURE 15-2 Insulin pump therapy may be used for better glucose control in clients with type 1 diabetes.

© iStock.com/MarkHatfield

Exploring
THE WEB

Search the Web for additional information on insulin therapies. What different types of therapies exist? Are there any experimental therapies currently being used and researched? What are some of the trial findings for these therapies?

exogenous insulin
insulin produced outside the body

endogenous insulin
insulin produced within the body

insulin reaction
hypoglycemia leading to insulin coma caused by too much insulin or too little food

coma
state of unconsciousness

HEALTH AND NUTRITION CONSIDERATIONS

Our nation needs to more carefully screen adults and children for pre-diabetes and support lifestyle changes to minimize chances they will convert to diabetes. It is important to point out to clients with diabetes that they can live a near-normal life by following their meal plan, taking medication as prescribed, and allowing time for sufficient exercise and rest. The dietitian must also stress the importance of eating all of the prescribed food, eating food at regular times to maintain the insulin–glucose balance, and carefully reading all labels on commercially prepared foods.

Adjustments must be made in shopping, cooking, and eating habits in order to follow the meal plan. Family meals can be simply adapted for the diabetic meal plan. The client with diabetes soon learns which exchange lists are to be included at each meal and at snack times and the foods within each exchange list. It is also important for the person's family to understand that the meal plan for diabetes is a very healthy way of eating. All members of the family could benefit from the portion control, lower fat content, and the awareness of everything being consumed.

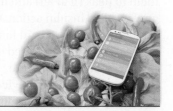

SUMMARY

The meal plan for diabetes is a key component in treating diabetes. Diabetes is a metabolic disease caused by the improper functioning of the pancreas that results in inadequate production or utilization of insulin. If the condition is left untreated, the body cannot use glucose properly, and then serious complications, even death, can occur. Treatment includes nutrition, medication, and exercise. Meal plans for diabetes are prescribed by the physician or dietitian in consultation with the client.

DISCUSSION TOPICS

1. Discuss the onset of type 1 and type 2 diabetes and list the symptoms.

2. Explain the difference between pre-diabetes, type 1 diabetes, and type 2 diabetes.

3. Name the risk factors for developing pre-diabetes, type 1 diabetes, and type 2 diabetes and discuss screening and diagnosis.

4. Discuss the treatment options for type 1 and type 2 diabetes.

5. Why would it be important for a client with diabetes to be educated about nutrition?

6. What are some of the complications that can occur if type 1 or type 2 diabetes is not well controlled or well managed?

7. True or False: It is necessary for clients with diabetes to purchase sugar-free and diabetic foods.

8. Discuss what the term *exchange* means in the meal plan for a client with diabetes.

9. Which of the following foods contain one carbohydrate exchange? More than one answer may be correct. (See Appendix F for more information.)
   a. 1 slice of bread
   b. ½ cup corn
   c. ½ cup black beans
   d. 1 tbsp butter
   e. 4 oz orange juice
   f. 8 oz milk
   g. 3 oz chicken
   h. 1 tsp olive oil

10. How is gestational diabetes different from type 1 or type 2 diabetes?

11. Name the four major complications that can occur long term in clients with diabetes.
   a. _____
   b. _____
   c. _____
   d. _____

12. Name two tips that can be done to help reduce calories while eating out.

SUGGESTED ACTIVITIES

1. Attend a local diabetes support group and listen to some of the topics the clients discuss. What are some of their difficulties, and how are they handling them?

2. Keep a food log for one week. Track in your log the time, the food, and the portion size of everything you eat. Use the respective food label to track calories, total carbohydrate, total fat, and protein consumed. If you don't have a food label, use the exchange list in Appendix E to estimate for those items consumed. At the week's end, answer these questions: How did you feel about writing down everything you ate? What difficulties did you encounter? Are there areas of your diet that could be modified to improve your health?

3. Visit a local grocery store. Find five foods that also offer a sugar-free option. Discuss the differences in the calories, carbohydrates, fats, and proteins in the regular verses the sugar-free version. What was the price difference between the two items? Did you find some foods where the sugar-free version would be better for a client with diabetes? Did you find some foods where it made little difference at all?

4. Identify someone you know who has diabetes. Ask to interview them. What are some of their challenges and frustrations in living with diabetes? What complications, if any, do they have? How often are they seeing their physician? Do they follow a meal plan? Have they ever had diabetes education or met with a registered dietitian or certified diabetes educator?

5. Investigate some of the resources available to clients with pre-diabetes and diabetes. Remember, we want clients to use credible and validated sources to obtain information about their health and caring for their diabetes. Make a list of some of the credible current resources. Can you find five books, five websites, five magazines/journals, and five smartphone applications that would be accurate, reliable, and helpful resources for clients with pre-diabetes and diabetes?

REVIEW

Multiple choice. Select the *letter* that precedes the best answer.

1. Which of the following statements is correct for type 1 diabetes?
   a. Most clients with diabetes (90–95%) have type 1.
   b. The pancreas continues to produce insulin; the body simply has difficulty using it.
   c. Clients with type 1 diabetes are often obese.
   d. Diabetes is caused by an autoimmune reaction.

2. Which of the following statements is correct for type 2 diabetes?
   a. Clients are usually diagnosed at a young age.
   b. Clients may not have obvious symptoms of type 2 diabetes.
   c. Insulin must be used to control blood sugars.
   d. The pancreas no longer produces any insulin.

3. Damage to the kidneys as a complication of diabetes is known as
   a. glycosuria
   b. polyuria
   c. nephropathy
   d. renal threshold

4. Insulin may be administered via which of the following routes?
   a. insulin pens
   b. insulin pumps
   c. insulin syringes
   d. by mouth
   e. only a, b, and c
   f. all

5. Oral medications for diabetes help improve blood sugars in all of the following ways except
   a. stimulating the pancreas to make more insulin
   b. helping the body use insulin more efficiently
   c. increasing appetite
   d. preventing the liver from releasing stored glucose

6. The American Diabetes Association recommends the A1C level for clients with diabetes to be below
   a. 7%   c. 3%
   b. 9%   d. 5%

7. Which of the following is NOT true of gestational diabetes?
   a. Foods high in concentrated sugars should be avoided.
   b. It is a risk factor for developing type 2 diabetes.
   c. Weight gain during the pregnancy should stop.
   d. Insulin injections may be used to control blood sugar.

8. Who should be tested for diabetes or pre-diabetes in adult populations?
   a. Anyone who is simply overweight and over age 45
   b. Only those who have a family history of diabetes
   c. Anyone who has started drinking more water
   d. Anyone who is overweight and has additional risk factors such as high blood pressure and lipids

CASE IN POINT

SIMONE: TYPE 2 DIABETES AND HEART HEALTH

Simone was diagnosed with type 2 diabetes 10 years ago. At the time of her diagnosis, her doctor had her attend classes to learn about monitoring her blood sugars and eating healthy. She went to the classes, but really didn't believe she had diabetes. She felt fine and she didn't have any family history of diabetes. In fact, her parents immigrated to the United States from France. The French have a very low incidence of diabetes. Surely her doctor had made a mistake. So, for the most part, Simone ate what she wanted and never worried about testing her blood sugars. She didn't have insurance to cover the cost of the test strips and they were just too expensive to purchase out of pocket. In addition, she decided not to go back to the doctor. She felt fine and he didn't know what he was talking about anyway.

Now that she is 50 years old, Simone has managed to all but forget about the diabetes. She is 5-ft and 5-in tall and weighs 134 lb. She is in her ideal body weight range and, up to this point, has no symptoms of diabetes. Then, while preparing breakfast one morning for her family, Simone experiences a sudden, sharp pain down her left arm and unbearable pressure on her chest. She falls to the floor and, in a state of panic, her husband calls 911.

Following emergent cardiac bypass surgery, Simone and her husband hear from the surgeon that she is lucky to be alive because the diabetes has greatly damaged her heart. The surgeon told Simone her A1C was 12.3%, and that if she didn't begin caring for her diabetes, she would certainly develop other complications in the near future.

ASSESSMENT

1. Why didn't Simone think she had diabetes?
2. Simone is 5 ft 5 in. and 134 lb. Is she within her ideal body weight range?
3. Simone's A1C is 12.3%. What is the normal range and the recommendation for someone with diabetes?
4. Why does the doctor think the diabetes has caused damage to Simone's heart?

DIAGNOSIS

5. Write a nursing diagnosis for Simone.

PLAN/GOAL

6. What resources do you think Simone's doctor should refer her to?
7. Simone's family needs to understand the severity of the situation and be supportive of her efforts. What could they do to support her efforts in gaining control of her diabetes and her health?
8. What is a primary goal in Simone's care?

IMPLEMENTATION

9. What could Simone begin doing to show she is beginning to accept her diagnosis and move toward a healthier lifestyle?

EVALUATION/OUTCOME CRITERIA

10. How would you determine the effectiveness of the plan and the goals?

THINKING FURTHER

11. Go to the website for the American Diabetes Association (http://www.diabetes.org) and look particularly at the food and fitness tab. What are some of the recommendations and resources they have available to clients? What information did you find useful?

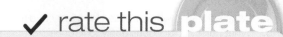
✔ rate this plate

Simone has met with a diabetes educator to learn about the importance of monitoring her blood sugar levels and eating healthy. Simone decides that carbohydrate counting would be the easiest way to plan her meals. The diabetes educator recommends a 1,500–1,600 calorie meal plan, which allows two to three carbohydrate choices per meal. Rate the plate that Simone plans for her breakfast:

1 toasted whole-grain English muffin

1 tsp margarine

1 tsp grape jelly

1 egg cooked over-easy

1 medium banana

8 oz low-fat milk

Does Simone have the correct number of carbohydrates for this meal? What should be added or subtracted from this plate?

CASE IN POINT

MICHAEL: MANAGING NEW-ONSET TYPE 1 DIABETES

Michael, age 15, is a freshman in high school, where he is very involved in athletics. During the basketball season, he develops an insatiable appetite. His mother is amazed at how much he can eat. At first, she assumes the overeating is due to a growth spurt and the increased activity level at daily basketball practice and games. At his last doctor's appointment, Michael measured 5 ft 10 in. and weighed 166 lb. Lately, however, his mother notices that Michael looks too thin, despite his increased food intake.

Michael has also been getting up frequently during the night to use the bathroom. When his mother questions him about this, Michael reports having a strong urge to go, but then can only void a small amount when in the bathroom. Michael is frustrated because the "false" urges are interrupting his sleep and, as a result, making him extremely tired throughout the school day. He states that he has been taking a water bottle to school daily and refilling it multiple times. He just thought he was dehydrated from basketball practice and his body just needed more water. He also assumed this was why he needed to get up in the night and go to the bathroom.

Michael and his mother are African American and have a strong family history of type 2 diabetes. His mother begins to piece together some of his symptoms and decides he needs to see his doctor. At the doctor's office, Michael's mother becomes very concerned. Michael only weighs 147 lb! After completing blood and urine tests, the doctor diagnoses Michael with type 1 diabetes and admits him to the hospital where insulin will be initiated to bring his blood sugar down. He and his mother will then be educated on nutrition, insulin, and blood sugar monitoring.

ASSESSMENT

1. List all the subjective information you have about Michael related to diabetes.
2. What objective data do you have about Michael?
3. What tests are necessary to confirm the diagnosis of diabetes?

DIAGNOSIS

4. What education will be needed for Michael's diagnosis?
5. What nursing diagnoses apply to Michael?

PLAN/GOAL

Complete the following goal statements:
6. Michael will verbalize and demonstrate his self-care measures related to _____.
7. Michael will verbalize and demonstrate survival skills for persons with diabetes and information by _____.

IMPLEMENTATION

The doctor has prescribed a long-acting insulin injection for Michael at bedtime and a dose of rapid-acting insulin at meals based on the amount of carbohydrate Michael will consume and his current pre-meal blood sugar level.

8. What topics are essential for Michael to learn?
9. What skills does he need to master before he goes home?
10. Who else needs to be in class with Michael?
11. What information does Michael's mother need to know about emergency situations?
12. What does Michael need to know about exercise?

EVALUATION/OUTCOME CRITERIA

13. What should Michael's fasting blood sugar be at his two-week follow-up appointment?
14. What should he be able to verbalize and demonstrate?
15. What should happen to his weight?

THINKING FURTHER

16. Why is it essential for Michael to manage his diabetes?
17. What challenges does Michael face in balancing between being a carefree teenager and managing a serious chronic disease?
18. What information will need to be provided to Michael's school, including his teachers and his coach?

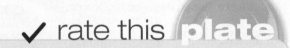 ✔ rate this **plate**

During his stay at the hospital, Michael receives a visit from a registered dietitian. The dietitian provides education on carbohydrate counting and how carbohydrates will affect his blood sugar levels. She also explains to Michael that exercise will have an effect on his blood sugar levels and that it is important to check his blood sugar regularly when engaging in basketball practice and games. Since Michael is an active, growing teenager, the dietitian recommends a 2,800 calorie diabetic meal plan. This meal plan allows for five to six carbohydrate choices per meal and two to three carbohydrate choices for snacks between meals. Rate the snack that Michael plans to eat before basketball practice.

2 mozzarella string cheese sticks

1 medium apple

1 oz cookie snack pack

8 oz low-fat milk

Will this snack provide him with enough carbohydrate servings to maintain his blood sugar levels through basketball practice? Does the mozzarella cheese contain carbohydrates? Why is it recommended to consume a protein source with a carbohydrate choice as a snack for the diabetic meal plan?

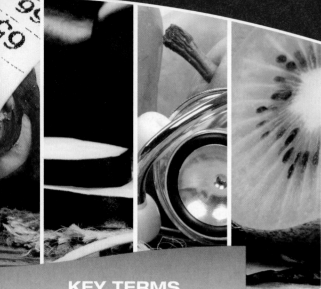

CHAPTER 16

KEY TERMS

angina pectoris
atherosclerosis
arteriosclerosis
cardiomyopathy
cardiovascular disease (CVD)
cerebrovascular accident (CVA)
compensated heart disease
congestive heart failure (CHF)
coronary artery disease (CAD)
Dietary Approaches to Stop
  Hypertension (DASH)
decompensated heart disease
endocardium
essential hypertension
hyperlipidemia
infarct
ischemia
lumen
myocardial infarction (MI)
myocardium
pericardium
peripheral vascular disease
  (PVD)
primary hypertension
secondary hypertension
serum cholesterol
thrombus
vascular disease

DIET AND CARDIOVASCULAR DISEASE

OBJECTIVES

After studying this chapter, you should be able to:

- Identify factors that contribute to heart disease
- Explain why cholesterol and saturated fats are limited in some cardiovascular conditions
- Identify foods to avoid or limit in a cholesterol-controlled diet
- Explain why sodium is limited in some cardiovascular conditions
- Identify foods that are limited or prohibited in sodium-controlled diets

Cardiovascular disease (CVD) affects the heart and blood vessels. It is the leading cause of death and permanent disability in the United States today. The grief and economic distress it causes are staggering. Organizations, especially the American Heart Association, are promoting programs designed to alert people to the risk factors for CVD and thereby reduce its frequency.

cardiovascular disease (CVD)
disease affecting heart and blood vessels

myocardial infarction (MI)
heart attack; caused by the blockage of an
artery leading to the heart

compensated heart disease
heart disease in which the heart is able to
maintain circulation to all body parts

decompensated heart disease
heart disease in which the heart cannot
maintain circulation to all body parts

myocardium
heart muscle

endocardium
lining of the heart

pericardium
outer covering of the heart

arteriosclerosis
thickening and hardening of the arteries

vascular disease
disease of the blood vessels

atherosclerosis
a form of arteriosclerosis affecting the intima
(inner lining) of the artery walls

lumen
the hollow area in a tube

ischemia
reduced blood flow causing an inadequate
supply of nutrients and oxygen to, and wastes
from, tissues

angina pectoris
pain in the heart muscle due to inadequate
blood supply

thrombus
blood clot

infarct
dead tissue resulting from blocked artery

cerebrovascular accident (CVA)
either a blockage or bursting of blood vessel
leading to the brain

**peripheral vascular disease
(PVD)**
narrowed arteries some distance from the
heart

hyperlipidemia
excessive amounts of fats in the blood

Cardiovascular disease can be acute (sudden) or chronic. **Myocardial infarction (MI)** is an example of the acute form. Chronic heart disease develops over time and causes the loss of heart function. If the heart can maintain blood circulation, the disease is classified as **compensated heart disease**. Compensation usually requires that the heart beat unusually fast. Consequently, the heart enlarges. If the heart cannot maintain circulation, the condition is classified as **decompensated heart disease**, and CHF occurs. The heart muscle (**myocardium**), the valves, the lining (**endocardium**), the outer covering (**pericardium**), or the blood vessels may be affected by heart disease.

ATHEROSCLEROSIS

Arteriosclerosis is the general term for **vascular disease** in which arteries harden (become thickened), making the passage of blood difficult and sometimes impossible. **Atherosclerosis** is the form of arteriosclerosis that most frequently occurs in developed countries. It is now believed to be a chronic inflammatory process, which begins in childhood and is considered one of the major causes of heart attack.

Atherosclerotic plaques are deposits of cholesterol, fats, and other substances that accumulate over time, thickening and weakening artery walls. Researchers now believe plaques develop within rather than on the artery wall and are driven by an inflammatory process (Figure 16-1). Plaque deposits gradually reduce the size of the **lumen** of the artery and, consequently, the amount of blood flow. The reduced blood flow causes an inadequate supply of nutrients and oxygen delivery to and waste removal from the tissues. This condition is called **ischemia**.

The reduced oxygen supply causes pain. When the pain occurs in the chest and radiates down the left arm, it is called **angina pectoris** and should be considered a warning. When the lumen narrows so that a blood clot (**thrombus**) occurs in a coronary artery and blood flow is cut off, a heart attack occurs. The dead tissue that results is called an **infarct**. The heart muscle that should have received the blood is the myocardium. Thus, such an attack is commonly called an acute MI. Some clients who experience an MI will require surgery to bypass the clogged artery. The procedure is a coronary artery bypass graft (CABG), which is commonly referred to as bypass surgery.

When blood flow to the brain is blocked in this way or blood vessels burst and blood flows into the brain, a stroke, or **cerebrovascular accident (CVA)**, results. When it occurs in tissue some distance from the heart, it is called **peripheral vascular disease (PVD)**.

Risk Factors

Risk factors for development of cardiovascular disease include:

- **Hyperlipidemia**
- Hypertension (high blood pressure)
- Smoking
- Obesity and unhealthy diet
- Diabetes, pre-diabetes
- Family history (heart disease in father or brother before age 55, or in mother or sister before age 65)

Normal artery

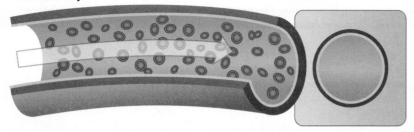

Partially blocked artery

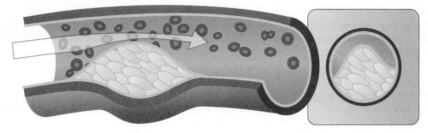

Occluded artery

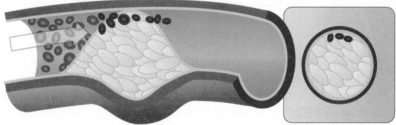

FIGURE 16-1 Progression of atherosclerosis.

- High stress levels
- Male sex
- Age (men age 45 or older, women age 55 or older)
- Physical inactivity

Although some of these factors are beyond one's control, some factors are not.

It is known that dietary cholesterol and triglycerides (fats in foods and in adipose tissue) contribute to hyperlipidemia. Foods containing saturated fats and trans fats increase **serum cholesterol**, whereas unsaturated fats tend to reduce it.

Lipoproteins carry cholesterol and fats in the blood to body tissues. Low-density lipoprotein (LDL) carries most of the cholesterol to the cells, and elevated blood levels of LDL are believed to contribute to atherosclerosis. High-density lipoprotein (HDL) carries cholesterol from the tissues to the liver for eventual excretion. It is believed that low serum levels of HDL can contribute to atherosclerosis.

It is important for clients to know their laboratory values of lipids in addition to monitoring of their blood pressure and weight. Table 16-1 offers a classification of serum lipid values. Heart disease progresses over years and often does not present with symptoms until the disease has progressed.

serum cholesterol
cholesterol in the blood

TABLE 16-1 Cholesterol and Triglyceride Classifications

TOTAL CHOLESTEROL	
Less than 200 mg/dl	Desirable
200–239 mg/dl	Borderline high
240 mg/dl and above	High
LDL CHOLESTEROL	
Less than 100 mg/dl	Optimal
100–129 mg/dl	Near optimal
130–159 mg/dl	Borderline high
160–189 mg/dl	High
190 mg/dl and above	Very high
HDL CHOLESTEROL	
Less than 40 mg/dl	Major heart disease risk factor
60 mg/dl and above	Gives some protection against heart disease
TRIGLYCERIDES	
<150 mg/dl	Optimal
150–199 mg/dl	Borderline high
>200 mg/dl	High

Adapted from the National Heart, Lung, and Blood Institute, NIH. "Your Guide to Lowering Cholesterol with TLC – Therapeutic Lifestyle Change." www.nhlbi.nih.gov

Diet can alleviate hypertension (discussed later in this chapter), reduce obesity, and help control diabetes mellitus. A sedentary lifestyle can be changed. Exercise can help the client lose weight, lower blood pressure, and increase the HDL ("good") cholesterol level. Exercise must be done in consultation with the physician and be increased gradually. Also, one can stop smoking. In sum, a person can considerably reduce the risk of atherosclerosis and thus an MI, CVA, and PVD.

MEDICAL NUTRITION THERAPY FOR HYPERLIPIDEMIA

Medical nutrition therapy is the primary treatment for hyperlipidemia. It involves reducing the quantity and types of fats and often calories in the diet. When the amount of dietary fat is reduced, there is typically a corresponding reduction in the amount of cholesterol and saturated fat ingested and a loss of weight. In overweight persons, weight loss alone will help reduce serum cholesterol levels.

The American Heart Association categorizes blood cholesterol levels of 200 mg/dl or less to be desirable, 200–239 mg/dl to be borderline high, and 240 mg/dl and greater to be high.

In an effort to prevent heart disease, the American Heart Association has developed guidelines in which it is recommended that adult diets contain less than 200 mg of cholesterol per day and that fats provide no more than 20–35% of calories, with a maximum of 7% of those fat calories coming from saturated fats. Carbohydrates should make up 50–55% of the calories and proteins from 12–20% of them. Currently, it is believed that nearly 40% of the calories in the average U.S. diet come from fats.

Some individuals may choose to follow a vegetarian, semi-vegetarian, or even vegan diet in response to learning they have heart disease. Others may choose to research the Mediterranean style of eating in which a higher percent of fat calories are consumed in the form of olive oil. Some may follow the DASH diet guidelines (discussed later in this chapter) or learn about foods recommended as part of the Omni Heart Study (see Exploring the Web).

One may find a heart-healthy diet challenging to adapt to, compared to the typical westernized diet. Some individuals whose taste buds are used to rich foods and restaurant eating may find it somewhat unpalatable and boring. The good news is that taste is malleable and over time adjusts to new food choices, flavors, and textures. For some, it takes approximately two or three months to adjust to a heart-healthy eating plan. In essence, a heart-healthy eating plan follows the Dietary Guideline advice for all Americans (Table 16-2).

Dietary counseling is an essential component in the primary prevention of heart disease as well as the treatment phase of all patients with established heart disease. Information about key diet concepts, the importance of cooking at home, and re-engineering the home environment to include physical activity must be a cornerstone of clinical support. The client must be taught to select whole, fresh foods and to prepare them with only minimal heart-healthy fat. Sodium and added sugars should be limited as part of a heart-healthy diet. Simple sugars can not only contribute to triglyceride raising but may also increase LDL cholesterol.

TABLE 16-2 Recommendations for a Heart-Healthy Diet

FOODS TO CHOOSE	THOSE TO AVOID
VEGETABLES, FRUITS, AND LEGUMES • Eat a variety of fresh, frozen, and canned vegetables and fruits without added salt or sugar • Eat more starchy beans (legumes) such as lentils and kidney beans	• Vegetables with high-fat sauces, fried, or salted • Fruit prepared with added sugars • Limit starchy beans prepared with pork fat
GRAINS • Choose fiber-rich whole grains for most grain servings (brown rice, barley, oats, cracked wheat, coarse bread, bran)	• Refined grains, such as white rice, white bread/bagels, low-fiber cereals, crackers, baked goods, buttery crackers, commercially prepared garlic bread, croissants, etc.
POULTRY, FISH, MEAT, AND EGGS • Choose poultry (white meat) and fish without skin • Fish—consume twice a week (especially those high in omega 3s, such as salmon, trout) • Lean red meat, preferably less than twice weekly • Eggs—Two to three times per week	• Fatty cuts of meat, dark poultry meat, or poultry with skin on • Fried meat, fish, or poultry • Salted, processed meats, such as bologna, hot dogs, bratwurst, bacon, etc. • Eggs: >four weekly
DAIRY • Fat-free (skim) and 1% dairy products, yogurt, low-fat cheese occasionally	• 2% and whole milk, cream, high fat cheeses, ice cream, cream soups, etc.
FATS AND OILS • Olive, canola oil, nuts, nut butters, seeds, in moderation • Mayo, oil/vinegar dressings used in moderation	• Butter, cream, lard, partially hydrogenated fats and trans fats • Commercially made creamy salad dressings—check labels
DESSERTS/BEVERAGES • Water, tea, and coffee • If you drink alcohol: One drink for women, two drinks for men • Prudent amounts of healthfully made desserts, small amount of dark chocolate	• Limit sugar sweetened beverages, such as soda, lemonade, punch, coffee drinks, energy drinks, etc. • Most regularly prepared desserts and sweets

TABLE 16-3 Sample Menus for a Heart-Healthy, Fat-Controlled Diet

BREAKFAST	LUNCH	DINNER
Orange	Low/reduced sodium tomato juice	3 oz salmon
Oatmeal	Homemade vegetable lentil soup	Baked sweet potato
1 tbsp raisins		Roasted broccoli with 2 tsp. olive oil
1 cup fat-free milk	6 high fiber crackers	
1 slice coarse whole-wheat toast	½ cup plain yogurt with 1 tsp honey	Leafy green salad with assorted vegetables and 2 tbsp olive oil vinaigrette
2 tsp peanut butter	½ cup blueberries	1 slice whole-wheat bread with 2 tsp with oil-based margarine
Coffee	2 tbsp granola	
	Tea	
		Canned peaches
		1 cup fat-free milk
		Tea

Exploring THE WEB

Search the Web for information on the Omni Heart Study. How does this diet differ from the American Heart Association guidelines or the DASH diet? Check out "a sample day's worth of eating" on the Omni Heart Diet from the Center for Science in the Public Interest.

In a fat-controlled diet, one must be particularly careful when using animal foods. Cholesterol is found only in animal tissue. Organ meats, egg yolks, and some shellfish are especially rich in cholesterol and should be used in limited quantities, if at all. Saturated fats are found in all animal foods and in coconut, chocolate, and palm oil. They tend to be solid at room temperature. Polyunsaturated fats are derived from plants and some fish and are usually soft or liquid at room temperature. Soft margarine containing mostly liquid vegetable oil is substituted for butter, and liquid vegetable oils are used in cooking.

Studies indicate that water-soluble fiber, such as that found in oats, oat bran, legumes (starchy beans such as lentils and kidney beans), and fruits (especially citrus, berries, apples, and bananas), binds with cholesterol-containing substances and prevents their reabsorption by the blood. The recommendation for total fiber per day is 38 g for men and 25 g for women. Research published by the National Institute of Health shows that people who increased their soluble fiber intake by 5–10 g each day had about a 5% drop in their LDL ("bad") cholesterol. If a client is able, a level of 10–25 g of soluble fiber is preferred. This is a large amount of fiber and must be introduced gradually to the diet along with increased fluids, or flatulence may result.

If appropriate blood lipid levels cannot be attained within three to six months by the use of a heart-healthy diet (see Table 16-3 for menus) teamed with increased physical activity, the physician may prescribe a cholesterol-lowering drug such as atorvastatin (Lipitor) or simvastatin (Zocor). Food and/or drug interactions can occur with cholesterol-lowering drugs, as well as with other cardiac drugs. For example, Zocor and Lipitor interact with grapefruit and its juice; therefore, total avoidance is necessary.

MYOCARDIAL INFARCTION

Myocardial infarction is caused by the blockage of a coronary artery supplying blood to the heart. The heart tissue is denied blood because of this blockage and dies (see Figure 16-2). Atherosclerosis is a primary cause, but hypertension, abnormal blood clotting, and infection such as that caused by rheumatic fever (which damages heart valves) are also contributory factors.

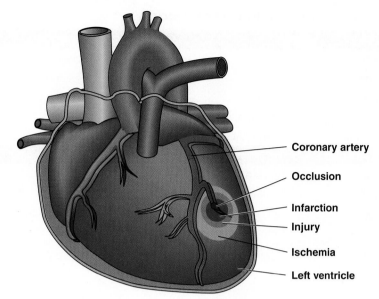

FIGURE 16-2 When a coronary artery is occluded, the heart muscle dies.

— Coronary artery

— Occlusion

— Infarction

— Injury

— Ischemia

— Left ventricle

After the attack, the client is in shock. This causes a fluid shift, and the client may feel thirsty. The client should be given nothing by mouth (NPO), however, until the physician evaluates the condition. If nausea remains after the period of shock, IV infusions are given to prevent dehydration.

After several hours, the client may begin to eat. A liquid diet may be recommended for the first 24 hours. Following that, a low-cholesterol–low-sodium diet is usually given, with the client regulating the amount eaten.

Foods should not be extremely hot or extremely cold. They should be easy to chew and digest and contain little roughage so that the work of the heart will be minimal. Both chewing and the increased activity of the gastrointestinal tract that follow ingestion of high-fiber foods cause extra work for the heart. The percentage of energy nutrients will be based on the particular needs of the client, but, in most cases, the types and amounts of fats will be limited. Sodium is usually limited to prevent fluid accumulation. Some physicians will order a restriction on the amount of caffeine for the first few days after an MI. The dual goal is to allow the heart to rest and its tissue to heal.

CONGESTIVE HEART FAILURE

Congestive heart failure (CHF) is an example of decompensation, or severe heart disease. Heart failure is caused by conditions that damage the heart muscle, including **coronary artery disease (CAD)**, heart attack, **cardiomyopathy**, valve disease, heart defects present at birth, diabetes mellitus, and chronic renal disease. Heart failure can also occur if several diseases or conditions are present. In this situation, when damage is extreme and the heart cannot provide adequate circulation, the amount of oxygen taken in is insufficient for body needs. Shortness of breath is common, and chest pain can occur on exertion.

Because of the reduced circulation, tissues retain fluid that would normally be carried off by the blood. Sodium builds up, and more fluid is retained, resulting in edema. In an attempt to compensate for this pumping deficit, the heart beats faster and enlarges. This adds to the heart's burden. In advanced cases when edema affects the lungs, death can occur.

congestive heart failure (CHF)
a form of decompensated heart disease

coronary artery disease (CAD)
severe narrowing of the arteries that supply blood to the heart

cardiomyopathy
damage to the heart muscle caused by infection, alcohol, or drug abuse

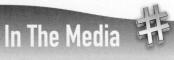

In The Media

Tricks Being Used by Scientists to Lower Sugar and Salt in Food

Since the early 2000s, companies have been trying to decrease the amount of sugar and salt in many popular food products in the name of health, yet still make them taste good. Campbell Soup Company slashed their salt content in their soups and recently announced they are phasing out monosodium glutamate (MSG) in their products. The flavor company FONA International has researched ways to use smells to trick the brain into thinking food contains more sugar and salt than it does. This new concept is called "phantom aroma." Researchers theorize that when the brain has a learned perception of a type of food, it fills in for the missing taste on its own. Very small amounts of vanillin and cherry/almond flavoring have been used to trick individuals into thinking a product is sweeter than it is, and ham flavoring helps trick individuals into thinking a product is saltier than it is. FONA has been able to achieve a 10% reduction in salt in food products through its phantom aroma studies.

Source: Adapted from Chen, Jenny. (2015, October 21). "Tasting Flavor That Doesn't Exist." *The Atlantic.* http://www.theatlantic.com/health/archive/2015/10/tasting-a-flavor-that-doesnt-exist/411454/

essential hypertension
high blood pressure with unknown cause; also called primary hypertension

primary hypertension
high blood pressure resulting from an unknown cause

secondary hypertension
high blood pressure caused by another condition such as kidney disease

TABLE 16-4 Potassium-Rich Foods

FRUITS		
Apricots	Dates	Kiwifruit
Oranges	Figs	Peaches
Bananas	Raisins	Pineapple
Avocados	Honeydew melon	Prunes
Cantaloupe	Grapefruit	Strawberries
VEGETABLES		
Asparagus	Squash	
Broccoli	Tomatoes	
Cabbage	Spinach	
Green beans	Potatoes, sweet potatoes, yams	
Pumpkin		

With the inadequate circulation, body tissues do not receive sufficient amounts of nutrients. This insufficiency can cause malnutrition and underweight, although the edema can mask these problems. In some cases, a fluid restriction may be ordered.

Diuretics to aid in the excretion of water and sodium and a sodium-restricted diet are typically prescribed. Because diuretics can cause an excessive loss of potassium, the client's blood potassium should be carefully monitored to prevent hypokalemia, which can upset the heartbeat. Fruits, especially oranges, bananas, and prunes, can be useful in such a situation because they are excellent sources of potassium and contain only negligible amounts of sodium (Table 16-4). When necessary, the physician will prescribe supplementary potassium.

HYPERTENSION

When blood pressure is chronically high, the condition is called hypertension (HTN). In 90% of hypertension cases, the cause is unknown, and the condition is called **essential hypertension** or **primary hypertension**. The other 10% of the cases are called **secondary hypertension** because the condition is caused by another problem. Some causes of secondary hypertension include kidney disease, problems of the adrenal glands, and use of oral contraceptives.

The blood pressure commonly measured is that of the artery in the upper arm. This measurement is made with an instrument called the sphygmomanometer. The top number is the systolic pressure, taken as the heart contracts. The lower number is the diastolic pressure, taken when the heart is resting. The pressure is measured in millimeters of mercury (mm Hg). Hypertension can be diagnosed when, on several occasions, the systolic pressure is 140 mm Hg or more and the diastolic pressure is 90 mm Hg or more. The blood pressure categories are the following:

- Normal: less than 120/less than 80 mm Hg
- Prehypertension: 120–139/80–88 mm Hg
- Stage 1 hypertension: 140–159/90–99 mm Hg
- Stage 2 hypertension: 160/100 mm Hg

Hypertension contributes to heart attack, stroke, heart failure, and kidney failure. It is sometimes called the *silent disease* because sufferers can be asymptomatic (without symptoms). Its frequency increases with age, and it is more prevalent among African Americans than others.

Heredity and obesity are predisposing factors in hypertension. Smoking and stress also contribute to hypertension. Weight loss usually lowers the blood pressure and, consequently, clients are often placed on weight reduction diets.

Excessive use of ordinary table salt also is considered a contributory factor in hypertension. Table salt consists of over 40% sodium plus chloride. Both are essential in maintaining fluid balance and thus blood pressure. When consumed in normal quantities by healthy people, they are beneficial.

When the fluid balance is upset and sodium and fluid collect in body tissue, causing edema, extra pressure is placed on the blood vessels. A sodium-restricted diet, often accompanied by diuretics, can be prescribed to alleviate this condition. When the sodium content in the diet is reduced, the water and salts in the tissues flow back into the blood to be excreted by the kidneys. In this way, the edema is relieved. The amount of sodium restricted is determined by the physician on the basis of the client's condition.

Previous research focused primarily on sodium as a primary factor in the development of hypertension, but as research continues, the effects of chloride also are receiving increasing scrutiny. In addition, the particular roles of calcium and magnesium in relation to hypertension are being studied.

Knowing that sodium raises blood pressure and that potassium lowers blood pressure, the NIH (National Institutes of Health) created the **Dietary Approaches to Stop Hypertension (DASH)** eating plan. The DASH plan has been clinically shown to reduce high blood pressure while increasing the serving of fruits and vegetables to 8–12 servings per day, depending upon calorie intake. In addition to the higher intake of fruits and vegetables with DASH, the hallmark of the diet is to ensure adequate calcium servings; to be prudent with protein portions; to include nuts, seeds, and legumes in diet three to four times per week; to limit fats and oils; and to keep sweets and added sugars down to five servings or fewer a week for adults.

Many fruits and vegetables are high in potassium levels, which will lower blood pressure. The newest guideline for potassium intake is 4.7 g, or 4,700 mg, per day to lower blood pressure. It is recommended that a physician be consulted if the DASH eating plan is undertaken and one is already on blood pressure-lowering medication.

Exploring THE WEB

Visit the American Heart Association's website (http://www.americanheart.org). Look for information on hypertension. Create a list of factors that may predispose people to hypertension. List ways to alleviate these risks and prevent hypertension and other serious heart conditions. How can diet play a role in alleviating some of these risk factors?

SUPERSIZE USA

Research presented at the American Heart Association's Scientific Session 2015 revealed that some obese children as young as 8 years old showed signs of heart disease and heart muscle abnormalities. Obese children were found to have increased muscle mass in the left ventricle of their hearts and thicker heart muscles, which are both indicators of heart disease. Thickened muscle in the heart can cause impaired pumping ability and was found in 40% of the obese child population in this study. Decreasing fat intake and increasing fruit and vegetable intake along with activity level at any age can help combat childhood obesity and further risks of developing diabetes, high cholesterol, and high blood pressure.

Source: Adapted from "Obese Kids as Young as Age 8 Show Signs of Heart Disease." (2015, November). American Heart Association Meeting Report – Abstract 15439. http://newsroom.heart.org/news/obese-kids-young-as-age-8-show-signs-of-heart-disease

DASH (Dietary Approaches to Stop Hypertension)
eating plan developed by the National Institutes of Health to reduce high blood pressure while increasing the serving of fruits and vegetables

Dietary Treatment for Hypertension

As indicated, weight loss for the obese client with hypertension usually lowers blood pressure, and thus a calorie-restricted diet might be prescribed. A sodium-restricted diet and DASH style eating plan frequently is prescribed for clients with hypertension. Certain ethnic groups, such as African Americans with new onset of HTN and those already diagnosed with HTN, should limit sodium intake to 1,500 mg/day. A discussion of this diet follows. When diuretics are prescribed together with a sodium-restricted diet, potassium may be lost via the urine and, thus, clients may be advised to increase the amount of potassium-rich foods in the diet (see Table 16-4). It is estimated that the average daily sodium intake for Americans is 3,400 mg.

Sodium-Restricted Diets

A sodium-restricted diet is a regular diet in which the amount of sodium is limited. Such a diet is used to alleviate edema and hypertension. Most people obtain far too much sodium from their diets. A committee of the Food and Nutrition Board recommends that the daily intake of sodium be limited to no more than 2,300 mg (2.3 g), and the board itself sets a safe minimum at 500 mg/day for adults (see Table 8-6). Sodium is found in food, water, and medicine.

It is impossible to have a diet totally free of sodium. Meats, fish, poultry, dairy products, and eggs all contain substantial amounts of sodium naturally. Cereals, vegetables, fruits, and fats contain small amounts of sodium naturally. Water contains varying amounts of sodium. However, sodium often is added to foods during processing and cooking and at the table. The food label should indicate the addition of sodium to commercial food products. In some of these foods, the addition of sodium is obvious because one can taste it, as in prepared dinners, potato chips, and canned soups. In others, it is not. Beyond salt (sodium chloride) used in cooking, in food products, and at the table, there are sodium-containing products frequently added to foods that the consumer may not notice:

- *Monosodium glutamate*—A flavor enhancer used in home, restaurant, and hotel cooking and in many packaged, canned, and frozen foods
- *Baking powder*—Used to leaven quick breads and cakes
- *Baking soda* (sodium bicarbonate)—Used to leaven breads and cakes
- *Brine* (table salt and water)—Used in freezing and canning certain foods; and for flavor, as in corned beef, pickles, and sauerkraut
- *Disodium phosphate*—Present in some quick-cooking cereals and processed cheeses
- *Sodium alginate*—Used in many chocolate milks and ice creams for smooth texture
- *Sodium benzoate*—Used as a preservative in many condiments such as relishes, sauces, and salad dressings
- *Sodium hydroxide*—Used in food processing to soften and loosen skins of ripe olives, hominy, and certain fruits and vegetables
- *Sodium propionate*—Used in pasteurized cheeses and in some breads and cakes to inhibit growth of mold
- *Sodium sulfite*—Used to bleach certain fruits and vegetables, also used as a preservative in some dried fruit, such as dried plums

SPOTLIGHT *on Life Cycle*

Sodium restrictions are a popular lifestyle prescription to help prevent hypertension and heart disease. While there has been debate over different levels of sodium intake and the effect on developing heart conditions, numerous medical studies support that mild sodium restriction can lower blood pressure. The guidelines established by the 2015 Dietary Guidelines for Americans and supported by the American Heart Association recommend no more than 1,500 mg of sodium per day for most middle-aged and older Americans. The 2015 Dietary Guidelines for Americans list 2,300 mg as the upper limit for healthy individuals. While the recommendation for 1,500 mg seems unrealistic for many Americans, it is still something to strive toward. Limiting the amount of processed foods and eliminating the salt shaker from the dinner table will assist in achieving the recommendation.

Because the amount of sodium in tap water varies from one area to another, the local department of health or the American Heart Association affiliate should be consulted if this information is needed. Softened water always has additional sodium. If the sodium content of the water is high, the client may have to use bottled water.

Some over-the-counter medicines contain sodium. Anyone on a sodium-restricted diet should obtain the physician's permission before using any medication or salt substitute. Many salt substitutes contain potassium, which can affect the heartbeat.

The amount of sodium allowed depends on the client's condition and is prescribed by the physician. A very low restriction limits sodium to 1½–2 g a day. A moderate restriction limits sodium to 2–3 g a day.

Adjustment to Sodium Restriction

Sodium-restricted diets range from "different" to "tasteless" because most people are accustomed to salt in their food. It can be difficult for one to understand the necessity for following such a diet, particularly if it must be followed for the remainder of his or her life. If the physician allows, it will help the client adjust if the sodium content of the diet can be reduced gradually.

A reminder of the numerous herbs, spices, and flavorings to be used in place of sodium will be beneficial (Table 16-5). It would also be useful to practice ordering from a menu so as to learn to choose those foods lowest in sodium content.

HEALTH AND NUTRITION CONSIDERATIONS

When one is given a new eating plan, it may take a long time for full compliance to be demonstrated. Asking one to make multiple changes at one time may result in poor compliance. Each task should be focused on separately, beginning with the most detrimental problem to you. The cardiac dietitian can help facilitate these changes and provide support along the way.

In The Media

Tips for Reducing Sodium Intake

Reducing your sodium intake can help prevent diseases such as heart attack, stroke, heart failure, kidney failure, and peripheral vascular disease. More than 75% of the sodium consumed is from processed foods. Replacing processed foods with fresh or frozen products is recommended. Other ways to reduce sodium intake include cooking with natural herbs and spices, purchasing "reduced sodium" products, avoiding the salt shaker when cooking and at the table, and avoiding most restaurant foods and processed foods.

Source: Adapted from "Reducing Sodium in a Salty World." (2015, August). American Heart Association. http://www.heart.org/HEARTORG/GettingHealthy/NutritionCenter/HealthyDietGoals/Reducing-Sodium-in-a-Salty-World_UCM_457519_Article.jsp#.VmBZZHarTIU

TABLE 16-5 Foods to Allow and Foods to Avoid on Sodium-Restricted Diets of 1–2 Grams

FOODS PERMITTED ON MOST SODIUM-RESTRICTED DIETS	FOODS TO LIMIT OR AVOID
Fruit juices without additives	Tomato juice and vegetable cocktail
Low-sodium vegetable juices	
Fresh fruits	Canned vegetables, if not salt-free
Fresh vegetables (except for those on the "Avoid" list), frozen vegetables prepared without salt	Sauerkraut, pickles, olives, frozen vegetables prepared with sodium
Dried peas or beans	Canned starchy beans
Fat-free milk	Dried, breaded, smoked, or canned fish or meats
Ready to eat breakfast cereals low in sodium	Cheeses; salted butter or margarine
Regular, cooked cereals without added salt, sugar, or flavorings	Salt-topped crackers or breads
Plain pasta or rice	Salty foods, such as potato chips, salted nuts, peanut butter, pretzels
Bread, english muffins, and bagels	Canned soups
Unsalted, uncoated popcorn	Ham, hot dogs, sausage, corned beef, lunch meats
Fresh fish	Prepared relishes, salad dressings, catsup, soy sauce
Fresh unsalted meats	Bouillon, baking soda, baking powder, MSG
Unsalted margarine	Commercially prepared meals
Oil	Fast foods, restaurant foods
Vinegar	
Spices containing no salt; herbs such as basil, oregano, garlic powder, etc.; lemon juice	
Unsalted nuts	
Jams, jellies, honey	
Coffee, tea	

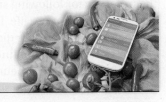

SUMMARY

Cardiovascular disease represents the leading cause of death in the United States. It may be acute, as in myocardial infarction, or chronic, as in hypertension and atherosclerosis. Hypertension may be a symptom of other disease. Weight loss, if the client is overweight, and a salt-restricted diet are typically prescribed.

Atherosclerosis is a vascular disease driven by chronic inflammation, in which the arteries are narrowed by fatty deposits, reducing blood flow. Angina pectoris, myocardial infarction, or stroke can result. Because cholesterol is associated with atherosclerosis, a low-cholesterol diet or a fat-restricted diet might be prescribed.

By maintaining one's weight and activities at a healthy level, limiting salt and fat intake, and avoiding smoking, one reduces the risks of heart disease.

DISCUSSION TOPICS

1. Why are sodium-restricted diets prescribed for clients with hypertension or heart failure?

2. What precautions might one take to prevent hypertension? To prevent atherosclerosis? Explain your answers.

3. What may occur in severe myocardial infarction? What causes myocardial infarction?

4. What are diuretics? How could they be harmful? How could this danger be avoided?

5. What is edema? How is it related to cardiovascular disease?

6. Why is it impossible to prepare a diet absolutely free of salt?

7. Why might a sodium-restricted diet be unpleasant for a client?

8. Name four snack items that would not be allowed on sodium-restricted diets.

9. For what heart condition might a fat-controlled diet be ordered?

10. What is cholesterol? How is it associated with atherosclerosis?

11. What is hyperlipidemia? How is it related to atherosclerosis?

12. Discuss known risk factors for the development of atherosclerosis. Which could be avoided? Explain.

SUGGESTED ACTIVITIES

1. Make a list of the foods eaten yesterday. Circle those foods that would not be allowed on a low-cholesterol diet and suggest satisfactory substitutions. Underline those not allowed on moderate sodium-restricted diets. Are any both circled and underlined?

2. Visit a local supermarket and, only checking foods along the outside walls, list the foods containing sodium compounds. Suggest substitutes for these foods for clients on sodium-restricted diets.

3. Marita Jiminez was placed on a fat-restricted diet containing no more than 70 g of fat. She wants to order the following breakfast:
   • Sliced avocado
   • Poached egg with ham in cheese sauce on English muffin
   • Coffee with cream

   Would this be acceptable? Explain your answer and, if necessary, suggest alternative foods that would be acceptable.

4. Justin Chen has been told that he has atherosclerosis and must follow a low-cholesterol diet. He is visiting his aunt who is serving the following meal:
   • Cream of broccoli soup
   • Roast chicken
   • Mashed potatoes with gravy
   • Lima beans with butter
   • Green salad with vinegar and oil dressing
   • Rolls and butter
   • Milk
   • Angel food cake with whipped cream and strawberries

   Which of the foods can Justin eat, and which must he avoid? Why? Can he eat certain parts of any of the foods? If so, which ones, and why?

5. Susan Smith has developed hypertension and has been placed on a mild sodium-restricted diet. She has planned the following dinner for her daughter's graduation party:
   • Fresh fruit cup
   • Baked ham
   • Potato chips
   • Fresh frozen broccoli chunks baked in canned cream of chicken soup
   • Homemade coleslaw
   • Rolls and butter
   • Dill pickles and olives
   • Chocolate cake with peppermint ice cream

   Which of the foods can she eat, and which must she avoid? Explain.

REVIEW

Multiple choice. Select the *letter* that precedes the best answer.

1. Some of the many risk factors for heart disease may include
   a. obesity, hypertension, and low milk intake
   b. high blood pressure, smoking, and hyperlipidemia
   c. inactivity, anemia, and diabetes
   d. insulin resistance, male over age 65, history of smoking

2. Sodium is commonly found in
   a. sugar
   b. fresh fruits
   c. baking soda and baking powder
   d. coffee and tea

3. A client with angina pectoris might be advised to follow a diet
   a. that contains limited sodium
   b. in which the calories are increased
   c. containing minimum amounts of proteins
   d. in which saturated fats are limited

4. Herbs, spices, and flavorings may
   a. be used in sodium-restricted diets
   b. never be used in sodium-restricted diets
   c. increase sodium in the diet
   d. be used only in the mild sodium-restricted diet

5. A sodium-restricted diet may be ordered for clients with
   a. mitral valve prolapse
   b. lipidemia
   c. congestive heart failure
   d. atherosclerosis

6. When water accumulates in body tissues
   a. the condition is called edema
   b. a fat-restricted diet may be prescribed
   c. it is a definite symptom of myocardial infarction
   d. salt is completely eliminated from the diet

7. It is thought that excessive fats in the blood over time contribute to
   a. congestive heart failure
   b. hypokalemia
   c. plaque
   d. edema

8. Table salt
   a. is 60% sodium
   b. is over 40% sodium
   c. contains only negligible amounts of sodium
   d. must be restricted in fat-restricted diets

9. In a low-cholesterol diet
   a. eggs are used freely
   b. vegetable oils are not permitted
   c. organ meats are permitted
   d. fat-free milk is used instead of whole milk

10. Cholesterol
    a. is found in food and in body tissue
    b. has no connection to lipoproteins
    c. is the primary cause of congestive heart failure
    d. is commonly found in fruits and vegetables

11. Foods allowed in a low-fat diet include
    a. cheese
    b. cooked vegetables
    c. sausage
    d. all soups

12. When preparing foods for the low-fat diet,
    a. small amounts of fat can be added
    b. visible fats must be removed from meats
    c. fat-free milk is never used
    d. butter is substituted for vegetable oil

13. On the low-cholesterol diet, saturated fats are
    a. reduced
    b. eliminated
    c. increased
    d. unchanged from the amount in the regular diet

14. Saturated fats are usually
    a. solid at room temperature
    b. liquid at room temperature
    c. found in fruits
    d. derived from plants

15. Polyunsaturated fats are usually
    a. solid at room temperature
    b. found in animal foods
    c. liquid at room temperature
    d. derived from dairy products

16. When the heart muscle reacts with pain because of inadequate blood supply after activity, the condition is called
    a. cerebral accident
    b. edema
    c. hypertension
    d. angina pectoris

17. Some examples of blood lipids are
    a. triglycerides
    b. polyunsaturated fats
    c. sterols
    d. plaques

18. Examples of foods particularly rich in potassium are
    a. milk and ice cream
    b. beef and lamb
    c. whole-grain breads and cereals
    d. bananas and oranges

CASE IN POINT

AYVION: CONGESTIVE HEART FAILURE

Ayvion is a manager for a large electronics distributor. He has been working long hours in preparation for the holiday season. For the past few days, he has noticed some tightening in his chest. Thinking it was indigestion, Ayvion started an over-the-counter antacid. The antacid has not provided him with much relief and today the pain seems to be radiating down his left arm. He also seems to be having difficulty catching his breath and is extremely tired. When he gets home from work, Ayvion is having so much trouble breathing, he asks his wife to take him to the emergency room.

When he arrives at the hospital, the doctor orders nasal oxygen and a series of blood tests for Ayvion, and admits him to the telemetry unit for further monitoring and assessment. The admitting nurse learns from Ayvion that his father suffered his first heart attack at age 36. Ayvion is currently 47 years old, is 5 ft 10-in tall, and weighs 215 lb. His current blood pressure is 208/98. The nurse knows that Ayvion's family history, age, weight, and African American ethnicity put him at risk for heart disease. Ayvion's blood work reveals an elevated cholesterol and LDL. It also shows that Ayvion has indeed suffered a minor heart attack. The doctor tells Ayvion he has some damage to his heart that would indicate he has had a previous heart attack that went undetected. The doctor tells Ayvion he is going to survive, but he needs to make some changes. His current problems coupled by his previous heart attack have caused him to develop a condition known as congestive heart failure. He tells Ayvion that his heart is weakened by the damage and cannot pump as strongly as it used to. As a result, Ayvion has fluid in his lungs that is causing the shortness of breath and the fatigue. The doctor orders medications to lower both his blood pressure and cholesterol. He orders diuretics to help control the fluid overload. He also refers Ayvion to a cardiac rehabilitation program in order to learn how to eat properly and exercise safely. Ayvion knows he needs to follow the doctor's recommendations. However, he is worried that his time away from work will cost him his job.

ASSESSMENT

1. What subjective data do you have about Ayvion and his health?
2. What objective data do you have?
3. How significant is his problem?
4. What are the potential consequences if Ayvion ignores his doctor's advice?

DIAGNOSIS

5. Write a diagnostic statement about Ayvion's lack of knowledge regarding his cardiac condition and his new diet.
6. What education is needed to help achieve improvement in his health?

PLAN/GOAL

7. What are several reasonable goals for Ayvion?

IMPLEMENTATION

8. What issues must Ayvion begin to comply with regarding his new diet?
9. What cardiac topics does Ayvion need to learn to understand his new diet?
10. What two food categories can Ayvion use that have almost no restriction in his new diet?
11. What other problems may Ayvion be at risk for?
12. How could the information at the American Heart Association website (http://www.americanheart.org) be helpful to Ayvion?

EVALUATION/OUTCOME CRITERIA

13. If diet and exercise are successful, what changes will be measurable in three to six months?

14. What will the dietitian be able to assess in an interview with Ayvion?

FURTHER THINKING

15. What are the possible consequences of noncompliance for Ayvion?

✔ rate this plate

Ayvion attended the cardiac rehabilitation program, with support from his wife, to learn about the importance of regular exercise, maintaining a healthy weight, and consuming meals that are low in cholesterol and sodium. Ayvion has decided to plan his meals on a weekly basis and to try and include meat, vegetables, fruits, and milk at every meal. Here is one of the meals he plans to prepare for dinner:

7 oz baked chicken breast in cream of broccoli soup

1 cup white rice with juices from the broccoli soup as dressing

1 cup of green beans with bacon bits

2 biscuits with butter

½ cup peaches and pears

8 oz 2%-milk

What foods are high in cholesterol and/or sodium, if any? Has Ayvion chosen the right portions and calories for weight loss? If not what should be changed?

CASE IN POINT

NANCY: ADHERING TO A CARDIAC DIET

Nancy is a 62-year-old retired paralegal. The year before she re- tired, she had several episodes of angina in which she thought she was having a heart attack. One of the episodes was so severe, her coworker called EMS. During her hospital visit, the doctor encouraged Nancy to attend a smoking cessation pro- gram and to meet with a dietitian to learn about a diet that was low in sodium and cholesterol. Nancy did quit smoking, but found the diet more difficult to adhere to than she imagined.

After she retired, she was attending her grandson's bas- ketball game when she suffered a similar event. This time it was an actual heart attack. Nancy was taken to the hospital and a cardiac catheterization was performed. It was noted that there was a significant amount of blockage. The doctor felt it was necessary to perform surgery immediately. Nancy underwent quadruple bypass.

The doctor requested that the hospital dietitian re- view Nancy's nutritional habits again. When the dieti- tian asks Nancy about her diet history she admits some changes need to be made. Since Nancy retired she has been able to cook breakfast instead of eating on the run. Her typical breakfast has been sausage or bacon and cheesy eggs. She has never been a coffee drinker so her breakfast caffeine is a diet cola. For lunch her favorite meal is a chicken salad croissant and potato chips. Supper is usually meat and potatoes with gravy. She will include a vegetable with supper, but typically purchases canned vegetables to save money. Once in a while, for variety, she will bake the vegetables in cheese. Throughout the course of the day, her main beverage is typically diet cola.

ASSESSMENT

1. What do you know about Nancy's health?
2. How significant is her health problem?
3. What would the consequences be if Nancy decided to ignore the doctor's advice?
4. What do you know about Nancy's willingness to comply?
5. List all the foods Nancy ate that contained sodium or that are usually restricted on a low-sodium diet.
6. List the foods Nancy likes to eat that are high in fat.

DIAGNOSIS

7. Write a diagnostic statement based on Nancy's condition.
8. What does Nancy need to understand about CHF and low-sodium diets?
9. Why does Nancy continue to retain fluid?

PLAN/GOAL

10. What are reasonable, measurable goals for Nancy?

IMPLEMENTATION

11. What are the main topics to teach Nancy about her diet?
12. Modify Nancy's food choices to reflect a low-sodium diet.
13. What food categories can Nancy eat without restrictions?
14. What else does Nancy need in order to control the edema?

EVALUATION/OUTCOME CRITERIA

15. At her two-week doctor's appointment, what changes can the doctor observe and measure as evidence of the effectiveness of the diet?

THINKING FURTHER

16. Can this disease be cured?
17. Why is managing the disease a constant challenge?

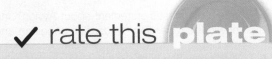

✔ rate this plate

Nancy enjoys preparing meals at home. She is trying to decrease her sodium and fat intake as the registered dietitian instructed. Nancy used a slow-cooker to make the following meal. Rate this plate:

- **4 oz beef roast made with cream of mushroom soup and dry onion soup mix**
- **3 oz cooked potatoes and carrots**
- **1 cup of salad greens with diced tomatoes, cucumbers, cheese, and croutons**
- **2 Tbsp low-fat salad dressing**
- **1 dinner roll with butter**
- **12 oz diet soda**

What changes would you make to her meal, if any? Is she eating according to her sodium restrictions? What do you think about her portion control?

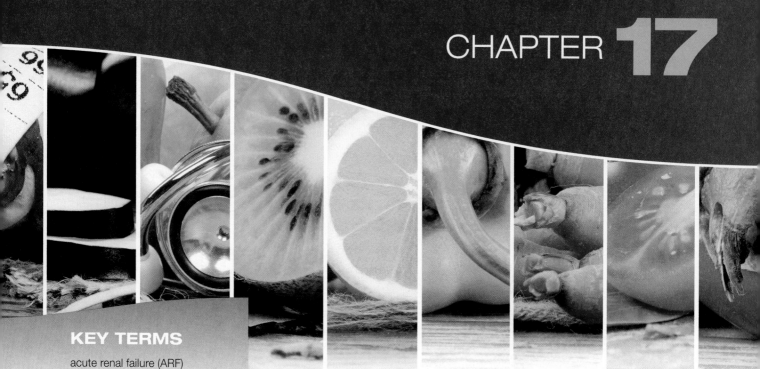

CHAPTER 17

KEY TERMS

acute renal failure (ARF)
chronic kidney disease
creatinine
cystine
cysts
dialysis
end-stage renal disease (ESRD)
glomerular filtration rate (GFR)
glomerulonephritis
glomerulus
hemodialysis
nephritis
nephrolithiasis
nephrons
nephrosclerosis
oliguria
peritoneal dialysis
polycystic kidney disease
purines
renal stones
urea
uremia
ureters
uric acid

DIET AND RENAL DISEASE

OBJECTIVES

After studying this chapter, you should be able to:

- Describe, in general terms, the work of the kidneys
- Discuss common causes of renal disease
- Explain why protein is restricted for renal clients
- Explain why sodium and water are sometimes restricted for renal clients
- Explain why potassium and phosphorus are sometimes restricted for renal clients

The kidneys are intricate and efficient processing systems that excrete wastes, maintain volume and composition of body fluids, and secrete certain hormones. To accomplish these tasks, they filter the blood, cleansing it of waste products, and recycle other usable substances so that the necessary constituents of body fluids are constantly available (Figure 17-1).

Each kidney contains approximately 1 million working parts called **nephrons**. Each nephron contains a filtering unit, called a **glomerulus**, in

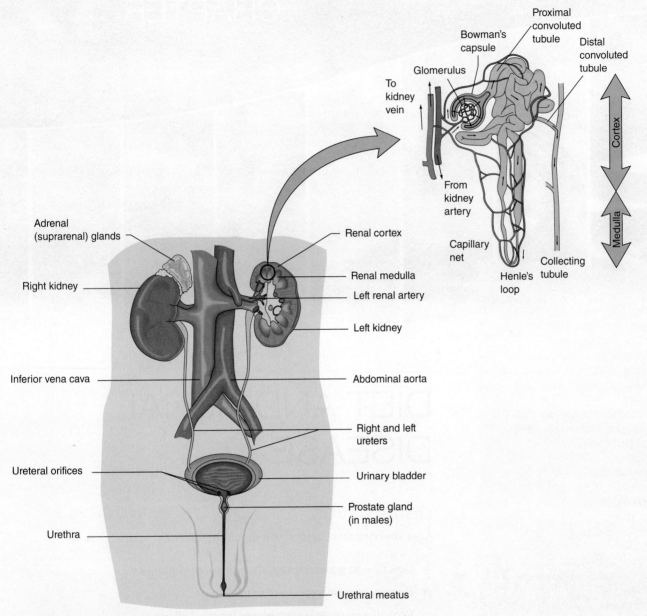

FIGURE 17-1 The urinary system with inset of a nephron.

nephrons
unit of the kidney containing a glomerulus

glomerulus
filtering unit in the kidneys

ureters
tubes leading from the kidneys to the bladder

urea
chief nitrogenous waste product of protein metabolism

uric acid
one of the nitrogenous waste products of protein metabolism

creatinine
an end (waste) product of protein metabolism

which there is a cluster of specialized capillaries (tiny blood vessels connecting veins and arteries). Approximately 180 L of ultrafiltrate is processed each day. As the filtrate passes through the nephrons, it is concentrated or diluted to meet the body's needs. In this way, the kidneys help maintain both the composition and the volume of body fluids and, consequently, they maintain fluid balance, acid–base balance, and electrolyte balance.

The liquid waste is sent via two tubes called **ureters** from the kidneys to the urinary bladder, from which they are excreted in approximately 1.5 L of urine per day. These waste materials include end products of protein metabolism (**urea, uric acid, creatinine**, ammonia, and sulfates), excess water and nutrients, dead renal cells, and toxic substances. When the urinary output is less than 500 mL/day, it is impossible for all the daily wastes to be eliminated. This condition is called **oliguria**. When the kidneys are unable to adequately eliminate nitrogenous waste (end products of protein metabolism), renal failure can result. The recycled materials are reabsorbed (taken back) by the blood. They include amino acids, glucose, minerals, vitamins, and water.

The kidneys synthesize and secrete certain hormones as needed. For example, it is the kidneys that make the final conversion of vitamin D. Active vitamin D promotes the absorption of calcium and the metabolism of calcium and phosphorus. The kidneys indirectly stimulate bone marrow to reproduce red blood cells by producing the hormone erythropoietin.

RENAL DISEASES

Etiology of Renal Disease

Kidney disorders can be initially caused by infection, degenerative changes, diabetes mellitus, high blood pressure, cysts, renal stones, or trauma (surgery, burns, poisons). When these conditions are severe, renal failure may develop. It may be acute or chronic. Acute renal failure (ARF) occurs suddenly and may last a few days or a few weeks. It can be caused by another medical problem such as a serious burn, a crushing injury, or cardiac arrest. It can be expected in some of these situations, so preventive steps should be taken.

Classification of Renal Disease

Chronic kidney disease develops slowly, causing the number of functioning nephrons to diminish. When renal tissue has been destroyed to a point at which the kidneys are no longer able to filter the blood, excrete wastes, or recycle nutrients as needed, uremia occurs. Uremia is a condition in which protein wastes that should normally have been excreted are instead circulating in the blood. Symptoms include nausea, headache, convulsions, and coma. Severe renal failure can result in death unless dialysis is begun or a kidney transplant is performed. The National Kidney Foundation has classified chronic kidney disease into five stages (see Table 17-1).

Nephritis is a general term referring to the inflammatory diseases of the kidneys. Nephritis can be caused by infection, degenerative processes, or vascular disease.

Glomerulonephritis is an inflammation affecting the capillaries in the glomeruli. It may occur acutely in conjunction with another infection and be self-limiting, or it may lead to serious renal deterioration.

oliguria
decreased output of urine to less than 500 mL/day

cysts
growths

renal stones
kidney stones

acute renal failure (ARF)
suddenly occurring failure of the kidneys

chronic kidney disease
slow development of kidney failure

uremia
condition in which protein wastes are circulating in the blood

dialysis
mechanical filtration of the blood; used when the kidneys are no longer able to perform normally

nephritis
inflammatory disease of the kidneys

glomerulonephritis
inflammation of the glomeruli of the kidneys

TABLE 17-1 Stages of Chronic Kidney Disease

STAGE	DESCRIPTION OF KIDNEY FUNCTION	GFR (mL/min/1.73 M2) (GLOMERULAR FILTRATION RATE)
1	Kidney damage, but normal to increased function	90–130
2	Mild decrease in function	60–89
3	Moderate decrease in function	30–59
4	Severe decrease in function	15–29
5	Kidney failure, defined as end-stage renal disease, dialysis usually initiated	<15

Source: The National Kidney Foundation. www.kidney.org

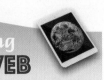
Nephrosclerosis is the hardening of renal arteries. It is caused by arteriosclerosis and hypertension. Although it usually occurs in older people, it sometimes develops in young diabetics.

Polycystic kidney disease is a relatively rare, hereditary disease. Cysts form and press on the kidneys. The kidneys enlarge and lose function. Although people with this condition have normal kidney function for many years, renal failure may develop near the age of 50.

Nephrolithiasis is a condition in which stones develop in the kidneys. The size of the stones varies from that of a grain of sand to much larger. Some remain at their point of origin, whereas others move. Although the condition is sometimes asymptomatic, symptoms include hematuria (blood in the urine), infection, obstruction, and, if the stones move, intense pain. The stones are classified according to their composition—calcium oxalate, uric acid, **cystine**, calcium phosphate, and magnesium ammonium phosphate (known as struvite). They are associated with metabolic disturbances and immobilization of the client.

SPECIAL CONSIDERATIONS FOR CLIENTS WITH RENAL DISEASES

Dietary Treatment of Renal Disease

Dietary treatment is intended to slow the buildup of waste in the bloodstream. Decreasing waste in the bloodstream will control symptoms of fluid retention, hyperkalemia, and nausea and vomiting. The goal is to reduce the amount of excretory work demanded of the kidneys while helping them maintain fluid, acid–base, and electrolyte balance. While sufficient protein is required to prevent malnutrition and muscle wasting, too much protein can contribute to uremia. Typically, one with chronic renal failure will have protein and sodium, and possibly potassium and phosphorus, restricted.

It is essential that renal clients receive sufficient calories (23–35 calories per kilogram of body weight) unless they are overweight. Energy requirements should be fulfilled primarily by carbohydrates and fat. The fats must be unsaturated to prevent or check hyperlipidemia. If the energy requirement is not met by carbohydrates and fat, ingested protein or body tissue will be metabolized for energy. Either would increase the work of the kidneys because protein increases the amount of nitrogen waste the kidneys must handle. During stage 3 or 4, the diet may limit protein to as little as 40 g for predialysis clients. On this lower protein diet, meat, fish, or poultry is limited to no more than 3 oz per day, and milk is not allowed, or limited to ½ cup day. Grains are limited to seven servings a day, fruit is limited to five servings a day (½ cup each), and vegetables are limited to two servings a day (½ cup). Low- and moderate-potassium fruit and vegetable choices likely will be used at this stage. Fat and sugar content of the diet can vary to meet total energy needs. The specific amount of protein allowed is calculated according to the client's **glomerular filtration rate (GFR)** and weight. Dietary counseling is vitally important for best outcome.

Fluids and sodium may be limited to prevent edema, hypertension, and congestive heart failure. Calcium supplements may be prescribed. In addition, vitamin D may be added and phosphorus limited to prevent osteomalacia (softening of the bones due to excessive loss of calcium). Phosphorus appears to be retained in clients with kidney disorders, and a disproportionately high ratio of phosphorus to calcium tends to increase calcium loss from bones.

nephrosclerosis
hardening of renal arteries

polycystic kidney disease
rare, hereditary kidney disease causing cysts or growths on the kidneys that can ultimately cause kidney failure in middle age

nephrolithiasis
development of stones in the kidney

cystine
a nonessential amino acid

glomerular filtration rate (GFR)
the rate at which the kidneys filter the blood

SUPERSIZE **USA**

Diabetes is the most common cause of kidney failure, with one-third of people with diabetes developing kidney disease, according to the National Kidney Foundation. Poor control of blood pressure, poor glucose control, inherited tendency, and diet are risk factors linked to increased risk of diabetic kidney disease. Serum creatinine and blood urea nitrogen (BUN) are checked as well as creatinine clearance, glomerular filtration rate (GFR), and urine albumin. About 30% of people with type 1 diabetes and 10–40% of people with type 2 diabetes will eventually develop end-stage kidney failure. African Americans, Hispanic Americans, and American Indian population groups have an increased risk of developing kidney failure from type 2 diabetes than do Caucasian Americans.

Source: Adapted from "Preventing Diabetic Kidney Disease: 10 Answers to Questions." The National Kidney Foundation. November 2015. http://www.kidney.org

Potassium may be restricted in some clients because hyperkalemia tends to occur in **end-stage renal disease (ESRD)**. Excess potassium can cause cardiac arrest. Because of this danger, renal clients should not use salt substitutes or low-sodium milk because the sodium in these products is replaced with potassium. Potassium restriction can be especially difficult. Potassium is particularly high in fruits—one of the few foods someone on a sodium-restricted diet may eat without concern. Table 17-2 summarizes typical diet recommendations in those with chronic kidney disease and those who have had transplantation.

end-stage renal disease (ESRD)
the stage at which the kidneys have lost most or all of their ability to function

TABLE 17-2 Typical Diet Recommendations for Chronic Kidney Disease and Transplant

DIET PARAMETER PER DAY	STAGES 1–4	STAGE 5 HEMODIALYSIS	STAGE 5 PERITONEAL	TRANSPLANT
Calories	23–35 kcals/kg	35 kcals/kg <60 years old; 30–35 kcals/kg >60 years old	30–35 kcals/kg, any age	30–35 kcals/kg
Protein	0.8–1.4 g/kg (stages 1 & 2) 0.6–0.8 g/kg (stages 3 & 4)	>1.2 g/kg body weight (50% high biologic value)	>1.2–1.3 g/kg body weight	1.3–2 g/kg
Phosphorus	800–1,000 mg if level is >4.6 mg/dl	800–1,200 mg	800–1,200 mg	Per dietary reference intake
Potassium	No limit unless serum levels elevated	2–3 g/day, adjusting based on serum values	2–4 g/day adjusting based on serum values	Varies depending on serum levels
Sodium	<2,400 mg	2,000–3,000 mg	2,000–3,000 mg	2,000–4,000 mg; restrict if blood pressure or fluid status dictates
Fluid	No restriction unless otherwise indicated	Individualized for fluid status, weight gain, and renal function	Maintain fluid balance	Maintain fluid balance

Source: Adapted from "Nutrition 411: Nutrition Care for Patients with Chronic Renal Failure." 2013. www.nutrition411.com

Renal clients often have an increased need for vitamins B, C, and D, and supplements are often given. Vitamin A should not be given because the blood level of vitamin A tends to be elevated in uremia. If a client is receiving antibiotics, a vitamin K supplement may be given. Otherwise, supplements of vitamins E and K are not necessary. Iron is commonly prescribed because anemia frequently develops. It is sometimes necessary to increase the amount of simple carbohydrates and unsaturated fats to ensure sufficient calories.

Dialysis

Dialysis is done by either **hemodialysis** or **peritoneal dialysis**. The most common is hemodialysis. Hemodialysis requires permanent access to the bloodstream through a fistula. Fistulas are unusual openings between two organs. They are often created near the wrist and connect an artery and a vein. Hemodialysis is done three times a week for approximately three to five hours each visit (Figure 17-2).

Peritoneal dialysis uses the peritoneal cavity as a semipermeable membrane and is less efficient than hemodialysis. Treatments usually last about 10–12 hours a day, three times a week (Figure 17-3). Some clients also use continuous ambulatory peritoneal dialysis (CAPD). The dialysis fluid is exchanged four or five times daily, making this a 24-hour treatment. Clients on CAPD have a

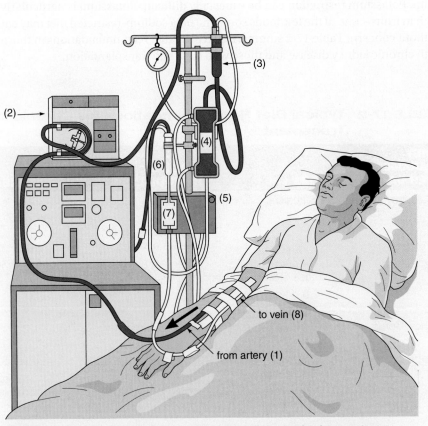

hemodialysis
cleansing the blood of wastes by circulating the blood through a machine that contains tubing of semipermeable membranes

peritoneal dialysis
removal of waste products from the blood by injecting the flushing solution into the abdomen and using the client's peritoneum as the semipermeable membrane

FIGURE 17-2 Hemodialysis. (1) Blood leaves the body via an artery. (2) Arterial blood passes through the blood pump. (3) Blood is filtered to remove any clots. (4) Blood passes through the dialyzer. (5) Blood passes into the venous blood line. (6) Blood is filtered to remove any clots. (7) Blood flows through the air detector. (8) Blood returns to the client through the venous blood line.

more normal lifestyle than do clients on either hemodialysis or peritoneal dialysis. Some complications associated with CAPD include peritonitis, hypotension, and weight gain.

Diet During Dialysis

Dialysis clients may need additional protein, but the amount must be carefully controlled to prevent the accumulation of protein waste between treatments.

A client on hemodialysis requires 1.2 g of protein per kilogram of body weight to make up for losses during dialysis. A client on peritoneal dialysis will require 1.2–1.3 g of protein per kilogram of body weight. The protein needs for clients on CAPD are 1.2 g per kilogram of body weight. Fifty percent of this protein should be high biological value (HBV) protein, which is found in eggs, meat, fish, poultry, milk, and cheese.

Potassium is usually restricted for dialysis clients. Healthy people ingest 2,000–6,000 mg per day. The daily intake allowed clients in renal failure is 2,000–4,000 mg. End-stage renal disease further reduces intake allowed to 1,500–2,500 mg per day. The physician will prescribe the milligrams of potassium needed by the client. Table 17-3 lists fruits and vegetables that are low, medium, and high in potassium.

Clients are taught to regulate their intake by making careful choices. Milk is normally restricted to ½ cup a day because it is high in potassium and high in methionine, an essential amino acid. A typical renal diet could be written as "80-3-3," which means 80 g of protein, 3 g of sodium, and 3 g of potassium a day. The day's allotment of food, for example, would be:

- 1 portion of milk or milk products/day (½ cup)
- 1 portion of milk substitutes/day
- 8 portions of meat or equivalent/day
- 3 portions of fruit or juices/day

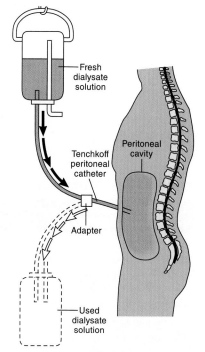

FIGURE 17-3 Peritoneal dialysis.

SPOTLIGHT on Life Cycle

For school-age children, receiving dialysis can be a challenge; however, there are home dialysis options that allow for more flexibility. Peritoneal dialysis (PD), whether through CAPD or automated peritoneal dialysis (APD), offers many advantages to children:

- Pain Free—Blood is cleaned inside the body and needles are not required as in hemodialysis.
- Flexible Treatment Schedule—Children are not required to visit a dialysis center to receive treatment, allowing them to attend school and participate in childhood activities.
- No Vascular Access Needed—Small blood vessels make it difficult to place a graft for hemodialysis; smaller-sized catheters work well in children.
- Ease of Travel—PD supplies can be shipped anywhere in the United States and PD devices are portable, making it easier for families with children receiving treatment to travel together.
- Fewer Dietary Restrictions—PD is done every day compared to hemodialysis which is done three times a week, therefore there are less restrictions.

Source: Adapted from DaVita. "Can Children Do Peritoneal Dialysis?" 2012. www.davita.com

- 8 portions of bread or starches/day
- 2 portions of vegetables/day
- Fats (polyunsaturated or unsaturated), such as oil, margarine, or mayonnaise, are not restricted

Vitamins and mineral supplements are sometimes indicated for clients receiving dialysis. Vitamin C and B complex may be given according to the dietary reference intake. Supplementation of iron and vitamin D is done when blood levels of those nutrients are low.

TABLE 17-3 Potassium Content of Selected Fruits and Vegetables

LOW POTASSIUM (<150 mg/SERVING*)	MEDIUM POTASSIUM (150–250 mg/SERVING*)	HIGH POTASSIUM (>250 mg/SERVING*)
Applesauce	Apple juice	Avocado, ½ fruit
Berries: blackberries, blueberries, boysenberries, gooseberries, raspberries, strawberries	Apple, raw, 1 large	Banana, ½ fruit
Cranberry sauce	Apricots, raw, 2 medium, canned	Dried fruits: figs, apricots, dates, prunes, raisins
Grape juice	Cherries, raw (15) or canned	Kiwifruit
Grapes, canned or raw	Grapefruit juice	Melons: cantaloupe, ¼ medium; casaba, ¾ cubed; honeydew, ⅛ medium; watermelon, 2 cups, cubed
Lemon or lime, 1 medium	Grapefruit sections	Nectarine, 1 medium
Mandarin oranges, canned	Mango	Orange, navel
Peaches, canned	Peach, raw, 1 medium	Orange juice, fresh, frozen, canned
Pears, canned	Pear, raw, 1 medium	Papaya
Plums, canned	Pineapple juice, raw or canned	Prune juice, canned or bottled
Rhubarb	Pineapple spears	Raisins, seedless
	Plums, raw, 2 medium	Tangelo
	Tangerine	
Bamboo shoots	Asparagus	Artichoke
Bean sprouts	Beets	Beet greens
Beans, green, wax, snap	Brussels sprouts	Dried beans and peas: kidney, lima, garbanzo, navy, and pinto beans; black-eyed peas
Broccoli	Carrots, cooked	Potato, ½ cup baked, boiled, or fried
Cabbage	Celery	Pumpkin
Cauliflower	Greens: collard, mustard, kale, dandelion, beet, turnip greens	Spinach
Corn, canned or small ear	Mixed vegetables	Sweet potato or yams
Cucumber	Okra	Tomato, raw or canned
Eggplant, cooked	Peas, green	Unsalted tomato juice
Hominy grits, cooked	Peppers	Winter squash: acorn, butternut, hubbard, spaghetti
Leek	Summer squash: yellow crookneck, white scallop, zucchini	
Lettuce: cos, romaine, iceberg, leaf, endive, watercress (1 cup shredded)		
Mushrooms		
Onion: green, red, yellow, white		
Peppers, sweet or hot		
Radishes, raw		
Rutabaga		
Summer squash		
Turnips		
Water chestnuts, canned		

*All portions are ½ cup unless otherwise noted.

The ability of the kidney to handle sodium and water in ESRD must be assessed often. Usually, the diet contains 3 g of sodium, which is the equivalent of a no-added-salt diet. Sodium and fluid needs may increase with perspiration, vomiting, fever, and diarrhea. The fluid content of foods, other than liquids, is not counted in fluid restriction. Clients on fluid restriction must be taught to measure their fluid intake and urine output, examine their ankles for edema, and weigh themselves regularly.

Diet After Kidney Transplant

After kidney transplant, there may be a need for extra protein or for the restriction of protein. Carbohydrates and sodium may be restricted. The appropriate amounts of these nutrients will depend largely on the medications given at that time.

Additional calcium and phosphorus may be necessary if there was substantial bone loss before the transplant. There may be an increase in appetite after transplants. Fats and simple carbohydrates may be limited to prevent excessive weight gain.

Dietary Treatment of Renal Stones

Because the causes of renal stones have not been confirmed, treatment of them may vary. In general, however, large amounts of fluid—at least half of it water—are helpful in diluting the urine, as is a well-balanced diet. Once the stones have been analyzed, specific diet modifications may be indicated.

Calcium Oxalate Stones

About 80% of the renal stones formed contain calcium oxalate. Recent studies provide no support for the theory that a diet low in calcium can reduce the risk of calcium oxalate renal stones. In fact, higher dietary calcium intake may decrease the incidence of renal stones for most people. Dietary intake of excessive animal protein has been shown to be a risk factor for stone formation in some clients.

Stones containing oxalate are thought to be partially caused by a diet especially rich in oxalate, which is found in beets, wheat bran, chocolate, tea, rhubarb, strawberries, and spinach (Table 17-4). Evidence also indicates that deficiencies of pyridoxine, thiamine, and magnesium may contribute to the formation of oxalate renal stones.

Exploring THE WEB

Search the Web for additional information on kidney dialysis, kidney transplant, and renal stones. Research the role diet plays in the treatment of these disorders. Could diet play a preventive role in these disorders? What is the morbidity and mortality of these disorders? Find some good resource material for clients with these disorders.

TABLE 17-4 Foods High in Oxalates

FOODS HIGH IN OXALATES	
Beets	Soy milk
Black tea and instant tea	Spinach
Chocolate	Sweet potatoes
Dried beans (black, navy, or Great Northern)	Tree nuts (almonds, cashews, hazelnuts)
Peanuts	Wheat bran
Rhubarb	Wheat germ
Soy beans	

purines
end products of nucleoprotein metabolism

Uric Acid Stones

When the stones contain uric acid, purine-rich foods are restricted. **Purines** are the end products of nucleoprotein metabolism and are found in all meats, fish, and poultry. Organ meats, anchovies, sardines, meat extracts, excessive alcohol, and broths are especially rich sources of purines. Uric acid stones are usually associated with gout, GI diseases that cause diarrhea, and malignant disease. Medication will prevent gout and other complications by decreasing the formation of uric acid.

Cystine Stones

Cystine is an amino acid. Cystine stones may form when the cystine concentration in the urine becomes excessive because of a hereditary metabolic disorder. The usual practice is to increase fluids and recommend an alkaline-ash diet.

Struvite Stones

Struvite stones are composed of magnesium ammonium phosphate. They are sometimes called infection stones because they develop following urinary tract infections caused by certain microorganisms. A low-phosphorus diet is often prescribed.

HEALTH AND NUTRITION CONSIDERATIONS

The client with renal disease has a lifelong challenge. Anger and depression are common among these clients. These feelings complicate management of the disease if they contribute to the client's unwillingness to learn about his or her nutritional needs. These complications then add to the client's problems.

It is extremely helpful for the health care professional to develop a trusting relationship with the client. Such a relationship can be established by listening to the client's complaints, needs, and concerns and responding with sincere understanding and sympathy. This approach can help motivate the client to learn how to manage his or her nutritional requirements with assistance from the dietitian.

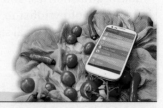

SUMMARY

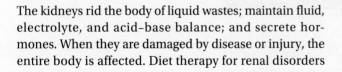

The kidneys rid the body of liquid wastes; maintain fluid, electrolyte, and acid–base balance; and secrete hormones. When they are damaged by disease or injury, the entire body is affected. Diet therapy for renal disorders can be extremely complex because of the multifaceted nature of the kidneys' functions. Untreated severe kidney disease can result in death unless dialysis or kidney transplant is undertaken.

DISCUSSION TOPICS

1. Discuss the three main tasks of the kidneys.
2. Define nephrons and explain what they do.
3. Discuss some causes of kidney disease.
4. What is nephritis? Glomerulonephritis? Nephrosclerosis?
5. Why is diet therapy for renal disease so complex?
6. Discuss why protein is typically decreased for clients with renal disease.
7. Why are sodium and water sometimes restricted in renal disease?
8. Why is potassium sometimes restricted in renal disease? What is hyperkalemia?
9. Why is phosphorus sometimes restricted in renal disease?
10. Why might calories be restricted in renal disease?
11. What is nephrolithiasis? How is it treated?

SUGGESTED ACTIVITIES

1. Invite a renal educator or dietitian to discuss renal disease with your class.
2. Invite a dialysis client to discuss her or his condition and reactions to dialysis.
3. Using outside sources, prepare a short report on the functions of the circulatory system, the liver, and the kidneys in eliminating nitrogenous waste products from the body.
4. Record your dietary intake for 24 hours. Analyze your choices to see which ones have the highest potassium.

REVIEW

Multiple choice. Select the *letter* that precedes the best answer.

1. The kidneys maintain the body's
   a. acid–base balance
   b. electrolyte balance
   c. fluid balance
   d. all of these

2. The specialized part within each nephron that actually filters the blood is called the
   a. ureter   c. glomerulus
   b. filter   d. capillary bunch

3. Kidney disorders may be caused by
   a. diabetes   c. burns
   b. infections   d. all of these

4. When renal tissue has been destroyed to a point at which it can no longer filter the blood, which of the following occurs?
   a. nephritis
   b. nephrosclerosis
   c. uremia
   d. nephrolithiasis

5. The general term referring to the inflammatory diseases of the kidneys is
   a. nephritis
   b. nephrosclerosis
   c. uremia
   d. nephrolithiasis

6. The term referring to the hardening of renal arteries is
   a. nephritis   c. uremia
   b. nephrosclerosis   d. nephrolithiasis

7. The rare hereditary disease causing cysts to develop on the kidneys is called
   a. nephritis
   b. glomerulonephritis
   c. renal stones
   d. polycystic kidney disease

8. The condition in which stones develop in the kidneys, ureters, or bladder is called
   a. nephritis
   b. nephrolithiasis
   c. polycystic kidney disease
   d. glomerulonephritis

9. Because its nitrogenous wastes contribute to uremia, which nutrient may be restricted in diets of renal clients?
   a. carbohydrate
   b. saturated fat
   c. protein
   d. vitamin A

10. Kidney dialysis
    a. is a means of filtering all protein from the blood
    b. is a means of removing toxic substances from the blood
    c. always requires the client be on a low-protein diet
    d. requires the client to increase his or her sodium intake

11. Sodium and water may be restricted in the diets of renal clients because they
    a. contribute to uremia
    b. increase hypercalcemia
    c. contribute to hyperlipidemia
    d. contribute to fluid retention

12. If osteomalacia occurs in renal clients, which nutrient may be prescribed?
    a. potassium
    b. protein
    c. calcium
    d. phosphorus

13. In a case of hyperkalemia, which nutrient may be restricted?
    a. potassium
    b. protein
    c. calcium
    d. phosphorus

14. Fruits are an especially rich source of
    a. protein
    b. potassium
    c. calcium
    d. phosphorus

15. The vitamins renal clients may have an increased need for are
    a. the water-soluble vitamins
    b. the fat-soluble vitamins
    c. vitamins B, C, and D
    d. vitamins E and A

16. An excess of which nutrient can compound bone loss in renal clients?
    a. phosphorus
    b. carbohydrate
    c. calcium
    d. iron

17. Purine-rich foods include
    a. organ meats and alcohol
    b. dairy foods
    c. vegetables, except corn and lentils
    d. fruits, except cranberries, plums, and prunes

18. An example of nitrogenous waste found in the urine is
    a. ureter
    b. uremia
    c. urea
    d. all of these

19. Which of the following recommendations has been proven to reduce the risk of calcium oxalate stones?
    a. higher whole grain intake
    b. higher dietary calcium intake
    c. increased intake of acetic acid
    d. increased intake of spinach

20. A typical renal diet that could be ordered by the doctor and written by the dietitian is a
    a. 90-2-2 diet
    b. 70-3-2 diet
    c. 80-3-3 diet
    d. 75-3-3 diet

CASE IN POINT

CHARLES: MANAGING DIET AFTER A KIDNEY STONE

Charles is a fourth-generation farmer from southern Indiana. He and his wife, Laura, have been married for 42 years. They both were raised on farms and have loved raising their family on a farm as well. At a young age, Charles and his wife learned that to survive as farmers you had to live a very modest lifestyle and let nothing go to waste. Laura is a good cook able to utilize every piece of the farm animals they butcher to provide food for the family. Laura cans the meats, fruits, and vegetables that were grown on the farm so the benefits of the harvest last all year long.

Charles is very consistent with his meals. For example, his breakfast always consists of bran flakes with strawberries on top and 2–3 cups of hot tea. As for other meals, he always enjoys a salad along with the main dish. He loves spinach and grew so much of it in the garden that his wife made a spinach salad with beets for supper daily. For dessert, his favorite is rhubarb pie, especially because Laura makes it just like his grandmother's recipe.

One morning, Charles wakes with a sharp, shooting pain in his abdomen. The intense pain radiates completely down his right side. By the time he meets Laura in the kitchen, he is doubled over in pain so severe he can barely move. Laura drives Charles to the emergency room. The doctor assesses Charles and discovers that Charles has a kidney stone. Once Charles is able to pass the stone, the doctor sends it to the lab for analysis. Charles learns that his kidney stone consists mainly of calcium oxalate. The doctor informs Charles that these types of stones can be related to a diet that is high in oxalate and animal proteins. The doctor advises Charles and Laura to meet with the hospital dietitian about Charles's diet.

ASSESSMENT

1. What do you know about Charles that put him at risk for kidney stones?
2. What were Charles's symptoms?
3. How will this condition affect Charles for the rest of his life?
4. How significant is this dietary change?

DIAGNOSIS

5. What is the cause of calcium oxalate stones?
6. Complete the following diagnostic statement: Charles's deficient knowledge is related to _____.

PLAN/GOAL

7. What are reasonable, measurable goals for Charles's change in health?

IMPLEMENTATION

8. What changes does Charles need to make in his diet?
9. What would the consequences be if Charles ignored the doctor's advice?
10. Could Charles have another stone?

EVALUATION/OUTCOME CRITERIA

11. How will the doctor know if the plan is effective?

THINKING FURTHER

12. What could someone else learn from Charles's experience?

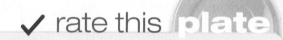 ✔ rate this **plate**

During his stay at the hospital, Charles spoke with a registered dietitian about his meal planning concerns. The dietitian told Charles that a diet rich in oxalates can lead to the formation of oxalate kidney stones. Charles provided the dietitian with a 24-hour recall of what he typically ate for lunch. Rate this plate:

5 oz grilled chicken sandwich on whole-grain bun

2 cups fresh spinach salad with strawberries, pecans, and cheese

2 Tbsp light vinaigrette salad dressing

1 medium orange

1 small slice of rhubarb pie

2 cups hot tea

What foods, if any, are high in oxalates? What nutrient deficiencies are common in clients who experience the formation of oxalate kidney stones? What can Charles include in his diet to hopefully prevent the formation of future kidney stones?

CASE IN POINT

LENA: DISCOVERING GLOMERULONEPHRITIS

Lena is a young mother of two boys. She has never considered herself a very healthy person. It seems she is constantly fighting off infections and colds. As far back as she can remember, people have referred to her as "sickly." Even as a child, her strong German mother could not understand why Lena was so pale and weak. After having children of her own, her illnesses continued. Every time the boys caught a cold at school or daycare, Lena was sure to end up with it. She had tried to eat healthy and take a regular multivitamin, but still her body just couldn't fight the infections. Recently, Lena has felt especially run-down, and she's been experiencing the need to urinate far more often than before. Her urine, too, appears a little darker than usual. Thinking she may be dehydrated, Lena started drinking a lot of water, but this made matters worse.

This morning her urine was a dark orange color and it even looked a little bubbly, like it was foaming. Her stomach ached and she had no appetite. Lena assumed she had yet another infection and made an appointment with her doctor for later in the day.

The nurse first gathered data for the doctor. She found Lena's blood pressure to be 148/98. She measured her at 5 ft and 7 in tall and 133 lb. After examining Lena, the doctor asked her to have some urine and blood work drawn. Upon reviewing the tests, Lena's doctor diagnosed her with glomerulonephritis. He told her that this was an inflammation of the capillaries in the glomeruli of her kidneys. Most likely, this had been caused by an infection. He told Lena that it would be necessary for her to start a blood pressure medication as well as a steroid to reduce the inflammation. He wanted her to begin decreasing the sodium, fluid, and protein she consumed. He told her other treatments might become necessary if her kidneys continue to worsen. He referred her to a registered dietitian to be educated regarding the changes necessary in her meal plan.

ASSESSMENT

1. What is the subjective data you have on Lena?
2. What is the objective data you have on Lena?
3. How will this condition affect Lena?

DIAGNOSIS

4. What is the cause of glomerulonephritis?
5. Write a nursing diagnosis for Lena.

PLAN/GOAL

6. What are reasonable, measurable goals for Lena?

IMPLEMENTATION

7. What changes does Lena need to make in her diet?
8. What would the consequences be if Lena did not follow doctor's advice?

EVALUATION/OUTCOME CRITERIA

9. How will the doctor know if the plan is effective?

THINKING FURTHER

10. What are some of the most effective ways to prevent infections?

✔ rate this plate

Lena met with a registered dietitian to discuss her concerns about preparing a healthy meal. The dietitian told Lena not to consume more than 48 oz of fluids per day to help control her blood pressure and lessen the workload on the kidneys. Sodium and potassium intake would be limited to improve blood pressure control and prevent fluid retention. Protein is also restricted to decrease the workload on the kidneys and prevent waste from building up in the blood. Lena's diet should be rich in complex carbohydrates and "good" fats until her body recovers. Rate the plate prepared for dinner.

- **4 oz breaded cod fillet**
- **¾ cup brown rice**
- **½ cup broccoli**
- **½ cup fruit salad containing apples, oranges, and grapes**
- **1 cup chocolate ice cream**
- **20 oz regular soda**

Does this meal meet the recommendations advised by the registered dietitian? If not, what can be improved?

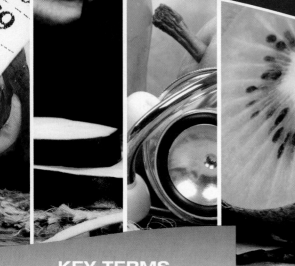

CHAPTER 18

KEY TERMS

ascites
celiac disease
cholecystectomy
cholecystitis
cholelithiasis
cirrhosis
colostomy
Crohn's disease
diaphragm
diverticulitis
diverticulosis
duodenal ulcer
dyspepsia
esophagitis
fibrosis
gastric ulcer
gastroesophageal reflux disease
  (GERD)
gluten
Helicobacter pylori
hepatitis
hiatal hernia
ileostomy
inflammatory bowel diseases
  (IBDs)
irritable bowel syndrome
jaundice
necrosis
pancreatitis
peptic ulcers
short bowel syndrome
stasis
steatorrhea
stoma
total parenteral nutrition (TPN)
ulcerative colitis

DIET AND GASTROINTESTINAL DISORDERS

OBJECTIVES

After studying this chapter, you should be able to:

- Explain the uses of diet therapy in gastrointestinal disturbances
- Identify the foods recommended and not recommended in the therapeutic diets discussed
- Adapt normal diets to meet the requirements of clients with these conditions

The gastrointestinal (GI) tract is where digestion and absorption of food occur. The primary organs include the mouth, esophagus, stomach, and small and large intestines. The liver, gallbladder, and pancreas are accessory organs that are also involved in these processes.

Numerous disorders of the gastrointestinal system can make absenteeism from work more prevalent. Some problems are physiologically caused; others can be psychological in origin. It is sometimes difficult to determine the cause(s) of a GI problem. There are numerous treatments and procedures to help identify GI problems and solutions.

DISORDERS OF THE PRIMARY ORGANS

Dyspepsia

Dyspepsia, or indigestion, is a condition of discomfort in the digestive tract that can be physical or psychological in origin. Symptoms include heartburn, bloating, pain, and sometimes regurgitation. If the cause is physical, it can be due to overeating or spicy foods, or it may be a symptom of another problem, such as appendicitis or a kidney, gallbladder, or colon disease, or possibly cancer. If the problem is organic in origin, treatment of the underlying cause will be the normal procedure.

Psychological stress can affect stomach secretions and trigger dyspepsia. Treatment should include counseling to help the client:

- Find relief from the underlying stress
- Allow sufficient time to relax and enjoy meals
- Learn to improve eating habits

Esophagitis

Esophagitis is caused by the irritating effect of acid reflux on the mucosa of the esophagus. Heartburn, regurgitation, and dysphagia (difficulty swallowing) are common symptoms. Acute esophagitis is caused by ingesting an irritating agent, or by **gastroesophageal reflux disease (GERD)**. This can be caused by a hiatal hernia, reduced lower esophageal sphincter (LES) pressure, abdominal pressure, recurrent vomiting, alcohol use, overweight, or smoking. Cancer of the esophagus and silent aspiration may be life-threatening for those with GERD.

Hiatal Hernia

Hiatal hernia is a condition in which a part of the stomach protrudes through the **diaphragm** into the thoracic cavity (Figure 18-1). The hernia prevents the food from moving normally along the digestive tract, although the food does mix somewhat with the gastric juices. Sometimes the food will move back into the esophagus, creating a burning sensation (heartburn), and sometimes food will be regurgitated into the mouth. This condition can be very uncomfortable.

Medical Nutrition Therapy

The symptoms can sometimes be alleviated by serving small, frequent meals (from a well-balanced diet) so that the amount of food in the stomach is never large. Avoid irritants to the esophagus such as carbonated beverages, chocolate, citrus fruits and juices, tomato products, spicy foods, coffee, pepper, and some herbs. Some foods can cause the lower esophageal sphincter to relax, and these should be avoided. Examples are fatty and fried foods, spicy foods, citrus food, tomato products, onions, chocolate, mint candy, caffeinated beverages, and alcohol. If obesity is present, weight loss may be recommended to reduce pressure on the abdomen. It may also be helpful if clients avoid late-night dinners and lying down for two to three hours after eating. When they do lie down, they may be more comfortable sleeping with their heads and upper torso somewhat elevated and wearing loose-fitting clothing. If discomfort cannot be controlled, surgery may be necessary.

dyspepsia
gastrointestinal discomfort of vague origin

esophagitis
inflammation of mucosal lining of the esophagus

gastroesophageal reflux disease (GERD)
backflow of stomach contents into the esophagus

hiatal hernia
condition wherein part of the stomach protrudes through the diaphragm into the chest cavity

diaphragm
thin membrane or partition

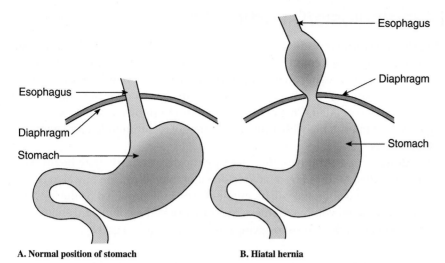

A. Normal position of stomach   B. Hiatal hernia

FIGURE 18-1 A hiatal hernia prevents food from moving through the diaphragm into the thoracic cavity.

Peptic Ulcers

An ulcer is an erosion of the mucous membrane (Figure 18-2). **Peptic ulcers** may occur in the stomach (**gastric ulcer**) or the duodenum (**duodenal ulcer**). The specific cause of ulcers is not clear, but some physicians believe that a number of factors—including genetic predisposition, abnormally high secretion of hydrochloric acid by the stomach, stress, excessive use of aspirin or ibuprofen (analgesics), cigarette smoking, and, in some cases, a bacterium called *Helicobacter pylori*—may contribute to their development.

A classic symptom is gastric pain, which is sometimes described as burning; in some cases, hemorrhage is also a symptom. The pain is typically relieved with food or antacids. A hemorrhage usually requires surgery.

Ulcers are generally treated with drugs such as antibiotics and cimetidine. The antibiotics kill the bacteria, and cimetidine inhibits acid secretion in the stomach and thus helps to heal the ulcer. Antacids containing calcium carbonate can also be prescribed to neutralize any excess acid. Stress management may also be beneficial in the treatment of ulcers.

Sufficient low-fat sources of protein should be provided but not in excess because of its ability to stimulate gastric acid secretion. It is recommended that clients receive no more than 0.8 g of protein per kilogram of body weight. However, if there has been blood loss, protein may be increased to 1–1.5 g per kilogram of body weight. Vitamin and mineral supplements, especially iron if there has been hemorrhage, may be prescribed.

Since fat delays the emptying of the stomach, an increased intake is beneficial. However, fat is only moderately increased since people suffering from peptic ulcers are more prone to atherosclerosis. Carbohydrates have little effect on gastric acid secretion.

Spicy foods may be eaten as tolerated. Coffee, tea, or anything else that contains caffeine or that seems to cause indigestion in the client or stimulates gastric secretion should be avoided. Alcohol and aspirin irritate the mucous membrane of the stomach, and cigarette smoking decreases the secretion of the pancreas that buffers gastric acid in the duodenum. Currently, a well-balanced diet of three meals a day consisting of foods that do not irritate the client is generally recommended.

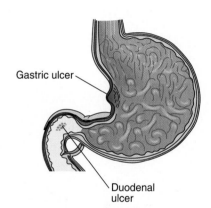

Gastric ulcer

Duodenal ulcer

FIGURE 18-2 Peptic ulcers are erosion of the mucous membrane in the stomach or the duodenum.

peptic ulcers
ulcers of the stomach or duodenum

gastric ulcer
ulcer in the stomach

duodenal ulcer
ulcer occurring in the duodenum

Helicobacter pylori
bacteria that can cause peptic ulcer

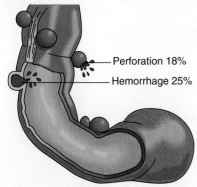

Perforation 18%

Hemorrhage 25%

FIGURE 18-3 Diverticulosis is a disorder characterized by little pockets forming in the sides of the large intestine. Rupture of the pockets may result in the need for corrective surgery.

Diverticulosis/Diverticulitis

Diverticulosis is an intestinal disorder characterized by little pockets in the sides of the large intestine (colon) (Figure 18-3). When fecal matter collects in these pockets instead of moving on through the colon, bacteria may breed, and inflammation and pain can result, causing **diverticulitis**. If a diverticulum ruptures, surgery may be needed. This condition is thought to be caused by a diet lacking sufficient fiber. A high-fiber diet is commonly recommended for clients with diverticulosis.

Along with antibiotics, diet therapy for diverticulitis may begin with a clear-liquid diet, followed by a low-residue diet that allows the bowel to rest and heal. Then a high-fiber diet will be initiated. The bulk provided by the high-fiber diet increases stool volume, reduces the pressure in the colon, and shortens the time the food is in the intestine, giving bacteria less time to grow.

Irritable Bowel Syndrome

Irritable bowel syndrome is a functional gastrointestinal disorder. The GI tract is not damaged; however, it does not function properly and causes a variety of symptoms. This disorder has both physical and mental causes and was previously called *spastic colon* or *colitis*. It is diagnosed when a person has abdominal pain or discomfort for the last three months, at least three times during those months. Some individuals may experience diarrhea, some constipation, and some a mixture of both. Cramping and bloating may occur.

The causes of this disorder are not well understood. Genetics, food sensitivity, bacterial infection or overgrowth, motility issues, altered neurotransmitters, or GI hormones or even psychological problems may be some of the root causes of this disorder.

Irritable bowel syndrome is treated by changes in diet, medication, probiotics, and therapies for mental health problems. Certain foods and drinks may aggravate symptoms in those with irritable bowel syndrome such as:

- Foods high in fat
- Some milk products
- Drinks with alcohol or caffeine
- Drinks with large amounts of artificial sweeteners
- Beans, cabbage, and other gas-producing foods

A newer diet therapy for individuals suffering from irritable bowel is to use the low FODMAP diet. FODMAP is an acronym for "fermentable oligo-, di-, mono-saccharides and polyols." A low FODMAP diet would restrict foods with constituents such as honey, high-fructose corn syrup, fruits with pits or seeds, milk, wheat, onions and garlic, starchy beans, and sugar alcohols.

Inflammatory Bowel Disease

Inflammatory bowel diseases (IBDs) are chronic conditions causing inflammation in the gastrointestinal tract. The inflammation causes malabsorption that often leads to malnutrition. The acute phases of these diseases occur at irregular intervals and are followed by periods in which clients are relatively free of symptoms. Neither cause nor cure for these conditions is known.

Two examples are **ulcerative colitis** and **Crohn's disease**. Ulcerative colitis causes inflammation and ulceration of the colon, the rectum, or sometimes

diverticulosis
intestinal disorder characterized by little pockets forming in the sides of the intestines; pockets are called *diverticula*

diverticulitis
inflammation of the diverticula

irritable bowel syndrome
functional gastrointestinal disorder

inflammatory bowel diseases (IBDs)
chronic condition causing inflammation in the gastrointestinal tract

ulcerative colitis
disease characterized by inflammation and ulceration of the colon, rectum, and sometimes entire large intestine

Crohn's disease
a chronic progressive disorder that causes inflammation, ulcers, and thickening of intestinal walls, sometimes causing obstruction

the entire large intestine. Crohn's disease, an autoimmune disease, is a chronic progressive disorder that can affect both the small and large intestines. The ulcers can penetrate the entire intestinal wall, and the chronic inflammation can thicken the intestinal wall, causing obstruction (Figure 18-4).

Both conditions cause bloody diarrhea, cramps, fatigue, nausea, anorexia, malnutrition, and weight loss. Electrolytes, fluids, vitamins, and other minerals are lost in the diarrhea, and the bleeding can cause loss of iron and protein. Clients with Crohn's disease are often thin and may be malnourished due to malabsorption of nutrients. Clients with ulcerative colitis usually experience weight loss related to the severity of the disease.

Treatment may involve anti-inflammatory drugs plus medical nutrition therapy. Usually a low-residue diet is required to avoid irritating the inflamed area and to avoid the danger of obstruction. When tolerated, the diet should include about 100 g of protein, additional calories, vitamins, and minerals.

In severe cases, **total parenteral nutrition (TPN)** (a process in which nutrients are delivered directly into the superior vena cava; see Chapter 21) may be necessary for a period. As the client begins to regain health, the diet may be increasingly liberalized to suit the client's tastes while maintaining good nutrition.

Ileostomy or Colostomy

Clients with severe ulcerative colitis or Crohn's disease frequently require a surgical opening from the body surface to the intestine for the purpose of defecation. The opening that is created is called a **stoma** and is about the size of a nickel. An **ileostomy** (from the ileum to abdomen surface) is required when the entire colon, rectum, and anus must be removed. A **colostomy** (from the colon to abdomen surface) can provide entrance into the colon if the rectum and anus are removed. This can be a temporary or a permanent procedure.

Crohn's Disease

Ulcerative Colitis

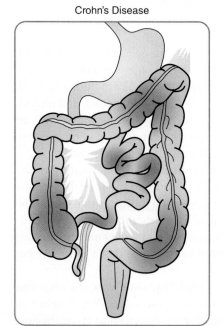
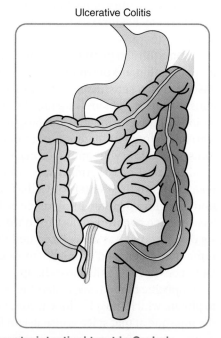

FIGURE 18-4 Affected sections of the gastrointestinal tract in Crohn's disease and ulcerative colitis.

total parenteral nutrition (TPN)
process of providing all nutrients intravenously

stoma
surgically created opening in the abdominal wall

ileostomy
opening from ileum to abdomen surface

colostomy
opening from colon to abdomen surface

When clients have had surgical removal of the small intestine (at least half of it), and/or dysfunction or removal of the colon, **short bowel syndrome** may result. Short bowel syndrome results when a patient lacks sufficient bowel length or function to support nutrient needs. This reduced intestinal length and decreased transit time results in nutrient malabsorption and fluid losses.

Even though parenteral or specialized enteral formulas may be used after surgery, it is very important to try to get the patient to eat food as soon as possible. Nutrients from food are the most potent stimuli to foster bowel adaptation. The ability of the gastrointestinal tract to adapt, as well as dietary and medication needs, depends on the length of the remaining small bowel and whether the colon is present. Successful adaptation is more likely in patients whose colon remains.

As excessive gastric secretions and intestinal hyper-motility are problematic in those with short bowel syndrome, medications to control these become an important part of treatment. Anti-diarrheal and anti-secretory medications are used in addition to pancreatic enzymes, oral rehydration solutions, and soluble fiber. The diet focus initially may be six small meals per day, with a low-fat, no concentrated sweet emphasis. Clients with ileostomies have a greater-than-normal need for salt and water because of excess losses. A vitamin C supplement is recommended and, in some cases, a B_{12} supplement may be needed as well as fat-soluble vitamins. Vitamin B_{12} can be given in monthly injections. To help maximize absorption, a liquid or chewable multivitamin with minerals can be given. Overall, the goal in short bowel syndrome is to achieve full nutritional autonomy. Larger health institutions have intestinal rehabilitation programs devoted to weaning individuals off parenteral nutrition and IV fluids.

Celiac Disease

Celiac disease, also known as **gluten**-sensitive enteropathy or sprue, is a chronic autoimmune disorder caused by intolerance to gluten. Gluten is a protein found in wheat, barley, and rye. Individuals with celiac disease produce antibodies that attack the intestine when they ingest gluten. Figure 18-5 shows the difference between healthy villi in the small intestine versus villi damage seen in celiac disease.

One-third of people carry the genes necessary for celiac disease; however, it appears that unknown environmental factors determine who gets celiac disease or gluten sensitivity and who does not. Symptoms may include diarrhea, constipation, weight loss or gain, abdominal cramping and bloating, and malnutrition. Joint pain, anemia, and fatigue are also common findings in individuals who have gluten intolerance, but not all people with celiac disease have symptoms. In children with untreated celiac disease, growth is compromised.

Nearly 1 of 133 Americans suffer from celiac disease, according to the research from the Center for Celiac Research. Coming to the forefront is how underdiagnosed gluten intolerance is. In fact, research indicates that celiac disease is twice as common as Crohn's disease, ulcerative colitis, and cystic fibrosis combined. It has been estimated that as many as 83% of celiac individuals remain undiagnosed or misdiagnosed. Some sources site that a 6- to 10-year lapse goes by before diagnosis happens.

Specific blood tests, called the "celiac panel," measure immune response to gluten, which must be done prior to the start of a gluten-free diet. A biopsy of the intestine at that stage is also useful for making the diagnosis of celiac disease. A strict gluten-free diet is absolutely necessary for the intestines to regenerate and heal.

short bowel syndrome
malabsorption caused by surgical removal or dysfunction of part of the small intestine and/or colon

celiac disease
a disorder of the gastrointestinal tract characterized by malabsorption; also called *gluten sensitivity*

gluten
protein found in wheat, rye, and barley

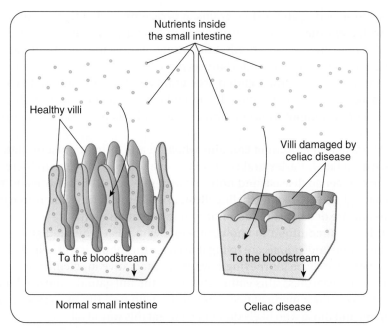

FIGURE 18-5 Celiac's damage.

Some individuals test negative for celiac but still have some degree of gluten sensitivity. Researchers believe this could be up to 6% of the population. At present, there is no serum biomarker for diagnosing gluten sensitivity. To assess non-celiac gluten intolerance, some clinicians recommend a trial of two to three weeks' of a gluten-free diet (an "elimination"), with then a "challenge" of returning back to gluten. Symptoms are then followed closely, recorded, and discussed with their doctor. Someone with non-celiac gluten sensitivity does not have the damage to the intestinal villi compared to someone with celiac disease.

- *Gluten-containing grains to avoid*: barley (including malt extract, beer, and ale), rye, wheat (all types of wheat flour and products made with wheat, bran, germ, starch), spelt, triticale, and farro.

- *Gluten-free grains and starches*: rice, wild rice, millet, amaranth, arrowroot, corn, flax, buckwheat, soy, teff, and flours made from nuts, beans, seeds, potato, tapioca, and sorghum.

Individuals with celiac disease can continue to meet their nutrition needs with naturally gluten-free foods: fruit, vegetables, dairy, eggs, nuts, beans and legumes, oils, butter, margarine, lean meats, and poultry (Table 18-1). When

TABLE 18-1 Sample Gluten-Free Menu

BREAKFAST	LUNCH	DINNER
Gluten-free oats	Tuna salad on spinach leaves	Chicken stir-fry (gluten-free soy sauce)
Fresh berries	Whole-grain gluten-free crackers with low-fat cheese	Brown rice
Gluten-free bagel with peanut butter	Gluten-free bran muffin	Fruit salad
Milk	Fresh fruit	Milk
SNACKS		
Hummus with raw vegetables		
Almonds with an apple		

it comes to selecting gluten-free grains, it is recommended that consumers be savvy with choosing the most nutritious high-fiber grains, which include brown rice, wild rice, quinoa, amaranth, buckwheat, gluten-free steel-cut oats, and rice bran. Label reading is important, as many gluten-free items sold in stores are made with very refined gluten-free grains with significant added sugars and fats and may not be fortified. It should be noted that commercially grown oats are contaminated in processing, so individuals must seek out certified gluten-free oats.

At present, if a product contains wheat in any form, it must be stated on the nutrition label. Barley and rye do not have to be listed. Due to increasing incidence of celiac disease and non-celiac gluten sensitivity, more and more foods have gluten-free food labeling. Restaurants are offering gluten-free menu options and are dedicated to preventing cross contamination.

It is not uncommon to know someone who has eliminated gluten from their diet. Some individuals are trying it because they think it will help them lose weight. Others may be journeying toward an integrative medicine approach to their health. Regardless, this eating style runs the full gamut—those who need to eat this way for a medical necessity, those who find themselves somewhat intolerant, and those who likely don't need to eat this way at all.

DISORDERS OF THE ACCESSORY ORGANS

Cirrhosis

The liver is of major importance to, and plays many roles in, metabolism. Except for a few of the fatty acids, all nutrients that are absorbed in the intestines are transported to the liver. The liver dismantles some of these nutrients, stores others, and uses some to synthesize other substances.

The liver determines where amino acids are needed and synthesizes some proteins, enzymes, and urea. It changes the simple sugars to glycogen, provides glucose to body cells, and synthesizes glucose from amino acids, if needed. It converts fats to lipoproteins and synthesizes cholesterol. It stores iron, copper, zinc, and magnesium as well as the fat-soluble vitamins and B vitamins. The liver synthesizes bile and stores it in the gallbladder. It detoxifies many substances such as barbiturates and morphine.

Liver disease may be acute or chronic. Early treatment can usually lead to recovery. **Cirrhosis** is a general term referring to all types of liver disease characterized by cell loss. Alcohol abuse is the most common cause of cirrhosis, but it can also be caused by congenital defects, infections, or other toxic chemicals.

Although the liver does regenerate, the replacement during cirrhosis does not match the loss. In addition to the cell loss during cirrhosis, there is fatty infiltration and **fibrosis**. These developments prevent the liver from functioning normally. Blood flow through the liver is upset, and a form of hypertension, anemia, and hemorrhage in the esophagus can occur. The normal metabolic processes will also be disturbed to such a degree that, in severe cases, death may result.

The dietary treatment of cirrhosis provides at least 25–35 calories or more and 0.8–1.0 g of protein per kilogram of weight each day, depending on the client's condition. If hepatic coma appears imminent, the lower amount is advocated. Supplements of vitamins and minerals are usually needed. In advanced cirrhosis, 50–60% of the calories should be from carbohydrates.

cirrhosis
generic term for liver disease characterized by cell loss

fibrosis
development of tough, stringy tissue

In some forms of cirrhosis, fat is not tolerated well, so it is restricted. In another form, protein may not be well tolerated, so it is restricted to 35–40 g a day. Sometimes cirrhosis causes ascites. In such a case, sodium and fluids may be restricted. If there is bleeding in the esophagus, fiber can be restricted to prevent irritation of the tissue. Smaller feedings will be better accepted than larger ones. No alcohol is allowed.

Hepatitis

Hepatitis is an inflammation of the liver. It is caused by viruses or toxic agents such as drugs and alcohol. Necrosis occurs, and the liver's normal metabolic activities are constricted. Hepatitis may be acute or chronic.

Hepatitis A virus (HAV) is contracted through contaminated drinking water, food, and sewage via a fecal–oral route. Hepatitis B virus (HBV) and hepatitis C virus (HCV) are transmitted through blood, blood products, semen, and saliva. Hepatitis B and C can lead to chronic active hepatitis (CAH), which is diagnosed by liver biopsy. Chronic active hepatitis can lead to liver failure and end-stage liver disease (ESLD).

In mild cases, the cells can be replaced. In severe cases, the damage can be so extensive that the necrosis leads to liver failure and death. There can be bile stasis and decreased blood albumin levels. Clients experience nausea, headache, fever, fatigue, tender and enlarged liver, anorexia, and jaundice. Weight loss can be pronounced.

Treatment is usually bed rest, plenty of fluids, and medical nutrition therapy. The diet should provide 35–40 calories per kilogram of body weight. Most of the calories should be provided by carbohydrates; there should be moderate amounts of fat and, if the necrosis has not been severe, up to 70–80 g of protein for cell regeneration. If the necrosis has been severe and the proteins cannot be properly metabolized, they must be limited to prevent the accumulation of ammonia in the blood. Small frequent meals may be better tolerated for those with liver disease.

Clients with liver disease require a great deal of encouragement because their anorexia and consequent feelings of general malaise can be severe. Their recovery takes patience, rest, and time.

Cholecystitis and Cholelithiasis

The dual function of the gallbladder is the concentration and storage of bile. After bile is formed in the liver, the gallbladder concentrates it to several times its original strength and stores it until needed. Fat in the duodenum triggers the gallbladder to contract and release bile into the common duct for the digestion of fat in the small intestine. If this flow is hindered, there may be pain.

The precise etiology of gallbladder disease is unknown, but heredity factors may be involved. Women develop gallbladder disease more often than men do. Obesity, TPN, very-low-calorie diets for rapid weight loss, the use of estrogen, and various diseases of the small intestine are frequently associated with gallbladder disease.

Cholecystitis (inflammation) and cholelithiasis (gallstones) may inhibit the flow of bile and cause pain. Cholecystitis can cause changes in the gallbladder tissue, which in turn can affect the cholesterol (a constituent of bile), causing it to harden and form stones. It is also thought that chronic overindulgence in fats may contribute to gallstones because the fat stimulates the liver to produce

ascites
abnormal collection of fluid in the abdomen

hepatitis
inflammation of the liver caused by viruses, drugs, or alcohol

necrosis
tissue death due to lack of blood supply

stasis
stoppage or slowing

jaundice
yellow cast of the skin and eyes

cholecystitis
inflammation of the gallbladder

cholelithiasis
gallstones

more cholesterol for the bile, which is necessary for the digestion of fat. In addition to pain, which can be severe, there may be indigestion and vomiting, particularly after the ingestion of fatty foods.

Treatment may include medication to dissolve the stones and diet therapy. If medication does not succeed, surgery to remove the gallbladder (**cholecystectomy**) may be indicated.

Medical nutrition therapy includes abstinence during the acute phase. This is followed by a clear-liquid diet and, gradually, a regular but fat-restricted diet. Amounts of fats allowed run from 40–45 g per day. In chronic cases, fat may be restricted on a permanent basis. For obese clients, weight loss is recommended in addition to a fat-restricted diet. (For information on fat-restricted diets, see Chapter 16.) Clients with chronic gallbladder conditions may require the water-miscible forms of fat-soluble vitamins.

Pancreatitis

In addition to the hormone insulin, the pancreas produces other hormones and enzymes that are important in the digestion of protein, fats, and carbohydrates. When food reaches the duodenum, the pancreas sends its enzymes to the small intestine to aid in digestion.

Pancreatitis is an inflammation of the pancreas. It may be caused by infections, surgery, alcoholism, biliary tract (includes bile ducts and gallbladder) disease, or certain drugs. It may be acute or chronic.

Abdominal pain, nausea, and **steatorrhea** are symptoms. Malabsorption (particularly of fat-soluble vitamins) and weight loss occur, and, in cases in which the islets of Langerhans are destroyed, diabetes mellitus may result.

Diet therapy is intended to reduce pancreatic secretions and bile. Just as fat stimulates the gallbladder to secrete bile, protein and hydrochloric acid stimulate the pancreas to secrete its juices and enzymes. During acute pancreatitis, the client is nourished strictly parenterally. Later, when the client can tolerate oral feedings, a liquid diet consisting mainly of carbohydrates is given because, of these three nutrients, carbohydrates have the least stimulatory effect on pancreatic secretions.

As recovery progresses, small, frequent feedings of carbohydrates and protein with little fat or fiber are given. The fat is restricted because of deficiencies of pancreatic lipase. The client is gradually returned to a less-restricted diet as tolerated. Vitamin supplements may be given. Alcohol is forbidden in all cases.

RESIDUE-CONTROLLED DIETS

Fiber is that part of food that is not broken down by digestive enzymes. It is called *dietary fiber*. Most dietary fiber is found in plant foods. Some are soluble, and some are insoluble (see Chapter 4). Examples of dietary fiber in plants include the outer shells of corn kernels, strings of celery, seeds of strawberries, and the connective tissue of citrus fruits.

Residue is the solid part of feces. Residue is made up of all the undigested and unabsorbed parts of food (including fiber), connective tissue in animal foods, dead cells, and intestinal bacteria and their products. Most of this residue is composed of fiber.

Diets can be adjusted to increase or decrease fiber and residue. The specific names of these diets vary among health care facilities. The specific foods allowed and thus the amount of fiber and residue allowed will depend on the physician's experience and the client's condition.

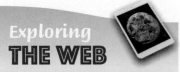

Exploring THE WEB

Choose one of the disorders discussed and thoroughly research it on the Internet. Create a list of the signs and symptoms, the possible causes, and the treatment choices for the disorder. Identify the nutritional needs for a person with this disorder. Can the disorder(s) be controlled through proper nutrition?

cholecystectomy
removal of the gallbladder

pancreatitis
inflammation of the pancreas

steatorrhea
abnormal amounts of fat in the feces

The High-Fiber Diet

High-fiber diets containing 30 g or more of dietary fiber are believed to help prevent diverticulosis, constipation, hemorrhoids, and colon cancer. They also are helpful in the treatment of diabetes mellitus (see Chapter 15) and atherosclerosis (see Chapter 16).

It is currently estimated that the normal diet in the United States contains about 15 g of dietary fiber each day. Recommendations for fiber intake include 38 g per day for men and 25 g per day for women, but not to exceed 50 g per day. The recommended foods for this diet include coarse- and whole-grain breads and cereals, bran, all fruits, vegetables (especially raw), and legumes. Milk, meats, and fats do not contain fiber (Table 18-2). The diet is nutritionally adequate. High-fiber diets must be introduced gradually to prevent the formation of gas and the discomfort that accompanies it. Eight 8-oz glasses of water also must be consumed along with the increased fiber.

The Low-Residue Diet

The low-residue diet of 5–10 g of dietary fiber a day is intended to reduce the normal work of the intestines by restricting the amount of dietary fiber and reducing

TABLE 18-2 Sample Menus for a High-Fiber Diet

BREAKFAST	LUNCH	DINNER
Medium orange	Fresh fruit cup	Baked pork chops
Oatmeal with ½ cup blueberries	Roast beef sandwich on cracked wheat bread	Red new potatoes with skin
Whole-wheat toast with marmalade	Coleslaw	Fresh broccoli
Coffee	Apple crisp with oat topping	Green salad with oil and vinegar dressing
	Fat-free milk	Whole-grain bread with margarine
	Coffee or tea	Fresh pineapple
		Fat-free milk
		Tea

SPOTLIGHT *on Life Cycle*

Here are some suggestions for helping adults increase fiber in the diet:

- Eat fresh fruits and vegetables in abundance. Consume a variety in both their cooked and raw state.
- Eat some of the skins of potatoes, apples, pears, and other fruits or vegetables. The outer portion of these foods contains fiber and valuable nutrients.
- Use coarse whole-grain breads and cereals instead of refined white bread and sugary cereals. Instead of meat, add beans (navy, lima, kidney, pinto), all of which are high in fiber and can also be a less expensive source of protein. Beans can also be used in casseroles, soups, stews, and other dishes.
- Try unbuttered air-popped popcorn or the reduced- or low-fat versions of microwave popcorn for a snack.
- Remember how important it is to increase the water in the diet when the fiber content is increased. At least 8 cups of liquid are needed each day.
- Keep moving: being active helps bowel regularity.

SUPERSIZE USA

High-fiber diets are believed to help prevent diverticulosis, constipation, hemorrhoids, and colon cancer, but new research has also found that fiber can promote satiety and weight control. A 2011 article in *Obesity Reviews* indicates that greater intakes of dietary fiber reduced appetite by 5% and lowered body weight by 1.3%. Fiber-rich foods tend to take more time to digest, therefore giving the sense of satiety or fullness after eating. The current average intake of daily fiber is only about half of the recommended amount. Consuming a variety of fruits and vegetables at each meal, starchy beans one to two times per week, and including more whole grains in the diet are a few ways people can help reach their daily fiber goals

Source: Adapted from Weisenberger, Jill. "Fiber: Fiber's Link with Satiety and Weight Control." *Todays Dietitian*, 17(2), p. 14. February 2015. http://www.todaysdietitian.com

food residue. Low-fiber or residue-restricted diets may be used in cases of severe diarrhea, diverticulitis, ulcerative colitis, and intestinal blockage and in preparation for and immediately after intestinal surgery.

In some facilities, these diets consist of foods that provide no more than 3 g of fiber a day and that do not increase fecal residue (Tables 18-3 and 18-4).

TABLE 18-3 Foods to Allow and to Avoid on Low-Residue Diets

FOODS TO ALLOW	FOODS TO AVOID
Milk, buttermilk (limited to 2 cups daily) if physician allows	Fresh or dried fruits and vegetables
Cottage cheese and some mild cheeses as flavorings in small amounts	Whole-grain breads and cereals,
Butter and margarine	Whole-grain pasta, brown/wild rice
Eggs, except fried	Legumes, coconut, and marmalade
Tender chicken, fish, ground beef, and ground lamb (meats must be baked, boiled, or broiled)	Tough meats
Soup broth	Rich pastries
Cooked, mild-flavored vegetables without coarse fibers; strained fruit juices (except for prune); applesauce; canned fruits including white cherries, peaches, and pears; pureed apricots; ripe bananas	Milk, unless physician allows
Refined breads and cereals, white crackers, macaroni, spaghetti, and noodles	Meats and fish with tough connective tissue
Custard, sherbet, vanilla ice cream; plain gelatin; angel food cake; sponge cake; plain cookies	Potato skin
Lettuce	Caffeine
Salt, sugar, small amount of spices as permitted by physician	Popcorn, nuts and seeds

TABLE 18-4 Sample Menus for a Low-Residue Diet

BREAKFAST	DINNER	LUNCH OR SUPPER
Strained orange juice	Chicken broth	Tomato juice
Cream of rice cereal with milk and sugar	Ground beef patty	Macaroni and cheese
White toast with margarine and jelly	Boiled potato, no skin	Green beans
Coffee with cream and sugar	Baked squash	White bread and butter
	Gelatin dessert	Lemon sherbet
	Milk	Tea with milk and sugar

HEALTH AND NUTRITION CONSIDERATIONS

Clients with gastrointestinal problems can be frustrated and irritable. Their problems can be psychologically caused; they may fear surgery or cancer; and they may suffer nausea, pain, or both. Some will want to eat foods that are not recommended; others will refuse foods they need.

Health care professionals who show respect and understanding for their clients will have the most success in helping them learn what they should and should not eat, and why.

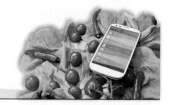

SUMMARY

Disturbances of the gastrointestinal tract require a wide variety of therapeutic diets. Peptic ulcers are treated with drugs, and diet therapy generally involves only the avoidance of alcohol and caffeine. Diverticulosis may be treated with a high-fiber diet, whereas diverticulitis is treated with a gradual progression from clear liquid to the high-fiber diet. Ulcerative colitis may require a low-residue diet combined with high protein and high calories. Celiac disease requires careful adherence to a gluten-free diet. Cirrhosis requires a substantial, balanced diet, with occasional restrictions of fat, protein, salt, or fluids. Diet therapy for hepatitis may include a full, well-balanced diet, although protein may be restricted, depending upon the client's condition. Cholecystitis and cholelithiasis clients require a fat-restricted diet and, in cases of overweight, a calorie-restricted diet as well. Pancreatitis diet therapy ranges from TPN to an individualized diet, as tolerated.

DISCUSSION TOPICS

1. Name the accessory organs in the gastrointestinal system and explain their roles in digestion and metabolism.

2. Discuss dyspepsia. Include its probable causes and the suggested therapy for it.

3. Describe hiatal hernia. Name its symptoms and possible treatment.

4. Define ulcers. Where are they found in the gastrointestinal system, and how are they treated? What substances should not be allowed for a person with an ulcer? Why?

5. Explain the difference between diverticulosis and diverticulitis. How are these conditions treated?

6. Discuss the high-fiber diet. For what conditions might it be used? Compare it with the low-fiber diet. Why is corn on the cob not allowed on the low-fiber diet? Name other foods that are not allowed on the low-fiber diet and tell why they would not be allowed.

7. Discuss ulcerative colitis. What is it? What causes it? How is it treated? How does it differ from other irritable bowel diseases?

SUGGESTED ACTIVITIES

1. Write a report on one or more of the gastrointestinal disturbances included in this chapter and the dietary treatment of them.

2. Create a PowerPoint presentation on celiac disease and gluten intolerance.

3. List 10 of your favorite foods. Circle those foods that would not be allowed on a low-residue diet. Underline the foods that are high in fiber.

4. Using activity 3, replace the low-fiber foods with choices containing high fiber.

REVIEW

Multiple choice. Select the *letter* that precedes the best answer.

1. Dyspepsia
   a. may be an indication of serious gastrointestinal disturbance
   b. is always psychological in origin
   c. cannot be overcome with improved eating habits
   d. is caused by high-fiber foods

2. Hiatal hernia
   a. occurs only in the small intestine
   b. is a typical sign of colon cancer
   c. causes weight loss in all clients
   d. may lead clients to be more comfortable with small, frequent meals

3. Peptic ulcers
   a. can occur in the stomach or the duodenum
   b. cannot be caused by stress
   c. are always treated with aspirin and a low-carbohydrate diet
   d. are usually treated with a low-protein diet

4. A person with celiac disease can eat
   a. barley soup, ham on rye, and a bag of chips
   b. flour burrito, rice, and beans
   c. chicken and rice soup, applesauce, and piece of chocolate
   d. lasagna, salad, and cheesecake

5. Diverticulosis
   a. is the inflammation of diverticula
   b. may be initially treated with a clear-liquid diet
   c. may be prevented with a high-fiber diet
   d. occurs in the liver

6. Food residue
   a. is ultimately evacuated in the feces
   b. always involves the small intestine
   c. never leaves the intestines
   d. results from incorrect cooking methods

7. Large amounts of food residue cause
   a. a decrease in fecal matter
   b. an increase in fecal matter
   c. weight gain
   d. diverticulosis

8. Which of the following would be recommended for the high-fiber diet?
   a. pretzels
   b. mashed potatoes
   c. rice pudding
   d. bran cereal

9. Which of the following would be allowed on a low-residue diet?
   a. fresh oranges
   b. corn on the cob
   c. macaroni and cheese
   d. fresh fruit cup

10. Ulcerative colitis
    a. affects the small intestine
    b. always requires parenteral feedings
    c. may be treated with a high-residue diet that is also high in calories and protein
    d. may cause malnutrition in clients

11. Which of the following foods would be recommended for an ulcerative colitis client, provided the client tolerates milk?
    a. fresh grapefruit
    b. chicken salad with chopped celery
    c. mashed potatoes with minced onion
    d. bisque tomato soup with crackers

12. The liver
    a. has no role in metabolism
    b. secretes insulin
    c. converts glucose to glycogen
    d. stores water-soluble vitamins

13. Cirrhosis
    a. is a liver disease characterized by cell loss
    b. is always caused by alcoholism
    c. inevitably results in death
    d. occurs only in the large intestine

14. Ascites
    a. is necessary for regeneration of liver cells
    b. is an accumulation of fluid in the abdomen
    c. requires the addition of sodium and water to the diet
    d. is caused by a shortage of iron

15. Hepatitis
    a. only occurs following exposure to HIV
    b. requires clients to follow very-low-carbohydrate diets
    c. is always fatal
    d. may be caused by viruses or toxic agents

16. Gallbladder problems may require
    a. the dietary restriction of dairy products
    b. cholecystectomy
    c. additional fat in the diet
    d. additional protein in the diet

17. Inflammation of the pancreas
    a. is called pancreatitis
    b. is asymptomatic
    c. can require a low-carbohydrate diet
    d. always signifies cancer

18. A client with celiac disease must avoid
    a. soy sauce and brown rice syrup
    b. corn chips and homemade salsa
    c. fruits and vegetables
    d. spinach salad with strawberries and pecans

19. Which IBD appears with a "cobblestoned" appearance in the colon?
    a. diverticulitis
    b. ulcerative colitis
    c. Crohn's disease
    d. celiac disease

20. Heartburn, regurgitation, and dysphagia are common symptoms of
    a. esophagitis
    b. peptic ulcers
    c. hiatal hernia
    d. duodenal ulcer

CASE IN POINT

CHARLOTTE: COPING WITH CELIAC DISEASE

Charlotte was diagnosed with type 1 diabetes at the age of 8. She has been in pretty good control overall. Her most recent A1C was 6.4%. Her doctor seemed very pleased with her control. She also developed thyroid disease in her early 20s. Her endocrinologist told her that people with type 1 diabetes are more at risk for developing other endocrine disorders and assured her that she did nothing to cause this to happen. Now 38, Charlotte jokes that she is celebrating her thirtieth anniversary with diabetes. She is otherwise healthy and has not developed any complications as of yet.

However, this week has been different for Charlotte. She is feeling very run down. She has had several bouts of diarrhea and a chronic stomachache. She loves milk with her breakfast, but barely made it to the bathroom after drinking a glass earlier this week. She is afraid she has an infection or a virus. So many things that she eats routinely have made her feel gassy or bloated or given her diarrhea. She stepped on the scale this morning to find that she has lost 10 lb. Charlotte is only 5-ft 3-in tall and weighed 115 lb prior to this last episode, so at 105 lb she now looks extremely thin. This morning her blood sugar is 258 mg/dL, which is higher than it has been in a long time. She is upset and feels very depressed. She makes an appointment to see her doctor.

After a battery of tests including blood work and an endoscopy of her gastrointestinal tract, her doctor informs Charlotte that she has celiac disease. He explains to her that it is not uncommon in people with type 1 diabetes and other endocrine disorders. He explains that foods containing gluten are causing inflammation and damage to her intestinal tract. She is going to need to begin following a gluten-free meal plan. He refers her to a registered dietitian to provide the education necessary for this new plan.

ASSESSMENT

1. What do you know about Charlotte that puts her at risk for celiac disease?
2. What symptoms did Charlotte have?
3. How will the disease alter her life?
4. How significant is this disease?

DIAGNOSIS

5. Write a diagnostic statement for Charlotte's potential alteration in nutrition.
6. Write a diagnosis for Charlotte's deficient knowledge related to the new diet.

PLAN/GOAL

7. What dietary goals are measurable and appropriate for Charlotte?
8. What education goals are specific and measurable for Charlotte?

IMPLEMENTATION

9. What information about celiac disease does Charlotte need to understand, to make necessary dietary changes?
10. What foods are going to be a problem for Charlotte?

EVALUATION/OUTCOME CRITERIA

11. At her follow-up doctor's appointment, what is her doctor likely to ask to determine if the plan was successful?

THINKING FURTHER

12. Can celiac disease be cured?
13. What medications are typically used to help manage this disease?

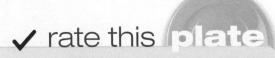

✔ rate this plate

Charlotte is overwhelmed by her new diagnosis of gluten sensitivity. As a diabetic, she has learned to control her blood sugar through counting carbohydrates, but following a gluten-free diet seems like a challenge. After receiving education from a registered dietitian, Charlotte feels more confident in preparing a healthy meal. Rate the plate she made for dinner:

2 slices gluten-free pepperoni pizza

1 cup Caesar side salad with croutons

20 oz iced tea

What types of food contain gluten? Is there anything in this plate that should be eliminated?

CASE IN POINT

ALEK: MANAGING AN ULCER THROUGH DIET

Alek is a stockbroker who has been working on Wall Street for nearly 20 years. His career has been high paced and high stress. Despite his demanding career, he has remained quite healthy. Alek is now 43 years old. His only health complaints through the years have been an ulcer and the occasional headache. The ulcer hasn't flared up in quite a while so he was hoping it had resolved. However, Alek has been working late hours and eating take-out food such as pizza, Mexican food, and spicy oriental chicken from the local restaurants nearby his office. The long, stressful hours have also brought

on many headaches. He has been treating these with a few doses of aspirin daily.

Recently while at work, Alek noticed a great amount of burning in his chest and abdomen. Then, throughout the night it became so severe he was sure his ulcer had flared up again. He went to the emergency room for assessment and was admitted for treatment. Upon discharge, Alek's doctor ordered medications to help treat his ulcer. The doctor also suggested that Alek follow a low-residue diet with no stimulants, spices, or alcohol.

ASSESSMENT

1. What put Alek at risk for his ulcer to bleed?
2. What symptoms did he have?
3. What could have been done to prevent this problem?
4. What impact did this health problem have on Alek?

DIAGNOSIS

5. Write two diagnoses for Alek's problems of diet and lack of knowledge.

PLAN/GOAL

6. What goals would be appropriate for Alek's education and nutrition?

IMPLEMENTATION

7. What does Alek need to learn about his new diet?
8. What does he need to learn about his ulcer and his new medications?
9. What challenges will he face in complying with the diet while at work?
10. Construct a meal that Alek would be likely to find at work.
11. Instead of aspirin, what can Alek use to treat his headaches that will not irritate his ulcer?

EVALUATION/OUTCOME CRITERIA

12. How will Alek's doctor know this plan is effective?

THINKING FURTHER

13. Diet, stress, and medications can contribute to ulcers and prevent them from healing. Can you list some of the other causes and treatments for ulcers?

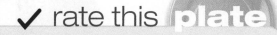

✔ rate this **plate**

Following a low-residue diet will allow Alek's ulcer to heal. Rate the plate that Alek ate while working late at the office:

3 Cajun chicken and steak fajitas with onions and peppers

¾ cup Spanish rice

½ cup refried beans

12 oz caffeine-free lemon-lime soda

How did Alek do with preparing his meal from what was catered in at the office? Can he eat everything? If not, what needs to be changed?

CHAPTER 19

KEY TERMS

anorexia
cachexia
carcinogens
chemotherapy
dysphagia
endometrium
genetic predisposition
hypoalbuminemia
Kaposi's sarcoma
malignant
metastasize
neoplasia
neoplasm
oncologist
oncology
phytochemicals
resection
xerostomia

DIET AND CANCER

OBJECTIVES

After studying this chapter, you should be able to:

- Discuss how nutrition can be related to the development or the prevention of cancer
- State the effects of cancer on the nutritional status of the host
- Describe nutritional problems resulting from the medical treatment of cancer
- Describe nutritional therapy for cancer clients

Cancer is the second leading cause of death in the United States. It is a disease characterized by abnormal cell growth and can occur in any organ. In some way, the genes lose control of cell growth, and reproduction becomes unstructured and excessive. The developing mass caused by the abnormal growth is called a *tumor*, or **neoplasm**. Cancer is also called **neoplasia**. Cancerous tumors are **malignant**, affecting the structure and consequently the function of organs. When cancer cells break away from their original site, move through the blood, and spread to a new site, they are said to **metastasize**. The mortality rate for cancer clients is high, but cancer does not always cause death. When it is found early in its development, prompt treatment can eradicate it. **Oncology** is the study of cancer, and a physician who specializes in cancer cases is called an **oncologist**.

THE CAUSES OF CANCER

The precise etiology of cancer is not known, but it is thought that heredity, viruses, environmental **carcinogens**, and possibly emotional stress contribute to its development. Cancer is not inherited, but some families appear to have a **genetic predisposition** for it. When such seems to be the case, environmental carcinogens should be carefully avoided and medical checkups made regularly. Environmental carcinogens include radiation (whether from x-rays, sun, or nuclear wastes), certain chemicals ingested in food or water, some chemicals that touch the skin regularly, and certain substances that are breathed in, such as tobacco smoke and asbestos.

Carcinogens are not known to cause cancer from one or even a few exposures, but after prolonged exposure. For example, skin cancer does not develop after one sunburn.

CLASSIFICATIONS OF CANCER

There are many types of cancer. A classification system was developed based on the type of cell that produced the cancer. The majority of all cancers fall under four headings: carcinomas, sarcomas, lymphomas, and leukemias.

- Carcinomas involve the epithelial cells (cells lining the body). These include the outer layer of the skin, the membranes lining the digestive tract, the bladder, the womb, and any duct or tube that goes through organs in the body.
- Sarcoma is cancer of the soft tissues of the body such as muscle, as well as fat, nerves, tendons, blood and lymph vessels, and any other tissues that support, surround, and protect the organs in the body. Soft tissue sarcomas are uncommon. Sarcomas can also occur in bone rather than soft tissue and primarily in the legs.
- Lymphomas are cancer of the lymphoid tissue. This includes the lymph nodes, bone marrow, spleen, and thymus gland.
- Leukemias develop from the white blood cells and also affect the bone marrow and spleen.

The site where the cancer is located will become part of the diagnosis, such as basal cell carcinoma.

Skin Cancer

Skin cancer is becoming more prevalent. There are three types of skin cancer: basal cell, squamous cell, and melanoma. Basal cell carcinoma is the most common form of skin cancer, affecting the outer skin layer and caused by exposure to sunlight. Those at high risk have fair skin, light hair, and blue, green, or gray eyes and spend considerable leisure time in the sun. Squamous cell carcinoma affects the squamous cells that are in the upper layer of the skin. Most cases arise from chronic exposure to sunlight, but may also occur where skin has been injured—burns, scars, or long-standing sores. Melanoma is the most serious and deadliest form of skin cancer and originates in the cells that produce the pigment melanin, which colors our skin, hair, and eyes. The majority of melanomas are black or brown, but some melanomas occasionally stop producing pigment and are skin colored, pink, red, or purple. If caught early, melanoma is almost 100% curable; therefore, a yearly exam by a dermatologist is recommended for early diagnosis of all skin cancers.

neoplasm
abnormal growth of new tissue

neoplasia
abnormal development of cells

malignant
life threatening

metastasize
spread of cancer cells from one organ to another

oncology
the study of cancer

oncologist
doctor specializing in the study of cancer

carcinogens
cancer-causing substances

genetic predisposition
inherited tendency

SUPERSIZE USA

According to the American Cancer Society, excess body weight contributes to as many as one out of five cancer-related deaths. Overweight and obesity can increase risks for many cancers, including cancer of the breast (in women past menopause), colon, rectum, endometrium, esophagus, kidney, and pancreas. Increased belly fat is linked to an increased risk of colon and rectal cancers. Being overweight or obese as a child may pose a higher risk for cancer compared to weight gain later in life. Excess body fat and the interplay with increased cancer risk is usually linked to too much visceral belly fat (abdominal fat) and elevated inflammatory hormones such as insulin, estrogen, and leptin. Losing weight results in improvement in hormone regulation and overall wellness and likely reduces risk for cancer.

Source: Adapted from *Does Body Weight Affect Cancer Risk.* American Cancer Society. (2015, April 24. http://www.cancer.org)

Viral Causes of Cancer

The following viruses have been linked to cancer: Epstein–Barr, hepatitis B, Kaposi sarcoma, herpes virus, retrovirus, and human papilloma virus (HPV). Epstein–Barr virus may cause nasopharyngeal cancer, T-cell lymphoma, Hodgkin's disease, and gastric carcinoma. There is an anticancer vaccine available to prevent hepatitis B and its serious consequences—that is, liver cancer. **Kaposi's sarcoma** is a cancerous tumor of the connective tissue and is often associated with the AIDS virus. More research is being conducted to determine the retroviral cause of cancer. A vaccine is now available to prevent cervical cancer caused by HPV. Cancer research is ongoing in these and other areas.

RELATIONSHIP AMONG LIFESTYLE HABITS, DIET, AND CANCER

In the last 25 years, researchers have shown that diet, physical activity, and body weight (overweight and obesity in particular) are major risk factors for developing certain types of cancer. In fact, studies demonstrate that one-third of all cancers could be prevented by lifestyle changes. The link between excess body fat (and its resultant chronic inflammation) and cancer has been one of the strongest findings in the cancer community. Approximately 117,000 cancer cases in the United States each year are linked to excess body fat. Obesity increases risk for at least seven types of cancer: colorectal, postmenopausal breast, kidney, pancreatic, **endometrium**, gallbladder, and esophageal cancer (adenocarcinoma).

The American Institute of Cancer Research recommends:

- Maintain body weight range within the normal BMI range, starting from the age of 21

- Avoid weight gain and increases in waist circumference through adulthood

- Consume energy-dense foods sparingly (sugary drinks, desserts, cookies, chips, fast food, hot dogs, etc.)

A sedentary way of life predisposes to obesity, which, as mentioned above, increases risk for some cancers. The American Cancer Society's Cancer Prevention Study II found that sitting more than six hours a day can elevate your

Kaposi's sarcoma
type of cancer common to individuals with AIDS

endometrium
mucous membrane of the uterus

chance of getting cancer and other chronic diseases. The link between physical activity and cancer prevention has been confirmed through decades of research. The recommendation is to:

- Be physically active for at least 30 minutes every day and limit sedentary habits. Physical activity may help improve tolerance of cancer treatment and the quality of life during and after cancer treatment.

Certain types of food and substances in foods are thought to contribute to cancer risk. Nitrites in cured and smoked foods such as bacon and ham can be changed to nitrosamines (carcinogens) during cooking. Regular ingestion of these foods is associated with cancers of the stomach and esophagus. These foods, along with a higher red meat intake, are thought to increase colorectal cancer risk. High-fat diets have been associated with cancers of the uterus, breast, prostate, and colon. Salty foods may increase risk of stomach cancer. People who drink alcohol immoderately appear to be at greater risk of cancers of the colon, rectum, breast, esophagus, mouth, and liver.

In summary, the recommendations are to:

- Limit consumption of red and processed meats. Beef, pork, lamb, and game should be limited to 18 oz or less per week. Processed meats such as cold cuts, bacon, sausage, and ham should be avoided.

- Limit consumption of salty foods and foods processed with salt.

- Limit alcoholic drinks. If they are consumed at all, limit them to two for men and one for women daily (one serving = 12 oz beer, 1.5 oz spirits, or 5 oz wine).

On the positive side, it is thought that diets higher in plant food may reduce the risk of cancer. Vitamins, minerals, and phytochemicals in plant foods demonstrate anticancer effects. However, it is the synergy of compounds working together in the overall diet that offers the strongest cancer protection.

Phytochemicals, substances that occur naturally in plant foods, are thought to be anticarcinogenic agents. Phytochemicals provide a plant with color, aroma, and flavor as well as protection from infection and predators. They have the potential to enhance the immune system, slow the growth rate of cancer cells, and prevent DNA damage that can contribute to cancer. Examples include flavonoids, phenols, and indoles. Consuming whole grains, legumes (starchy beans), nuts, seeds, and a variety of colorful fruits and vegetables is the best way to provide the body with phytochemicals. It is recommended to:

- Fill at least two-thirds of your plate with vegetables, fruits, whole grains, legumes, and nuts, while devoting less than one-third of it to animal proteins. Some may choose to go meatless some or all of the time.

- Eat 2 ½ cups of vegetables and 2 cups of fruit daily (for an average 2,000-calorie diet) and include a wide variety especially from the cruciferous family (broccoli, cabbage, etc.), dark-green leafy vegetables, berries, citrus, and yellow/orange vegetable family.

And related to general cancer preventative recommendations, it is important to:

- Breastfeed exclusively for up to 6 months, then add other liquids and foods.

- Not rely on dietary supplements to replace nutrient-rich foods in diet.

- Not smoke or chew tobacco.

phytochemicals
substances occurring naturally in plant foods

THE EFFECTS OF CANCER

One of the first indications of cancer may be unexplained weight loss because the tumor cells use for their own metabolism and development the nutrients the host has taken in. The host may suffer from weakness, and anorexia may occur, which compounds the weight loss. Anorexia is typically present in 15% to 25% of all cancer patients at diagnosis and may also occur as a side effect of their treatment. The weight loss includes the loss of muscle tissue and hypoalbuminemia, and anemia may develop. The sense of taste and smell may be affected. Some foods may taste different: they may not have much taste, or everything may taste the same. Cancer clients, after chemotherapy, may experience a metallic taste when eating protein foods. Many clients complain of food tasting too sweet. Radiation to the neck and head can cause damage to the taste buds and could also affect taste and smell, causing loss of appetite and weight loss.

Cancer clients become satiated earlier than normal, possibly because of decreased digestive secretions. Insulin production may be abnormal, and hyperglycemia can delay the stomach's emptying and dull the appetite. Some cancers cause hypercalcemia. If this is chronic, renal stones and impaired kidney function can occur.

The effects of cancer on the host are particularly determined by the location of a tumor. For example, an esophageal or intestinal tumor can cause blockage in the gastrointestinal tract, causing malabsorption. If the cancer is untreated, the continued anorexia and weight loss will create a state of malnutrition, which in turn can lead to cachexia and, ultimately, death.

THE TREATMENT OF CANCER

Medical treatment of cancer can include surgical removal, radiation, chemotherapy, or a combination of these methods. These treatments, unfortunately, have side effects that can further undermine nutritional status. The nutritional effects of surgery in general are discussed in Chapter 21. Cancer surgery, however, can have some additional effects. Surgery on the mouth, for example, might well affect the ability to chew or swallow. Gastric or intestinal resection can affect absorption and result in nutritional deficiencies. The removal of the pancreas will result in diabetes mellitus.

Exploring THE WEB

Choose one particular type of cancer. Research the relationship of food to this type of cancer using the Internet. Can alterations in diet prevent, cure, or help combat this type of cancer?

In The Media

Sniffing Out Cancer

Research is being conducted in Britain to further understand the ability of dogs to use their sense of smell to identify cancer. Lucy, a Lab and Irish water spaniel mix, has been able to detect bladder, kidney, and prostate cancers with 95% accuracy. A dog's sense of smell is 10,000 to 100,000 stronger than that of humans. The first study on this topic was published in *The Lancet* in 1989, which featured a dog identifying malignant melanoma when he continued to lick a mole on his owner. More research is being done to evaluate this as an adjunct to screening for cancer.

Source: Adapted from Savoy, Christian. (2015, November 22). "Dogs That Smell Cancer Being Tested in Order to Determine Their Effectiveness". *Inquisitr.* http://www.inquisitr.com/2582581/dogs-that-smell-cancer-being-tested-in-britain-in-order-to-determine-their-effectiveness/

anorexia
a loss of appetite, especially as a result of a disease

hypoalbuminemia
abnormally low amounts of protein in the blood

cachexia
severe malnutrition and body wasting caused by chronic disease

chemotherapy
treatment of diseased tissue with chemicals

resection
reduction

Radiation of the head or neck can cause a decrease in salivary secretions, which causes dry mouth (**xerostomia**) and difficulty in swallowing (**dysphagia**). This reduction in saliva also causes tooth decay and sometimes the loss of teeth. Severe weight loss from not eating enough can also result from radiation therapy. Radiation reduces the amount of absorptive tissue in the small intestine. In addition, it can cause bowel obstruction or diarrhea.

Chemotherapy reduces the ability of the small intestine to regenerate absorptive cells, and it can cause hemorrhagic colitis. Both radiation and chemotherapy depress appetite. They may cause nausea, vomiting, and diarrhea, leading to fluid and electrolyte imbalances, which can lead to fluid retention. Weight loss may result with some chemotherapy treatments; however, with breast cancer, there may be some weight gain due to the inclusion of steroids in some of the chemotherapeutic agents. Nevertheless, when the therapy is completed and a well-balanced diet is resumed, these problems may disappear.

NUTRITIONAL CARE OF THE CANCER CLIENT

Nutrition therapy plays a major role in treatment of the cancer patient. Good nutrition can help maintain weight and the body's nutrition stores, thereby increasing the patient's chances of responding positively to treatment. Healthy food and beverage options need to be carefully planned into the cancer patient's diet to supply the proper nutrients to nourish, repair, and heal. Poor nutrition practices, which result in undernutrition, may contribute to the incidence and severity of treatment side effects. This could increase risk of infection, which affects mortality rate. Often a high-protein, high-calorie (and nutrient-dense) diet is prescribed to prevent protein calorie malnutrition, which is the most common secondary diagnosis in individuals diagnosed with cancer.

Anorexia, cachexia, and an early satiety sensation can result. These manifest as a range of reactions, from altered tastes to a physical inability to take in or digest food, leading to reduced eating. It is particularly difficult to combat because cancer clients tend to develop strong food aversions that are thought to be caused by the effects of chemotherapy. Receiving chemotherapy near mealtime may cause an association between food served and the nausea caused by the chemotherapy, which can often lead to food aversions. These aversions result in limited acceptance of food and contribute further to the client's malnutrition. It is recommended that chemotherapy be withheld for two to three hours before and after meals. The appetite and absorption usually improve after chemotherapy has been completed. A dietitian, having obtained the likes and dislikes, will create a diet plan containing nutrient- and calorie-dense foods. Comfort foods should be included liberally.

xerostomia
sore, dry mouth caused by a reduction of salivary secretions; may be caused by radiation for treatment of cancer

dysphagia
difficulty in swallowing

SPOTLIGHT *on Life Cycle*

Children receiving chemotherapy may experience nausea and vomiting, putting their nutrition status at risk. Giving chemotherapy at bedtime may help alleviate nausea and vomiting in children. It may allow them to sleep through the emetic effects. Playing soft music, such as lullabies, or playing a recording of a caregiver singing soft songs is soothing and distracting and may alleviate symptoms of nausea and vomiting.

Early recognition and detection of risk for malnutrition through nutrition screening followed by a comprehensive assessment is a gold standard for quality care in these patients. Diet plans for the cancer client require special attention. A dietitian at the hospital or oncology center will obtain the client's weight and height to calculate calorie needs. The dietitian will compile a list of nutrient-rich foods and comfort foods to encourage nutrient intake and appetite. It is essential that favorite foods, prepared in familiar ways, be included in the meal plan. If chewing is a problem, a soft diet may be helpful. If diarrhea is a problem, a low-residue diet may help. Table 19-1 offers helpful diet tips when patients experience changes to their eating, digestion, or absorption as a result of cancer treatment.

If the client is scheduled to undergo radiation or chemotherapy, these factors must be included in the diet planning. High-protein, high-calorie diets may be recommended. Energy demands are high because of the hypermetabolic state often caused by cancer. Calorie needs are individualized, but 30–35 calories per kilogram of body weight may be recommended.

TABLE 19-1 Diet Therapy Tips During Cancer Treatment

SYMPTOM	DIET TIP
Nausea and Vomiting	• Small amounts of food more frequently are better tolerated than large portions. • Sip on beverages between meals so fluids are not so filling at meals. • Foods and clear liquids at room temperature or cooler may be easier to handle. • Avoid foods with strong odors, and those that are spicy, fatty, or overly sweet. • Keep in upright position for an hour after eating. • Don't eat or drink until vomiting is controlled, then sip on clear liquids (cranberry juice, broth) and nibble as tolerated on plain, starchy foods such as crackers or pretzels. • Follow your doctor's orders for prescribed anti-nausea meds.
Change in Taste and Smell	• Cooler foods have less aroma and therefore their taste may be more appealing than hot foods. • A small amount of sugar may mask a food's bitter or salty taste. • Frozen melon balls, grapes, and oranges that are juicy and naturally sweet may be desirable as may tart foods and beverages. • If there is a taste aversion to red meat, use starchy beans, poultry, fish, eggs, and nutbutters as protein sources. • Marinades and spices can mask unpleasant tastes. • Keep mouth clean by brushing and rinsing often. Dilute salt and baking soda solutions are an effective mouth rinse (1 quart water with 1 tsp salt, 1 tsp baking soda).
Sore Mouth or Throat	• Soft, moist foods that have extra gravy, sauce, or dressings go down easier. • Alcohol, spicy or acidic foods, and caffeine may cause irritation as may dry, coarse, or rough foods. • Find the temperature of food that soothes the irritated throat or mouth best (warm, cool, or icy). • Drink plenty of fluids—warm or cool milk-based beverages, non-acidic fruit drinks (extra water if needed), flat soda, and cream or broth-based soups. • Rinse mouth several times a day with dilute salt and baking soda solution as described above.
Poor Appetite	• Eat your main meal when you are the hungriest and start with your high protein offering when your appetite is the strongest. • Try five or six smaller meals per day. • Keep nutritious, high-calorie foods and beverages within easy access—homemade energy bars, hummus, egg salad with mayo, peanut butter and crackers, high-protein shakes and smoothies. • Work with a loved one to help buy groceries and prepare nutritious meals.

(continues)

TABLE 19-1 *(continued)*

SYMPTOM	DIET TIP
Diarrhea	• Keep hydrated with water, dilute clear juices, sports drinks, weak tea or electrolyte or rehydration solutions available at your local pharmacies. • Eat soft, bland foods that have soluble fiber, such as bananas, boiled potatoes, oatmeal, cooked apple, etc. Rice, yogurt, plain toast, and tea may also help. • Pass on high-fiber foods for now, such as popcorn, high-fiber, cereal and breads, nuts and seeds, and raw vegetables, skin on fruit. • Eat small amounts of food throughout day and take an anti-diarrhea med if it is prescribed.
Constipation	• Keep up an excellent fluid intake, such as water (even fruit-infused waters), warm juices, teas, hot lemon water, and a small amount of prune juice. • Increase intake of high-fiber foods—starchy beans such as kidney beans, garbanzo beans, whole grains; high-fiber cereals such as bran flakes and oatmeal; and fresh fruits and vegetables, dried fruit, and nuts. • Increase physical activity as able as prescribed by your health care team.

Source: Adapted from "Heal Well—A Cancer Nutrition Guide." American Institute for Cancer Research.

Carbohydrates and fat will be needed to provide this energy and spare protein for tissue building and the immune system. Clients with good nutritional status will need 1.0–1.2 g of protein per kilogram of body weight per day. Malnourished clients may need 1.3–2.0 g of protein per kilogram of body weight per day. Vitamins and minerals are essential for metabolism and tissue maintenance and may be supplied in supplemental form. Some dietary supplements contain levels of antioxidants, such as vitamins C and E, which could be much greater than those recommended for optimal health. During chemotherapy or radiation, oncologists advise against taking higher doses of antioxidant supplements. It is best for cancer clients receiving treatment to avoid dietary supplements that give more than 100% of the Daily Value for antioxidants, according to the American Cancer Society. Fluids are important to help the kidneys eliminate the metabolic wastes and the toxins from drugs.

Oral feedings are always preferred for a variety of reasons (especially for proper immune response); however, enteral or total parenteral nutrition may become necessary if an oral diet is not tolerated and cachexia is extreme. Sometimes an oral diet with a nutritional supplement may be used in conjunction with total parenteral nutrition (see Chapter 21). When appetite is poor, a high-calorie, high-protein liquid supplement may be given. As the client improves, calorie and nutritional content of the diet should be gradually increased.

HEALTH AND NUTRITION CONSIDERATIONS

A healthy lifestyle that includes regular physical activity, a nutrient-rich diet liberal in plant foods, and an appropriate body weight can help limit someone's chances of getting cancer. If cancer is discovered, care needs to be taken to ensure that the full complement of nutrients is received daily to the best extent possible. It is important that the dietitian establish a good relationship with the cancer client as well as encourage and monitor food intake. Working hand in hand, the dietitian can help the client find creative ways to bolster intake for best nourishment and healing.

Exploring
THE WEB

Search the Internet for the nutritional needs of the chemotherapy client. How do these needs change as the client progresses through therapy? Once therapy is complete, how do nutritional needs change? Plan some sample menus for the chemotherapy client. Check for protein and vitamins that are contraindicated for chemotherapy clients. Check out http://www.cancer.org for more information.

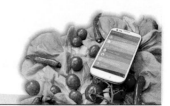

If the prognosis for the client is not good, nutritional care will not be as important as the client's feelings and immediate comfort.

SUMMARY

Cancer is a disease characterized by abnormal cell growth. It can strike any body tissue. Energy needs may increase because of the hypermetabolic state and the tumor's needs for energy nutrients. At the same time, anorexia occurs in the client. It causes severe wasting, anemia, and various metabolic problems. Treatment of cancer includes surgery, radiation, and chemotherapy. Improving the client's nutritional state is difficult because of the illness and anorexia. Parenteral or enteral nutrition may be necessary.

DISCUSSION TOPICS

1. Discuss how cancer has affected you, your family, or your friends.

2. Explain why some cancer clients lose weight and others may gain weight when undergoing chemotherapy.

3. Why is the anorexia of cancer clients especially difficult to combat? What causes it? Are there any ways it can be prevented?

4. Are supplemental feedings of liquid foods useful in the nutritional rehabilitation of a cancer client? Explain.

5. Discuss enteral and parenteral nutrition in relation to cancer clients.

SUGGESTED ACTIVITIES

1. Invite an oncology nurse to speak to the class.

2. Write an essay about how you might feel if you had just been told that you had a malignant tumor.

3. Plan a day's menus for a cancer client who will eat only the following foods:

Sweetened orange juice	Soda crackers
Bananas	Milkshakes
Applesauce	Eggnog
Cooked pears	Cottage cheese
Puffed rice cereal	Cream of chicken
Rice pudding	soup
White toast with jelly	Poached eggs
	Bouillon

REVIEW

Multiple choice. Select the *letter* that precedes the best answer.

1. Cancer
   a. is characterized by reduced cell growth
   b. growth called a tumor can also be called a neoplasm
   c. inevitably causes death
   d. can metastasize only in clients 50 years and older

2. Carcinogens may include
   a. viruses
   b. certain green vegetables
   c. gluten-containing foods
   d. salmonella

3. Carcinogens
   a. cause cancer after only limited exposure
   b. include some chemical substances
   c. are never found in food or water
   d. are found only in meats and fish

4. Cancer clients
   a. seldom experience weight loss
   b. usually experience an increase in appetite
   c. seldom suffer from anorexia
   d. may suffer from cachexia

5. Radiation and chemotherapy
   a. seldom affect cancer clients' nutritional status
   b. may increase appetite
   c. have no connection to electrolyte imbalance
   d. may create food aversions

6. It is thought that cancer may be caused by
   a. frequent ingestion of smoked meats over a long period
   b. moderate use of alcohol
   c. high-fiber diets
   d. excessive use of vitamin A-rich foods

7. High-fat diets
   a. usually are harmless
   b. have been associated with breast and prostate cancer
   c. provide large amounts of fiber and vitamin C
   d. contribute to the health of the immune system

8. Phytochemicals are
   a. abundantly supplied in fruits and vegetables
   b. widely known carcinogens
   c. most prevalent in carbohydrates and fats
   d. plentifully supplied in proteins

9. It is recommended to cancer clients to take
   a. two multivitamins per day
   b. fish oil and flax seed oil daily
   c. a multivitamin with only 100% of the antioxidants
   d. none of these, as no supplements are required

10. Cachexia
    a. is the result of continued anorexia and weight loss
    b. is inevitable in all cancer clients
    c. occurs only in clients with mouth and throat cancers
    d. does not seem to appear in untreated cancer

CASE IN POINT

KATE: ADJUSTING TO LIFE WITH A COLOSTOMY

Kate turned 50 years old last year. Her family threw a huge party to celebrate. This was a tradition her large, but close-knit Greek family started years ago. Kate always felt they didn't need much of an excuse to celebrate with a party. Shortly after her birthday, Kate went for her routine physical to mark her birthday celebration like she had for many years. Her doctor had told her that now that she was 50, it was time to have a colonoscopy. He explained that it would assess the health of her colon and detect any problems before they could start. He told Kate it was recommended for everyone her age, but he was particularly concerned about her because her father had died from colon cancer years ago. Kate had heard so many horror stories about colonoscopies. Several of her friends had had the procedure done already and warned Kate about how bad the prep was. She even remembered her parents discussing this when her dad was so sick. Every time he had a colonoscopy, he received more bad news. Kate just wasn't sure she could go through with it. Over the past year, Kate has found numerous excuses as to why she couldn't get the colonoscopy and kept putting it off.

Lately, Kate hasn't been feeling herself. She has been very tired and her stomach seems to always be cramping up in knots. She has had a lot of diarrhea and is pretty sure that she has a hemorrhoid because she has seen blood in the toilet from time to time. She wishes she felt better, then she could be more excited about the 15 lb she has lost. Finally, Kate decides to schedule the colonoscopy. The prep was pretty bad, but the procedure was easy. She wakes up remembering nothing about what happened. The doctor meets with Kate after the colonoscopy and informs Kate that they found cancerous tumors in her colon. The doctor explains to Kate that her cancer has only progressed to stage 2, but due to the location of the tumor, she will need a colostomy, at least temporarily. Kate's doctor asks her to meet with the nurse educator and dietitian in his practice group following her surgery. The nurse will train Kate on how to change her bag and care for her new colostomy. The dietitian will help Kate find foods that are not irritants to her colon and monitor her weight. He is concerned that because Kate is 5-ft 9-in tall and currently weighs only 132 lb, she may be at risk for malnutrition if she continues to lose weight. He asks the dietitian to also work with Kate to find high-protein snacks or supplements that will aid in her healing and prevent further weight loss or wasting.

ASSESSMENT

1. What do you know about Kate?
2. What barriers does she have to balance nutrition?
3. What resources does she have to overcome these barriers?
4. How important is her nutrition to her current health? How about to her future treatments?

DIAGNOSIS

5. Write a diagnosis about potential alteration in nutrition.
6. Write a diagnosis about her deficient knowledge.

PLAN/GOAL

7. What is the immediate goal for Kate's nutrition?
8. What is the long-term goal?

IMPLEMENTATION

9. What does Kate need to learn?
10. List strategies to increase what Kate eats at home.
11. How important is nutrition to her healing?
12. What can a home health care nurse do to enhance Kate's nutrition? What can a dietitian do?

EVALUATION/OUTCOME CRITERIA

13. What can the home health nurse observe and measure as evidence of the success of the plan?

THINKING FURTHER

14. Why is it important to use nutrition to reduce your risk of cancer?

✔ rate this plate

The dietitian meets with Kate to discuss protein sources and foods she can include in her diet to help decrease bowel irritation. Everyone's body acts differently to various types of food, so Kate would have to experiment to see what her intestines could tolerate. In order to prevent additional weight loss, the dietitian recommends a protein supplement drink for Kate if she is unable to obtain sufficient protein from her meals and snacks. Rate the plate she plans to eat for lunch, taking into consideration any possible irritants and protein sources:

2 cups spinach salad with mandarin oranges and pecans

3 oz crispy chicken on top of the salad

¾ cup tomato soup made with water, not milk

½ cup cottage cheese

½ cup sliced peaches

Are there any parts to this meal that may cause Kate some intestinal discomfort? What foods in this meal are rich in protein? Will Kate need to drink the supplement with this meal or does it provide enough protein alone?

CASE IN POINT

DAVE: APPETITE AND WEIGHT LOSS DURING CHEMOTHERAPY

Dave is a 56-year-old Asian man who is currently undergoing chemotherapy. Dave was diagnosed with lymphoma three months ago. His initial course of chemotherapy consisted of 10 treatments. Through the first three treatments, Dave experienced a lot of anxiety and fear about how his body would respond to the medications. He had seen people who had undergone chemotherapy and he always thought they appeared very frail and weak. Dave had been trying to maintain as much normalcy in his life as possible while undergoing the chemotherapy. He continued to work as much as he was able. He tried to eat many of his favorite foods to help keep up his strength and prevent a large amount of weight loss. So far, his weight has remained fairly stable.

The oncologist has informed Dave that the treatments will become more difficult each time. He advises him that if he begins losing weight then he will have to prescribe an appetite stimulant for Dave to take during the next few rounds of treatment. He also suggests that Dave meet with a registered dietitian to assess his daily caloric needs.

The dietitian recommends a nutritional supplement for Dave to use between meals if his appetite is poor. She also suggests he weighs himself weekly and notify her if he begins to lose weight. Hopefully, in working with the dietitian, he can avoid having to take one more medication.

ASSESSMENT

1. What has Dave's response to the chemotherapy been so far?
2. What does the doctor suspect will happen to Dave's nutrition during round four of chemotherapy?
3. What can the dietitian assess to measure how Dave is eating?

DIAGNOSIS

4. Write a diagnostic statement describing the nutrition problems Dave could have with chemotherapy.

PLAN/GOAL

5. What is the major nutrition goal for Dave?
6. What is the rationale for aggressive proactive nutrition between rounds of chemotherapy?
7. What does Dave need to know related to the nutritional demands of ongoing chemotherapy?

IMPLEMENTATION

8. List four strategies the dietitian can use to encourage Dave to eat.
9. List three strategies that his family can use to help him eat.
10. If Dave eats only 5–10% of his normal food volume, what foods should be a priority? How are fluids important?
11. In preparation for round five of chemotherapy, what could Dave do to enhance his nutrition once his appetite returns?
12. How can other cancer clients undergoing chemotherapy and their families help Dave?
13. How can the Internet be of help? Check out the American Cancer Society at http://www.cancer.org.

EVALUATION/OUTCOME CRITERIA

14. How would the doctor evaluate the success of the diet plan?

THINKING FURTHER

15. Why is nutrition so important in the successful treatment of cancer?

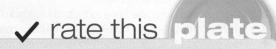
✔ rate this **plate**

Dave has done a good job at eating healthy and maintaining his weight while receiving chemotherapy treatments. Dave will be seeing the dietitian a few times a month to review his food intake and weight status. Using the meal he made for lunch as an example, will Dave be able to maintain his weight? Rate this plate:

- **4 oz salmon fillet**
- **1 cup mashed potatoes**
- **¾ cup sautéed vegetables, including red peppers, broccoli, and zucchini**
- **1 cup romaine salad with dried cranberries and cherries**
- **2 Tbsp light poppy seed dressing**
- **1 toffee nut cookie**

Cancer patients need additional protein because cancer tends to deplete protein stores. Has Dave planned enough protein for this meal? If not, how could he adjust this meal to include more protein?

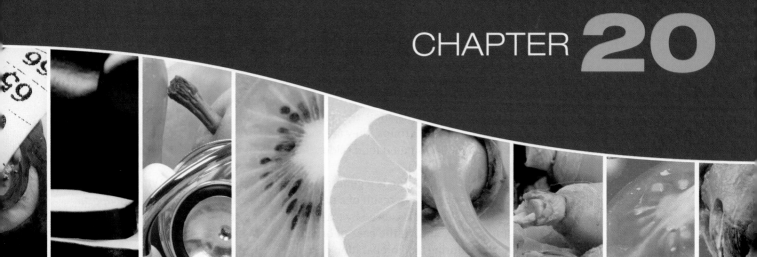

CHAPTER 20

KEY TERMS

abstinence
allergens
allergic reactions
allergy
anaphylaxis
botulism
carriers
cross-contamination
dermatitis
desensitized
dysentery
elimination diet
enterotoxins
food poisoning
hypersensitivity
insecticides
mold
neurotoxins
pathogens
Salmonella
skin tests
Staphylococcus (staph)
urticaria

FOODBORNE ILLNESS, ALLERGIES, AND INTOLERANCES

OBJECTIVES

After studying this chapter, you should be able to:

- Identify diseases caused by contaminated food, their signs, and the means by which they are spread
- List signs of food contamination
- State precautions for protecting food from contamination
- Describe allergies and elimination diets and their uses
- Distinguish between a food allergy and an intolerance

The most nutritious food can cause illness if it is contaminated with **pathogens** (disease-causing agents) or certain chemicals. Some of the pathogens that can cause foodborne illness include certain bacteria, viruses, molds, worms, and protozoa. The chemicals may be a natural component of specific foods, intentionally added during production or processing or accidentally added through carelessness or pollution.

There are always microorganisms in the environment. Some are useful, such as the bacteria used to make yogurt and certain cheeses. Others are pathogens. Pathogens may be in the air, on equipment, in food, on the skin, or in mucus and feces. Food is a particularly good breeding place for them because it provides nutrients, moisture, and often warmth. Although pathogens can be found in all food groups, they are most commonly found in foods from animal sources. Contaminated food seldom smells, looks, or tastes different from non-contaminated food.

Food poisoning is a general term for foodborne illness. When food poisoning develops as a result of a pathogen's infecting someone, it is a *foodborne infection*. When it is caused by toxins produced by the pathogen, it is called *food intoxication* and, in the case of botulism, can kill. Toxins can be produced by bacteria during food preparation or storage or by bacteria in one's digestive tract. **Enterotoxins** affect mucous membranes in the digestive tract, and **neurotoxins** affect the nervous system.

It is thought that as many as one in six Americans may experience food poisoning each year. Its typical symptoms include vomiting, diarrhea, headache, and abdominal cramps. Many never know they are suffering from food poisoning and assume they have the flu. Others, especially young children, the elderly, pregnant women, or those with compromised immune systems (such as people who are HIV positive) may become very ill, and some may die.

BACTERIA THAT CAUSE FOODBORNE ILLNESS

Campylobacter jejuni, Clostridium botulinum, Clostridium perfringens, Cyclospora Cayetanensis, Escherichia coli 0157:H7, Listeria monocytogenes, Salmonella, Shigella, and *Staphylococcus aureus* are examples of bacteria that can cause foodborne illness. Refer to Table 20-1.

Campylobacter jejuni

Campylobacter jejuni is believed to be one of the most prevalent causes of diarrhea. It is commonly found in the intestinal tracts of cattle, pigs, sheep, chickens, turkeys, dogs, and cats and can contaminate meat during slaughter. It is caused by the ingestion of live bacteria.

It can take two to five (or more) days to develop after infection and may last up to seven days. Symptoms include diarrhea (sometimes bloody), fever, headache, and muscle and abdominal pain. It can be transmitted to humans via unpasteurized milk; contaminated water; and raw or undercooked meats, poultry, and shellfish.

Clostridium botulinum

Clostridium botulinum is found in soil and water, on plants, and in the intestinal tracts of animals and fish. The spores of these bacteria can divide and produce toxin in the absence of oxygen. (Spores are single cells that are produced asexually, each of which is able to develop into a new organism. They have thick, protective walls that allow them to survive unfavorable conditions.) This means that the toxin can be produced in sealed containers such as cans, jars, and vacuum-packaged foods.

pathogens
disease-causing agents

food poisoning
foodborne illness

enterotoxins
toxins affecting mucous membranes

neurotoxins
toxins affecting the nervous system

TABLE 20-1 Foodborne Illnesses

BACTERIA	ASSOCIATED FOODS	SYMPTOMS AND POTENTIAL IMPACT	PREVENTION
Campylobacter jejuni	Contaminated water, raw or unpasteurized milk, and raw or undercooked meat, poultry, or shellfish.	Diarrhea (sometimes bloody), cramping, abdominal pain, and fever that appear two to five days after eating; may last seven days. May spread to bloodstream and cause a life-threatening infection.	Cook meat and poultry to a safe minimum internal temperature; do not drink or consume unpasteurized milk or milk products; wash your hands after coming in contact with feces.
Clostridium botulinum	Improperly canned foods, garlic in oil, vacuum-packed and tightly wrapped food.	Bacteria produce a nerve toxin that causes illness, affecting the nervous system. Toxin affects the nervous system. Symptoms usually appear 18–36 hours, but can sometimes appear as few as six hours or as many as 10 days after eating; double vision, blurred vision, drooping eyelids, slurred speech, difficulty swallowing, dry mouth, and muscle weakness. If untreated, these symptoms may progress causing muscle paralysis and even death.	Do not use damaged canned foods or canned foods showing signs of swelling, leakage, punctures, holes, fractures, extensive deep rusting, or crushing/denting severe enough to prevent normal stacking. Follow safety guidelines when home canning food. Boil home canned foods for 10 minutes before eating to ensure safety. (Note: Safe home canning guidelines may be obtained from State University or County Extension Office.)
Clostridium perfringens	Meats, meat products, and gravy called "the cafeteria germ" because many outbreaks result from food left for long periods in steam tables or at room temperature.	Intense abdominal cramps, nausea, and diarrhea may appear 6–24 hours after eating; usually last about one day, but for immune-comprised individuals, symptoms may last one to two weeks. Complications and/or death can occur only very rarely.	Keep hot foods hot and cold foods cold! Once food is cooked, it should be held hot, at an internal temperature of 140°F or above. Use a food thermometer to make sure. Discard all perishable foods left at room temperature longer than two hours; one hour in temperatures above 90°F.
Cryptosporidium	Soil, food, water, contaminated surfaces. Swallowing contaminated water, including that from recreational sources, (e.g., a swimming pool or lake); eating uncooked or contaminated food; placing a contaminated object in the mouth.	Dehydration, weight loss, stomach cramps or pain, fever, nausea, and vomiting; respiratory symptoms may also be present. Symptoms begin 2–10 days after becoming infected, and may last one to two weeks. Immune-comprised individuals may experience a more serious illness.	Wash your hands before and after handling raw meat products and after changing diapers, going to the bathroom, or touching animals. Avoid water that might be contaminated. (Do not drink untreated water from shallow wells, lakes, rivers, springs, ponds, and streams.)
Escherichia coli O157:H7	Uncooked beef (especially ground beef), unpasteurized milk and juices (e.g., "fresh" apple cider); contaminated raw fruits and vegetables, or water. Person-to-person contamination can also occur.	Severe diarrhea (often bloody diarrhea), abdominal cramps, and vomiting. Usually little or no fever. Can begin two to eight days, but usually three to four days after consumption of contaminated food or water and last about five to seven days, depending on severity. Children under 5 are at greater risk of developing hemolytic uremic syndrome (HUS), which causes acute kidney failure.	Cook hamburgers and ground beef to a safe minimum internal temperature of 160°F. Drink only pasteurized milk, juice, or cider. Rinse fruits and vegetables under running tap water, especially those that will not be cooked. Wash your hands with warm water and soap after changing diapers, using the bathroom, handling pets, or having any contact with feces.

(continues)

TABLE 20-1 *(continued)*

BACTERIA	ASSOCIATED FOODS	SYMPTOMS AND POTENTIAL IMPACT	PREVENTION
Listeria monocytogenes	Ready-to-eat foods such as hot dogs, luncheon meats, cold cuts, fermented or dry sausage, and other deli-style meat and poultry. Also, soft cheeses made with unpasteurized milk. Smoked seafood and salads made in the store such as ham salad, chicken salad, or seafood salad.	Fever, muscle aches, and sometimes gastrointestinal symptoms such as nausea or diarrhea. If infection spreads to the nervous system, symptoms such as headache, stiff neck, confusion, loss of balance, or convulsions can occur. Those at risk (including pregnant women and newborns, older adults, and people with weakened immune systems) may later develop more serious illness; death can result from Listeria. Can cause severe problems with pregnancy, including miscarriage or death in newborns.	Cook raw meat, poultry, and seafood to a safe minimum internal temperature; prevent cross-contamination, separating ready-to-eat foods from raw eggs, and raw meat, poultry, seafood, and their juices; wash your hands before and after handling raw meat, poultry, seafood, and egg products. Those with a weakened immune system should avoid eating hot dogs and deli meats, unless they are reheated to 165°F or steaming hot. Do not drink raw (unpasteurized) milk or foods that have unpasteurized milk in them (e.g., soft cheeses). Do not eat deli salads made in store, such as ham, egg, tuna, or seafood salad.
Salmonella (over 2,300 types)	Raw or undercooked eggs, poultry, and meat; unpasteurized milk and juice; cheese and seafood; and contaminated fresh fruits and vegetables.	Diarrhea, fever, and abdominal cramps usually appear 12–72 hours after eating; may last four to seven days. In people with weakened immune system, the infection may be more severe and lead to serious complications, including death.	Cook raw meat, poultry, and egg products to a safe temperature. Do not eat raw or undercooked eggs. Avoid consuming raw or unpasteurized milk or other dairy products. Produce should be thoroughly washed before consuming.
Shigella (over 30 types)	Person-to-person by fecal-oral route; fecal contamination of food and water. Most outbreaks result from food, especially salads, prepared and handled by workers using poor personal hygiene.	Disease referred to as "shigellosis" or bacillary dysentery. Diarrhea (watery or bloody), fever, abdominal cramps; one to two days from ingestion of bacteria and usually resolves in five to seven days.	Hand washing is a very important step to prevent shigellosis. Always wash your hands with warm water and soap before handling food and after using the bathroom, changing diapers, or having contact with an infected person.
Staphylococcus aureus	Commonly found on the skin and in the noses of up to 25% of healthy people and animals. Person-to-person through food from improper food handling. Multiply rapidly at room temperature to produce a toxin that causes illness. Contaminated milk and cheeses.	Severe nausea, abdominal cramps, vomiting, and diarrhea occur 30 minutes to six hours after eating; recovery from one to three days—longer if severe dehydration occurs.	Because the toxins produced by this bacterium are resistant to heat and cannot be destroyed by cooking, preventing the contamination of food before the toxin can be produced is important. Keep hot foods hot (over 140°F) and cold foods cold (40°F or under); wash your hands with warm water and soap and wash kitchen counters with hot water and soap before and after preparing food.
Vibrio vulnificus	Uncooked or raw seafood (fish or shellfish); oysters.	In healthy persons, symptoms include diarrhea, stomach pain, and vomiting. May result in a blood infection and death for those with a weakened immune system, particularly with underlying liver disease.	Do not eat raw oysters or other raw shellfish; cook shellfish (oysters, clams, mussels) thoroughly. Prevent cross-contamination by separating cooked seafood and other foods from raw seafood and its juices. Refrigerate cooked shellfish within two hours after cooking.

Source: United States Departments of Agriculture. Food Safety and Inspection Service. "Foodborne Illness: What Consumers Need to Know." Reviewed August 7, 2013. Accessed January 8, 2016. http://www.fsis.usda.gov

The spores are extremely heat resistant and must be boiled for six hours before they will be destroyed. Such a lengthy time will, of course, destroy the food they have infected. Home canned goods should be boiled for 10 minutes to ensure safety. **Botulism** is perhaps the rarest but most deadly of all food poisonings. Symptoms usually appear within 18–36 hours after eating and include double vision, speech difficulties, inability to swallow, and respiratory paralysis. The disease can be fatal in 5–10% of cases. Great care must be taken to prevent botulism when canning foods at home. The Centers for Disease Control and Prevention (CDC) reported that an average of 145 cases of botulism occur annually. If a can bulges, *Clostridium botulinum* may be present and can be fatal. A good rule of thumb is "If in doubt, throw it out" where children and animals cannot reach it.

Clostridium perfringens

Clostridium perfringens is often called the "cafeteria" or "buffet germ" because it tends to infect those who eat food that has been standing on buffets or steam tables for long periods. *C. perfringens* is found in soil dust, sewage, and the intestinal tracts of animals. It is a spore-forming pathogen that needs little oxygen. The bacteria are destroyed by cooking, but the spores can survive it.

Clostridium perfringens is transmitted by eating heavily contaminated food. Symptoms include nausea, diarrhea, and inflammation of the stomach and intestines. Symptoms may appear within 6–24 hours of ingestion and last approximately 24 hours. The CDC estimates that about 10,000 actual cases occur annually in the United States.

To best prevent it, hot foods should be kept at or above 140°F and cold foods below 40°F. Leftovers should be heated to 165°F before serving. Foods should be stored at temperatures of 40°F or lower. People with compromised immune systems should be very cautious concerning *C. perfringens*.

Cryptosporidium

Cryptosporidium is a parasite that causes cryptosporidiosis in the intestines of humans and animals. It can live outside of the body for long periods of time and is commonly found in infected stool of animals or humans. "Crypto" is commonly found in contaminated soil, food, and water, as well as in recreational water sources including swimming pools, lakes, rivers, and hot tubs.

The most common symptom of Crypto is watery diarrhea. Other symptoms include stomach cramps, fever, nausea, vomiting, and dehydration. Symptoms usually begin 2–10 days after becoming infected with the parasite and may last 1–2 weeks. Practicing good hygiene such as washing hands after going to the bathroom and handling raw meat can prevent infection. Contaminated water from wells, lakes, springs, and ponds should also be avoided.

Escherichia coli (E. coli 0157:H7)

Escherichia coli, commonly called *E. coli*, is a group of bacteria that can cause illness in humans. *E. coli* 0157:H7 is a highly infectious strain of this group. These bacteria can be found in the intestines of some mammals (including humans and animals used for food), in raw milk, and in water contaminated by animal or human feces.

E. coli are transmitted to humans through contaminated water, unpasteurized milk or apple juice, raw or rare ground beef products, unwashed fruits

botulism
deadliest of food poisonings; caused by the bacteria *Clostridium botulinum*

or vegetables, and directly from person-to-person. Plant foods can be contaminated by fertilization with raw manure or irrigation with contaminated water. The CDC estimates 70,000 cases of infection with *E. coli* 0157:H7 occur in the United States every year.

Symptoms include severe abdominal cramps, diarrhea that may be watery or bloody, and nausea. Symptoms may occur within three to eight days of ingestion with most people recovering within 10 days. Sometimes, however, *E. coli* 0157:H7 can cause hemorrhagic colitis (inflammation of the colon). This in turn can result in *hemolytic uremic syndrome* (HUS) in children, which can damage the kidneys.

E. coli can be controlled by careful choice and cooking of foods. All meats and poultry should be cooked thoroughly. Ground beef, veal, and lamb should be cooked to 160°F and ground poultry to at least 165°F. Fruits and vegetables should be carefully washed, and unpasteurized milk and other dairy products and vegetable and fruit juices should be avoided. People with compromised immune systems should be especially vigilant.

Listeria monocytogenes

Listeria monocytogenes is a bacterium often found in human and animal intestines and in milk, leafy vegetables, and soil. It can grow in the refrigerator and can be transmitted to humans by unpasteurized dairy foods such as milk, soft cheeses, and ice creams and via raw leafy vegetables and processed meats.

Listeria monocytogenes can affect a person from 12 hours to eight days after ingestion. Symptoms include fatigue, fever, chills, headache, backache, abdominal pain, and diarrhea. It can develop into more serious conditions and cause respiratory distress, spontaneous abortion, or meningitis.

To prevent infection by *Listeria monocytogenes*, meats and poultry should be thoroughly cooked and salad greens carefully washed. Attention must be paid to all dairy products—especially the unfamiliar from new sources—to be certain they have been pasteurized.

Salmonellosis

Salmonellosis (commonly called Salmonella) is an infection caused by the *Salmonella* bacteria. Salmonella can be found in raw eggs, poultry, and meat; unpasteurized milk and juice; cheese and seafood; and contaminated fruits and vegetables. It is transmitted by eating contaminated food or by contact with a carrier. Salmonellosis is characterized by headache, vomiting, diarrhea, abdominal cramps, and fever. Symptoms generally begin from 12–72 hours after eating. In severe cases, it can result in death. One species of *Salmonella* causes typhoid fever. Those who suffer the most severe cases are typically the very young, the elderly, and the weak or incapacitated.

Refrigeration (40°F or lower) inhibits the growth of these bacteria, but they can remain alive in the freezer and in dried foods. Heating foods to 145–165°F will render *Salmonella* bacteria, making it safe to ingest. To prevent contamination, thaw poultry and meats in the refrigerator or microwave and cook immediately. Avoid cross-contamination of raw and cooked foods by carefully cleaning utensils and counter surfaces that were in contact with raw food. Raw or undercooked eggs, or foods that contain them, should not be eaten. Even a taste of raw cookie dough or Caesar salad dressing made with raw egg yolk can cause contamination. People with compromised immune systems should be especially careful.

Salmonella
an infection caused by the *Salmonella* bacteria

Shigella

Shigella bacteria are found in the intestinal tract and thus the feces of infected individuals. The disease they cause is called *shigellosis*. These bacteria are typically passed on by an infected food handler who did not practice proper hand washing after using the toilet. They are also found on plants that were fertilized with untreated animal feces or given contaminated water. According to the Association for Dressings and Sauces, research has found that commercially prepared mayonnaise is not the common culprit for foodborne illnesses in cold salads. *Shigella* are destroyed by heat, but infected cold foods such as tuna, chicken, or egg salads are common carriers and should be kept on ice when served.

Shigellosis can occur from one day to one week following infection. Symptoms include diarrhea (sometimes with blood and mucus), fever, chills, headache, nausea, and abdominal cramps and can lead to dehydration. Some people, however, experience no symptoms. Foods must be cooked to 145–165°F to make them safe for consumption.

Staphylococcus aureus

Staphylococcus aureus bacteria are found on human skin, in infected cuts and pimples, and in noses and throats. Staphylococcal poisoning is commonly called **Staphylococcus (staph)**. These bacteria grow in meats; poultry; fish; egg dishes; salads such as potato, egg, macaroni, and tuna; and cream-filled pastries. This poisoning is transmitted by carriers and by eating foods that contain the toxin these bacteria create.

Symptoms, which include vomiting, diarrhea, and abdominal cramps, begin within 30 minutes to six hours after ingestion of the toxin and last from 24–72 hours. Staph is considered a mild illness.

The growth of these bacteria is inhibited if foods are kept at temperatures above 140°F or below 40°F. Their toxin can be destroyed by boiling the food for several hours or by heating it in a pressure cooker at 240°F for 30 minutes. Both of these methods would destroy the appeal and nutrient content of the infected foods. It is more practical to safely discard foods suspected of being contaminated.

OTHER SUBSTANCES THAT CAUSE FOOD POISONING

Mold is a type of fungus. Its roots go down, into the food, and it grows a stalk upward on which spores form. The green "fuzzy" part that can be seen by the naked eye is where the spores are found. Some spores cause respiratory problems and allergic reactions for some people. For this reason, moldy food should never be smelled.

Some molds produce a dangerous mycotoxin called aflatoxin that can cause cancer. It can develop in spoiled peanuts and peanut butter, soybeans, grains, nuts, and spices. Symptoms of such an infection include abdominal pain, vomiting, and diarrhea, and may occur from one day to several months after ingestion. It can cause liver and skin damage and, ultimately, cancer.

The Food and Drug Administration monitors the aflatoxin content of foods closely, and although this toxin cannot as yet be totally eradicated, foods containing more than a very minute amount of it cannot be sold by one state to another.

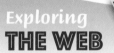

Exploring THE WEB

Choose one of the pathogens in the text that causes foodborne illness. Research this pathogen using the Web. What sources can you find on the pathogen? Create a fact sheet listing the signs and symptoms of the illness, the foods commonly infected with the pathogen, assessment of the client for the presence of the illness, and treatment. Also include tips on prevention of the illness.

Staphylococcus (staph)
genus of bacteria causing food poisoning called "staph" or "staphylococcal poisoning"

mold
a type of fungus

Neither cooking nor refrigeration destroys this toxin. Cheese may develop mold, and that part should be cut away to a depth of at least 1 in. (Cheeses such as bleu or Roquefort that were intentionally ripened by harmless molds are safe to eat.) Fruits and vegetables showing signs of mold should not be purchased.

Trichinella spiralis is a parasitic worm that causes trichinosis. This disease is transmitted by eating inadequately cooked pork from pigs that are infected with the *T. spiralis* parasite. Wild game, especially bear, has been found to carry this parasite. Symptoms include abdominal pain, vomiting, fever, chills, and muscle pain. Symptoms occur about 24 hours after ingesting infected pork. Due to increased regulation of feed and products given to pigs, this infection is less common than it used to be. Cooking whole cuts of pork to an internal temperature of at least 145°F kills the organism (ground meat to 160°F) and prevents this disease. It can also be destroyed by freezing.

Dysentery is a disease caused by protozoa (tiny, one-celled animal). The protozoa are introduced to food by carriers or contaminated water. They cause severe diarrhea that can occur intermittently until the client is treated appropriately.

TREATMENT AND PREVENTION OF FOODBORNE ILLNESSES

The primary treatment needed for most foodborne illness is replacing lost fluids and electrolytes to prevent dehydration. Clear liquids such as fruit juice, broth, sports drinks and so forth, can be given as tolerated, starting with small sips. Older adults and those with weakened immune systems may need oral rehydration solutions. Gradually reintroducing bland, easy-to-digest foods such as potatoes, rice, toast, applesauce, and bananas is a good starting point when solids are ready to be consumed. Children may need to be given commercial oral rehydration solutions to prevent dehydration, with transition to food as soon as tolerated. Infants will need breast milk or formula along with their rehydration solutions.

Anti-diarrheal medications such as loperamide and bismuth subsalicylate can help stop diarrhea in adults; however, those who have bloody diarrhea, which is a sign of bacterial or parasitic infection, should not use these medications. Children and infants usually are not prescribed these medications; however, this would be evaluated by the physician on a case by case basis.

If deemed appropriate, a health care provider may prescribe other medications such as antibiotics to treat the illness. Hospitalization may be needed to treat complications of foodborne illness such as severe dehydration, paralysis, or hemolytic uremic syndrome.

Strict federal, state, and local laws regulate the commercial production of food in the United States, and dairies, canneries, bakeries, and meatpacking plants are all subject to government inspection. Individuals that work in food service receive food handler training. Nevertheless, errors and accidents can and do occur, and illness can result. *Most foodborne illnesses occur because of the ignorance or carelessness of people who handle food.* People can introduce pathogens to food, prevent them from reaching it, or kill them with appropriate cooking temperatures.

Cleanliness is especially important in preventing foodborne illness. When kitchen equipment, such as a cutting board, meat grinder, or countertop, is used for preparing pathogen-infected foods and not cleaned properly afterward, non-infected food that is subsequently prepared with this equipment can become

dysentery
disease caused by microorganism; characterized by diarrhea

infected by the same pathogen(s). This is called cross-contamination. Dishes used to hold uncooked meat, poultry, fish, or eggs must always be washed before cooked foods are placed on them.

There are four easy ways to reduce foodborne illness following these principles: clean, separate, cook, and chill (Figure 20-1).

- *Clean*—Wash hands often. Wet hands with clean running water and apply soap. Scrub all parts of the hands for 20 seconds. Rinse thoroughly under running water and dry hands with clean paper towel.

- *Separate*—Keep raw meats and ready-to-eat foods separate as you prepare and store them. Store raw fish, meat, and poultry on a shelf below ready-to-eat foods. Use separate cutting boards for raw meat, poultry, and seafood and one for ready-to-eat foods (color coded cutting boards are helpful).

- *Cook*—Cook to proper temperatures. Fish, meat, poultry, and egg dishes should be cooked to the recommended safe minimum internal temperature to destroy any potentially harmful bacteria. A food thermometer is helpful.

- *Chill*—Refrigerate leftovers promptly to 40°F or below. Foods are no longer safe to eat if they have been in the danger zone of 40–140°F for more than two hours (one hour if temperature is over 90°F). Keep refrigerator at 40°F or below and freezer at 0°F or below.

Even though we think of meat, seafood, and poultry as harboring harmful bacteria, fruits and vegetables may be contaminated as well. Produce needs to be washed before peeling to make sure dirt and bacteria aren't transferred from the knife to your produce. Using commercial produce wash is not necessary.

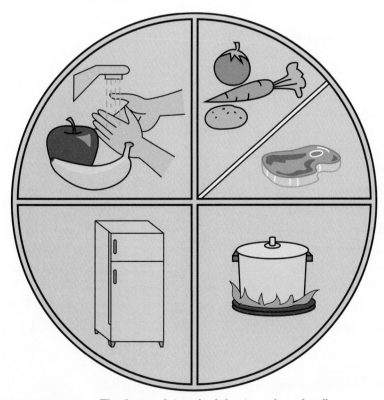

FIGURE 20-1 The four safety principles to reduce foodborne illness are clean, separate, cook, and chill.

In The Media

E. coli in a Popular Mexican Grill

In October 2015, an *E. coli* outbreak sickened more than 50 people after they consumed meals from Chipotle Mexican Grill. The outbreak originated in Washington and Oregon with customers reporting signs and symptoms of illness one week after eating at Chipotle. In December 2015, a different strain of *E. coli* was reported from at least five people in Kansas, North Dakota, and Oklahoma. No deaths have been linked to the outbreak and no ingredient was found as a direct cause. Since then, the company is making many changes to ensure the safety and quality of their food products. Some changes include receiving pre-shredded cheese, adding lemon juice to ingredients like onions to kill germs, testing meats before they are sent to stores, as well as conducting preparation of ingredients such as tomatoes and cilantro at centralized locations so they can be tested.

Adapted from NY Daily News. (2015, December 23). "Chipotle Tweaks Cooking Methods After E. coli Outbreak Sickens More Than 50 People." Accessed January 2016. http://www.nydailynews.com/life-style/health/chipotle-tweaks-cooking-methods-e-coli-outbreak-article-1.2475395

Cross-contamination
unintentional transfer of harmful bacteria from one food or object to another

Tap water removes bacteria sufficiently. Farm produce can be scrubbed with a clean produce brush. It's best to avoid produce with mold, bruises, or cuts. Some produce does not need refrigeration until peeled or cut, such as bananas and potatoes. Produce that needs refrigeration should be stored in a refrigerator within 2 hours of purchase.

When food workers fail to wash their hands after blowing their noses or using the toilet, they can "share" their germs very easily. Mucus and feces are favorite breeding areas of pathogens.

Food workers who have even small cuts on their hands must wear gloves because a wound could carry a pathogen. Foods must be covered and stored properly to keep dust, insects, and animals from reaching and possibly contaminating them. Water from unknown sources should not be used for cooking because it, too, can carry pathogens.

Temperatures during preparation and storage of food must be carefully observed. When infected foods are undercooked, the pathogen is not destroyed and can be passed to consumers (Table 20-2). Foods allowed to stand at temperatures between 40°F and 140°F provide an ideal breeding place for pathogens (Figure 20-2).

Leftover food should always be refrigerated as soon as the meal is finished and covered when it is cold. It should not be allowed to cool to room temperature before it is refrigerated. Frozen food should be either cooked from the frozen

TABLE 20-2 Cooking Temperatures

PRODUCT	FAHRENHEIT
Eggs and Egg Dishes	
• Eggs	Cook until yolk and white are firm
• Egg dishes	160°
Fresh Beef, Veal, Lamb	
• Ground products like hamburger (prepared as patties, meatloaf, meatballs, etc.)	160°
• Roasts, steaks, and chops	
○ Medium rare	145°
○ Medium	160°
○ Well done	170°
Fresh Pork	
• Whole cuts	145°
• Ground pork	160°
Poultry	
• Ground chicken, turkey	165°
• Whole chicken, turkey (well done)	180°
• Whole bird with stuffing (stuffing must reach 165°F)	180°
• Poultry breasts, roasts	170°
• Thighs, wings	Cook until juices run clear
Ham	
• Fresh (raw)	160°
• Fully cooked, to reheat	140°

Source: U.S. Department of Agriculture, Food Safety and Inspection Service, Washington, DC. http://www.fsis.usda.gov

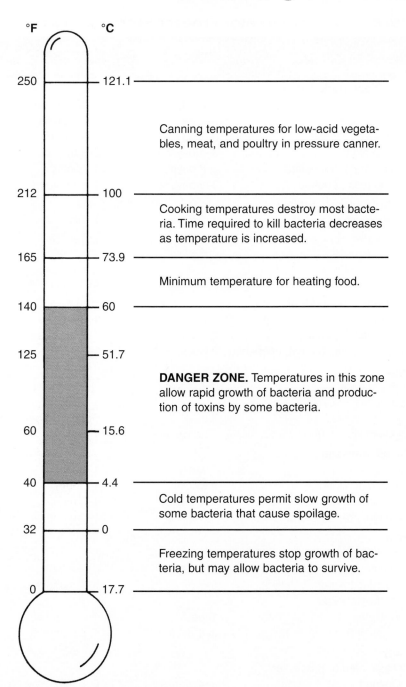

°F   °C

250 — 121.1 ——————————————————

Canning temperatures for low-acid vegetables, meat, and poultry in pressure canner.

212 — 100 ——————————————————

Cooking temperatures destroy most bacteria. Time required to kill bacteria decreases
as temperature is increased.

165 — 73.9 ——————————————————

Minimum temperature for heating food.

140 — 60 ——————————————————

125 — 51.7

DANGER ZONE. Temperatures in this zone
allow rapid growth of bacteria and production of toxins by some bacteria.

60 — 15.6

40 — 4.4 ——————————————————

Cold temperatures permit slow growth of
some bacteria that cause spoilage.

32 — 0 ——————————————————

Freezing temperatures stop growth of bacteria, but may allow bacteria to survive.

0 — 17.7 ——————————————————

FIGURE 20-2 Temperatures of food for control of bacteria.

state or thawed in the refrigerator. (When cooked from the frozen state, cooking time will generally increase by at least 50%.) Frozen food should not be thawed at room temperature. Food must always be protected from dust, insects, and animals. Table 20-3 offers useful information on how long perishable meats and cheeses can be stored in the refrigerator and freezer.

Carriers are people (or animals) capable of transmitting infectious (disease-causing) organisms. Often the carrier suffers no effects from the organism and therefore is unaware of the danger she or he represents. Food workers should be tested regularly to confirm that they are not carriers of communicable diseases.

carriers
those who are capable of transmitting an infectious organism

TABLE 20-3 Refrigerator/Freezer Storage Chart

PERISHABLE FOOD	REFRIGERATOR (BELOW 40°F)	FREEZER (AT OR BELOW 0°F)
Meat (beef, pork, lamb)		
Steaks	3–5 days	6–12 months
Chops	3–5 days	4–6 months
Roasts	3–5 days	6–9 months
Cooked meat	3–4 days	2–3 months
Ground meat, uncooked	1–2 days	4 months
Ground meat, cooked	3–4 days	4 months
Poultry (chicken, turkey)		
Poultry, whole	1–2 days	1 year
Poultry, pieces	1–2 days	9 months
Poultry, cooked	3–4 days	4 months
Ground poultry, uncooked	1–2 days	4 months
Ground poultry, cooked	3–4 days	4 months
Hot Dogs, Lunch Meat		
Hot dogs, opened	1 week	1–2 months
Lunch meat, opened	3–5 days	1–2 months
Hot dogs or lunch meat, unopened	2 weeks	1–2 months
Eggs		
Fresh, in shell	3–5 weeks	Do not freeze
Egg whites and yolks	2–4 days	1 year
Egg substitutes, opened	3 days	Does not freeze well
Egg substitutes, unopened	10 days	1 year
Bacon, Sausage		
Bacon, opened	1 week	1 month
Bacon, unopened	2 weeks	1 month
Sausage, raw	1–2 days	1–2 months
Sausage, pre-cooked/smoked	1 week	1–2 months
Ham		
Fresh ham, uncooked		
Uncured	3–5 days	6 months
Cured (cook before eating)	5–7 days	3–4 months
Ham, fully cooked		
Whole	1 week	1–2 months
Slices or half	3–4 days	1–2 months
Dairy		
Cheese, hard or processed		
Opened	3–4 weeks	6 months
Unopened	6 months	6 months
Cheese, soft	1 week	6 months
Cottage or ricotta	1 week	Do not freeze
Cream cheese	2 weeks	Do not freeze
Butter	1–3 months	6–9 months

Source: Adapted from "Keep It Cool: Refrigerator/Freezer Food Storage Chart."
www.homefoodsafety.org

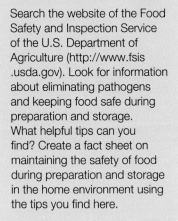

Exploring THE WEB

Search the website of the Food Safety and Inspection Service of the U.S. Department of Agriculture (http://www.fsis.usda.gov). Look for information about eliminating pathogens and keeping food safe during preparation and storage. What helpful tips can you find? Create a fact sheet on maintaining the safety of food during preparation and storage in the home environment using the tips you find here.

Selection of food should be made with great care. Packages and jars should be properly sealed. Cans should not bulge. Foods that look or smell at all unusual and foods showing signs of mold should be left in the store. Only pasteurized milk and dairy products should be used (Table 20-4).

TABLE 20-4 Ways to Prevent Food Poisoning

- Keep kitchen and equipment thoroughly clean.
- Wash hands after blowing nose or using the bathroom.
- Wear gloves if cooking with any hand wound.
- Cover and store foods to prevent microbes or animals from reaching it.
- Cook foods to appropriate temperatures.
- Limit standing time at temperatures between 40°F and 140°F.
- Prevent known carriers from preparing foods.
- Select only packages and jars that were sealed by the manufacturer.
- Avoid bulging cans, foods that look or smell odd, and foods showing signs of mold.

MISCELLANEOUS FOOD POISONINGS

Occasionally, food poisoning is caused by ingesting certain plants or animals that contain poison. Examples are plants such as poisonous mushrooms, rhubarb leaves, and fish from polluted water.

Poisoning also can result from ingesting cleaning agents, insecticides, or excessive amounts of a drug. Children may swallow cleaning agents or medicines. The cook may mistakenly use a poison instead of a cooking ingredient. Sometimes insecticides cling to fresh fruits and vegetables. It is essential that all potential poisons be kept out of the reach of young children and kept separate from all food supplies. Fresh fruits and vegetables should be thoroughly washed before being eaten.

FOOD ALLERGIES

An allergy is an altered reaction of the tissues of some individuals to substances that, in similar amounts, are harmless to other people. The substances causing hypersensitivity are called allergens. Some common allergens are pollen, dust, animal dander (bits of dried skin), drugs, cosmetics, and certain foods. This discussion will be limited to allergic reactions to foods. A food allergy occurs when the immune system reacts to a food substance, usually a protein. When such a reaction occurs, antibodies form and cause allergic symptoms. An altered reaction to a specific food that does not involve the immune system is called (the specific food) *intolerance*.

Food allergy is a growing public health concern. The Centers for Disease Control and Prevention released a study in 2013 stating that food allergies among children increased by 50% between 1997 and 2011. Some sources feel the growing allergy problem is related to changes in hygiene. Compared to the past, when more of us worked in farm and labor situations, we are exposed to less bacteria and endotoxins, especially with the advent of anti-bacterial products. Further, some also speculate there may be a relationship between overuse of antibiotics and allergy increase. Approximately 8% of children and 4% of adults are known to have food allergies; many of these allergies began in the first year of life

Types of Allergic Reactions

Sometimes allergic reactions are immediate, and sometimes several hours elapse before signs occur. Allergic individuals seem most prone to allergic reactions during periods of stress. Typical signs of food allergies include hay fever, urticaria, edema, headache, dermatitis, nausea, dizziness, and asthma (which causes breathing difficulties).

insecticides
agents that destroy insects

allergy
sensitivity to specific substance(s)

hypersensitivity
abnormally strong sensitivity to certain substance(s)

allergens
substance causing allergy

urticaria
hives; common allergic reaction

dermatitis
inflammation of the skin

TABLE 20-5 Common Food Allergens

TOP EIGHT ALLERGENS
Milk
Wheat
Eggs
Tree nuts
Peanuts
Soybeans
Fish
Shellfish

OTHER ALLERGENIC FOODS
Corn
Citrus fruit
Tomatoes
Strawberries
Legumes
Chocolate
Pork

allergic reactions
adverse physical reactions to specific substances

anaphylaxis
serious allergic reaction that involves more than one body system

skin tests
allergy tests using potential allergens on scratches on the skin

elimination diet
limited diet in which only certain foods are allowed; intended to find the food allergen causing reaction

Allergic reactions are uncomfortable and can be detrimental to health. When breathing difficulties are severe, they are life-threatening. **Anaphylaxis** is a serious allergic reaction that involves more than one body system and is usually related to food, latex, medicines, and insect stings. Related to food, peanuts, treenuts, seafood, and shellfish are the most likely foods to cause these severe reactions. Symptoms of anaphylaxis include:

- *Mouth*—itching, swelling of lips and/or tongue
- *Throat*—itching, tightness/closure, hoarseness
- *Skin*—itching, hives, redness, swelling
- *Gut*—vomiting, diarrhea, cramps
- *Lung*—shortness of breath, coughing, wheezing
- *Heart*—weak pulse, dizziness, passing out

Only a few symptoms may be present. Severity of symptoms can change quickly. Reactions to the throat, lung, and heart can be life threatening. Injectable epinephrine needs to be given quickly with a call to 911. An emergency action plan is important for those at risk of anaphylaxis.

Allergic reactions to the same food can differ in two individuals. For example, the fact that someone gets hives from eating strawberries does not mean that an allergic reaction to strawberries will appear as hives in another member of the same family. Allergic reactions can even differ from time to time with the same individual.

Treatment for Allergies

The simplest treatment for allergies is to remove the item that causes the allergic reaction. However, because of the variety of allergic reactions, finding the allergen can be difficult.

When food allergies are suspected, it is wise for the client to keep a food diary for several days and to record all food and drink ingested as well as allergic reactions and the time of their onset. Such records can help pinpoint specific allergens. Some common food allergens are listed in Table 20-5. Eight foods cause 90% of the allergic reactions. It is common for other foods in the same class as the allergens to cause allergic reactions as well. Cooking sometimes alters the foods and can eliminate allergic reactions in some people.

Blood tests may be used to find the allergen or allergens. **Skin tests** are sometimes used to detect allergies. However, food allergies can be difficult to determine from skin tests.

After completion of the allergy testing, the client is usually placed on an **elimination diet**. For several weeks the client does not eat any of the tested compounds that gave a positive reaction. The client includes in the diet the foods that almost no one reacts to, such as rice, fresh meats and poultry, noncitrus fruits, and vegetables. Sometimes, these diets allow only a limited number of foods and can be nutritionally inadequate. If that is the case, vitamin and mineral supplements may be prescribed.

When relief is found from the allergic symptoms, the client is continued on the diet, and gradually other foods are added to the diet at a rate of only one every four to seven days. Those foods most likely to produce allergic reactions are added last until an allergic reaction occurs. The allergy can then be pinpointed, and the offending foods eliminated from the diet. Knowing the cause of the allergy enables the client to lead a healthy, normal life, provided that eliminating these foods does not affect her or his nutrition.

SPOTLIGHT *on Life Cycle*

The National Institute of Allergy and Infectious Disease published *Guidelines for the Diagnosis and Management of Food Allergy in the United States* for physicians and other health care professionals as well as clients, families, and caregivers. Families with children who have food allergies can access the guideline summary to learn more about how to manage the disorder and start conversations with their doctors about allergy care options for their children. The guidelines provide the following information:

- Definitions of food allergy and disorders associated with food allergy
- Descriptions of the development of food allergy and conditions associated with food allergy
- Recommendations on how to diagnose, manage life-threatening reactions and food-induced anaphylaxis, and other acute reactions

Definitions, common food allergens, how food allergies develop, and ways to manage food allergies after diagnosis are some of the numerous topics discussed within the guidelines. Being knowledgeable about allergies and the care for them will make discussions with a health professional more understandable and easier.

Source: Adapted from National Institute of Allergy and Infectious Diseases, Department of Health and Human Services, National Institutes of Health. May 2011.

If the elimination of the allergen results in a diet deficient in certain nutrients, suitable substitutes for those nutrients must be found. For example, if a client is allergic to citrus fruits, other foods rich in vitamin C to which the client is not allergic must be found. If the allergy is to milk, soybean milk may be substituted.

The client must be taught the food sources of the nutrient or nutrients lacking so that other foods can be substituted that are nutritionally equal to those causing the allergy. It is essential that the client be taught to read the labels on commercially prepared foods and to check the ingredients of restaurant foods carefully. The Food Allergen Labeling and Consumer Protection Act of 2004 (FALCPA) mandates that the label clearly state if a product contains any of the top eight allergens. This is usually listed after the ingredient list on the nutrition facts label.

Sometimes, however, the allergies require such a restriction of foods that the diet does become nutritionally inadequate. As in all cases of allergy, and particularly in such cases, it is hoped that the client can become **desensitized** to the allergens so that a nutritionally balanced diet can be restored. The client is desensitized by eating a minute amount of food allergen after a period of complete **abstinence** from it. The amount of the allergen is gradually increased until the client can tolerate it.

FOOD INTOLERANCES

A food intolerance is often called a nonallergic food hypersensitivity. Unlike a food allergy, which involves an immune system response, a food intolerance doesn't involve the immune system and is more common in nature. Food intolerances or sensitivities can be a result of a missing enzyme (such as lactose

Exploring
THE WEB

Go to the website for the International Food Information Council Foundation (http://www.ific.org). Search for information on allergic reactions and foods. What types of illnesses can be caused by food allergies? How are these allergies detected? Can you locate a recipe source online for individuals with food allergies?

desensitized
having gradually reduced the body's sensitivity (allergic reaction) to specific items

abstinence
avoidance

intolerance) or they may be due to an issue with a food preservative or an additive. Food sensitivities can take anywhere from 72–96 hours to produce a symptom; therefore, it is often problematic for individuals to identify food intolerances on their own.

Depending on the type and severity of symptoms identified, some clinicians, especially those involved in functional medicine, may recommend a food sensitivity test followed by an elimination diet. The common food intolerances are lactose, gluten (celiac disease or gluten intolerance), histamine and tyramine (aged cheese, processed meats, beer, wine), salicyclate (a type of salt contained in some foods), tartrazine (artificial food color), benzoates, BHA, BHT, sulfites (preservatives), MSG (monosodium glutamate—a flavor enhancer), and other food dyes.

HEALTH AND NUTRITION CONSIDERATIONS

Some clients will need simple instructions from the health care professional about avoiding microbial contamination of food supplies at home. Many, if not most, should be warned not to thaw food at room temperature. Others should be reminded that leftover foods should *not* be cooled at room temperature before being refrigerated.

Clients with food allergies will require careful training to avoid their specific allergens. They must be taught to read food labels carefully and to ask for the ingredients of foods in restaurants and at friends' homes. Role-playing is an effective way to help such clients.

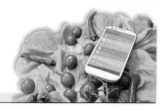

SUMMARY

Infection or poisoning traced to food is usually caused by human ignorance or carelessness. The serving of safe meals is essentially the responsibility of the cook. Food should not be prepared by anyone who has or carries a contagious disease. All fresh fruits and vegetables should be washed before being eaten. Meats, poultry, fish, eggs, and dairy products should be refrigerated. Pork should always be cooked to the well-done stage. Food should be covered to prevent contamination by dust, insects, or animals. Garbage should also be covered so that it does not attract insects. Hands that prepare foods should be clean and free of cuts or wounds. Kitchen equipment should be spotless. Finally, the food itself should be safe. People should avoid foods containing natural poisons.

Food allergies can cause many different and unpleasant symptoms. Elimination diets are used to determine the food allergen. Some of the most common food allergens have been found to be milk, eggs, fish, shellfish, peanuts, treenuts, soy, and wheat.

DISCUSSION TOPICS

1. Name four types of foodborne illness. If any class member has suffered from one, ask the person to describe the symptoms.

2. How does food become contaminated?

3. Why should foods be refrigerated?

4. What are allergies? What can cause them?

5. What are some common allergic reactions to food? How can they be avoided?

6. Do people inherit allergies? Explain.

7. Of what use is a food diary in relation to allergies? What about food intolerances? What are elimination diets, and when are they used? What is the most difficult part of treating food allergies?

8. How can an allergic client be desensitized?

9. Is an elimination diet always nutritious? Explain.

10. Research the Food Allergen Labeling and Consumer Protection Act and note the allergen statements on common food products that cover the top eight food allergens.

SUGGESTED ACTIVITIES

1. Ask a doctor or registered nurse to explain skin tests to the class. Discuss these tests after the lecture.

2. Ask someone with food allergies to speak to the class. Follow this talk with questions from the audience.

3. Visit a restaurant kitchen. Look for practices that may lead to potential food poisoning. Note the practices and uses of equipment designed to prevent food poisoning.

4. Ask the class if anyone has had a foodborne illness. What food caused the illness? What were the symptoms? How long were you sick?

REVIEW

Multiple choice. Select the *letter* that precedes the best answer.

1. A microorganism is
   a. a unit of measurement
   b. sometimes pathogenic
   c. a component of a microscope
   d. an individual human cell

2. Which of the following refrigeration temperatures inhibits the growth of *Salmonella*?
   a. 42°F
   b. 41°F
   c. 39°F
   d. 50°F

3. Someone who is capable of spreading an infectious organism but is not sick is called a
   a. food handler
   b. carrier
   c. transport
   d. fomite

4. When an organism is infectious, it is
   a. disease-causing
   b. prone to infections
   c. not contagious
   d. always fatal

5. Most cases of food poisoning in the United States are caused by
   a. careless processing in commercial factories
   b. lack of government inspection
   c. careless handling of food in the kitchen
   d. house pets

6. Food poisoning symptoms generally include
   a. joint pain
   b. constipation
   c. abdominal upset and headache
   d. swelling of the feet

7. Salmonella infections and staphylococcal poisoning are caused by
   a. a virus
   b. bacteria
   c. protozoa
   d. parasites

8. The deadliest of the bacterial food poisonings is
   a. staphylococcal poisoning
   b. salmonellosis
   c. botulism
   d. perfringens poisoning

9. The disease caused by a parasite sometimes found in pork is
   a. tularemia
   b. dysentery
   c. avitaminosis
   d. trichinosis

10. The disease caused by a protozoan and characterized by severe diarrhea is
    a. salmonellosis
    b. botulism
    c. dysentery
    d. infectious hepatitis

11. Foods may be contaminated by
    a. people
    b. overcooking them
    c. refrigeration
    d. all of the above

12. The temperatures in the danger zone that encourage bacterial growth are from
    a. 0–32°F
    b. 32–60°F
    c. 40–140°F
    d. 125–212°F

13. Leftover foods should be
    a. put in the refrigerator immediately after meals
    b. cooled to room temperature before refrigerating
    c. cooled in the refrigerator for at least an hour before freezing
    d. stored unwrapped in the refrigerator

14. Frozen foods should be
    a. thawed at room temperature
    b. refrozen if not used immediately after thawing
    c. thawed in the refrigerator
    d. any of the above

15. An adverse physical reaction to a food is called a food
    a. refusal
    b. allergy
    c. symptom
    d. allergen

16. Substances that cause altered physical reactions are called
    a. symptoms
    b. allergies
    c. allergens
    d. abstinence

17. One of the typical symptoms of food allergies is
    a. hives
    b. colitis
    c. dry mouth
    d. diarrhea

18. The simplest treatment for a food allergy is
    a. a skin test
    b. allergy shots
    c. elimination of the allergen
    d. the use of penicillin

19. In cases of food allergy, an elimination diet may be prescribed to
    a. desensitize the client
    b. avoid medication
    c. avoid surgery
    d. find the allergen

20. Some foods that frequently cause an allergic reaction are
    a. milk, eggs, and wheat
    b. lamb, rice, and sugar
    c. chocolate and strawberries
    d. rice and pears

CASE IN POINT

ALAMEDA: LISTERIA INFECTION DURING PREGNANCY

Alameda is eight months pregnant with her second child. She has been very busy trying to get ready for the new baby and balance life with a toddler. She has been very tired lately. In an effort to save money and free up a little extra time, she has not been cooking as she usually does. Alameda and her husband are Native Americans and she still loves to cook many of the same foods they ate growing up. While she knows her children will probably be influenced by many American customs and foods, she likes to keep the Native American culture and cuisine within their home. Recently, Alameda and her family have been eating quite a number of simple meals such as lunchmeat sandwiches, raw vegetables with ranch dressing, salads, and fresh fruit. Cutting down on food prep and cooking has given Alameda time for an extra nap here and there, too.

This morning Alameda awoke to flu-like symptoms. She aches all over her body and also has a stiff neck. Since she is currently 32 weeks pregnant she thought she should give her doctor a call. After examining Alameda, the doctor runs a blood test to confirm his suspicions. After the blood work is completed, the doctor tells Alameda she has Listeria. He tells Alameda that pregnant women are 13 times more susceptible to Listeria infections than the average population. He explains that raw meats such as lunchmeats, raw fruits and vegetables, and unpasteurized products often cause Listeria infections. He prescribes an antibiotic for Alameda and requests that she follow up with him again next week. He also instructs Alameda to make sure she heats any meats and vegetables she consumes thoroughly.

ASSESSMENT

1. What is Listeria?
2. What food sources may contain Listeria?
3. What are the symptoms of Listeria?
4. How can Listeria infection be prevented?

DIAGNOSIS

5. Write a nursing diagnosis for Alameda.

PLAN/GOAL

6. What should Alameda know about Listeria infections during pregnancy?
7. Are there any medications that are recommended for Listeria infection?

IMPLEMENTATION

8. Why is it important for Alameda to follow the recommended guidelines for preventing Listeria?

EVALUATION/OUTCOME CRITERIA

9. How will Alameda's doctor know she is following the recommended guidelines?

THINKING FURTHER

10. Aside from pregnant women, who may be at increased risk for Listeria infections?

✔ rate this plate

Alameda takes the doctor's advice and takes extra precaution when eating luncheon meats and fresh produce. Alameda's family recently hosted a baby shower for her, where a lunch buffet was prepared by friends and family. The buffet consisted of the following items.

Cold cut tray consisting of turkey, ham, roast beef, and cheeses (served over ice)

Relish tray with pickles, olives, and condiments

Baked cheesy potato salad

Green salad with egg and tomato

Macaroni salad

Pretzels and potato chips

Cold cheese ball with crackers

Previously baked crab dip

Vegetable tray

Fruit salad

Cupcakes and cookies

Make a plate that would be safe for Alameda to eat, telling why you chose what you did.

CASE IN POINT

CARSON: DISCOVERING A SHELLFISH ALLERGY

Carson is a 9-year-old boy from Indiana. He is very excited about the long-awaited summer vacation his family has been planning. His family is headed to Bar Harbor, Maine, to relax and enjoy some deep-sea fishing. Carson has often been fishing with his grandparents at their lake home, but he has never been deep-sea fishing. He is very excited and anxious to try his hand at helping to clean and cook his catch! Many of the local restaurants allow people to clean and cook their catch on site.

Carson and his dad are very excited to begin their fishing trip. While at sea, Carson caught many fish and even caught a lobster, some clams, and a few oysters. Carson had never had seafood other than fish. Fresh seafood in Indiana is a little harder to come by. Carson really enjoyed trying the seafood he caught on the boat that day. He loved the lobster in butter sauce and of course the fried clams. The oysters weren't his favorite, but he liked getting to try them anyway. Later that evening they returned to the hotel. During the night, Carson awoke with severe stomach pains. He was nauseous and dizzy as well. He woke up his parents to inform them of his situation. When he began having difficulty breathing, his parents rushed him to the ER at the local hospital for assessment.

ASSESSMENT

1. What complaints did Carson have during the night?
2. What would you expect to be the problem?
3. Which foods are most likely the cause of the problem?

DIAGNOSIS

4. Carson's abdominal pain and nausea could have been caused by _____.
5. What information should be gathered during his initial assessment?

PLAN/GOAL

6. What is the immediate goal for Carson?
7. What is the long-range goal?

IMPLEMENTATION

8. In the ER, what should Carson and his parents discuss with the physicians?
9. Does it appear that Carson may have a food allergy?
10. Is the doctor able to verify that this is an allergy?
11. What is the most likely recommendation for Carson?
12. What should Carson be cautioned about in the future about dining out?

EVALUATION/OUTCOME CRITERIA

13. When the intervention is complete, how will Carson know it has been effective?

THINKING FURTHER

14. What information could be obtained on the Internet?

✔ rate this plate

Carson was so excited about his catch of the day and wanted to try everything for dinner. Is this a good idea? Rate this plate.

- **2 oz lobster in butter sauce**
- **3 oz fried clams**
- **1 oz oysters on the half shell**
- **1 small order of French fries**
- **1 small Caesar salad made with homemade dressing containing a raw egg**
- **12 oz regular soda**

Since Carson had not tried shellfish before, should he have been given so many different choices to taste? Would it have been better for Carson to have been served only one shellfish item and no raw eggs?

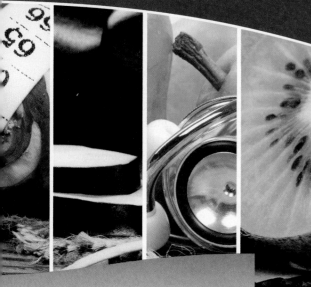

NUTRITIONAL CARE OF CLIENTS WITH SPECIAL NEEDS

OBJECTIVES

After studying this chapter, you should be able to:

- Describe the body's reactions to stress as it relates to nutrition

- Explain the special nutrition needs of clients undergoing surgery and those with burns, fever, or infection

- Discuss enteral and parenteral nutrition

- Explain the special dietary needs of AIDS clients

- Identify special nutrition considerations in elderly clients who need long-term care

Illness and surgery can have devastating effects on nutritional status. Normally, the human body operates in a state of homeostasis. When the body experiences the trauma of surgery, severe burns, or infections, this balance is upset. The body reacts in an attempt to restore itself to homeostasis.

During its response to physical stress, the body signals the endocrine system, which activates a self-protective, **hypermetabolic** response. This increases energy output. The intensity of the response depends on the severity of the condition.

Catabolism occurs, causing the rapid breakdown of energy reserves to provide glucose and other substances necessary for the anabolic phase of wound healing and tissue maintenance. Proteins, fats, and minerals are lost in the catabolic phase just when there is an increased need for them to rebuild tissue. When the condition includes hemorrhage and vomiting, these losses are compounded.

Sufficient nutrients, fluids, and calories are required as soon as possible to replace the losses, build and repair tissue, and return the body to homeostasis. Obviously, nutrition plays an important role in the lives of clients undergoing surgery or of those who suffer from burns or infections.

THE CLIENT WITH PROTEIN-ENERGY MALNUTRITION

When the increased needs for energy and protein are not met by food intake, the body must use its stores of glycogen and fat. When they have been used, the body breaks down its own protein stores to provide energy. Protein-energy malnutrition, commonly called PEM, can be a problem among hospitalized clients, especially the elderly. It can delay wound healing, contribute to anemia, depress the immune system, and increase susceptibility to infections. Symptoms of PEM include weight loss and dry, pale skin. When malnutrition occurs as a result of hospitalization, it is called **iatrogenic malnutrition**.

THE SURGICAL CLIENT
Presurgery Nutritional Care

Elective surgery stresses the client prior to the procedure. Prior to surgery, the client's nutritional status should be evaluated and if improvement is needed, it should be undertaken immediately. A good nutritional status before surgery enhances recovery. A nutritional assessment of the client before surgery will be helpful to the dietitian in providing nutrition that will be accepted by the client after surgery, when appetite is poor.

Improvement of nutritional status will usually mean providing extra protein, carbohydrates, vitamins, and minerals. The extra protein is needed for wound healing, tissue building, and blood regeneration. Extra carbohydrates will be converted to glycogen and stored to help provide energy after surgery, when needs are high and when clients may be unable to eat normally. The B vitamins are needed for the increased metabolism, vitamins A and C and zinc for wound healing, vitamin D for the absorption of calcium, and vitamin K for proper clotting of the blood. Iron is necessary for blood building, calcium and phosphorus for bones, and the other minerals for maintenance of acid–base, electrolyte, and fluid balance in the body.

In cases of overweight, improved nutritional status includes weight reduction before surgery whenever possible. Excess fat is a surgical hazard because the extra tissue increases the chances of infection, and fatty tissue tends to retain the anesthetic longer than other tissue.

Many physicians order their clients to be NPO (nothing by mouth) after midnight the night before surgery. Withholding food ensures that the stomach contains no food, which could be regurgitated and then **aspirated** into the lungs

hypermetabolic
higher-than-normal rate of metabolism

iatrogenic malnutrition
caused by treatment or diagnostic procedures

aspirated
inhaled or suctioned

during surgery. If there is to be gastrointestinal surgery, a low-residue diet may be ordered for a few days before surgery (see Chapter 18), to reduce intestinal residue.

Postsurgery Nutritional Care

The postsurgery diet is intended to provide calories and nutrients in amounts sufficient to fulfill the client's increased metabolic needs and to promote healing and subsequent recovery. In general, during the 24 hours immediately following major surgery, most clients will be given intravenous solutions only. These solutions will contain water, 5–10% dextrose, electrolytes, vitamins, and medications as needed. The maximum calories supplied by intravenous solutions are 400–500 calories per 24-hour period. The estimated daily calorie requirement for adults after surgery is 35–45 calories per kilogram of body weight. A 110-lb individual would require at least 2,000 calories a day. Obviously, until the client can take food, there will be a considerable calorie deficit each day. Body fat will be used to provide energy and to spare body protein, but the calorie intake must be increased to meet energy demands as soon as possible.

Because protein losses following surgery can be significant and because protein is especially needed then to rebuild tissue, control edema, avoid shock, resist infection, and transport fats, a high-protein diet may be recommended. Protein requirements for postsurgical clients can range from 1.5–2.0 g/kg of body weight per day. In addition, extra minerals and vitamins are needed. When peristalsis returns, ice chips may be given; if they are tolerated, a clear-liquid diet can follow. (Peristalsis is evidenced by the presence of bowel sounds.)

Normally in postoperative cases, clients proceed from the clear-liquid diet to the regular diet. Sometimes this change is done directly and sometimes by way of the full-liquid diet, depending on the client and the type of surgery. The average client will be able to take food within one to four days after surgery. If the client cannot take food then, parenteral or enteral feeding may be necessary.

Sometimes following gastric surgery, **dumping syndrome** occurs within 15–30 minutes after eating. This is characterized by dizziness, weakness, cramps, vomiting, and diarrhea. It is caused by food moving too quickly from the stomach into the small intestine.

To prevent dumping syndrome, smaller more frequent meals should be eaten and sugary drinks, sweets, and dried fruits should be avoided. Fluids should be limited to 4 oz at meals, or restricted completely, so as not to fill up the stomach with fluids instead of nutrients. Fluids can be taken 30 minutes after meals. Some clients do not tolerate milk well after gastric surgery, so its inclusion in the diet will depend on the client's tolerance.

The food habits of the postoperative client should be closely observed because they will affect recovery. When the client's appetite fails to improve, the physician and the dietitian should be notified, and efforts should be made to offer nutritious foods and supplements (either in liquid or solid form) that the client will ingest. The client should be encouraged to eat slowly to avoid swallowing air, which can cause abdominal distension and pain.

THE CLIENT RECEIVING ENTERAL NUTRITION

The term **enteral nutrition** means the forms of feeding that bring nutrients directly into the digestive tract (Figure 21-1). Oral feeding is the usual method and should be used whenever possible; however, when clients cannot or will not

dumping syndrome
nausea and diarrhea caused by food moving too quickly from the stomach to the small intestine

enteral nutrition
feeding by tube directly into the client's digestive tract

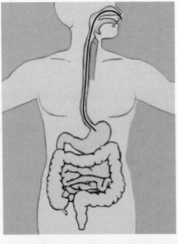

Nasogastric Route

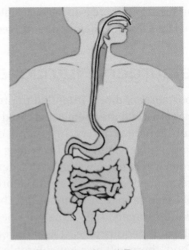

Nasoduodenal Route

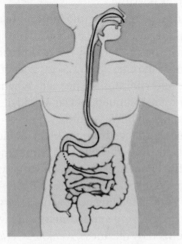

Nasojejunal Route

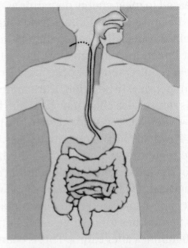

Esophagostomy Route

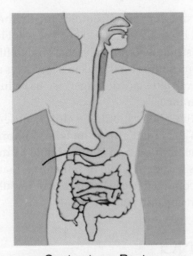

Gastrostomy Route

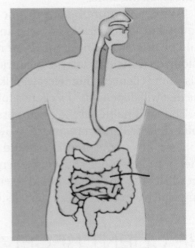

Jejunostomy Route

FIGURE 21-1 Enteral feeding routes.

take food by mouth but their gastrointestinal tract is working, they will be given a **tube feeding (TF)**. Enteral feedings are preferred over parenteral nutrition because there are many physiologic benefits of keeping the gut functioning, such as improved immune status. Tube feedings may be necessary because of unconsciousness, surgery, stroke, severe malnutrition, or extensive burns.

Usually, for periods that do not exceed six weeks, tube feeding is administered through a **nasogastric (NG) tube** inserted through the nose and into the stomach or small intestine. When the tube cannot be placed in the nose or when tube feedings will be required for more than four to six weeks, an opening called an enterostomy may be surgically created in either the esophagus (an esophagostomy), the stomach (**gastrostomy**), or the intestine (**jejunostomy**).

A percutaneous endoscopic gastrostomy tube (PEG) may be placed at the stomach if the patient is not at risk for aspiration. An esophagostomy tube might be placed at the side of the neck, at the level of the cervical spine after head and neck surgeries. A percutaneous endoscopic jejunostomy (sometimes referred to as JPEG) is a weighted feeding tube (from PEG insertion) passed into the duodenum. This is indicated for patients who cannot tolerate gastric feedings due to a history of reflux or aspiration or those who may have gastric obstruction or functional problems of the stomach. Sometimes, there is direct tube placement at the jejunum.

The tubes used for these feedings are soft, flexible, and as small as they can be and still allow the feeding to pass through. Although some tubes are weighted to keep them in place in the stomach or intestine, the use of weighted tubes has not been proved to be better than unweighted.

Numerous commercial formulas are available, with varying types and amounts of nutrients. Clients who are able to digest and absorb nutrients can be given **polymeric formulas** (1–2 calories/mL) containing intact proteins, carbohydrates, and fats that require digestion. Clients who have limited ability to digest or absorb nutrients may be given **elemental** or **hydrolyzed formulas** (1 calorie/mL) that contain the products of digestion of proteins, carbohydrates, and fats, and are lactose free. **Modular formulas** (3.8–4.0 calories/mL) can be used as supplements to other formulas or for developing customized formulas for certain clients (such as those with extensive wound-healing needs). The use of modular formulas has been decreasing due to the development of high-protein formulas. Disease-specific formulas have been developed to be used in the acute setting and for a short period of time. Clients admitted to the hospital with renal failure, respiratory failure, or liver failure have been shown to benefit from these specialized formulas.

There are three methods for administering tube feedings: continuous, intermittent, and bolus. Intermittent means to only administer tube feeding at night, with solid foods eaten during the day. If there is a food–drug interaction, such as with phenytoin (Dilantin), the TF should be stopped 1 hour before and be restarted one hour after administration of the medication via tube.

For bolus feedings, daily calorie needs of the client are usually divided into six servings per day (not to exceed 400 cc at a time). These feedings are given over a 15-minute time span and followed by 25–60 mL of water, hence the term *bolus*. This method is usually done when a client has a PEG tube, but it could also be done with an NG tube.

Usually the feedings are administered by a pump. This means the feeding is continuous during a 16- to 24-hour period. Tube feedings need to start slowly, such as 20–25 mL per hour. This rate may be increased by 10–25 mL every four hours until tolerance has been established and the client is at their goal rate to meet calorie needs. Early signs of intolerance may be abdominal

Exploring THE WEB

Search the Web for information on the various types of enteral nutrition formulas discussed in the text. What are the makeups of these formulas? Are any nutrients lacking in these formulas? Is there the potential for side effects of or allergies to these formulas that clients should be aware of and monitored for?

tube feeding (TF)
feeding by tube directly into the stomach or intestine or via a vein

nasogastric (NG) tube
tube leading from the nose to the stomach for tube feeding

gastrostomy
opening created by the surgeon directly into the stomach for enteral nutrition

jejunostomy
opening created by the surgeon into the intestine for enteral nutrition

polymeric formulas
commercially prepared formulas for tube feedings that contain intact proteins, carbohydrates, and fats that require digestion

elemental formulas
those formulas containing products of digestion of proteins, carbohydrates, and fats; also called hydrolyzed formulas

hydrolyzed formulas
contain products of digestion of proteins, carbohydrates, and fats; also called elemental formulas; used for clients who have difficulty digesting food

modular formulas
made by combining specific nutrients

distention, or if the client is verbal, verbalization of issues with cramping or nausea. Some may experience diarrhea. Patients in critical care may have delayed GI motility, therefore often have a pro-motility medication given. Gastric residuals are checked by nursing staff and newer protocols are suggesting that tube feedings do not need to be held until residuals reach 500 mL. When clients are ready to return to oral feedings, the transfer must be done gradually.

Possible Complications with Enteral Nutrition

The osmolality of a liquid substance indicates the number of particles per kilogram of solution. Solutions with more particles (high osmolality) exert more pressure than solutions with fewer particles. Solutions with high osmolality attract water from nearby fluids that contain lower osmolality. When a formula with high osmolality reaches the intestine, the body may draw fluid from the blood to dilute the formula. This process can cause weakness and diarrhea. However, diarrhea should be attributed to the tube feeding only when all other causes have been ruled out. Liquid medications containing sorbitol or *Clostridium difficile* (C-diff) (the bacterium that causes dysentery) are two possible causes of diarrhea.

Aspiration can occur (some of the formula enters the lung), causing the client to develop pneumonia. The tube may become clogged, or the client may pull the tube out. The placement of the feeding tube should be checked with an x-ray to decrease the possibility of aspiration. Before beginning the tube feeding, the health care provider must administer the flush solution according to the physician's order and raise the head of the bed. If the feeding is continuous, then the head of the bed needs to remain elevated. Some facilities, to verify correct placement of the NG tube in the stomach, will check the gastric pH before each use.

Clients requiring tube feeding may need a great deal of reassurance and support. The health care team should be patient and understanding during the care of tube-fed clients.

THE CLIENT RECEIVING PARENTERAL NUTRITION

Parenteral nutrition is the provision of nutrients intravenously. It is used if the gastrointestinal tract is not functional or if normal feeding is not adequate for the client's needs. It can be used alone or as part of a dietary plan that includes oral or tube feeding as well. When parenteral nutrition is used to provide total nutrition not using the GI tract, it is called total parenteral nutrition (TPN) or hyperalimentation. The TPN solution is a combination of dextrose (carbohydrate), amino acids (protein), lipids (fats), in addition to electrolytes and trace elements.

Nutrient solutions are prescribed by the physician and dietitian and are prepared by a pharmacist. They can be administered via a central vein or, for a period of two weeks or less, a **peripheral vein**. This solution is not combined until just before entry into the vein because the components do not form a stable solution.

Total parenteral nutrition that is required for an extended period is provided via a central vein. A catheter is surgically inserted, under sterile conditions, by a physician or an IV nurse. It is inserted into a subclavian vein or the superior vena cava. The vena cava is used because the high blood flow there facilitates the quick dilution of the highly concentrated TPN solution. Dilution reduces the possibility of **phlebitis** and **thrombosis**.

peripheral vein
a vein that is near the surface of the skin

phlebitis
inflammation of a vein

thrombosis
blockage, as a blood clot

When parenteral nutrition is no longer necessary, the client must be transferred gradually to an oral diet. Sometimes clients are given a tube feeding before oral feeding as they are weaned from TPN. Prior to weaning, the daily oral fluid and calorie goal must be close to being met. In weaning, the parenteral nutrition infusion volume may be decreased on a daily basis or there may be a reduction in the number of days of the week the infusion takes place. Assessment is done via the oral intake, stool, and urine output analysis along with monitoring of weight, electrolytes, and other laboratory parameters. The health care team works together to form an optimized diet and medication plan.

Possible Complications with Parenteral Nutrition

Infection can occur at the site of the catheter and enter the bloodstream, causing an infection of the blood, called **sepsis**. Bacterial or fungal infections can develop in the solution if it is unrefrigerated for over 24 hours. Abnormal electrolyte levels may develop, as can phlebitis or blood clots. Careful monitoring of the client is essential.

THE CLIENT WITH BURNS

In cases of serious burns, the loss of skin surface leads to enormous losses of fluids, electrolytes, and proteins. Water moves from other tissues to the burn site in an effort to compensate for the loss, but this only compounds the problem. This fluid loss can reduce the blood volume and thus blood pressure, as well as urine output.

Fluids and electrolytes are replaced by intravenous therapy immediately to prevent shock. Glucose is not included in these fluids for the first two to three days after the burn to avoid hyperglycemia.

The hypermetabolic state after a serious burn continues until the skin is largely healed, so there is an enormous increase in energy needed for the healing process. Calorie requirements are based on weight (size) and the total burned surface, including depth of burns, although most adult calorie needs are calculated at 35–40 kcal/kg per day. Protein needs for adults are as high as 1.5–2.0 g/kg of body weight. Children will need additional protein for healing at 2.5–3.0 g/kg per day. It is reasonable to provide 12–15% of nonprotein calories from fat. A high-protein, high-calorie diet is used. There is an increased need for vitamin C and zinc for healing and B vitamins for the metabolism of the extra nutrients. Vitamin A is important for the immune system and the epithelial tissues. The amino acids arginine and glutamine help increase immune functioning and wound healing. Arginine assists in wound healing by aiding in collagen formation and nitrogen retention. Some of glutamine's functions are to help prevent bacterial infections, improve immune function, and preserve gut integrity.

Also, it is essential that severely burned clients have sufficient fluids to help the kidneys hold the unusual load of wastes in solution and to replace those lost.

If the client is able to eat, oral feedings are advisable. Liquid commercial formulas may be used at first, and solid food may be added during the second week after the burn. If the client is unable to eat, tube feedings should be started immediately (Figure 21-2). In some cases, parenteral feeding is required. The foods served should be those the client likes and is willing to eat. To determine this, a registered dietitian must perform an individualized assessment for each burn victim. The best assessment of the adequacy of the nutrients provided is wound healing.

Exploring THE WEB

Search the Web for additional information on parenteral nutrition. What types of formulas are used for TPN? Are there nutrients lacking from this form of nutritional support? What possible side effects or allergies should the client be monitored for?

sepsis
infection of the blood

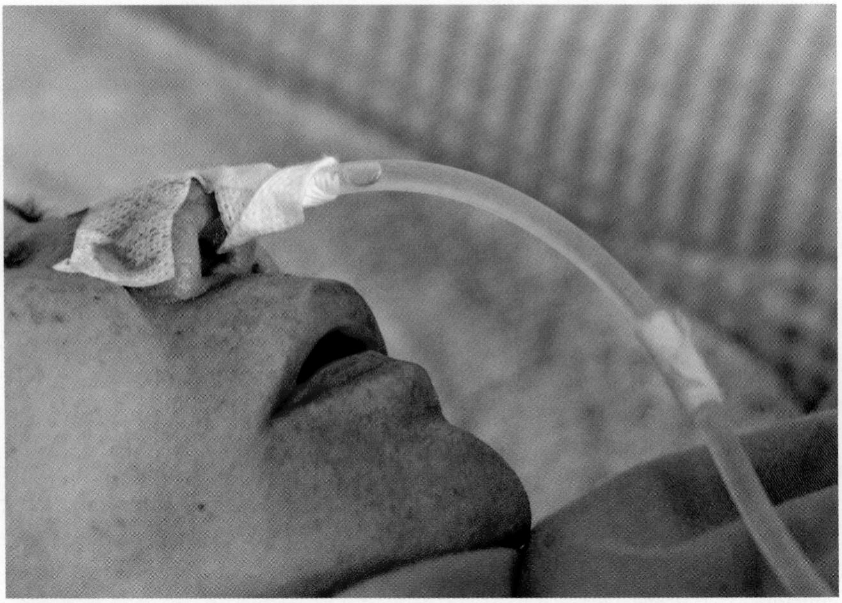

FIGURE 21-2 Adequate nutrition and assistance is essential for clients with severe burns.

Burn clients need a great deal of encouragement. They are in pain; are worried about disfigurement; and know they face a long, costly, and painful hospital stay with the possibility of surgery.

THE CLIENT WITH INFECTION

Fever typically accompanies an infection. Fevers and infections may be acute or chronic. Fever is a hypermetabolic state in which each degree of fever on the Fahrenheit scale raises the basal metabolic rate (BMR) by 7%. If extra calories are not provided during fever, the body first uses its supply of glycogen, then its stored fat, and finally its own muscle tissue for energy.

Protein intake should be increased because of infections (sepsis) and the amounts required need to be individualized. Protein is needed to replace body tissue and to produce **antibodies** to fight the infection. Minerals are needed to help build and repair body tissue and to maintain acid–base, electrolyte, and fluid balance. Extra calories are needed for the increased metabolic rate. Extra vitamins are also necessary for the increased metabolic rate and to help fight the infection causing the fever. Extra fluid is needed to replace that lost through perspiration, vomiting, or diarrhea, which often accompany infection.

Clients with fever usually have very poor appetites, but they will often accept ice water, fruit juice, and carbonated beverages. Some will accept broth, jello, or popsicles. Usually, the diet during fever and infection progresses from the liquid to the regular diet, with frequent, small meals recommended. It should be high in protein, calories, and vitamins. In some cases, parenteral and enteral feedings are necessary.

High doses of antibiotics or long-term use during infections can lead to oral **thrush**, a yeast infection caused by the *Candida* bacteria (Figure 21-3). Although the bacteria naturally exist in healthy individuals, it can only grow if a client has a compromised immune system. Clients with thrush usually experience decreased appetite due to pain on the tongue during eating. Treatment is not usually needed in oral thrush. Clients can take acidophilus capsules or eat yogurt containing acidophilus to speed recovery.

antibodies
substances produced by the body in reaction to foreign substance; neutralize toxins from foreign bodies

thrush
a yeast infection of the mucous membrane lining the mouth and tongue

THE CLIENT WITH AIDS

A virus is a microscopic parasite that invades and lives in or on, and thus infects, another organism, called the host. The virus obtains nourishment from the host and duplicates itself countless times. There are many viruses that infect humans. Some, like those of the common cold, make the host only mildly ill. Others, like the human immunodeficiency virus (HIV), are deadly.

HIV invades the T cells, which are white blood cells that protect the body from infections. When the T cells cannot function normally, the body has no resistance to opportunistic infections. Opportunistic infections are caused by other microorganisms that are present but do not affect people who have healthy immune systems.

Persons infected with HIV are said to be HIV positive. HIV infection ultimately leads to acquired immune deficiency syndrome (AIDS), which is incurable and fatal.

HIV can affect anyone exposed to it, regardless of age, sex, or physical condition. HIV infection cannot be cured, but it can be prevented. The virus is not transmitted through casual contact, such as shaking hands. It is transmitted via body fluids.

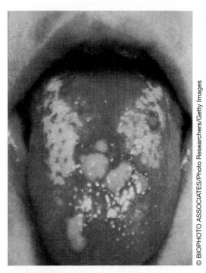

FIGURE 21-3 Thrush is very painful.

The Relationship of HIV Infection and Nutrition

A healthful diet is essential for a healthy immune system, which may delay the onset of AIDS. Persons diagnosed as being HIV positive should have a baseline nutrition and diet assessment by a registered dietitian. Unhealthful eating habits can be corrected at an early stage of the disease, and future nutritional needs can be explained.

As the condition progresses, the client begins to experience fatigue, skin rashes, headache, night sweats, diarrhea, weight loss, oral lesions, cough, fevers, and so forth. Infections increase the metabolic rate and nutrient and calorie needs and, at the same time, decrease the appetite and often the body's ability to absorb nutrients (Table 21-1).

Medications may further reduce the appetite and cause nausea. When there are oral infections, taste may change, and swallowing can become painful. Fever, pain, and depression can depress appetite. Dysphagia and dementia can also contribute to anorexia.

AIDS clients experience serious protein-energy malnutrition (PEM) and, thus, body wasting. This may be referred to as HIV wasting syndrome, which results in hypoalbuminemia and weight loss. The immune system is further damaged by insufficient amounts of protein and calories, thus hastening death.

human immunodeficiency virus (HIV)
a virus that weakens the body's immune system and ultimately leads to AIDS

opportunistic infections
caused by microorganisms that are present but that do not normally affect people with healthy immune systems

acquired immune deficiency syndrome (AIDS)
caused by the human immunodeficiency virus (HIV), which weakens the body's immune system, leaving it susceptible to fatal infections

hypoalbuminemia
abnormally low amounts of protein in the blood

TABLE 21-1 Causes of Nutrient Loss in AIDS Clients

- Anorexia
- Cancer
- Diarrhea
- Increased metabolism due to fever
- Certain medications
- Malabsorption caused by cancer or diarrhea
- Protein-energy malnutrition

TABLE 21-2 Methods to Improve the Appetite of an AIDS Client

- Give medications *after* meals.
- Offer soft food.
- Avoid spicy, acidic, and extremely hot or cold foods.
- Serve frequent, small meals.
- Add sugar and flavorings to liquid supplements.
- Take advantage of the "good" days and offer any food the client tolerates.
- Talk with the client to help ease concerns about finances, family, and friends.

In The Media

Managing Stress Is Key for Individuals with HIV and AIDS

Increased stress can have a number of negative effects on the physical body. Such negative effects include digestive and sleep disorders, headaches, depression, anxiety, and immune system suppression. For individuals with HIV and AIDS, managing stress can be especially beneficial. Stress reduces the production of T cells, which are produced to help fight infections. T cells are lowered in HIV/AIDS individuals. Participating in muscle relaxation, deep breathing, meditation, low-impact exercise, massage, acupuncture, and maintaining a healthy diet can help reduce stress levels and promote overall mental and physical health.

Source: Adapted from Scrivani, Joseph Robert. (2016, January 7). "The Importance of Stress Management for People with HIV/AIDS." Accessed January 2016. www.goodtherapy.org

Problems Related to Feeding AIDS Clients

Just when an AIDS client most needs a nutrient- and calorie-rich diet, he or she is most apt to refuse it. It may be useful to discuss nutritional care with the client and offer methods to improve appetite (Table 21-2).

Because of the nausea and diarrhea, sufficient fluids are essential. If the client has difficulty swallowing or simply cannot eat, tube feeding may be imperative. If the tube causes pain or if severe diarrhea or malabsorption is present, parenteral nutrition may be necessary.

IMPROVING CLIENT'S NUTRITIONAL STATUS IN THE HOSPITAL SETTING

The importance of improving a client's nutritional status is obvious. Formal nutritional assessments of clients should be made on a regular basis, but all members of the health care team should be alert to signs of malnutrition on a daily basis. The nurse or nursing assistant who sees the client regularly is in the best position to help the client. The nurse will inform the dietitian of decreased intake. The dietitian may implement the following:

1. The client may need information about nutritional needs.
2. The client may need a supplement.
3. The client may want other foods.

If not contraindicated by the client's health condition, it can be helpful to invite friends and relatives to bring the client some of his or her favorite foods.

Serving the Meal

More and more hospitals across the nation are using a "room service" menu whereby a patient is allowed to make reasonable selections, within a flexible time frame, from the menu provided. Therapeutic diets are still served; however, if at all possible, a liberalized menu plan is used to facilitate a good intake. When a meal is served at the bedside, the tray should be lined with a pretty cloth or paper liner. Attractive dishes that fit the tray conveniently without crowding it should be used. The food should be arranged attractively on the plate with a garnish. Utensils must be arranged conveniently. Water should be served as well as another beverage (unless it is prohibited by the physician). Foods must be served at proper temperatures.

When the client is on complete bed rest, special preparations are required before the meal is served. The client should be given the opportunity to use the bedpan and to wash before the meal is served. The client should be helped to a comfortable position, and any unpleasant sights should be removed before the meal is served. Pleasant conversation during the preparations can improve the client's mood considerably. Certain topics of conversation can help stimulate the client's interest in eating. Appropriate remarks on the client's progress, whenever possible, are helpful.

At meal time, the tray should be placed on the bedside table and positioned for easy feeding or if necessary, convenient for someone else to do the feeding. If the client needs help, the napkin should be opened and placed, the bread spread, the meat cut, and the straw offered. The client should be encouraged to eat and be allowed sufficient time.

If the client complains of too much food on the tray, then one might try serving one to two dishes at a time. Many older clients find it disturbing to waste food and therefore may benefit from smaller portions at meal times. The physician may note a poor intake and may request a calorie and protein count, which is an accurate report of the types and amounts of food eaten.

Feeding the Client Who Requires Assistance

If the client is unable to self-feed, the person doing the feeding should sit near the side of the bed (Figure 21-4). Small amounts of food should be placed toward the back of the mouth with a slight pressure on the tongue with the spoon or fork. The client must be allowed to self-help as much as possible. If the client begins to choke, assist in sitting up straight. Food or water obviously should not be given while the client is choking. The client's mouth should be wiped as needed. A client diagnosed with dysphagia will require a specialized diet. Depending upon the swallowing abnormality, the client may need pureed foods with either thin or thickened (to a nectar or honey consistency) liquids. A dysphagic client should not use straws.

Feeding the Blind Client

Special care must be taken in serving a meal to a client who is blind. An appetizing description of the meal can help create a desire to eat. To help the client who is blind self-feed, arrange the food as if the plate were the face of a clock

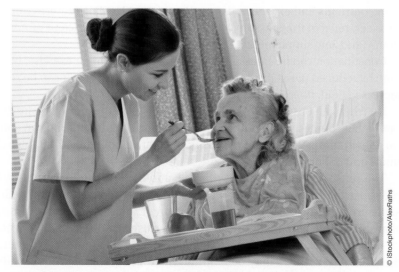

FIGURE 21-4 Some clients require assistance when eating.

Exploring THE WEB

Search the Web for information on nutritional status during acute or chronic illness. Why is appetite affected by illness? For what length of time is it normal to have a decreased appetite when ill? What can be done to improve appetite and maintain nutritional balance when ill?

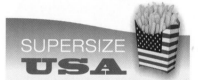

SUPERSIZE USA

According to a new study published in the journal *eLife*, frequent late-night snacking can alter brain physiology, causing a deficiency in the hippocampal area of the brain, which controls learning and memory. Current studies, which were conducted on mice, tested the ability of mice to recognize a novel object. Nerve impulses to the hippocampus were reduced when food was offered to mice during a six-hour window in the middle of their sleep time as opposed to their daytime window. Eating at the wrong time can not only impair cognition but also disrupt sleep patterns. Researchers have yet to confirm their findings in humans, but have found that night shift workers have shown to perform less well on cognitive tests.

Source: Adapted from *Science Daily* (2015, December 23). "Midnight Munchies Mangle Memory." Accessed January 2016. www.sciencedaily.com

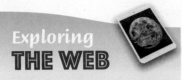

Exploring
THE WEB

Search the Web for adaptive devices that may help a client with a disability self-feed. Become familiar with the operation of these devices so that you can aid in teaching clients how to help themselves.

(Figure 21-5). The meat might be put at 6 o'clock, vegetables at 9 o'clock, salad at 12, and bread at 3 o'clock. The person who regularly arranges the meal should remember to use the same pattern for all meals. Plate guards should be placed around the plate to assist with feeding and prevent food from spilling. People who are blind usually feel better when they can help themselves.

Transition to Home

When a client is discharged from the hospital to go home, the dietitian may be asked to give the client a diet plan. Examples of diet plans include low-sodium, low-cholesterol, and low-residue diets. In the home, the family menu should be adapted and serve as the basis of the client's meal when possible.

LONG-TERM CARE OF THE ELDERLY

Because of increasing longevity, the number of elderly people requiring long-term care is increasing. The changes people undergo with age that can affect their nutritional status are discussed in Chapter 13.

Physical Problems of the Elderly in Long-Term Care

It is estimated that the majority of people 85 and above have at least one chronic disease, such as arthritis, osteoporosis, diabetes mellitus, cardiovascular disease, or mental disorder. These conditions affect their attitudes, physical activities, appetites, and, thus, nutritional status. PEM is a major concern for this population.

Anemia can develop if the client has insufficient iron intake. It can contribute to confusion and depression but may go unnoticed because one of its major symptoms, fatigue, may be simply thought to be a characteristic of old age. It is helpful to make sure there is sufficient animal protein and vitamin C (an iron enhancer) in the client's diet.

Pressure ulcers (bedsores) can develop in bedridden clients. The ulcers develop in areas where unrelieved pressure on the skin prevents the blood from bringing nutrients and oxygen and removing wastes. Healing requires treatment of the ulcer, relief of the pressure, a high-calorie diet with sufficient protein, and vitamin C and zinc supplements. Prevention is a must.

Constipation can be caused by inadequate fiber, fluid, or exercise; by medication; by reduced peristalsis; or by former abuse of laxatives. It can be relieved by increased fluid, fiber, and exercise (if possible).

Diarrhea can be caused by digestive disorders, medications, viruses, bacteria, and other sources. It will reduce the absorption of nutrients and can contribute to dehydration. An increase of fiber in the diet combined with supplemental vitamins and minerals may be helpful.

The sense of smell declines with age, and the appetite diminishes. A reduced sense of taste can be caused by medications, disease, mineral deficiencies, or xerostomia (dry mouth). The addition of spices, herbs, salt, and sugar (if allowed) can be helpful. Xerostomia can be caused by disease or medications. Drinking water, eating frequent small meals, and chewing sugar-free gums or sucking on hard candies may be helpful. The inadequate amount of saliva in these clients contributes to increased tooth decay.

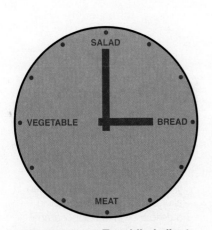

FIGURE 21-5 To a blind client, a plate of food can be pictured as the face of a clock.

pressure ulcers
bedsores

Dysphagia (difficulty in swallowing) can result from a stroke, closed head trauma, head or neck cancer, surgery, or Alzheimer's and other diseases. A swallow study needs to be done to determine the consistency of diet needed by clients with dysphagia. A swallow study is done by a speech therapist using a video fluoroscope. While being videotaped, the client is given liquids, semiliquids, pureed food, and solid food to determine the consistency of the bolus (food mass) that he or she is able to swallow without aspirating. Many dysphagia clients must have thickened liquids. Dysphagia clients should always be in an upright position with their chin tucked toward their chest when eating. This will prevent aspiration. Nursing staff must be sure swallowing is complete for at-risk patients. If patient can tolerate foods of regular consistency, care needs to be taken to ensure food is cut up into small pieces prior to consumption.

Some individuals may become more sedentary in long-term care than they were in their home setting, and they may have a lack of appetite. Activity and exercise may be offered in the facility; however, many are not able to participate due to physical limitations. Menu advancements have been made in many of the long-term care establishments to improve intake and general nutrition, but some facilities still lag behind. All care-giving staff and nurses should advocate for optimum conditions for our elderly. They all need, respond to, and deserve warmth and respect from their caregivers in addition to excellent care.

HEALTH AND NUTRITION CONSIDERATIONS

Clients who fall within the categories of conditions discussed in this chapter can be a challenge for the health care professional. Clients experiencing illness, hospitalization, and/or surgery may seem to make excessive demands due to pain, uncertainty, or anxiety.

The health care professional can help herself or himself as well as the client by thinking positively and using therapeutic communication with the client and family. Enhancing the nutrition status of the patient, whether it be by assisting with menu selections, ensuring supplementation, or providing parenteral or enteral nutrition, is of paramount importance in recovery and rehabilitation. Healing is facilitated when there is optimum nutrition provided.

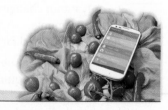

SUMMARY

Surgery, burns, fevers, and infections are traumas that cause the body to respond hypermetabolically. This response creates the need for additional nutrients at the same time that the injury causes a loss of nutrients. Care must be taken to provide extra fluid, proteins, calories, vitamins, minerals, and carbohydrates as needed in these situations. When surgery is elective, nutritional status should be improved before surgery, if necessary. When food cannot be taken orally, enteral or parenteral nutrition may be used. Elderly clients requiring long-term care may be at risk from several nutrition-related health problems that, with proper treatment, can sometimes be relieved. The health care team should work together to improve the clients' nutritional status.

DISCUSSION TOPICS

1. In what ways might a diet history of a presurgical client be helpful?

2. Why must a client's stomach be empty at the time of surgery?

3. Explain why intravenous dextrose solutions are not sufficient to fulfill nutritional requirements after surgery.

4. Describe parenteral nutrition. What is it? How is it delivered? What are some dangers related to it?

5. How do illness and surgery affect one's nutrition?

6. What is iatrogenic malnutrition? How might it develop?

7. In what ways might the nurse help improve the client's nutrition?

8. How can the behavior and attitude of the attending person affect the appetite of the client?

9. Why is anemia so easily overlooked in elderly clients?

10. Discuss how a diminished sense of smell might affect one's appetite.

SUGGESTED ACTIVITIES

1. Ask a certified nutrition support dietitian (CNSD) to visit the class and discuss tube feedings, telling why and when they are used and problems associated with them.

2. Invite a nurse from a local hospital to discuss burns and the nutritional challenges facing clients with burns.

3. If a class member has experienced any of the traumas discussed in this chapter, ask that person to recount it and describe her or his reactions, appetite, and recovery.

4. Role-play a situation in which a client is five days' postsurgery and cannot eat and the nurse is trying to convince her to eat.

5. Invite a nurse who works in a nursing home to talk to the class. Ask the nurse to describe techniques with client feeding. Ask the nurse about the dietitian's role at his health facility.

REVIEW

Multiple choice. Select the *letter* that precedes the best answer.

1. During trauma, there is usually
   a. reduced need for protein and minerals
   b. a hypermetabolic response in the body
   c. only minor changes in nutritional requirements
   d. decreased need for calories

2. Wound healing, tissue building, and blood regeneration all require
   a. extra fat
   b. extra cholesterol
   c. megadoses of vitamin C
   d. additional protein

3. Protein is needed after major surgery to
   a. provide calories
   b. resist infection
   c. control fat metabolism during trauma
   d. aid in healing

4. Dumping syndrome is characterized by
   a. migraine headache
   b. hypertension and tremors
   c. reduced clotting time
   d. dizziness and cramps

5. TPN for more than two weeks is given through
   a. a nasogastric tube
   b. a peripheral vein in the ankle
   c. the superior vena cava
   d. an esophagostomy

6. Normal absorption of nutrients
   a. is not affected by chemotherapy
   b. is unaffected by diarrhea
   c. can be decreased after surgery
   d. is unaffected by PEM

7. Iatrogenic malnutrition
   a. is the inevitable result of surgery
   b. can be a result of hospitalization
   c. is commonly caused by low-grade fevers
   d. has no effect on wound healing

8. Dysphagia
   a. means memory loss
   b. is common following bone surgery
   c. can safely be ignored
   d. sufferers should not be fed in the supine position

9. Feeding the client who requires assistance involves
   a. placing small amount of food toward the back of the mouth
   b. feeding in the supine position
   c. giving sips of fluid between bites
   d. cutting food into bite-size pieces

10. Favorite foods brought to hospitalized clients from home
    a. should not be allowed
    b. have no effect on the client's nutritional status
    c. should be approved by the dietitian before being given to the client
    d. are neither helpful nor harmful

CASE IN POINT

BETTY: TRANSITIONING FROM PARENTERAL NUTRITION

Betty and her husband Kenny were recently in a car accident on the way to visit their daughter. The weather took a turn for the worse and Kenny hit a patch of black ice. The car slid off the road and flipped into a ditch. Kenny wasn't seriously injured in the accident, but Betty had to be airlifted to the trauma center at a local hospital. She was found to have leg and ankle fractures, rib fractures with abdominal injuries, and head injuries. She was sedated for over a week while she underwent numerous surgeries in an attempt to save her life. During this time, Betty's nutritional needs were being provided via hyperalimentation. Kenny and Betty are both 83 years old, and Kenny is worried that she will not survive the surgeries. Although she was seriously injured, the doctor assured Kenny that his wife is responding well.

The hospital dietitian monitored Betty's nutritional status, including weight and lab values, closely. After three weeks, she was able to transition to oral nutrition. The doctor estimates that Betty will be hospitalized for a few more weeks, followed by several weeks of rehab and therapy for her fractures. When she began eating again, the nurses noted she was eating only 30–40% of her meals. The doctor was afraid her poor intake would inhibit her wounds from healing properly. The physical therapist noted that her tolerance for activity was low and her fatigue came rapid and easily. The dietitian requested the nurses document all foods Betty consumes. She also ordered a high-protein supplement for Betty to have between meals.

ASSESSMENT

1. What information do you have about Betty and her nutrition?
2. What deficit does the dietitian suspect?
3. What does the physician suspect?
4. How significant is the problem?
5. If Betty were 5-ft 2-in tall and weighed 110 lb before the accident, what would be her daily protein requirements?
6. What two benefits of protein is Betty missing?

DIAGNOSIS

7. What is the cause of Betty's nutritional problem?
8. Complete the following nursing diagnosis statement: Betty's imbalanced nutrition less than body requirements, related to _____.

PLAN/GOAL

9. What is your goal for Betty?

IMPLEMENTATION

10. What will the calorie count reveal?
11. What do you need to know about Betty's food preferences?
12. What could Kenny do to help during meals?
13. What should be the size and frequency of Betty's meals?
14. Should appetite stimulants be used?
15. Should liquid nutritional supplements be used?
16. Which proteins could provide the highest quality per bite?

EVALUATION/OUTCOME CRITERIA

17. What criteria would the doctor, physical therapist, and dietitian use to evaluate the effectiveness of the plan?
18. Would weight gain be an effective criterion? If not, why?

THINKING FURTHER

19. How could the lessons from this case be used in other situations?

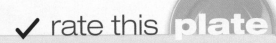

✔ rate this plate

Along with offering a protein supplement between meals, the dietitian encouraged Betty to include protein sources in her meals and snacks. Increased protein intake will provide her with additional energy and assist in healing her fractures. Rate the plate she ate for breakfast:

½ cup oatmeal

¼ cup blueberries

1 slice whole-wheat toast with butter

4 oz strawberry yogurt

4 oz orange juice

Sips of coffee

How many calories and grams of protein did Betty receive from this meal? Was this meal sufficient in calories and protein? What foods can be added to this meal, if any, to increase protein? What can be done to encourage Betty to eat more than 50% of her plate at meal time?

CASE IN POINT

LOUIS: SUFFERING FROM WEIGHT LOSS AND SKIN BREAKDOWN

Louis is a 79-year-old African American man. He had been married for 47 years until his wife passed away six months ago. Since her death, things just haven't been the same for Louis. He finds himself very lonely and at a loss for what to do. He never was a good cook, but now he has no desire to prepare meals at all. He spends most of his days sitting in his recliner watching television. Louis's brother, Lenny, who's also single, has been worried about Louis. He has decided to move in with him, at least temporarily, to help support his brother physically and emotionally.

When Lenny arrives at Louis's house, he notices Louis has lost quite a bit of weight since he last saw him. His skin looks very thin and dry. Lenny begins to prepare meals for Louis. Louis is thankful for the meals, but still has very little appetite. Lenny complies with Louis's request to stay in his recliner for meals. Louis states his gait has become increasingly unsteady and he prefers to just stay put.

Now that Lenny has been with Louis about a week, he realizes that Louis is even sleeping in his recliner. In fact, Louis really only gets up when he needs to use the bathroom. Lenny decides he needs to assist his brother in getting a shower and a little activity. While assisting Louis, his brother notices a large pressure ulcer on his tailbone. Lenny is very concerned and decides to take Louis to the doctor. Louis's doctor determines he needs to have surgery to clean and repair the ulcer, and then Louis must keep off his tailbone for several weeks. Louis is also instructed to increase his protein intake, to assist in wound healing. Louis's doctor asks the two men to meet with a dietitian to review a meal plan that would facilitate wound healing and help Louis regain some of the weight he has lost over the past several months.

ASSESSMENT

1. What do you know about Louis and his nutrition?
2. Did he eat a balanced diet?
3. What barriers were there to his healing?
4. What foods are priorities for healing?
5. How significant is nutrition to this problem?

DIAGNOSIS

6. Write at least two diagnoses that apply to Louis's problem.

PLAN/GOAL

7. What is the priority goal for Louis?

IMPLEMENTATION

8. What does the dietitian need to know about Louis to help?
9. What is the dietitian likely to recommend?
10. How could vitamin supplements help?
11. Who else can help?
12. What strategies could be helpful to get Louis to eat?
13. What could a home health nurse do?
14. What does Louis need to do to help himself?
15. If Louis is unable to eat enough food to maintain his weight, what alternatives does the doctor have?

EVALUATION/OUTCOME CRITERIA

16. What needs to happen for Louis to avoid having a feeding tube?
17. What criteria will the doctor use to determine if the plan is effective?

THINKING FURTHER

18. How are Louis's needs similar to those of any other surgical client?
19. What are the most serious consequences if Louis is unable to heal, even with tube feedings?

✔ rate this plate

Lenny made the following meal for Louis. Rate this plate on protein quality:

6 oz baked meatloaf

1 medium baked potato with shredded cheese and butter

¾ cup mixed vegetables

1 dinner roll with butter

4 oz custard cup

How many grams of protein are in this meal? Is it enough to support the healing of Louis' ulcer?

DIETARY GUIDELINES FOR AMERICANS, 2015–2020: ESTIMATED CALORIE NEEDS PER DAY BY AGE, SEX, AND PHYSICAL ACTIVITY LEVEL[a]

Reprinted from *Dietary Guidelines for Americans, 2015-2020* (8th ed.), by the U.S. Department of Health and Human Services and U.S. Department of Agriculture, 2015, Washington, DC: U.S. Government Printing Office.

Gender/ Activity level[b]	Male/ Sedentary	Male/ Moderately active	Male/ Active	Female[c]/ Sedentary	Female[c]/ Moderately active	Female[c]/ Active
Age (years)						
2	1,000	1,000	1,000	1,000	1,000	1,000
3	1,000	1,400	1,400	1,000	1,200	1,400
4	1,200	1,400	1,600	1,200	1,400	1,400
5	1,200	1,400	1,600	1,200	1,400	1,600
6	1,400	1,600	1,800	1,200	1,400	1,600
7	1,400	1,600	1,800	1,200	1,600	1,800
8	1,400	1,600	2,000	1,400	1,600	1,800
9	1,600	1,800	2,000	1,400	1,600	1,800
10	1,600	1,800	2,200	1,400	1,800	2,000
11	1,800	2,000	2,200	1,600	1,800	2,000
12	1,800	2,200	2,400	1,600	2,000	2,200
13	2,000	2,200	2,600	1,600	2,000	2,200
14	2,000	2,400	2,800	1,800	2,000	2,400
15	2,200	2,600	3,000	1,800	2,000	2,400
16	2,400	2,800	3,200	1,800	2,000	2,400
17	2,400	2,800	3,200	1,800	2,000	2,400
18	2,400	2,800	3,200	1,800	2,000	2,400
19–20	2,600	2,800	3,000	2,000	2,200	2,400
21–25	2,400	2,800	3,000	2,000	2,200	2,400
26–30	2,400	2,600	3,000	1,800	2,000	2,400
31–35	2,400	2,600	3,000	1,800	2,000	2,200
36–40	2,400	2,600	2,800	1,800	2,000	2,200

(continues)

(continued)

Gender/ Activity level[b]	Male/ Sedentary	Male/ Moderately active	Male/ Active	Female[c]/ Sedentary	Female[c]/ Moderately active	Female[c]/ Active
Age (years)						
41–45	2,200	2,600	2,800	1,800	2,000	2,200
46–50	2,200	2,400	2,800	1,800	2,000	2,200
51–55	2,200	2,400	2,800	1,600	1,800	2,200
56–60	2,200	2,400	2,600	1,600	1,800	2,200
61–65	2,000	2,400	2,600	1,600	1,800	2,000
66–70	2,000	2,200	2,600	1,600	1,800	2,000
71–75	2,000	2,200	2,600	1,600	1,800	2,000
76+	2,000	2,200	2,400	1,600	1,800	2,000

[a]Based on Estimated Energy Requirements (EER) equations, using reference heights (average) and reference weights (healthy) for each age–gender group. For children and adolescents, reference height and weight vary. For adults, the reference man is 5 ft 10 in tall and weighs 154 lb. The reference woman is 5 ft 4 in tall and weighs 126 lb. EER equations are from the Institute of Medicine. Dietary Reference Intakes for Energy, Carbohydrate, Fiber, Fat, Fatty Acids, Cholesterol, Protein, and Amino Acids. Washington (DC): The National Academies Press; 2002.

[b]Sedentary means a lifestyle that includes only the light physical activity associated with typical day-to-day life. Moderately active means a lifestyle that includes physical activity equivalent to walking about 1.5–3 miles per day at 3–4 miles per hour, in addition to the light physical activity associated with typical day-to-day life. Active means a lifestyle that includes physical activity equivalent to walking more than 3 miles per day at 3–4 miles per hour, in addition to the light physical activity associated with typical day-to-day life.

[c]Estimates for females do not include women who are pregnant or breastfeeding.

DIETARY GUIDELINES FOR AMERICANS, 2015–2020: FOOD SOURCES OF SELECTED NUTRIENTS

Selected Foods from *Dietary Guidelines for Americans, 2015–2020* (8th ed.), by the U.S. Department of Health and Human Services and U.S. Department of Agriculture, 2016, Washington, DC: U.S. Government Printing Office.

Appendix B-1　　Potassium

Selected food sources ranked by amounts of potassium and calories per standard food portion.

Food	Standard portion size	Calories in standard portion[a]	Potassium in standard portion (mg)[a]
Potato, baked, flesh and skin	1 medium potato	163	941
Prune juice, canned	1 cup	182	707
Carrot juice, canned	1 cup	94	689
Tomato paste	¼ cup	54	664
Beet greens, cooked	½ cup	19	654
White beans, canned	½ cup	149	595
Tomato juice, canned	1 cup	41	556
Plain yogurt, nonfat or low-fat	8 ounces	127	579
Tomato puree	½ cup	48	549
Sweet potato, baked in skin	1 medium	103	542
Clams, canned	3 ounces	121	534
Orange juice, fresh	1 cup	112	496
Halibut, cooked	3 ounces	94	449
Soybeans, green, cooked	½ cup	127	485
Tuna, yellowfin, cooked	3 ounces	111	448
Lima beans, cooked	½ cup	108	478
Soybeans, mature, cooked	½ cup	149	443
Rockfish, Pacific, cooked	3 ounces	93	397
Chocolate milk (1%, 2%, and whole)	1 cup	178–208	418–425
Bananas	1 medium	105	422
Spinach, cooked	½ cup	21–25	370–419
Tomato sauce	½ cup	30	364
Peaches, dried, uncooked	¼ cup	96	399
Prunes, stewed	½ cup	133	398
Skim milk (nonfat)	1 cup	83	382

(continues)

(continued)

Food	Standard portion size	Calories in standard portion[a]	Potassium in standard portion (mg)[a]
Rainbow trout, wild or farmed, cooked	3 ounces	128–143	381–383
Apricots, dried, uncooked	¼ cup	78	378
Pinto beans, cooked	½ cup	123	373
Low-fat milk (1%)	1 cup	98–102	366–370
Lentils, cooked	½ cup	115	365
Plantains, cooked	½ cup	89	358
Kidney beans, cooked	½ cup	113	357

[a]Source: U.S. Department of Agriculture, Agricultural Research Service, Nutrient Data Laboratory. 2014. USDA National Nutrient Database for Standard Reference, Release 27. Available at: http://www.ars.usda.gov/nutrientdata.

Appendix B-2   Dietary Fiber

Selected food sources ranked by amounts of dietary fiber and calories per standard food portion.

Food	Standard portion size	Calories in standard portion[a]	Dietary fiber in standard portion (g)[a]
Beans (navy, pinto, black, kidney, white, great northern, lima), cooked	½ cup	108–149	5.7–9.6
High fiber bran ready-to-eat cereal	⅓–¾ cup	60–81	9.1–14.3
Split peas, lentils, chickpeas, or cowpeas, cooked	½ cup	99–176	5.6–8.1
Artichoke, Globe or French, cooked	½ cup	45	7.2
Pear	1 medium	101	5.5
Soybeans, cooked	½ cup	149	5.2
Plain rye wafer crackers	2 wafers	73	5.0
Wheat bran ready-to-eat cereals (various)	¾ cup	90–98	4.9–5.5
Quinoa, cooked	½ cup	111	2.6
Green peas, cooked (fresh, frozen, canned)	½ cup	59–67	3.5–4.4
Peanuts, oil roasted	1 ounce	92	2.7
Bulgur, cooked	½ cup	76	4.1
Mixed vegetables, cooked from frozen	½ cup	59	4.0
Raspberries	½ cup	32	4.0
Sweet potato, baked in skin	1 medium	103	3.8
Blackberries	½ cup	31	3.8
Soybeans, green, cooked	½ cup	127	3.8
Prunes, stewed	½ cup	133	3.8
Shredded wheat ready-to-eat cereal (various)	1–1¼ cup	155–220	5.0–9.0
Figs, dried	¼ cup	93	3.7
Apple, with skin	1 medium	95	4.4
Pumpkin, canned	½ cup	42	3.6
Collards, cooked	½ cup	32	3.8
Almonds	1 ounce	163	3.5
Popcorn	3 cups	93	3.5
Whole wheat spaghetti, cooked	½ cup	87	3.2
Banana	1 medium	105	3.1
Orange	1 medium	69	3.1
Guava	1 fruit	37	3.0
Potato, baked, with skin	1 medium	163	3.6

(continues)

(continued)

Food	Standard portion size	Calories in standard portion[a]	Dietary fiber in standard portion (g)[a]
Oat bran muffin	1 small	178	3.0
Pearled barley, cooked	½ cup	97	3.0
Dates	¼ cup	104	2.9
Winter squash, cooked	½ cup	38	2.9
Parsnips, cooked	½ cup	55	2.8

[a]Source: U.S. Department of Agriculture, Agricultural Research Service, Nutrient Data Laboratory. 2014. USDA National Nutrient Database for Standard Reference, Release 27. Available at: http://www.ars.usda.gov/nutrientdata.

Appendix B-3   Calcium

Selected food sources ranked by amounts of calcium and calories per standard food portion.

Food	Standard portion size	Calories in standard portion[a]	Calcium in standard portion[a] (mg)
Fortified ready-to-eat cereals (various)	¾–1¼	100–210	250–1,000
Orange juice, calcium fortified	1 cup	117	349
Plain yogurt, nonfat	8 ounces	127	452
Romano cheese	1½ ounces	165	452
Pasteurized process Swiss cheese	2 ounces	189	438
Evaporated milk	½ cup	170	329
Tofu, regular, prepared with calcium sulfate	½ cup	94	434
Plain yogurt, low-fat	8 ounces	143	415
Fruit yogurt, low-fat	8 ounces	238	383
Ricotta cheese, part skim	½ cup	171	337
Swiss cheese	1½ ounces	162	336
Sardines, canned in oil, drained	3 ounces	177	325
Pasteurized process American cheese food	2 ounces	187	387
Provolone cheese	1½ ounces	149	321
Mozzarella cheese, part-skim	1½ ounces	128	304
Cheddar cheese	1½ ounces	173	287
Low-fat milk (1%)	1 cup	102	305
Muenster cheese	1½ ounces	156	305
Skim milk (nonfat)	1 cup	83	299
Soymilk, original and vanilla, with added calcium	1 cup	109	340
Reduced fat milk (2%)	1 cup	122	293
Low-fat chocolate milk (1%)	1 cup	178	290
Whole buttermilk	1 cup	152	282
Rice milk, with added calcium	1 cup	113	283
Whole chocolate milk	1 cup	208	280
Whole milk	1 cup	149	276
Reduced fat chocolate milk (2%)	1 cup	190	273
Ricotta cheese, whole milk	½ cup	216	257
Tofu, raw, regular, prepared with calcium sulfate	½ cup	94	434

[a]Source: U.S. Department of Agriculture, Agricultural Research Service, Nutrient Data Laboratory. 2014. USDA National Nutrient Database for Standard Reference, Release 27. Available at: http://www.ars.usda.gov/nutrientdata.

Appendix B-4   Vitamin D

Selected food sources ranked by amounts of vitamin D and calories per standard food portion.

Food	Standard portion size	Calories in standard portion[a]	Vitamin D in standard portion[a,b] (mcg)
Salmon, sockeye, canned	3 ounces	142	17.9
Salmon, Chinook, smoked	3 ounces	99	14.5
Salmon, pink, canned	3 ounces	117	12.3
Rockfish, Pacific, mixes species, cooked	3 ounces	93	3.9
Tuna, light, canned in oil, drained	3 ounces	168	5.7
Orange juice,[c] fortified	1 cup	117	2.5
Sardine, canned in oil, drained	3 ounces	177	4.1
Yogurt (various types and flavors)[c]	8 ounces	98–254	2.0–3.0
Whole milk[c]	1 cup	149	3.2
Whole chocolate milk[c]	1 cup	208	3.2
Reduced fat chocolate milk (2%)[c]	1 cup	190	3.0
Milk (nonfat, 1% and 2%)[c]	1 cup	83–122	2.9
Low-fat chocolate milk (1%)[c]	1 cup	178	2.8
Soymilk[c]	1 cup	109	2.9
Almond milk (all flavors)[c]	1 cup	91–120	2.4
Flatfish (flounder and sole), cooked	3 ounces	73	3.0
Fortified ready-to-eat cereals (various)[c]	⅓–1¼ cup	74–247	0.2–2.5
Rice drink[c]	1 cup	113	2.4
Herring, Atlantic, cooked	3 ounces	173	4.7
Pork, cooked (various cuts)	3 ounces	122–390	0.2–2.2
Margarine (various)[c]	1 tbsp	75–100	1.5
Egg, hard-boiled	1 large	78	1.1
Mushrooms, Chanterelle, raw	½ cup	10	1.4

[a]Source: U.S. Department of Agriculture, Agricultural Research Service, Nutrient Data Laboratory. 2014. USDA National Nutrient Database for Standard Reference, Release 27. Available at: http://www.ars.usda.gov/nutrientdata.

[b]1 mcg of vitamin D is equivalent to 40 IU.

[c]Vitamin D fortified.

DIETARY GUIDELINES FOR AMERICANS, 2015–2020: EATING PATTERNS

Reprinted from *Dietary Guidelines for Americans, 2015–2020* (8th ed.), by the U.S. Department of Health and Human Services and U.S. Department of Agriculture, 2016, Washington, DC: U.S. Government Printing Office.

Appendix C-1

Healthy U.S.-Style Eating Pattern: Recommended Amounts of Food from Each Food Group at 12 Calorie Levels
The Healthy U.S.-Style Pattern is the base USDA Food Pattern. While the Healthy U.S.-Style Pattern is substantially unchanged from the base USDA Food Pattern of the 2010 edition of the Dietary Guidelines, *small changes in the recommended amounts reflect updating the Patterns based on current food consumption and composition data. The Healthy U.S.-Style Pattern includes 12 calorie levels to meet the needs of individuals across the lifespan. To follow this Pattern, identify the appropriate calorie level, choose a variety of foods in each group and subgroup over time in recommended amounts, and limit choices that are not in nutrient-dense forms so that the overall calorie limit is not exceeded.*

Calorie level of pattern[a]	1,000	1,200	1,400	1,600	1,800	2,000	2,200	2,400	2,600	2,800	3,000	3,200
Food Group[b]	Daily Amount[c] of Food from Each Group (vegetable and protein foods subgroup amounts are per week)											
Fruits (c-eq)	1 c	1 c	1½ c	1½ c	1½ c	2 c	2 c	2 c	2 c	2½ c	2½ c	2½ c
Vegetables (c-eq)	1 c	1½ c	1½ c	2 c	2½ c	2½ c	3 c	3 c	3½ c	3½ c	4 c	4 c
Dark-green vegetables	½ c/wk	1 c/wk	1 c/wk	1½ c/wk	1½ c/wk	1½ c/wk	2 c/wk	2 c/wk	2½ c/wk	2½ c/wk	2½ c/wk	2½ c/wk
Red and orange vegetables	2½ c/wk	3 c/wk	3 c/wk	4 c/wk	5½ c/wk	5½ c/wk	6 c/wk	6 c/wk	7 c/wk	7 c/wk	7½ c/wk	7½ c/wk
Beans and peas (legumes)	½ c/wk	½ c/wk	½ c/wk	1 c/wk	1½ c/wk	1½ c/wk	2 c/wk	2 c/wk	2½ c/wk	2½ c/wk	3 c/wk	3 c/wk
Starchy vegetables	2 c/wk	3½ c/wk	3½ c/wk	4 c/wk	5 c/wk	5 c/wk	6 c/wk	6 c/wk	7 c/wk	7 c/wk	8 c/wk	8 c/wk
Other vegetables	1½ c/wk	2½ c/wk	2½ c/wk	3½ c/wk	4 c/wk	4 c/wk	5 c/wk	5 c/wk	5½ c/wk	5½ c/wk	7 c/wk	7 c/wk
Grains	3 oz-eq	4 oz-eq	5 oz-eq	5 oz-eq	6 oz-eq	6 oz-eq	7 oz-eq	8 oz-eq	9 oz-eq	10 oz-eq	10 oz-eq	10 oz-eq
Whole grains[d]	1½ oz-eq	2 oz-eq	2½ oz-eq	3 oz-eq	3 oz-eq	3 oz-eq	3½ oz-eq	4 oz-eq	4½ oz-eq	5 oz-eq	5 oz-eq	5 oz-eq
Enriched grains	1½ oz-eq	2 oz-eq	2½ oz-eq	2 oz-eq	3 oz-eq	3 oz-eq	3½ oz-eq	4 oz-eq	4½ oz-eq	5 oz-eq	5 oz-eq	5 oz-eq
Protein foods	2 oz-eq	3 oz-eq	4 oz-eq	5 oz-eq	5 oz-eq	5½ oz-eq	6 oz-eq	6½ oz-eq	6½ oz-eq	7 oz-eq	7 oz-eq	7 oz-eq
Seafood	3 oz/wk	4 oz/wk	6 oz/wk	8 oz/wk	8 oz/wk	8 oz/wk	9 oz/wk	10 oz/wk	10 oz/wk	10 oz/wk	10 oz/wk	10 oz/wk
Meat, poultry, eggs	10 oz/wk	14 oz/wk	19 oz/wk	23 oz/wk	23 oz/wk	26 oz/wk	28 oz/wk	31 oz/wk	31 oz/wk	33 oz/wk	33 oz/wk	33 oz/wk
Nuts, seeds, soy products	2 oz/wk	2 oz/wk	3 oz/wk	4 oz/wk	4 oz/wk	5 oz/wk	5 oz/wk	5 oz/wk	5 oz/wk	6 oz/wk	6 oz/wk	6 oz/wk

(continues)

(continued)

Calorie level of pattern[a]	1,000	1,200	1,400	1,600	1,800	2,000	2,200	2,400	2,600	2,800	3,000	3,200
Food Group[b]	Daily Amount[c] of Food from Each Group (vegetable and protein foods subgroup amounts are per week)											
Dairy	2 c	2½ c	2½ c	3 c	3 c	3 c	3 c	3 c	3 c	3 c	3 c	3 c
Oils	15 g	17 g	17 g	22 g	24 g	27 g	29 g	31 g	34 g	36 g	44 g	51 g
Limit on calories for other uses, calories (% of calories)[e,f]	150 (15%)	100 (8%)	110 (8%)	130 (8%)	170 (9%)	270 (14%)	280 (13%)	350 (15%)	380 (15%)	400 (14%)	470 (16%)	610 (19%)

[a]Food intake patterns at 1,000, 1,200, and 1,400 calories are designed to meet the nutritional needs of 2- to 8-year-old children. Patterns from 1,600 to 3,200 calories are designed to meet the nutritional needs of children 9 years and older and adults. If a child 4–8 years of age needs more calories and, therefore, is following a pattern at 1,600 calories or more, his/her recommended amount from the dairy group should be 2.5 cups per day. Children 9 years and older and adults should not use the 1,000-, 1,200-, or 1,400-calorie patterns.

[b]Foods in each group and subgroup are:

- **Vegetables**
  - Dark-green vegetables: All fresh, frozen, and canned dark-green leafy vegetables and broccoli, cooked or raw: for example, broccoli, spinach, romaine, kale, collard, turnip, and mustard greens.
  - Red and orange vegetables: All fresh, frozen, and canned red and orange vegetables or juice, cooked or raw: for example, tomatoes, tomato juice, red peppers, carrots, sweet potatoes, winter squash, and pumpkin.
  - Legumes (beans and peas): All cooked from dry or canned beans and peas: for example, kidney beans, white beans, black beans, lentils, chickpeas, pinto beans, split peas, and edamame (green soybeans). Does not include green beans or green peas.
  - Starchy vegetables: All fresh, frozen, and canned starchy vegetables: for example, white potatoes, corn, green peas, green lima beans, plantains, and cassava.
  - Other vegetables: All other fresh, frozen, and canned vegetables, cooked or raw: for example, iceberg lettuce, green beans, onions, cucumbers, cabbage, celery, zucchini, mushrooms, and green peppers.
- **Fruits**
  - All fresh, frozen, canned, and dried fruits and fruit juices: for example, oranges and orange juice, apples and apple juice, bananas, grapes, melons, berries, and raisins.
- **Grains**
  - Whole grains: All whole-grain products and whole grains used as ingredients: for example, whole-wheat bread, whole-grain cereals and crackers, oatmeal, quinoa, popcorn, and brown rice.
  - Refined grains: All refined-grain products and refined grains used as ingredients: for example, white breads, refined grain cereals and crackers, pasta, and white rice. Refined grain choices should be enriched.
- **Dairy**
  - All milk, including lactose-free and lactose-reduced products and fortified soy beverages (soymilk), yogurt, frozen yogurt, dairy desserts, and cheeses. Most choices should be fat-free or low-fat. Cream, sour cream, and cream cheese are not included due to their low calcium content.
- **Protein foods**
  - All seafood, meats, poultry, eggs, soy products, nuts, and seeds. Meats and poultry should be lean or low-fat and nuts should be unsalted. Legumes (beans and peas) can be considered part of this group as well as the vegetable group, but should be counted in one group only.

[c]Food group amounts shown in cup-(c) or ounce-equivalents (oz-eq). Oils are shown in grams (g). Quantity equivalents for each food group are:

- Vegetables and fruits, 1 cup-equivalent is: 1 cup raw or cooked vegetable or fruit, 1 cup vegetable or fruit juice, 2 cups leafy salad greens, ½ cup dried fruit or vegetable.
- Grains, 1 ounce-equivalent is: ½ cup cooked rice, pasta, or cereal; 1 ounce dry pasta or rice; 1 medium (1 ounce) slice bread; 1 ounce of ready-to-eat cereal (about 1 cup of flaked cereal).
- Dairy, 1 cup-equivalent is: 1 cup milk, yogurt, or fortified soymilk; 1½ ounces natural cheese such as cheddar cheese or 2 ounces of processed cheese.
- Protein foods, 1 ounce-equivalent is: 1 ounce lean meat, poultry, or seafood; 1 egg; ¼ cup cooked beans or tofu; 1 tbsp peanut butter; ½ ounce nuts or seeds.

[d]Amounts of whole grains in the Patterns for children are less than the minimum of 3 oz-eq in all Patterns recommended for adults.

[e]All foods are assumed to be in nutrient-dense forms, lean or low-fat and prepared without added fats, sugars, refined starches, or salt. If all food choices to meet food group recommendations are in nutrient-dense forms, a small number of calories remain within the overall calorie limit of the Pattern (i.e., limit on calories for other uses). The number of these calories depends on the overall calorie limit in the Pattern and the amounts of food from each food group required to meet nutritional goals. Nutritional goals are higher for the 1,200- to 1,600-calorie Patterns than for the 1,000-calorie Pattern, so the limit on calories for other uses is lower in the 1,200- to 1,600-calorie Patterns. Calories up to the specified limit can be used for added sugars, added refined starches, solid fats, alcohol, or to eat more than the recommended amount of food in a food group. The overall eating Pattern also should not exceed the limits of less than 10% of calories from added sugars and less than 10% of calories from saturated fats.

(continues)

(continued)

At most calorie levels, amounts that can be accommodated are less than these limits. For adults of legal drinking age who choose to drink alcohol, a limit of up to 1 drink per day for women and up to 2 drinks per day for men within limits on calories for other uses applies. Alcohol and calories from protein, carbohydrate, and total fats should be within the Acceptable Macronutrient Distribution Ranges (AMDRs).

[f]Values are rounded.

Source: U.S. Department of Agriculture and U.S. Department of Health and Human Services. Dietary Guidelines for Americans, 2015–2020. 8th Edition, Washington, DC: U.S. Government Printing Office, December 2015.

Appendix C-2

Composition of the Healthy Mediterranean-Style and Healthy Vegetarian Eating Patterns at the 2,000-Calorie Level,[a] With Daily or Weekly Amounts From Food Groups, Subgroups, and Components

Food group[b]	Healthy mediterranean-style eating pattern	Healthy vegetarian-style eating pattern
Vegetables	2½ c-eq/d	2½ c-eq/d
Dark green	1½ c-eq/wk	1½ c-eq/wk
Red and orange	5½ c-eq/wk	5½ c-eq/wk
Legumes (beans and peas)	1½ c-eq/wk	3 c-eq/wk[c]
Starchy	5 c-eq/wk	5 c-eq/wk
Other	4 c-eq/wk	4 c-eq/wk
Fruits	2½ c-eq/d	2 c-eq/d
Grains	6 oz-eq/d	6½ oz-eq/d
Whole grains	≥3 oz-eq/d	≥3½ oz-eq/d
Refined grains	≤3 oz-eq/d	≤3 oz-eq/d
Dairy	2 c-eq/d	3 c-eq/d
Protein foods	6½ oz-eq/d	3½ oz-eq/d[c]
Seafood	15 oz-eq/wk[d]	–
Meats, poultry, eggs	26 oz-eq/wk	3 oz-eq/wk (eggs)
Nuts, seeds, soy products	5 oz-eq/wk	14 oz-eq/wk
Oils	27 g/d	27 g/d
Limit on calories for other uses (% of calories)[e]	260 kcal/d (13%)	290 kcal/d (15%)

[a]Food group amounts shown in cup-(c) or ounce-equivalents (oz-eq). Oils are shown in grams (g). Amounts will vary for those who need less than 2,000 or more than 2,000 calories per day. See Dietary Guidelines 2015–2020 for all 12 calorie levels of the patterns.

[b]Definitions for each food group and subgroup are provided in the prior Appendix.

[c]Vegetarian patterns include 1½ cups per week of legumes as a vegetable subgroup, and an additional 6 oz-eq (1½ cups) per week of legumes as a protein food. The total amount is shown here as legumes in the vegetable group.

[d]The FDA and EPA provide additional guidance regarding seafood consumption for women who are pregnant or breastfeeding and young children. For more information, see the FDA or EPA websites www.FDA.gov/fishadvice;www.EPA.gov/fishadvice.

[e]Assumes food choices to meet food group recommendations are in nutrient-dense forms. Calories from added sugars, solid fats, added refined starches, alcohol, and/or to eat more than the recommended amount of nutrient-dense foods are accounted for under this category.

Note: The eating pattern should not exceed *Dietary Guidelines* limits for intake of added sugars, saturated fats, alcohol, and the AMDR for calories from protein, carbohydrate, and total fats. For some calorie patterns, there are not enough calories available after meeting food group needs to consume 10% of calories from added sugars and 10% of calories from saturated fats and still stay within calorie limits. Values are rounded.

Source: U.S. Department of Agriculture and U.S. Department of Health and Human Services. Dietary Guidelines for Americans, 2015–2020. 8th Edition, Washington, DC: U.S. Government Printing Office, December 2015.

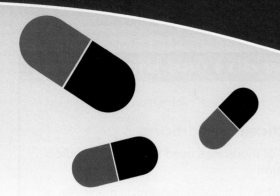

Avoid **Food–Drug** Interactions

A Guide from the National Consumers League and
U.S. Food and Drug Administration

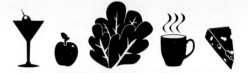

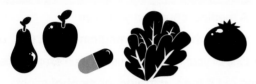

What you eat and drink can affect the way your medicines work. Use this guide to alert you to possible "food–drug interactions" and to help you learn what you can do to prevent them.

In this guide, a food–drug interaction is a change in how a medicine works caused by **food**, **caffeine**, or **alcohol**.

A food–drug interaction can:

- prevent a medicine from working the way it should

- cause a side effect from a medicine to get worse or better

- cause a new side effect

A medicine can also change the way your body uses a food. Any of these changes can be harmful.

This guide covers interactions between some common prescription and over-the-counter medicines and food, caffeine, and alcohol. These interactions come from medicine labels that FDA has approved. This guide uses the generic names of medicines, never brand names.

What Else Can Affect How My Medicines Work?

Your age, weight, and sex; medical conditions; the dose of the medicine; other medicines; and vitamins, herbals, and other dietary supplements can affect

how your medicines work. Every time you use a medicine, carefully follow the information on the label and directions from your doctor or pharmacist.

Does It Matter If I Take a Medicine on a Full Or Empty Stomach?

Yes, with some medicines. Some medicines can work faster, slower, better, or worse when you take them on a full or empty stomach. On the other hand, some medicines can upset your stomach, and if there is food in your stomach, that can help reduce the upset. If you don't see directions on your medicine labels, ask your doctor or pharmacist if it is best to take your medicines on an empty stomach (1 hour before eating, or 2 hours after eating), with food, or after a meal (full stomach).

Does It Matter If I Take My Medicine with Alcohol?

Yes, the way your medicine works can change when:

- you swallow your medicine with alcohol

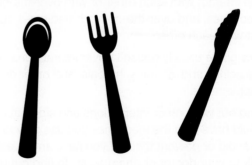

- you drink alcohol after you've taken your medicine
- you take your medicine after you've had alcohol

Alcohol can also add to the side effects caused by medicines. You should talk to your doctor about any alcohol you use or plan to use.

How Do I Know If Caffeine Is in My Food or Drinks?

Check the labels on your foods and drinks to see if they have caffeine. Some foods and drinks with caffeine are coffee, cola drinks, teas, chocolate, some high-energy drinks, and other soft drinks. For more information about caffeine go to: www.fda.gov /downloads/UCM200805.pdf

Remember!

This guide should never take the place of the advice from your doctor, pharmacist, or other health care professionals. Always ask them if there are any problems you could have when you use your medicines with other medicines; with vitamins, herbals and other dietary supplements; or with food, caffeine, or alcohol.

What Isn't in This Guide?

This guide won't include every medicine and every type of medicine that's used to treat a medical condition. And just because a medicine is listed here, doesn't mean you should or shouldn't use it.

This guide only covers food-drug interactions with medicines you should swallow. It doesn't cover, for example, medicines that you put on the skin, inject through the skin, drop in your eyes and ears, or spray into your mouth.

This guide also doesn't cover drug–drug interactions, which are changes in the way your medicines work caused by other medicines. Prescription medicines can interact with each other or with over-the-counter medicines, and over-the-counter medicines can interact with each other.

This guide usually doesn't cover interactions between medicines and vitamins, herbals, and other dietary supplements.

Find out what other interactions and side effects you could have with the medicines you use so you can try to avoid or prevent them. If you have any questions, talk to your doctor or pharmacist. To find out more

about how to use your medicines safely, visit the websites listed on the back panel of this guide.

How do I use this guide?

This guide arranges information by:

Medical conditions

Types of medicines used to treat the medical condition

Examples of active ingredients in medicines of this type

Interactions are listed by

Food, Caffeine, and Alcohol.

If you see...

- A medical condition you have
- **One of the types of medicines you use, or**
- One of your medicines used as an example here,

find out if **food, caffeine,** or **alcohol** might change the way your medicine works.

Allergies

Antihistamines

Antihistamines treat or relieve symptoms of colds and allergies, such as sneezing, runny nose, stuffy nose, and itchy eyes. They block the histamine your body releases when a substance (allergen) causes the symptoms of an allergic reaction. Some antihistamines you can buy over-the-counter and some you can buy only with a prescription from your doctor or other health care professional who can write a prescription. Some antihistamines can cause drowsiness.

Examples

brompheniramine

cetirizine

chlorpheniramine

clemastine

desloratadine

diphenhydramine

fexofenadine

levocetirizine

triprolidine

Interactions

Alcohol: Avoid alcohol because it can add to any drowsiness caused by these medicines.

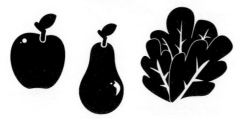

Arthritis, Pain, and Fever

Analgesics/Antipyretics (Pain Relievers/ Fever Reducers)

Analgesics/antipyretics relieve mild to moderate pain and lower fever.

Example

acetaminophen

Acetaminophen relieves from mild to moderate headaches, muscle aches, toothaches, backaches, menstrual cramps, the common cold, pain of arthritis, and lowers fever.

Interactions

Alcohol: If you drink three or more alcoholic drinks every day, ask your doctor if you should use medicines with acetaminophen or other pain reliever/fever reducers. Acetaminophen can cause liver damage. The chance for severe liver damage is higher if you drink three or more alcoholic drinks every day.

Nonsteroidal Anti-Inflammatory Drugs (NSAIDs)

NSAIDs relieve pain, fever, and inflammation. Some NSAIDs you can buy over-the-counter and some you can buy only with a prescription. The over-the-counter NSAIDs give short term relief from minor aches and pains from headaches, muscle aches, toothaches, backaches, menstrual cramps, and minor aches and pain of arthritis. NSAIDs may be prescribed for conditions such as osteoarthritis (arthritis caused by the breakdown of the lining of the joints). NSAIDS can cause stomach bleeding.

Examples

aspirin

celecoxib

diclofenac

ibuprofen

ketoprofen

naproxen

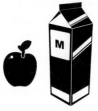

Interactions

Food: Take these medicines with food or milk if they upset your stomach.

Alcohol: If you drink three or more alcoholic drinks every day, ask your doctor if you should use medicines with NSAIDs or other pain relievers/ fever reducers. NSAIDs can cause stomach bleeding and the chance is higher if you drink three or more alcoholic drinks every day.

Narcotic Analgesics

Narcotic analgesics treat moderate to severe pain. Codeine can also help you cough less. Some of these medicines are mixed with other medicines that aren't narcotics, such as acetaminophen, aspirin, or cough syrups. You can only buy narcotic analgesics with a prescription. Follow your doctor's or pharmacist's advice carefully because these medicines can be habit forming and can cause serious side effects if not used correctly.

Examples

codeine + acetaminophen

hydrocodone + acetaminophen

meperidine

morphine

oxycodone + acetaminophen

Interactions

Alcohol: Don't drink alcohol while using narcotics. Alcohol can increase the chance of dangerous side effects, such as coma, or death.

Asthma

Bronchodilators

Bronchodilators treat and prevent breathing problems from bronchial asthma, chronic bronchitis, emphysema, and chronic obstructive pulmonary disease (COPD). These medicines relax and open the air passages to the lungs to relieve wheezing, shortness of breath, troubled breathing, and chest tightness.

Take these medicines only as directed. If your symptoms get worse or you need to take the medicine more often than usual, you should talk to your doctor right away.

Examples

albuterol

theophylline

Interactions

Food: Food can have different effects on different forms of theophylline (some forms are regular release, sustained release, and sprinkles). Check with your pharmacist to be sure you know which form of the medicine you use and if food can affect your medicine.

Follow directions for sprinkle forms of the medicine. You can swallow sprinkle capsules whole or open them and sprinkle them on soft foods, such as applesauce or pudding. Swallow the mixture without chewing, as soon as it is mixed. Follow with a full glass of cool water or juice.

Caffeine: Using bronchodilators with foods and drinks that have caffeine can increase the chance of side effects, such as excitability, nervousness, and rapid heartbeat.

Alcohol: Avoid alcohol if you're using theophylline medicines because alcohol can increase the chance of side effects, such as nausea, vomiting, headache, and irritability.

Cardiovascular Disorders

These medicines prevent or treat disorders of the cardiovascular system, such as high blood pressure, angina (chest pain), irregular heartbeat, heart failure, blood clots, and high cholesterol. Some types of medicines can treat many conditions. For example, beta-blockers can treat high blood pressure, angina (chest pain), and irregular heartbeats.

ACE Inhibitors (Angiotensin Converting Enzyme Inhibitors)

ACE inhibitors alone or with other medicines lower blood pressure or treat heart failure. They relax blood vessels so blood flows more smoothly and the heart can pump blood better.

Examples

captopril

enalapril

lisinopril

moexipril

quinapril

ramipril

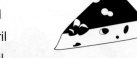

Interactions

Food: Take captopril and moexipril 1 hour before meals.

ACE inhibitors can increase the amount of potassium in your body. Too much potassium can be harmful and can cause an irregular heartbeat and heart palpitations (rapid heartbeats). Avoid eating large amounts of foods high in potassium, such as bananas, oranges, green leafy vegetables, and salt substitutes that contain potassium. They can raise the level of potassium even higher. Tell your doctor if you are taking salt substitutes with potassium, potassium supplements, or diuretics (water pills) because these can add to the amount of potassium in your body.

Beta-Blockers

Beta-blockers can be used alone or with other medicines to treat high blood pressure. They are also used to prevent angina (chest pain) and treat heart attacks. They work by slowing the heart rate and relaxing the blood vessels so the heart doesn't have to work hard to pump blood.

Don't suddenly stop taking a beta-blocker without talking to your doctor. If you stop a beta-blocker suddenly, you can get chest pain, an irregular heartbeat, or a heart attack. Your doctor might tell you to decrease your dose gradually.

Examples

carvedilol

metoprolol

Interactions

Food: Take carvedilol with food to decrease the chance that it will lower your blood pressure too much. Take carvedilol extended release capsules in the morning with food; don't crush, chew, or divide the capsule. Take metoprolol with a meal or right after a meal.

Diuretics

Sometimes called "water pills," diuretics help remove water, sodium, and chloride from the body. Diuretics reduce sodium and the swelling and excess fluid caused by some medical problems such as heart or liver disease. Diuretics can also treat high blood pressure.

Examples

bumetanide

furosemide

hydrochlorothiazide

metolazone

triamterene

triamterene + hydrochlorothiazide

Interactions

Food: Take your diuretic with food if it upsets your stomach.

Some diuretics cause loss of the minerals such as potassium, calcium, and magnesium from the body.

Other diuretics, like triamterene (not with hydro-chlorothiazide), lower the kidneys' ability to remove potassium, which can cause high levels of potassium in the blood stream (hyperkalemia). Too much potassium can be harmful and can cause an irregular or rapid beating of the heart. When you use diuretics that can increase potassium in your body, avoid eating large amounts of foods high in potassium, such as bananas, oranges, and green leafy vegetables, and salt substitutes that contain potassium. They can raise the level of potassium even higher. Tell your doctor if you are taking salt substitutes with potassium or potassium supplements because they can add to the amount of potassium in your body.

Glycosides

Glycosides treat heart failure and abnormal heart rhythms. They help control the heart rate and help the heart work better.

Example

digoxin

Interactions

Food: Take digoxin 1 hour before or 2 hours after eating food. Try to take it at the same time(s) every day and carefully follow the label and directions from your doctor. Foods high in fiber may decrease the digoxin in your body, so take digoxin at least 2 hours before or 2 hours after eating foods high in fiber (such as bran).

Avoid taking digoxin with senna and St. John's wort since they may decrease the amount and action of digoxin in your body.

Avoid taking digoxin with black licorice (which contains the glycyrrhizin used in some candies, cakes and other sweets). Digoxin with glycyrrhizin can cause irregular heartbeat and heart attack.

Lipid-Altering Agents (also called Statins)

Statins lower cholesterol by lowering the rate of production of LDL (low-density lipoproteins, or sometimes called "bad cholesterol"). Some of these medicines also lower triglycerides. Some statins can raise HDL-C (high-density lipoproteins, or sometimes called "good cholesterol"), and lower the chance of heart attack, stroke, or small strokes.

Examples

atorvastatin

fluvastatin

lovastatin

pravastatin

simvastatin

rosuvastatin

Interactions

Food: You can take most statins on a full or empty stomach. Some statins will work better if you take them with an evening meal. Don't drink more than one quart of grapefruit juice a day if you are taking atorvastatin, lovastatin, or simvastatin. Large amounts of grapefruit juice can raise the levels of those statins in your body and increase the chance of side effects. Some statins don't interact with grapefruit juice. Ask your doctor or pharmacist if you have any questions.

Alcohol: Avoid alcohol because it can increase the chance of liver damage.

Vasodilators—Nitrates

Nitrates prevent or treat chest pain (angina). They work by relaxing the blood vessels to the heart, which improves the blood and oxygen flow to the heart.

Examples

isosorbide dinitrate or mononitrate

nitroglycerin

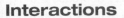

Interactions

Food: You can take all forms of nitrates on a full or empty stomach.

Alcohol: Avoid alcohol. Alcohol may add to the blood vessel-relaxing effect of nitrates and lead to a dangerously low blood pressure.

Vitamin K Agonists/Anticoagulants

Anticoagulants are also called "blood thinners." They lower the chance of blood clots forming or growing larger in your blood or blood vessels. Anticoagulants are used to treat people with certain types of irregular heartbeat, people with prosthetic (replacement or mechanical) heart valves, and people who have had a heart attack. Anticoagulants also treat blood clots that have formed in the veins of the legs or lungs.

Example

warfarin

Interactions

Food: You can take warfarin on a full or empty stomach. Vitamin K in food can make the medicine less effective. Eat a normal balanced diet with a steady amount of leafy green vegetables, and talk to your doctor before making changes in your diet. Foods high in vitamin K include broccoli, cabbage, collard greens, spinach, kale, turnip greens, and brussel sprouts. Avoid cranberry juice or cranberry products while using anticoagulants because they can change the effects of warfarin. Many dietary supplements and vitamins can interact with anticoagulants and can reduce the benefit or increase the risk of warfarin. Avoid garlic, ginger, glucosamine, ginseng, and ginkgo because they can increase the chance of bleeding.

Alcohol: Tell your doctor and pharmacist if you drink alcohol or have problems with alcohol abuse. Avoid alcohol because it can affect your dose of warfarin.

Gastroesophageal Reflux Disease (GERD) and Ulcers

Proton Pump Inhibitors

Proton Pump Inhibitors (PPIs) work by decreasing the amount of acid made in the stomach. They treat conditions when the stomach produces too much acid. Some of these medicines you can buy over-the-counter

to treat frequent heartburn, such as omeprazole and lansoprazole. Some of these medicines you can only buy with a prescription to treat conditions such as ulcers, gastroesophageal reflux disease, and to reduce the risk of stomach ulcers in people taking nonsteroidal antiinflammatory drugs (NSAIDs). (See Arthritis, Pain and Fever-Nonsteroidal Anti-inflammatory Drugs section aforementioned.) Proton pump inhibitors are also used along with antibiotics to stop infections in the stomach that cause ulcers.

Proton pump inhibitors come in different forms (such as delayed-release tablets, delayed-release disintegrating tablets, immediate release). Don't change your dose or stop using these without talking to your doctor first.

Examples

dexlansoprazole

esomeprazole

lansoprazole

omeprazole

pantoprazole

rabeprazole

Interactions

Food: You can take dexlansoprazole and pantoprazole on a full or empty stomach. Esomeprazole should be taken at least 1 hour before a meal. Lansoprazole and omeprazole should be taken before eating. Ask your doctor or pharmacist how you should take rabeprazole.

Tell your doctor if you cannot swallow delayed-release medicines whole because you shouldn't split, crush, or chew them. Some of these medicines can be mixed with food but you must carefully follow the label and directions from your doctor or pharmacist.

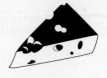

Hypothyroidism

Hypothyroidism is a condition where the thyroid gland doesn't produce enough thyroid hormone. Without this hormone, the body cannot function properly, so there is poor growth, slow speech, lack of energy, weight gain, hair loss, dry thick skin, and increased sensitivity to cold.

Thyroid Medicines

Thyroid medicines control hypothyroidism but they don't cure it. They reverse the symptoms of hypothyroidism. Thyroid medicine is also used to treat congenital hypothyroidism (cretinism), autoimmune hypothyroidism, other causes of hypothyroidism (such as after thyroid surgery), and goiter (enlarged thyroid gland). It may take several weeks before you notice a change in your symptoms. Don't stop taking the medicine without talking to your doctor.

Example

levothyroxine

Interactions

Foods: Tell your doctor if you are allergic to any foods. Take levothyroxine once a day in morning on an empty stomach, at least 1.5–1 hour before eating any food. Tell your doctor if you eat soybean flour (also found in soybean infant formula), cotton seed meal, walnuts, and dietary fiber; the dose of the medicine may need to be changed.

Infections

Be sure to finish all of your medicine for an infection, even if you are feeling better. All of the medicine is needed to kill the cause of infection. If you stop the medicine early, the infection may come back; the next time, the medicine may not work for the infection. Ask your doctor if you should drink more fluids than usual when you take medicine for an infection.

Antibacterials

Medicines known as antibiotics or antibacterials are used to treat infections caused by bacteria. None of these medicines will work for infections that are caused by viruses (such as colds and flu).

Quinolone Antibacterials

Examples

ciprofloxacin

levofloxacin

moxifloxacin

Interactions

Food: You can take ciprofloxacin and moxifloxacin on a full or empty stomach. Take levofloxacin *tablets* on a full or empty stomach. Take levofloxacin *oral solution* 1 hour before eating or 2 hours after eating.

Don't take ciprofloxacin with dairy products (like milk and yogurt) or calcium-fortified juices alone, but you can take ciprofloxacin with a meal that has these products in it.

Caffeine: Tell your doctor if you take foods or drinks with caffeine when you take ciprofloxacin, because caffeine may build up in your body.

Tetracycline Antibacterials

Examples

doxycycline

minocycline

tetracycline

Interactions

Food: Take these medicines 1 hour before a meal or 2 hours after a meal, with a full glass of water.

You can take tetracycline with food if it upsets your stomach, but avoid dairy products (such as milk, cheese, yogurt, ice cream) 1 hour before or 2 hours after. You can take minocycline and some forms of doxycycline with milk if the medicine upsets your stomach.

Oxazolidinone Antibacterials

Example

linezolid

Interactions

Food: Avoid large amounts of foods and drinks high in tyramine while using linezolid. High levels of tyramine can cause a sudden, dangerous increase in your blood pressure. Follow your doctor's directions very carefully.

Foods with Tyramine

Foods that are spoiled or not refrigerated, handled, or stored properly, and aged, pickled, fermented, or smoked foods may contain tyramine. Some of these are:

- cheeses, especially strong, aged, or processed cheese, such as American processed, cheddar, colby, blue, brie, mozzarella, and parmesan cheese; yogurt; sour cream (you can eat cream and cottage cheese)

- beef or chicken liver, dry sausage (including Genoa salami, hard salami, pepperoni, and

Lebanon bologna), caviar, dried or pickled herring, anchovies, meat extracts, meat tenderizers and meats prepared with tenderizers

- avocados, bananas, canned figs, dried fruits (raisins, prunes), raspberries, overripe fruit, sauerkraut, soy beans and soy sauce, yeast extract (including brewer's yeast in large quantities)
- broad beans (fava)
- excessive amounts of chocolate

Caffeine: Many foods and drinks with caffeine also contain tyramine. Ask your doctor if you should avoid or limit caffeine.

Alcohol: Avoid alcohol while using linezolid. Many alcoholic drinks contain tyramine, including tap beer, red wine, sherry, and liqueurs. Tyramine can also be in alcohol-free and reduced alcohol beer.

Metronidazole Antibacterials

Example

metronidazole

Interactions

Alcohol: Don't drink alcohol while taking metronidazole and for at least one full day after finishing the medicine; together alcohol and metronidazole can cause nausea, stomach cramps, vomiting, flushing, and headaches.

Antifungals

Antifungals are medicines that treat or prevent fungal infections. Antifungals work by slowing or stopping the growth of fungi that cause infection.

Examples

fluconazole

itraconazole

posaconazole

voriconazole

griseofulvin

terbinafine

Interactions

Food: Itraconazole *capsules* will work better if you take it during or right after a full meal. Itraconazole *solution* should be taken on an empty stomach. Posaconazole will work better if you take it with a meal, within 20 minutes of eating a full meal, or with a liquid nutritional supplement. Don't mix voriconazole suspension with any other medicines, water, or any other liquid. Griseofulvin works better when taken with fatty food.

You can take the rest of the antifungals listed here on a full or empty stomach.

Alcohol: Avoid alcohol while you are taking griseofulvin because griseofulvin can make the side effects of alcohol worse. For example, together they can cause the heart to beat faster and can cause flushing.

Antimycobacterials

Antimycobacterials treat infections caused by mycobacteria, a type of bacteria that causes tuberculosis (TB), and other kinds of infections.

Examples

ethambutol

isoniazid

rifampin

rifampin + isoniazid

rifampin + isoniazid + pyrazinamide

Interactions

Food: Ethambutol can be taken with or without food. Take the rest of these medicines 1 hour before a meal or 2 hours after a meal, with a full glass of water.

Avoid foods and drinks with tyramine and foods with histamine if you take isoniazid alone or combined with other antimycobacterials. High levels of tyramine can cause a sudden, dangerous increase in your blood pressure. Foods with histamine can cause headache, sweating, palpitations (rapid heartbeats), flushing, and hypotension (low blood pressure). Follow your doctor's directions very carefully.

Foods that contain tyramine are listed on page 21, under **"Foods with Tyramine."**

Foods with histamine include skipjack, tuna, and other tropical fish.

Caffeine: Many foods and drinks with caffeine also contain tyramine. Ask your doctor if you should avoid or limit caffeine.

Alcohol: Avoid alcohol. Many alcoholic drinks contain tyramine, including tap beer, red wine, sherry, and liqueurs. Tyramine can also be in alcohol-free and reduced alcohol beer. If you drink alcohol every day while using isoniazid you may have an increased risk of isoniazid hepatitis.

Antiprotozoals

Antiprotozoals treat infections caused by certain protozoa (parasites that can live in your body and can cause diarrhea).

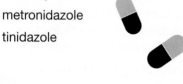

Examples

metronidazole

tinidazole

Interactions

Alcohol: Together alcohol and these medicines can cause nausea, stomach cramps, vomiting, flushing, and headaches. Avoid drinking alcohol while taking metronidazole and for at least one full day after finishing the medicine. Avoid drinking alcohol while taking tinidazole and for 3 days after finishing the medicine.

Psychiatric Disorders

Depression, bipolar disorder, general anxiety disorder, social phobia, panic disorder, and schizophrenia are a few examples of common psychiatric (mental) disorders. Use the amount of medicine that your doctor tells you to use, even if you are feeling better. In some cases it can take several weeks before you see your symptoms get better. Don't stop these medicines until you talk to your doctor. You may need to stop your medicine gradually to avoid getting side effects. Some of these medicines can affect your thinking, judgment, or physical skills. Some may cause drowsiness and can affect how alert you are and how you respond. Don't do activities like operating machinery or driving a car, until you know how your medicine affects you.

Anti-Anxiety and Panic Disorder Medicines

Examples

alprazolam

clonazepam

diazepam

lorazepam

Interactions

Alcohol: Avoid alcohol. Alcohol can add to the side effects caused by these medicines, such as drowsiness.

Antidepressants

Antidepressants treat depression, general anxiety disorder, social phobia, obsessive–compulsive disorder, some eating disorders, and panic attacks. The medicines below work by increasing the amount of serotonin, a natural substance in the brain that helps maintain mental balance.

Never stop an antidepressant medicine without first talking to a doctor. You may need to stop your medicine gradually to avoid getting side effects.

Examples

citalopram

escitalopram

fluoxetine

paroxetine

sertraline

Interactions

Food: You can take these medicines on a full or empty stomach. Swallow paroxetine whole; don't chew or crush it.

Alcohol: Avoid alcohol. Alcohol can add to the side effects caused by these medicines, such as drowsiness.

Antidepressants—Monoamine Oxidase Inhibitors (MAOIs)

MAOIs treat depression in people who haven't been helped by other medicines. They work by increasing the amounts of certain natural substances that are needed for mental balance.

Examples

phenelzine

tranylcypromine

Interactions

Food: Avoid foods and drinks that contain tyramine when you use MAOIs. High levels of tyramine can cause a sudden, dangerous increase in your blood pressure. Follow your doctor's directions very carefully.

Foods that contain tyramine are listed on page 21, under **"Foods with Tyramine."**

Caffeine: Many foods and drinks with caffeine also contain tyramine. Ask your doctor if you should avoid or limit caffeine.

Alcohol: Don't drink alcohol while using these medicines. Many alcoholic drinks contain tyramine, including tap beer, red wine, sherry, and liqueurs. Tyramine also can be in alcohol-free and reduced alcohol beer. Alcohol also can add to the side effects caused by these medicines.

Antipsychotics

Antipsychotics treat the symptoms of schizophrenia and acute manic or mixed episodes from bipolar disorder. People with schizophrenia may believe things that are not real (delusions) or see, hear, feel, or smell things that are not real (hallucinations). They can also have disturbed or unusual thinking and strong or inappropriate emotions. These medicines work by changing the activity of certain natural substances in the brain.

Examples

aripiprazole

clozapine

olanzapine

quetiapine

risperidone

ziprasidone

Interactions

Food: Take ziprasidone capsules with food. You can take the rest of these medicines on a full or empty stomach.

Caffeine: Avoid caffeine when using clozapine because caffeine can increase the amount of medicine in your blood and cause side effects.

Alcohol: Avoid alcohol. Alcohol can add to the side effects caused by these medicines, such as drowsiness.

Sedatives and Hypnotics (Sleep Medicines)

Sedative and hypnotic medicines treat people who have problems falling asleep or staying asleep. They work by slowing activity in the brain to allow sleep. Some of these medicines you can buy over-the-counter and some you can only buy with a prescription.

Tell your doctor if you have ever abused or have been dependent on alcohol, prescription medicines, or street drugs before starting any sleep medicine.

You could have a greater chance of becoming addicted to sleep medicines.

Examples

eszopiclone

zolpidem

Interactions

Food: To get to sleep faster, don't take these medicines with a meal or right after a meal.

Alcohol: Don't drink alcohol while using these medicines. Alcohol can add to the side effects caused by these medicines.

Bipolar Disorder Medicines

People with bipolar disorder experience mania (abnormally excited mood, racing thoughts, more talkative than usual, and decreased need for sleep) and depression at different times during their lives. Bipolar disorder medicines help people who have mood swings by helping to balance their moods.

Examples

carbamazepine

divalproex sodium

lamotrigine

lithium

Interactions

Food: Take divalproex with food if it upsets your stomach. Take lithium immediately after meal or with food or milk to avoid stomach upset. Lithium can cause you to lose sodium, so maintain a normal diet, including salt; drink plenty of fluids (8–12 glasses a day) while on the medicine.

Alcohol: Avoid alcohol. Alcohol can add to the side effects caused by these medicines, such as drowsiness.

Osteoporosis

Bisphosphonates (Bone Calcium Phosphorus Metabolism)

Bisphosphonates prevent and treat osteoporosis, a condition in which the bones become thin and weak and break easily. They work by preventing bone breakdown and increasing bone thickness.

Examples

alendronate sodium

alendronate sodium + cholecalciferol

ibandronate sodium

risedronate sodium

risedronate sodium + calcium carbonate

Food: These medicines work only when you take them on an empty stomach. Take the medicine first thing in the morning with a full glass (6–8 ounces) of plain water while you are sitting or standing up. Don't take with mineral water. Don't take antacids or any other medicine, food, drink, calcium, or any vitamins or other dietary supplements for at least 30 minutes after taking alendronate or risedronate, and for at least 60 minutes after taking ibandronate. Don't lie down for at least 30 minutes after taking alendronate or risedronate and for at least 60 minutes after taking ibandronate. Don't lie down until you eat your first food of the day.

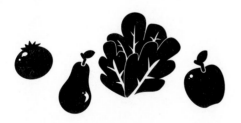

More About Using Medicines Safely

Read the Label Before You Use Any Medicine

Over-the-counter medicines

Over-the-counter medicine has a label called **_Drug Facts_** on the medicine container or packaging. The label is there to help you choose the right medicine for you and your problem and use the medicine

safely. Some over-the-counter medicines also come with a consumer information leaflet which gives more information.

Prescription Medicines

Medication Guide (also called Med Guide):

This is one kind of information written for consumers about prescription medicines. The pharmacist must give you a Medication Guide each time you fill your prescription when there is one written for your medicine. Medication Guides are made for certain medicines that have serious risks. The information tells about the risks and how to avoid them. Read the information carefully before you use the medicine. If you have any questions, ask a doctor or pharmacist.

For more information on Medication Guides, visit: www.fda.gov/drugs

Patient Package Insert (also called "PPI" or patient information):

This is another kind of information written for consumers about prescription medicines. Your pharmacist might give this to you with your medicine. It gives you information about the medicine and how to use it. The pharmacist must give you a PPI with birth control pills or any medicine with estrogen.

Resources

http://www.fda.gov/usemedicinesafely
Consumer education on how to choose and use medicine, from the FDA.

http://www.medlineplus.gov
Health information for consumers, from the government's National Library of Medicine (NLM).

http://dailymed.nlm.nih.gov
FDA-approved drug labeling written for healthcare professionals, from the government's National Institutes of Health (NIH); sometimes this labeling will also have a "Patient Package Insert" or PPI or a "Medication Guide," written for patients.

http://www.accessdata.fda.gov/scripts/cder /drugsatfda/index.cfm
Drugs@FDA website with FDA-approved labeling written for healthcare professionals; sometimes this labeling will also have a "Patient Package Insert" or PPI, or a "Medication Guide," written for patients. The site may have a "Drug Safety Communication," or "Other Important Information from FDA," if there has been new information about the medicine that has not made it to the label yet.

http://www.fda.gov/drugs/ucm079489.htm
A personal medicine record can help you keep
track of your prescription and over-the-counter
medicines and vitamins, herbals, and other dietary
supplements you use. If you keep a written record,
it can make it easy to share this information with all
your healthcare professionals—at office, clinic and
hospital visits, and in emergencies.

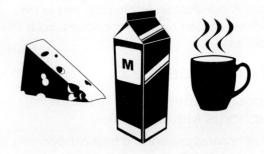

National Consumers League

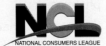

A 501(c)(3) nonprofit membership
organization
Phone: 202-835-3323
Fax: 202-835-0747
Email: info@nclnet.org
Web: www.nclnet.org

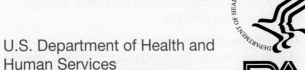

U.S. Department of Health and
Human Services

Food and Drug Administration

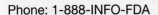

Phone: 1-888-INFO-FDA
Email questions: druginfo@fda.hhs.gov
Web: www.fda.gov/drugs

For an online version of this guide, visit:
www.nclnet.org or www.fda.gov/drugs

Publication no. (FDA) CDER 10-1933

APPENDIX **E**

EXCHANGE LISTS FOR MEAL PLANNING

Balanced Energy: A healthy weight is the result of balancing energy in and energy out of the body. You get energy from the food you eat. Energy is measured in calories. You use energy when you breathe, sit, walk, and move. You stay at the same weight when energy in—the food you eat—is the same as the energy you use. You gain weight when you take in more energy (calories) than your body uses. This extra energy is stored as unwanted weight. You can lose weight by taking in fewer calories than your body needs or burning off more than you take in. Then your body uses stored energy to meet your needs. Ask your RD to estimate how much energy your body needs. When you balance energy from food and energy used for exercise, you can maintain a healthy weight.

Starch

One starch exchange equals 15 g carbohydrate, 3 g protein, 0–1 g fat, and 80 calories

Bread

	Food	Serving Size
	Bagel, large (about 4 oz)	¼ (1 oz)
▽!	Biscuit, 2½ inches across	1
	Bread	
☺	reduced-calorie	2 slices (1½ oz)
	with whole-grain, pumpernickel, rye, unfrosted raisin	1 slice (1 oz)
	Chapatti, small, 6 inches across	1
▽!	Cornbread, 1¾ inch cube	1 (1½ oz)
	English muffin	½
	Hot dog bun or hamburger bun	½ (1 oz)
	Naan, 8 inches by 2 inches	¼
	Pancake, 4 inches across, ¼ inch thick	1
	Pita, 6 inches across	½
	Roll, plain, small	1 (1 oz)
▽!	Stuffing, bread	⅓ cup
▽!	Taco shell, 5 inches across	2
	Tortilla, corn, 6 inches across	1
	Tortilla, flour, 6 inches across	1
	Tortilla, flour, 10 inches across	⅓ tortilla
▽!	Waffle, 4-inch square or 4 inches across	1

Source: Reproduction of the Exchange Lists in whole or part, without permission of the American Dietetic Association or the American Diabetes Association, Inc., is a violation of federal law. This material has been modified from Choose Your Foods: Exchange Lists for Diabetes, which is the basis of a meal planning system designed by a committee of the American Diabetes Association and the American Dietetic Association. While designed primarily for people with diabetes and others who must follow special diets, the Exchange Lists are based on principles of good nutrition that apply to everyone. Copyright © 2008 by the American Diabetes Association and Academy of Nutrition and Dietetics (formerly American Dietetic Association)

Cereals and Grains

	Food	Serving Size
	Barley, cooked	⅓ cup
	Bran, dry	
☺	oat	¼ cup
☺	wheat	½ cup
☺	Bulgur (cooked)	½ cup

(continues)

☺ = More than 3 grams of dietary fiber per serving.

▽! = Extra fat, or prepared with added fat (Count as 1 starch 1 fat.).

Cereals and Grains *(continued)*

Food	Serving Size
Cereals	
☺ bran	½ cup
cooked (oats, oatmeal)	½ cup
puffed	1½ cups
shredded wheat, plain	½ cup
sugar-coated	½ cup
unsweetened, ready-to-eat	¾ cup
Couscous	⅓ cup
Granola	
low-fat	¼ cup
⚠ regular	¼ cup
Grits, cooked	½ cup
Kasha	½ cup
Millet, cooked	⅓ cup
Muesli	¼ cup
Pasta, cooked	⅓ cup
Polenta, cooked	⅓ cup
Quinoa, cooked	⅓ cup
Rice, white or brown, cooked	⅓ cup
Tabbouleh (tabouli), prepared	½ cup
Wheat germ, dry	3 Tbsp
Wild rice, cooked	½ cup

Tip: An open handful is equal to about 1 cup or 1–2 oz of snack food.

Source: Reproduction of the Exchange Lists in whole or part, without permission of the American Dietetic Association or the American Diabetes Association, Inc., is a violation of federal law. This material has been modified from Choose Your Foods: Exchange Lists for Diabetes, which is the basis of a meal planning system designed by a committee of the American Diabetes Association and the American Dietetic Association. While designed primarily for people with diabetes and others who must follow special diets, the Exchange Lists are based on principles of good nutrition that apply to everyone. Copyright © 2008 by the American Diabetes Association and Academy of Nutrition and Dietetics (formerly American Dietetic Association)

Crackers and Snacks

Food	Serving Size
Animal crackers	8
Crackers	
⚠ round-butter type	6
⚠ saltine-type	6
sandwich-style, cheese or peanut butter filling	3
⚠ whole-wheat regular	2–5 (¾ oz)
☺ whole-wheat lower fat or crispbreads	2–5 (¾ oz)

(continues)

☺ = More than 3 grams of dietary fiber per serving.

⚠ = Extra fat, or prepared with added fat (Count as 1 starch 1 fat.).

Crackers and Snacks *(continued)*

Food	Serving Size
Graham cracker, 2½-inch square	3
Matzoh	¾ oz
Melba toast, about 2-inch by 4-inch piece	4 pieces
Oyster crackers	20
Popcorn	3 cups
⚠️ with butter	3 cups
☺ no fat added	3 cups
☺ lower fat	3 cups
Pretzels	¾ oz
Rice cakes, 4 inches across	2
Snack chips	
fat-free or baked (tortilla, potato), baked pita chips	15–20 (¾ oz)
⚠️ regular (tortilla, potato)	9–13 (¾ oz)

Note: For other snacks, see the **Sweets, Desserts, and Other Carbohydrates**.

Source: Reproduction of the Exchange Lists in whole or part, without permission of the American Dietetic Association or the American Diabetes Association, Inc., is a violation of federal law. This material has been modified from Choose Your Foods: Exchange Lists for Diabetes, which is the basis of a meal planning system designed by a committee of the American Diabetes Association and the American Dietetic Association. While designed primarily for people with diabetes and others who must follow special diets, the Exchange Lists are based on principles of good nutrition that apply to everyone. Copyright © 2008 by the American Diabetes Association and Academy of Nutrition and Dietetics (formerly American Dietetic Association)

Fruits

Fruit

The weight listed includes skin, core, seeds, and rind.

Food	Serving Size
Apple, unpeeled, small	1 (4 oz)
Apples, dried	4 rings
Applesauce, unsweetened	½ cup
Apricots	
canned	½ cup
dried	8 halves
☺ fresh	4 whole (5½ oz)
Banana, extra small	1 (4 oz)
☺ Blackberries	¾ cup
Blueberries	¾ cup
Cantaloupe, small	⅓ melon or 1 cup cubed (11 oz)
Cherries	
sweet, canned	½ cup
sweet fresh	12 (3 oz)

(continues)

☺ = More than 3 grams of dietary fiber per serving.

⚠️ = Extra fat, or prepared with added fat (Count as 1 starch 1 fat.).

Fruit *(continued)*

Food	Serving Size
Dates	3
Dried fruits (blueberries, cherries, cranberries, mixed fruit, raisins)	2 Tbsp
Figs	
dried	1½
☺ fresh	1½ large or 2 medium (3½ oz)
Fruit cocktail	½ cup
Grapefruit	
large	½ (11 oz)
sections, canned	¾ cup
Grapes, small	17 (3 oz)
Honeydew melon	1 slice or 1 cup cubed (10 oz)
☺ Kiwi	1 (3½ oz)
Mandarin oranges, canned	¾ cup
Mango, small	½ fruit (5½ oz) or ½ cup
Nectarine, small	1 (5 oz)
☺ Orange, small	1 (6½ oz)
Papaya	½ fruit or 1 cup cubed (8 oz)
Peaches	
canned	½ cup
fresh, medium	1 (6 oz)
Pears	
canned	½ cup
fresh, large	½ (4 oz)
Pineapple	
canned	½ cup
fresh	¾ cup
Plums	
canned	½ cup
dried (prunes)	3
small	2 (5 oz)
☺ Raspberries	1 cup
☺ Strawberries	1¼ cup whole berries
☺ Tangerines, small	2 (8 oz)
Watermelon	1 slice or 1¼ cups cubes (13½ oz)

Source: Reproduction of the Exchange Lists in whole or part, without permission of the American Dietetic Association or the American Diabetes Association, Inc., is a violation of federal law. This material has been modified from *Choose Your Foods: Exchange Lists for Diabetes*, which is the basis of a meal planning system designed by a committee of the American Diabetes Association and the American Dietetic Association. While designed primarily for people with diabetes and others who must follow special diets, the Exchange Lists are based on principles of good nutrition that apply to everyone. Copyright © 2008 by the American Diabetes Association and Academy of Nutrition and Dietetics (formerly American Dietetic Association)

☺ = More than 3 grams of dietary fiber per serving.

Fruit Juice

Food	Serving Size
Apple juice/cider	½ cup
Fruit juice blends, 100% juice	⅓ cup
Grape juice	⅓ cup
Grapefruit juice	½ cup
Orange juice	½ cup
Pineapple juice	½ cup
Prune juice	⅓ cup

Source: Reproduction of the Exchange Lists in whole or part, without permission of the American Dietetic Association or the American Diabetes Association, Inc., is a violation of federal law. This material has been modified from Choose Your Foods: Exchange Lists for Diabetes, which is the basis of a meal planning system designed by a committee of the American Diabetes Association and the American Dietetic Association. While designed primarily for people with diabetes and others who must follow special diets, the Exchange Lists are based on principles of good nutrition that apply to everyone. Copyright © 2008 by the American Diabetes Association and Academy of Nutrition and Dietetics (formerly American Dietetic Association)

Milk

Milk and Yogurts

Food	Serving Size	Count as
Fat-free or low-fat (1%)		
Milk, buttermilk, acidophilus milk, Lactaid	1 cup	1 fat-free milk
Evaporated milk	½ cup	1 fat-free milk
Yogurt, plain or flavored with an artificial sweetener	⅔ cup (6 oz)	1 fat-free milk
Reduced-fat (2%)		
Milk, acidophilus milk, kefir, Lactaid	1 cup	1 reduced-fat milk
Yogurt, plain	⅔ cup (6 oz)	1 reduced-fat milk
Whole		
Milk, buttermilk, goat's milk	1 cup	1 whole milk
Evaporated milk	½ cup	1 whole milk
Yogurt, plain	8 oz	1 whole milk

Source: Reproduction of the Exchange Lists in whole or part, without permission of the American Dietetic Association or the American Diabetes Association, Inc., is a violation of federal law. This material has been modified from Choose Your Foods: Exchange Lists for Diabetes, which is the basis of a meal planning system designed by a committee of the American Diabetes Association and the American Dietetic Association. While designed primarily for people with diabetes and others who must follow special diets, the Exchange Lists are based on principles of good nutrition that apply to everyone. Copyright © 2008 by the American Diabetes Association and Academy of Nutrition and Dietetics (formerly American Dietetic Association)

Dairy-like Foods

Food	Serving Size	Count as
Chocolate milk		
fat-free	1 cup	1 fat-free milk + 1 carbohydrate
whole	1 cup	1 whole milk + 1 carbohydrate
Eggnog, whole milk	½ cup	1 carbohydrate + 2 fats

(continues)

Dairy-like Foods *(continued)*

Food	Serving Size	Count as
Rice drink		
flavored, low-fat	1 cup	2 carbohydrates
plain, fat-free	1 cup	1 carbohydrate
Smoothies, flavored, regular	10 oz	1 fat-free milk + 2½ carbohydrates
Soy milk		
light	1 cup	1 carbohydrate + ½ fat
regular, plain	1 cup	1 carbohydrate + 1 fat
Yogurt		
and juice blends	1 cup	1 fat-free milk + 1 carbohydrate
low carbohydrate (less than 6 g carbohydrate per choice)	⅔ cup (6 oz)	½ fat-free milk
with fruit, low-fat	⅔ cup (6 oz)	1 fat-free milk + 1 carbohydrate

Note: Coconut milk is on the **Fats** list.

Source: Reproduction of the Exchange Lists in whole or part, without permission of the American Dietetic Association or the American Diabetes Association, Inc., is a violation of federal law. This material has been modified from Choose Your Foods: Exchange Lists for Diabetes, which is the basis of a meal planning system designed by a committee of the American Diabetes Association and the American Dietetic Association. While designed primarily for people with diabetes and others who must follow special diets, the Exchange Lists are based on principles of good nutrition that apply to everyone. Copyright © 2008 by the American Diabetes Association and Academy of Nutrition and Dietetics (formerly American Dietetic Association)

Sweets, Desserts, and other Carbohydrates

Beverages, Soda, and Energy/Sports Drinks

Food	Serving Size	Count as
Cranberry juice cocktail	½ cup	1 carbohydrate
Energy drink	1 can (8.3 oz)	2 carbohydrates
Fruit drink or lemonade	1 cup (8 oz)	2 carbohydrates
Hot chocolate		
regular	1 envelope added to 8 oz water	1 carbohydrate + 1 fat
sugar-free or light	1 envelope added to 8 oz water	1 carbohydrate
Soft drink (soda), regular	1 can (12 oz)	2½ carbohydrates
Sports drink	1 cup (8 oz)	1 carbohydrate

Source: Reproduction of the Exchange Lists in whole or part, without permission of the American Dietetic Association or the American Diabetes Association, Inc., is a violation of federal law. This material has been modified from Choose Your Foods: Exchange Lists for Diabetes, which is the basis of a meal planning system designed by a committee of the American Diabetes Association and the American Dietetic Association. While designed primarily for people with diabetes and others who must follow special diets, the Exchange Lists are based on principles of good nutrition that apply to everyone. Copyright © 2008 by the American Diabetes Association and Academy of Nutrition and Dietetics (formerly American Dietetic Association)

Brownies, Cake, Cookies, Gelatin, Pie, and Pudding

Food	Serving Size	Count as
Brownie, small, unfrosted	1¼-in square, ⅞-in high (about 1 oz)	1 carbohydrate + 1 fat
Cake		
angel food, unfrosted	1⁄12 of cake (about 2 oz)	2 carbohydrates
frosted	2-in square (about 2 oz)	2 carbohydrates + 1 fat
unfrosted	2-in square (about 2 oz)	1 carbohydrate + 1 fat
Cookies		
chocolate chip	2 cookies (2¼ in across)	1 carbohydrate + 2 fats
gingersnap	3 cookies	1 carbohydrate
sandwich, with crème filling	2 small (about ⅔ oz)	1 carbohydrate + 1 fat
sugar-free	3 small or 1 large (¾–1 oz)	1 carbohydrate + 1–2 fats
vanilla wafer	5 cookies	1 carbohydrate + 1 fat
Cupcake, frosted	1 small (about 1¾ oz)	2 carbohydrates + 1–1½ fats
Fruit cobbler	½ cup (3½ oz)	3 carbohydrates + 1 fat
Gelatin, regular	½ cup	1 carbohydrate
Pie		
commercially prepared fruit, 2 crusts	⅙ of 8-in pie	3 carbohydrates + 2 fats
pumpkin or custard	⅛ of 8-in pie	1½ carbohydrates + 1½ fats
Pudding		
regular (made with reduced-fat milk)	½ cup	2 carbohydrates
sugar-free or sugar- and fat-free (made with fat-free milk)	½ cup	1 carbohydrate

Source: Reproduction of the Exchange Lists in whole or part, without permission of the American Dietetic Association or the American Diabetes Association, Inc., is a violation of federal law. This material has been modified from Choose Your Foods: Exchange Lists for Diabetes, which is the basis of a meal planning system designed by a committee of the American Diabetes Association and the American Dietetic Association. While designed primarily for people with diabetes and others who must follow special diets, the Exchange Lists are based on principles of good nutrition that apply to everyone. Copyright © 2008 by the American Diabetes Association and Academy of Nutrition and Dietetics (formerly American Dietetic Association)

Candy, Spreads, Sweets, Sweeteners, Syrups, and Toppings

Food	Serving Size	Count as
Candy bar, chocolate/peanut	2 "fun size" bars (1 oz)	1½ carbohydrates + 1½ fats
Candy, hard	3 pieces	1 carbohydrate
Chocolate "kisses"	5 pieces	1 carbohydrate + 1 fat
Coffee creamer		
dry, flavored	4 tsp	½ carbohydrate + ½ fat
liquid, flavored	2 Tbsp	1 carbohydrate
Fruit snacks, chewy (pureed fruit concentrate)	1 roll (¾ oz)	1 carbohydrate
Fruit spreads, 100% fruit	1½ Tbsp	1 carbohydrate
Honey	1 Tbsp	1 carbohydrate
Jam or jelly, regular	1 Tbsp	1 carbohydrate
Sugar	1 Tbsp	1 carbohydrate
Syrup		
chocolate	2 Tbsp	2 carbohydrates
light (pancake type)	2 Tbsp	1 carbohydrate
regular (pancake type)	1 Tbsp	1 carbohydrate

(continues)

Candy, Spreads, Sweets, Sweeteners, Syrups, and Toppings *(continued)*

Source: Reproduction of the Exchange Lists in whole or part, without permission of the American Dietetic Association or the American Diabetes Association, Inc., is a violation of federal law. This material has been modified from Choose Your Foods: Exchange Lists for Diabetes, which is the basis of a meal planning system designed by a committee of the American Diabetes Association and the American Dietetic Association. While designed primarily for people with diabetes and others who must follow special diets, the Exchange Lists are based on principles of good nutrition that apply to everyone. Copyright © 2008 by the American Diabetes Association and Academy of Nutrition and Dietetics (formerly American Dietetic Association)

Condiments and Sauces

Food	Serving Size	Count as
Barbeque sauce	3 Tbsp	1 carbohydrate
Cranberry sauce, jellied	¼ cup	1½ carbohydrates
Gravy, canned or bottled	½ cup	½ carbohydrate + ½ fat
Salad dressing, fat-free, low-fat, cream-based	3 Tbsp	1 carbohydrate
Sweet and sour sauce	3 Tbsp	1 carbohydrate

Source: Reproduction of the Exchange Lists in whole or part, without permission of the American Dietetic Association or the American Diabetes Association, Inc., is a violation of federal law. This material has been modified from Choose Your Foods: Exchange Lists for Diabetes, which is the basis of a meal planning system designed by a committee of the American Diabetes Association and the American Dietetic Association. While designed primarily for people with diabetes and others who must follow special diets, the Exchange Lists are based on principles of good nutrition that apply to everyone. Copyright © 2008 by the American Diabetes Association and Academy of Nutrition and Dietetics (formerly American Dietetic Association)

Doughnuts, Muffins, Pastries, and Sweet Breads

Food	Serving Size	Count as
Banana nut bread	1-inch slice (1 oz)	2 carbohydrates + 1 fat
Doughnut		
cake, plain	1 medium (1½ oz)	1½ carbohydrates + 2 fats
yeast type, glazed	3¾ inches across (2 oz)	2 carbohydrates + 2 fats
Muffin (4 oz)	¼ muffin (1 oz)	1 carbohydrate + ½ fat
Sweet roll or Danish	1 (2½ oz)	2½ carbohydrates + 2 fats

Note: You can also check the **Fats** list and **Free Foods** list for other condiments.

Source: Reproduction of the Exchange Lists in whole or part, without permission of the American Dietetic Association or the American Diabetes Association, Inc., is a violation of federal law. This material has been modified from Choose Your Foods: Exchange Lists for Diabetes, which is the basis of a meal planning system designed by a committee of the American Diabetes Association and the American Dietetic Association. While designed primarily for people with diabetes and others who must follow special diets, the Exchange Lists are based on principles of good nutrition that apply to everyone. Copyright © 2008 by the American Diabetes Association and Academy of Nutrition and Dietetics (formerly American Dietetic Association)

Frozen Bars, Frozen Desserts, Frozen Yogurt, and Ice Cream

Food	Serving Size	Count as
Frozen pops	1	½ carbohydrate
Fruit, juice bars, frozen, 100% juice	1 bar (3 oz)	1 carbohydrate

(continues)

⊙ = 480 mg or more of sodium per serving.

Frozen Bars, Frozen Desserts, Frozen Yogurt, and Ice Cream *(continued)*

Food	Serving Size	Count as
Ice cream		
fat-free	½ cup	1½ carbohydrates
light	½ cup	1 carbohydrate + 1 fat
no sugar added	½ cup	1 carbohydrate + 1 fat
regular	½ cup	1 carbohydrate + 2 fats
Sherbet, sorbet	½ cup	2 carbohydrates
Yogurt, frozen		
fat-free	⅓ cup	1 carbohydrate
regular	½ cup	1 carbohydrate + 0–1 fat

Source: Reproduction of the Exchange Lists in whole or part, without permission of the American Dietetic Association or the American Diabetes Association, Inc., is a violation of federal law. This material has been modified from Choose Your Foods: Exchange Lists for Diabetes, which is the basis of a meal planning system designed by a committee of the American Diabetes Association and the American Dietetic Association. While designed primarily for people with diabetes and others who must follow special diets, the Exchange Lists are based on principles of good nutrition that apply to everyone. Copyright © 2008 by the American Diabetes Association and Academy of Nutrition and Dietetics (formerly American Dietetic Association)

Granola Bars, Meal Replacement Bars/Shakes, and Trail Mix

Food	Serving Size	Count as
Granola or snack bar, regular or low-fat	1 bar (1 oz)	1½ carbohydrates
Meal replacement bar	1 bar (1⅓ oz)	1½ carbohydrates + 0–1 fat
Meal replacement bar	1 bar (2 oz)	2 carbohydrates + 1 fat
Meal replacement shake, reduced-calorie	1 can (10–11 oz)	1½ carbohydrates + 0–1 fat
Trail mix		
candy/nut-based	1 oz	1 carbohydrate + 2 fats
dried fruit-based	1 oz	1 carbohydrate + 1 fat

Source: Reproduction of the Exchange Lists in whole or part, without permission of the American Dietetic Association or the American Diabetes Association, Inc., is a violation of federal law. This material has been modified from Choose Your Foods: Exchange Lists for Diabetes, which is the basis of a meal planning system designed by a committee of the American Diabetes Association and the American Dietetic Association. While designed primarily for people with diabetes and others who must follow special diets, the Exchange Lists are based on principles of good nutrition that apply to everyone. Copyright © 2008 by the American Diabetes Association and Academy of Nutrition and Dietetics (formerly American Dietetic Association)

Vegetables

Beans, Peas, and Lentils

The choices on this list count as 1 starch 1 1 lean meat.

	Food	Serving Size
☺	Baked beans	⅓ cup
☺	Beans, cooked (black, garbanzo, kidney, lima, navy, pinto, white)	½ cup
☺	Lentils, cooked (brown, green, yellow)	½ cup
☺	Peas, cooked (black-eyed, split)	½ cup
🧂 ☺	Refried beans, canned	½ cup

(continues)

☺ = More than 3 g of dietary fiber per serving.

🧂 = 480 mg or more of sodium per serving.

Beans, Peas, and Lentils *(continued)*

Starchy Vegetables

Food	Serving Size
Cassava	⅓ cup
Corn	½ cup
on cob, large	½ cob (5 oz)
☺ Hominy, canned	¾ cup
☺ Mixed vegetables with corn, peas, or pasta	1 cup
☺ Parsnips	½ cup
☺ Peas, green	½ cup
Plantain, ripe	⅓ cup
Potato	
baked with skin	¼ large (3 oz)
boiled, all kinds	½ cup or ½ medium (3 oz)
⚠ mashed, with milk and fat	½ cup
French fried (oven-baked)	1 cup (2 oz)
☺ Pumpkin, canned, no sugar added	1 cup
Spaghetti/pasta sauce	½ cup
☺ Squash, winter (acorn, butternut)	1 cup
☺ Succotash	½ cup
Yam, sweet potato, plain	½ cup

Nonstarchy Vegetables

Amaranth or Chinese spinach			Beets
Artichoke		ⓢ	Borscht
Artichoke hearts			Broccoli
Asparagus		☺	Brussels sprouts
Baby corn			Cabbage (green, bok choy, Chinese)
Bamboo shoots		☺	Carrots
Bean sprouts			Cauliflower
Beans (green, wax, Italian)			Celery

(continues)

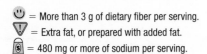

☺ = More than 3 g of dietary fiber per serving.

⚠ = Extra fat, or prepared with added fat.

ⓢ = 480 mg or more of sodium per serving.

Nonstarchy Vegetables *(continued)*

☺ Chayote

Coleslaw, packaged, no dressing

Cucumber

Eggplant

Gourds (bitter, bottle, luffa, bitter melon)

Green onions or scallions

Greens (collard, kale, mustard, turnip)

Hearts of palm

Jicama

Kohlrabi

Leeks

Mixed vegetables (without corn, peas, or pasta)

Mung bean sprouts

Mushrooms, all kinds, fresh

Okra

Onions

Oriental radish or daikon

Pea pods

☺ Peppers (all varieties)

Radishes

Rutabaga

🧂 Sauerkraut

Soybean sprouts

Spinach

Squash (summer, crookneck, zucchini)

Sugar pea snaps

☺ Swiss chard

Tomato

🧂 Tomato sauce

Tomatoes, canned

⚠ Tomato/vegetable juice

Turnips

Water chestnuts

Yard-long beans

Note: Salad greens (like chicory, endive, escarole, lettuce, romaine, spinach, arugula, radicchio, watercress) are on the **Free Foods**.

Source: Reproduction of the Exchange Lists in whole or part, without permission of the American Dietetic Association or the American Diabetes Association, Inc., is a violation of federal law. This material has been modified from Choose Your Foods: Exchange Lists for Diabetes, which is the basis of a meal planning system designed by a committee of the American Diabetes Association and the American Dietetic Association. While designed primarily for people with diabetes and others who must follow special diets, the Exchange Lists are based on principles of good nutrition that apply to everyone. Copyright © 2008 by the American Diabetes Association and Academy of Nutrition and Dietetics (formerly American Dietetic Association)

Meat and Meat Substitutes

	Carbohydrate (g)	Protein (g)	Fat (g)	Calories
Lean meat	—	7	0–3	45
Medium-fat meat	—	7	4–7	75
High-fat meat	—	7	81	100
Plant-based protein	Varies	7	Varies	varies

Source: Reproduction of the Exchange Lists in whole or part, without permission of the American Dietetic Association or the American Diabetes Association, Inc., is a violation of federal law. This material has been modified from Choose Your Foods: Exchange Lists for Diabetes, which is the basis of a meal planning system designed by a committee of the American Diabetes Association and the American Dietetic Association. While designed primarily for people with diabetes and others who must follow special diets, the Exchange Lists are based on principles of good nutrition that apply to everyone. Copyright © 2008 by the American Diabetes Association and Academy of Nutrition and Dietetics (formerly American Dietetic Association)

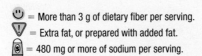

☺ = More than 3 g of dietary fiber per serving.

⚠ = Extra fat, or prepared with added fat.

🧂 = 480 mg or more of sodium per serving.

Portion Sizes: Portion size is an important part of meal planning. The **Meat and Meat Substitute** list is based on cooked weight (4 oz of raw meat is equal to 3 oz of cooked meat) after bone and fat have been removed. Try using the following comparisons to help estimate portion sizes:

- 1 oz cooked meat, poultry, or fish is about the size of a matchbox.
- 3 oz cooked meat, poultry, or fish is about the size of a deck of playing cards.
- 2 Tbsp peanut butter is about the size of a golf ball.
- The palm of a woman's hand is about 3–4 oz of cooked, boneless meat. The palm of a man's hand is a larger serving.
- 1 oz cheese is about the size of 4 dice.

Lean Meats and Meat Substitutes

	Food	Amount
	Beef: Select or Choice grades trimmed of fat: ground round, roast (chuck, rib, rump), round, sirloin, steak (cubed, flank, porterhouse, T-bone), tenderloin	1 oz
Ⓢ	Beef jerky	1 oz
	Cheeses with 3 g of fat or less per oz	1 oz
	Cottage cheese	¼ cup
	Egg substitutes, plain	¼ cup
	Egg whites	2
	Fish, fresh or frozen, plain: catfish, cod, flounder, haddock, halibut, orange roughy, salmon, tilapia, trout, tuna	1 oz
Ⓢ	Fish, smoked: herring or salmon (lox)	1 oz
	Game: buffalo, ostrich, rabbit, venison	1 oz
Ⓢ	Hot dog with 3 g of fat or less per oz	1
	(8 dogs per 14 oz package)	
	Note: May be high in carbohydrate	
	Lamb: chop, leg, or roast	1 oz
	Organ meats: heart, kidney, liver	1 oz
	Note: May be high in cholesterol	
	Oysters, fresh or frozen	6 medium
	Pork, lean	
Ⓢ	Canadian bacon	1 oz
	rib or loin chop/roast, ham, tenderloin	1 oz
	Poultry, without skin: Cornish hen, chicken, domestic duck or goose (well drained of fat), turkey	1 oz
	Processed sandwich meats with 3 g of fat or less per oz: chipped beef, deli thin-sliced meats, turkey ham, turkey kielbasa, turkey pastrami	1 oz
	Salmon, canned	1 oz
	Sardines, canned	2 medium
Ⓢ	Sausage with 3 g of fat or less per oz	1 oz
	Shellfish: clams, crab, imitation shellfish, lobster, scallops, shrimp	1 oz
	Tuna, canned in water or oil, drained	1 oz
	Veal, lean chop, roast	1 oz
		(continues)

Ⓢ = 480 mg or more of sodium per serving (based on the sodium content of a typical 3-oz serving of meat, unless 1 or 2 oz is the normal serving size).

Lean Meats and Meat Substitutes *(continued)*

Medium-Fat Meat and Meat Substitutes

Food	Amount
Beef: corned beef, ground beef, meatloaf, Prime grades trimmed of fat (prime rib), short ribs, tongue	1 oz
Cheeses with 4–7 g of fat per oz: feta, mozzarella, pasteurized processed cheese spread, reduced-fat cheeses, string	1 oz
Egg	1
Note: High in cholesterol, so limit to 3 per week	
Fish, any fried product	1 oz
Lamb: ground, rib roast	1 oz
Pork: cutlet, shoulder roast	1 oz
Poultry: chicken with skin; dove, pheasant, wild duck, or goose; fried chicken; ground turkey	1 oz
Ricotta cheese	2 oz or ¼ cup
Ⓢ Sausage with 4–7 g of fat per oz	1 oz
Veal, cutlet (no breading)	1 oz

High-Fat Meat and Meat Substitutes

These foods are high in saturated fat, cholesterol, and calories and may raise blood cholesterol levels if eaten on a regular basis. Try to eat 3 or fewer servings from this group per week.

Food	Amount
Bacon	
Ⓢ pork	2 slices (16 slices per lb or 1 oz each, before cooking)
Ⓢ turkey	3 slices (½ oz each before cooking)
Cheese, regular: American, bleu, brie, cheddar, hard goat, Monterey jack, queso, and Swiss	1 oz
Ⓢ ▽ Hot dog: beef, pork, or combination (10 per lb-sized package)	1
Ⓢ Hot dog: turkey or chicken (10 per lb-sized package)	1

(continues)

▽ = Extra fat, or prepared with added fat.

Ⓢ = 480 mg or more of sodium per serving (based on the sodium content of a typical 3-oz serving of meat, unless 1 or 2 oz is the normal serving size).

High-Fat Meat and Meat Substitutes *(continued)*

Food	Amount
Pork: ground, sausage, spareribs	1 oz
Processed sandwich meats with 8 g of fat or more per oz: bologna, pastrami, hard salami	1 oz
⑤ Sausage with 8 g fat or more per oz: bratwurst, chorizo, Italian, knockwurst, Polish, smoked, summer	1 oz

Source: Reproduction of the Exchange Lists in whole or part, without permission of the American Dietetic Association or the American Diabetes Association, Inc., is a violation of federal law. This material has been modified from Choose Your Foods: Exchange Lists for Diabetes, which is the basis of a meal planning system designed by a committee of the American Diabetes Association and the American Dietetic Association. While designed primarily for people with diabetes and others who must follow special diets, the Exchange Lists are based on principles of good nutrition that apply to everyone. Copyright © 2008 by the American Diabetes Association and Academy of Nutrition and Dietetics (formerly American Dietetic Association)

Plant-Based Proteins

Because carbohydrate content varies among plant-based proteins, you should read the food label.

	Food	Amount	Count as
	"Bacon" strips, soy-based	3 strips	1 medium-fat meat
☺	Baked beans	⅓ cup	1 starch + 1 lean meat
☺	Beans, cooked: black, garbanzo, kidney, lima, navy, pinto, white	½ cup	1 starch + 1 lean meat
☺	"Beef" or "sausage" crumbles, soy-based	2 oz	½ carbohydrate + 1 lean meat
	"Chicken" nuggets, soy-based	2 nuggets (1½ oz)	½ carbohydrate + 1 medium- fat meat
☺	Edamame	½ cup	½ carbohydrate + 1 lean meat
	Falafel (spiced chickpea and wheat patties)	3 patties (about 2 inches across)	1 carbohydrate + 1 high-fat meat
	Hot dog, soy-based	1 (1½ oz)	½ carbohydrate + 1 lean meat
☺	Hummus	⅓ cup	1 carbohydrate + 1 high-fat meat
☺	Lentils, brown, green, or yellow	½ cup	1 carbohydrate + 1 lean meat
☺	Meatless burger, soy-based	3 oz	½ carbohydrate + 2 lean meats
☺	Meatless burger, vegetable- and starch-based	1 patty (about 2½ oz)	1 carbohydrate + 2 lean meats
	Nut spreads: almond butter, cashew butter, peanut butter, soy nut butter	1 Tbsp	1 high-fat meat
☺	Peas, cooked: black-eyed and split peas	½ cup	1 starch + 1 lean meat
☺	Refried beans, canned	½ cup	1 starch + 1 lean meat
	"Sausage" patties, soy-based	1 (1½ oz)	1 medium-fat meat
	Soy nuts, unsalted	¾ oz	½ carbohydrate + 1 medium-fat meat
	Tempeh	¼ cup	1 medium-fat meat
	Tofu	4 oz (½ cup)	1 medium-fat meat
	Tofu, light	4 oz (½ cup)	1 lean meat

Note: Beans, peas, and lentils are also found on the **Starch** list. Nut butters in smaller amounts are found in the **Fats** list.

 = More than 3 g of dietary fiber per serving.

 = 480 mg or more of sodium per serving (based on the sodium content of a typical 3-oz serving of meat, unless 1 or 2 oz is the normal serving size).

Plant-Based Proteins *(continued)*

Source: Reproduction of the Exchange Lists in whole or part, without permission of the American Dietetic Association or the American Diabetes Association, Inc., is a violation of federal law. This material has been modified from Choose Your Foods: Exchange Lists for Diabetes, which is the basis of a meal planning system designed by a committee of the American Diabetes Association and the American Dietetic Association. While designed primarily for people with diabetes and others who must follow special diets, the Exchange Lists are based on principles of good nutrition that apply to everyone. Copyright © 2008 by the American Diabetes Association and Academy of Nutrition and Dietetics (formerly American Dietetic Association)

Fats

1 fat choice equals:

- 1 teaspoon of regular margarine, vegetable oil, butter
- 1 tablespoon of regular salad dressing

Unsaturated Fats—Monounsaturated Fats

Food	Serving Size
Avocado, medium	2 Tbsp (1 oz)
Nut butters (trans fat-free): almond butter, cashew butter, peanut butter (smooth or crunchy)	1½ tsp
Nuts	
almonds	6 nuts
brazil	2 nuts
cashews	6 nuts
filberts (hazelnuts)	5 nuts
Macadamia	3 nuts
mixed (50% peanuts)	6 nuts
peanuts	10 nuts
pecans	4 halves
pistachios	16 nuts
Oil: canola, olive, peanut	1 tsp
Olives	
black (ripe)	8 large
green, stuffed	10 large

Polyunsaturated Fats

Food	Serving Size
Margarine: lower-fat spread (30%–50% vegetable oil, *trans* fat-free)	1 Tbsp
Margarine: stick, tub (*trans* fat-free), or squeeze (*trans* fat-free)	1 tsp
Mayonnaise	
reduced-fat	1 Tbsp
regular	1 tsp
Mayonnaise-style salad dressing	
reduced-fat	1 Tbsp
regular	2 tsp
Nuts	
pignolia (pine nuts)	1 Tbsp
walnuts, English	4 halves
Oil: corn, cottonseed, flaxseed, grape seed, safflower, soybean, sunflower	1 tsp

(continues)

Polyunsaturated Fats *(continued)*

Food	Serving Size
Oil: made from soybean and canola oil—Enova	1 tsp
Plant stanol esters	
light	1 Tbsp
regular	2 tsp
Salad dressing	
🧂 reduced-fat	2 Tbsp
Note: May be high in carbohydrate.	
🧂 regular	1 Tbsp
Seeds	
flaxseed, whole	1 Tbsp
pumpkin, sunflower	1 Tbsp
sesame seeds	1 Tbsp
Tahini or sesame paste	2 tsp

Source: Reproduction of the Exchange Lists in whole or part, without permission of the American Dietetic Association or the American Diabetes Association, Inc., is a violation of federal law. This material has been modified from Choose Your Foods: Exchange Lists for Diabetes, which is the basis of a meal planning system designed by a committee of the American Diabetes Association and the American Dietetic Association. While designed primarily for people with diabetes and others who must follow special diets, the Exchange Lists are based on principles of good nutrition that apply to everyone. Copyright © 2008 by the American Diabetes Association and Academy of Nutrition and Dietetics (formerly American Dietetic Association)

Saturated Fats

Food	Serving Size
Bacon, cooked, regular or turkey	1 slice
Butter	
reduced-fat	1 Tbsp
stick	1 tsp
whipped	2 tsp
Butter blends made with oil	
reduced-fat or light	1 Tbsp
regular	1½ tsp
Chitterlings, boiled	2 Tbsp (½ oz)
Coconut, sweetened, shredded	2 Tbsp
Coconut milk	
light	⅓ cup
regular	1½ Tbsp
Cream	
half and half	2 Tbsp
heavy	1 Tbsp
light	1½ Tbsp
whipped	2 Tbsp
whipped, pressurized	¼ cup

(continues)

🧂 = 480 mg or more of sodium per serving.

Saturated Fats *(continued)*

Food	Serving Size
Cream cheese	
reduced-fat	1½ Tbsp (¾ oz)
regular	1 Tbsp (½ oz)
Lard	1 tsp
Oil: coconut, palm, palm kernel	1 tsp
Salt pork	¼ oz
Shortening, solid	1 tsp
Sour cream	
reduced-fat or light	3 Tbsp
regular	2 Tbsp

Source: Reproduction of the Exchange Lists in whole or part, without permission of the American Dietetic Association or the American Diabetes Association, Inc., is a violation of federal law. This material has been modified from Choose Your Foods: Exchange Lists for Diabetes, which is the basis of a meal planning system designed by a committee of the American Diabetes Association and the American Dietetic Association. While designed primarily for people with diabetes and others who must follow special diets, the Exchange Lists are based on principles of good nutrition that apply to everyone. Copyright © 2008 by the American Diabetes Association and Academy of Nutrition and Dietetics (formerly American Dietetic Association)

Free Foods

Selection Tips

- Most foods on this list should be limited to three servings (as listed here) per day.
- Food and drink choices listed here without a serving size can be eaten whenever you like.

Low Carbohydrate Foods

Food	Serving Size
Cabbage, raw	½ cup
Candy, hard (regular or sugar-free)	1 piece
Carrots, cauliflower, or green beans, cooked	¼ cup
Cranberries, sweetened with sugar substitute	½ cup
Cucumber, sliced	½ cup
Gelatin	
dessert, sugar-free	
unflavored	
Gum	
Jam or jelly, light or no sugar added	2 tsp
Rhubarb, sweetened with sugar substitute	½ cup
Salad greens	
Sugar substitutes (artificial sweeteners)	
Syrup, sugar-free	2 Tbsp

(continues)

Low Carbohydrate Foods *(continued)*

Modified Fat Foods with Carbohydrate

Food	Serving Size
Cream cheese, fat-free	1 Tbsp (½ oz)
Creamers	
nondairy, liquid	1 Tbsp
nondairy, powdered	2 tsp
Margarine spread	
fat-free	1 Tbsp
reduced-fat	1 tsp
Mayonnaise	
fat-free	1 Tbsp
reduced-fat	1 tsp
Mayonnaise-style salad dressing	
fat-free	1 Tbsp
reduced-fat	1 tsp
Salad dressing	
fat-free or low-fat	1 Tbsp
fat-free, Italian	2 Tbsp
Sour cream, fat-free or reduced-fat	1 Tbsp
Whipped topping	
light or fat-free	2 Tbsp
regular	1 Tbsp

Condiments

Food	Serving Size
Barbecue sauce	2 tsp
Catsup (ketchup)	1 Tbsp
Honey mustard	1 Tbsp
Horseradish	
Lemon juice	

(continues)

Condiments *(continued)*

Food	Serving Size
Miso	1½ tsp
Mustard	
Parmesan cheese, freshly grated	1 Tbsp
Pickle relish	1 Tbsp
Pickles	
dill	1½ medium
sweet, bread and butter	2 slices
sweet, gherkin	¾ oz
Salsa	¼ cup
Soy sauce, light or regular	1 Tbsp
Sweet and sour sauce	2 tsp
Sweet chili sauce	2 tsp
Taco sauce	1 Tbsp
Vinegar	
Yogurt, any type	2 Tbsp

Free Food List

A *free food* is any food or drink that contains less than 20 calories or less than 5 gm of carbohydrate per serving. Foods with a serving size listed should be limited to three servings per day. Be sure to spread them out throughout the day. Eating all three servings at one time could affect your blood glucose level. Foods listed without a serving size can be eaten as often as you like.

Artificial Sweeteners: Sugar substitutes, alternatives, or replacements that are approved by the Food and Drug Administration (FDA) are safe to use. Common brand names include:

- Equal and Nutrasweet (aspartame)
- Splenda (sucralose)
- Sugar Twin, Sweet-10, Sweet'N Low, and Sprinkle Sweet (saccharin)
- Sweet One (acesulfame K)

Although each sweetener is tested for safety before it can be marketed and sold, use a variety of sweeteners and in moderate amounts.

= 480 mg or more of sodium per serving.

Fat-Free or Reduced-Fat Foods

Cream cheese, fat-free	1 Tbsp
Creamers, nondairy, liquid	1 Tbsp
Creamers, nondairy, powdered	2 tsp
Mayonnaise, fat-free	1 Tbsp
Mayonnaise, reduced-fat	1 tsp
Margarine, fat-free	4 Tbsp
Margarine, reduced-fat	1 tsp
Miracle Whip, nonfat	1 Tbsp
Miracle Whip, reduced-fat	1 tsp
Nonstick cooking spray	
Salad dressing, fat-free	1 Tbsp
Salad dressing, fat-free, Italian	2 Tbsp
Salsa	¼ cup
Sour cream, fat-free, reduced-fat	1 Tbsp
Whipped topping, regular light	2 Tbsp

Source: Reproduction of the Exchange Lists in whole or part, without permission of the American Dietetic Association or the American Diabetes Association, Inc., is a violation of federal law. This material has been modified from Choose Your Foods: Exchange Lists for Diabetes, which is the basis of a meal planning system designed by a committee of the American Diabetes Association and the American Dietetic Association. While designed primarily for people with diabetes and others who must follow special diets, the Exchange Lists are based on principles of good nutrition that apply to everyone. Copyright © 2008 by the American Diabetes Association and Academy of Nutrition and Dietetics (formerly American Dietetic Association)

Sugar-Free or Low-Sugar Foods

Candy, hard, sugar-free	1 candy
Gelatin dessert, sugar-free	
Gelatin, unflavored	
Gum, sugar-free	
Jam or jelly, low-sugar or light	2 tsp
Syrup, sugar-free	2 Tbsp

Sugar substitutes, alternatives, or replacements that are approved by the Food and Drug Administration (FDA) are safe to use. Common brand names include:

Equal (aspartame)

Sprinkle Sweet (saccharin)

Sweet One (acesulfame K)

Sweet-10 (saccharin)

Sugar Twin (saccharin)

Sweet'N Low (saccharin)

Source: Reproduction of the Exchange Lists in whole or part, without permission of the American Dietetic Association or the American Diabetes Association, Inc., is a violation of federal law. This material has been modified from Choose Your Foods: Exchange Lists for Diabetes, which is the basis of a meal planning system designed by a committee of the American Diabetes Association and the American Dietetic Association. While designed primarily for people with diabetes and others who must follow special diets, the Exchange Lists are based on principles of good nutrition that apply to everyone. Copyright © 2008 by the American Diabetes Association and Academy of Nutrition and Dietetics (formerly American Dietetic Association)

Drinks

Bouillon, broth, consommé*	
Bouillon or broth, low sodium	
Carbonated or mineral water	
Club soda	
Cocoa powder, unsweetened	1 Tbsp
Coffee	
Diet soft drinks, sugar-free	
Drink mixes, sugar-free	
Tea	
Tonic water, sugar-free	

* = 400 mg or more of sodium per exchange.

Source: Reproduction of the Exchange Lists in whole or part, without permission of the American Dietetic Association or the American Diabetes Association, Inc., is a violation of federal law. This material has been modified from Choose Your Foods: Exchange Lists for Diabetes, which is the basis of a meal planning system designed by a committee of the American Diabetes Association and the American Dietetic Association. While designed primarily for people with diabetes and others who must follow special diets, the Exchange Lists are based on principles of good nutrition that apply to everyone. Copyright © 2008 by the American Diabetes Association and Academy of Nutrition and Dietetics (formerly American Dietetic Association)

Condiments

Catsup	1 Tbsp
Horseradish	
Lemon juice	
Lime juice	
Mustard	
Pickles, dill*	1½ large
Soy sauce, regular or light*	
Taco sauce	1 Tbsp
Vinegar	

Source: Reproduction of the Exchange Lists in whole or part, without permission of the American Dietetic Association or the American Diabetes Association, Inc., is a violation of federal law. This material has been modified from Choose Your Foods: Exchange Lists for Diabetes, which is the basis of a meal planning system designed by a committee of the American Diabetes Association and the American Dietetic Association. While designed primarily for people with diabetes and others who must follow special diets, the Exchange Lists are based on principles of good nutrition that apply to everyone. Copyright © 2008 by the American Diabetes Association and Academy of Nutrition and Dietetics (formerly American Dietetic Association)

Drinks/Mixes

Any food on this list—without a serving size listed—can be consumed in any moderate amount.

- Bouillon, broth, consommé
- Bouillon or broth, low-sodium
- Carbonated or mineral water
- Club soda
- Cocoa powder, unsweetened (1 Tbsp)
- Coffee, unsweetened or with sugar substitute

- Diet soft drinks, sugar-free
- Drink mixes, sugar-free
- Tea, unsweetened or with sugar substitute
- Tonic water, diet
- Water
- Water, flavored, carbohydrate-free

Seasonings

Any food on this list can be consumed in any moderate amount.

- Flavoring extracts (for example, vanilla, almond, peppermint)
- Garlic
- Herbs, fresh or dried
- Nonstick cooking spray

- Pimento
- Spices
- Hot pepper sauce
- Wine, used in cooking
- Worcestershire sauce

Read the label, and choose those seasonings that do not contain sodium or salt.

Basil (fresh)	Garlic	Onion powder
Celery seeds	Garlic powder	Oregano
Cinnamon	Herbs	Paprika
Chili powder	Hot pepper sauce	Pepper
Chives	Lemon	Pimento
Curry	Lemon juice	Spices
Dill	Lemon pepper	Soy sauce
Flavoring extracts	Lime	Soy sauce, low sodium ("lite")
(vanilla, almond, walnut, peppermint, lemon, butter, etc.)	Lime juice	Wine, used in cooking (¼ cup)
	Mint	Worcestershire sauce

 Be careful with seasonings that contain sodium or are salts, such as garlic salt, celery salt, and lemon pepper.

 = 480 mg or more of sodium per serving.

Combination Foods

Entrees

Food	Serving Size	Count as
Casserole type (tuna noodle, lasagna, spaghetti with meatballs, chili with beans, macaroni and cheese)	1 cup (8 oz)	2 carbohydrates + 2 medium-fat meats
Stews (beef/other meats and vegetables)	1 cup (8 oz)	1 carbohydrate + 1 medium-fat meat 1 0–3 fats
Tuna salad or chicken salad	½ cup (3½ oz)	½ carbohydrate + 2 lean meats 1 1 fat

Source: Reproduction of the Exchange Lists in whole or part, without permission of the American Dietetic Association or the American Diabetes Association, Inc., is a violation of federal law. This material has been modified from Choose Your Foods: Exchange Lists for Diabetes, which is the basis of a meal planning system designed by a committee of the American Diabetes Association and the American Dietetic Association. While designed primarily for people with diabetes and others who must follow special diets, the Exchange Lists are based on principles of good nutrition that apply to everyone. Copyright © 2008 by the American Diabetes Association and Academy of Nutrition and Dietetics (formerly American Dietetic Association)

Frozen Meals/Entrees

Food	Serving Size	Count as
Burrito (beef and bean)	1 (5 oz)	3 carbohydrates + 1 lean meat + 2 fats
Dinner-type meal	generally 14–17 oz	3 carbohydrates + 3 medium-fat meats + 3 fats
Entree or meal with less than 340 calories	about 8–11 oz	2–3 carbohydrates + 1–2 lean meats
Pizza		
cheese/vegetarian, thin crust	¼ of a 12 inch (4½–5 oz)	2 carbohydrates + 2 medium-fat meats
meat topping, thin crust	¼ of a 12 inch (5 oz)	2 carbohydrates + 2 medium-fat meats + 1½ fats
Pocket sandwich	1 (4½ oz)	3 carbohydrates + 1 lean meat + 1–2 fats
Pot pie	1 (7 oz)	2½ carbohydrates + 1 medium-fat meat + 3 fats

Salads (Deli-Style) Food	Serving Size	Count as
Coleslaw	½ cup	1 carbohydrate + 1½ fats
Macaroni/pasta salad	½ cup	2 carbohydrates + 3 fats
Potato salad	½ cup	1½–2 carbohydrates + 1–2 fats

Source: Reproduction of the Exchange Lists in whole or part, without permission of the American Dietetic Association or the American Diabetes Association, Inc., is a violation of federal law. This material has been modified from Choose Your Foods: Exchange Lists for Diabetes, which is the basis of a meal planning system designed by a committee of the American Diabetes Association and the American Dietetic Association. While designed primarily for people with diabetes and others who must follow special diets, the Exchange Lists are based on principles of good nutrition that apply to everyone. Copyright © 2008 by the American Diabetes Association and Academy of Nutrition and Dietetics (formerly American Dietetic Association)

Soups

Food	Serving Size	Count as
Bean, lentil, or split pea	1 cup	1 carbohydrate + 1 lean meat
Chowder (made with milk)	1 cup (8 oz)	1 carbohydrate + 1 lean meat + 1½ fats
Cream (made with water)	1 cup (8 oz)	1 carbohydrate + 1 fat
Instant	6 oz prepared	1 carbohydrate
with beans or lentils	8 oz prepared	2½ carbohydrates + 1 lean meat
Miso soup	1 cup	½ carbohydrate + 1 fat
Oriental noodle	1 cup	2 carbohydrates + 2 fats
Rice (congee)	1 cup	1 carbohydrate
Tomato (made with water)	1 cup (8 oz)	1 carbohydrate
Vegetable beef, chicken noodle, or other broth type	1 cup (8 oz)	1 carbohydrate

(continues)

 = More than 3 g of dietary fiber per serving.

 = 600 mg or more of sodium per serving (for fast food main dishes/meals)

Soups *(continued)*

Source: Reproduction of the Exchange Lists in whole or part, without permission of the American Dietetic Association or the American Diabetes Association, Inc., is a violation of federal law. This material has been modified from Choose Your Foods: Exchange Lists for Diabetes, which is the basis of a meal planning system designed by a committee of the American Diabetes Association and the American Dietetic Association. While designed primarily for people with diabetes and others who must follow special diets, the Exchange Lists are based on principles of good nutrition that apply to everyone. Copyright © 2008 by the American Diabetes Association and Academy of Nutrition and Dietetics (formerly American Dietetic Association)

Fast Foods

The choices in the Fast Foods list are not specific fast food meals or items, but are estimates based on popular foods. You can get specific nutrition information for almost every fast food or restaurant chain. Ask the restaurant or check its website for nutrition information about your favorite fast foods.

Breakfast Sandwiches

	Food	Serving Size	Count as
Ⓢ	Egg, cheese, meat, English muffin	1 sandwich	2 carbohydrates + 2 medium-fat meats
Ⓢ	Sausage biscuit sandwich	1 sandwich	2 carbohydrates + 2 high-fat meats + 3½ fats

Source: Reproduction of the Exchange Lists in whole or part, without permission of the American Dietetic Association or the American Diabetes Association, Inc., is a violation of federal law. This material has been modified from Choose Your Foods: Exchange Lists for Diabetes, which is the basis of a meal planning system designed by a committee of the American Diabetes Association and the American Dietetic Association. While designed primarily for people with diabetes and others who must follow special diets, the Exchange Lists are based on principles of good nutrition that apply to everyone. Copyright © 2008 by the American Diabetes Association and Academy of Nutrition and Dietetics (formerly American Dietetic Association)

Main Dishes/Entrees

	Food	Serving Size	Count as
Ⓢ ☻	Burrito (beef and beans)	1 (about 8 oz)	3 carbohydrates + 3 medium-fat meats + 3 fats
Ⓢ	Chicken breast, breaded and fried	1 (about 5 oz)	1 carbohydrate + 4 medium-fat meats
Ⓢ	Chicken drumstick, breaded and fried	1 (about 2 oz)	2 medium-fat meats
Ⓢ	Chicken nuggets	6 (about 3½ oz)	1 carbohydrate + 2 medium-fat meats + 1 fat
Ⓢ	Chicken thigh, breaded and fried	1 (about 4 oz)	½ carbohydrate + 3 medium-fat meats + 1½ fats
Ⓢ	Chicken wings, hot	6 (5 oz)	5 medium-fat meats +½ fats

Source: Reproduction of the Exchange Lists in whole or part, without permission of the American Dietetic Association or the American Diabetes Association, Inc., is a violation of federal law. This material has been modified from Choose Your Foods: Exchange Lists for Diabetes, which is the basis of a meal planning system designed by a committee of the American Diabetes Association and the American Dietetic Association. While designed primarily for people with diabetes and others who must follow special diets, the Exchange Lists are based on principles of good nutrition that apply to everyone. Copyright © 2008 by the American Diabetes Association and Academy of Nutrition and Dietetics (formerly American Dietetic Association)

Oriental

	Food	Serving Size	Count as
Ⓢ	Beef/chicken/shrimp with vegetables in sauce	1 cup (about 5 oz)	1 carbohydrate + 1 lean meat + 1 fat
Ⓢ	Egg roll, meat	1 (about 3 oz)	1 carbohydrate + 1 lean meat + 1 fat
Ⓢ	Fried rice, meatless	½ cup	1½ carbohydrates + 1½ fats
Ⓢ	Meat and sweet sauce (orange chicken)	1 cup	3 carbohydrates + 3 medium-fat meats + 2 fats
Ⓢ ☻	Noodles and vegetables in sauce (chow mein, lo mein)	1 cup	2 carbohydrates + 1 fat

Source: Reproduction of the Exchange Lists in whole or part, without permission of the American Dietetic Association or the American Diabetes Association, Inc., is a violation of federal law. This material has been modified from Choose Your Foods: Exchange Lists for Diabetes, which is the basis of a meal planning system designed by a committee of the American Diabetes Association and the American Dietetic Association. While designed primarily for people with diabetes and others who must follow special diets, the Exchange Lists are based on principles of good nutrition that apply to everyone. Copyright © 2008 by the American Diabetes Association and Academy of Nutrition and Dietetics (formerly American Dietetic Association)

☻ = More than 3 g of dietary fiber per serving.

Ⓢ = 600 mg or more of sodium per serving (for fast food main dishes/meals).

Pizza

	Food	Serving Size	Count as
🔲	Pizza		
	cheese, pepperoni, regular crust	½ of a 14 inch (about 4 oz)	2½ carbohydrates + 1 medium-fat meat + 1½ fats
🔲	cheese/vegetarian, thin crust	¼ of a 12 inch (about 6 oz)	2½ carbohydrates + 2 medium-fat meats + 1½ fats

Source: Reproduction of the Exchange Lists in whole or part, without permission of the American Dietetic Association or the American Diabetes Association, Inc., is a violation of federal law. This material has been modified from Choose Your Foods: Exchange Lists for Diabetes, which is the basis of a meal planning system designed by a committee of the American Diabetes Association and the American Dietetic Association. While designed primarily for people with diabetes and others who must follow special diets, the Exchange Lists are based on principles of good nutrition that apply to everyone. Copyright © 2008 by the American Diabetes Association and Academy of Nutrition and Dietetics (formerly American Dietetic Association)

Sandwiches

	Food	Serving Size	Count as
🔲	Chicken sandwich, grilled	1	3 carbohydrates + 4 lean meats
🔲	Chicken sandwich, crispy	1	3½ carbohydrates + 3 medium-fat meats + 1 fat
	Fish sandwich with tartar sauce	1	2½ carbohydrates + 2 medium-fat meats + 2 fats
	Hamburger		
🔲	large with cheese	1	2½ carbohydrates + 4 medium-fat meats + 1 fat
	regular	1	2 carbohydrates + 1 medium-fat meat + 1 fat
🔲	Hot dog with bun	1	1 carbohydrate + 1 high-fat meat + 1 fat
	Submarine sandwich		
🔲	less than 6 g fat	6-inch sub	3 carbohydrates + 2 lean meats
🔲	regular	6-inch sub	3½ carbohydrates + 2 medium-fat meats + 1 fat
	Taco, hard or soft shell (meat and cheese)	1 small	1 carbohydrate + 1 medium-fat meat + 1½ fats

Source: Reproduction of the Exchange Lists in whole or part, without permission of the American Dietetic Association or the American Diabetes Association, Inc., is a violation of federal law. This material has been modified from Choose Your Foods: Exchange Lists for Diabetes, which is the basis of a meal planning system designed by a committee of the American Diabetes Association and the American Dietetic Association. While designed primarily for people with diabetes and others who must follow special diets, the Exchange Lists are based on principles of good nutrition that apply to everyone. Copyright © 2008 by the American Diabetes Association and Academy of Nutrition and Dietetics (formerly American Dietetic Association)

Salads

	Food	Serving Size	Count as
🔲 🙂	Salad, main dish (grilled chicken type, no dressing or croutons)	Salad	1 carbohydrate + 4 lean meats
	Salad, side, no dressing or cheese	Small (about 5 oz)	1 vegetable

Source: Reproduction of the Exchange Lists in whole or part, without permission of the American Dietetic Association or the American Diabetes Association, Inc., is a violation of federal law. This material has been modified from Choose Your Foods: Exchange Lists for Diabetes, which is the basis of a meal planning system designed by a committee of the American Diabetes Association and the American Dietetic Association. While designed primarily for people with diabetes and others who must follow special diets, the Exchange Lists are based on principles of good nutrition that apply to everyone. Copyright © 2008 by the American Diabetes Association and Academy of Nutrition and Dietetics (formerly American Dietetic Association)

Sides/Appetizers

	Food	Serving Size	Count as
⚠️	French fries, restaurant style	Small	3 carbohydrates + 3 fats
		Medium	4 carbohydrates + 4 fats
		Large	5 carbohydrates + 6 fats

(continues)

 = Extra fat, or prepared with added fat.

 = 600 mg or more of sodium per serving (for fast food main dishes/meals).

Sides/Appetizers *(continued)*

	Food	Serving Size	Count as
🧂	Nachos with cheese	Small (about 4½ oz)	2½ carbohydrates + 4 fats
🧂	Onion rings	1 serving (about 3 oz)	2½ carbohydrates + 3 fats

Desserts

Food	Serving Size	Count as
Milkshake, any flavor	12 oz	6 carbohydrates + 2 fats
Soft-serve ice cream cone	1 small	2½ carbohydrates + 1 fat

Note: See the **Starch** list and **Sweets, Desserts, and Other Carbohydrates** list for foods such as bagels and muffins.

Alcohol

Food	Serving Size	Count as
Beer		
light (4.2%)	12 fl oz	1 alcohol equivalent + ½ carbohydrate
regular (4.9%)	12 fl oz	1 alcohol equivalent + 1 carbohydrate
Distilled spirits: vodka, rum, gin, whiskey 80 or 86 proof	1½ fl oz	1 alcohol equivalent
Liqueur, coffee (53 proof)	1 fl oz	1 alcohol equivalent + 1 carbohydrate
Sake	1 fl oz	½ alcohol equivalent
Wine		
dessert (sherry)	3½ fl oz	1 alcohol equivalent + 1 carbohydrate
dry, red or white (10%)	5 fl oz	1 alcohol equivalent

🧂 = 600 mg or more of sodium per serving (for fast food main dishes/meals).

ENGLISH AND METRIC UNITS AND CONVERSIONS

Units of Measure in the English System

Unit	Abbreviation	Equivalent
Dash		less than 1/8 teaspoon
few grains	f.g.	less than 1/8 teaspoon
drop		—
15 drops		—
1 teaspoon	tsp	1/3 tablespoon
1 tablespoon	Tbsp	3 teaspoons
1 fluid ounce	oz	2 tablespoons
1 cup	c	8 fluid ounces or 16 tablespoons
1 pint	pt	2 cups
1 quart	qt	2 pints or 4 cups
1 gallon	gal	4 quarts
1 peck	pk	2 gallons
1 bushel	bu	4 pecks
1 pound	lb	16 ounces

Units of Measure in the Metric System

Basic unit of *weight* is the *gram* (g)
Basic unit of *volume* is the *liter* (l)
Basic unit of *length* is the *meter* (m)
Temperature is measured in degrees *Celsius* (°C)

kilo: (*key*-low) = 1,000
deci: (*dess*-ee) = 0.1 (1/10)
centi: (*sent*-ee) = 0.01 (1/100)
milli: (*mill*-ee) = 0.001 (1/1000)

Unit Relationships within the Metric System

Weight			Volume		
1,000 grams	=	1 *kilo*gram	1000 liters	=	1 *kilo*liter*
100 grams	=	1 *hecto*gram*	100 liters	=	1 *hecto*liter*
10 grams	=	1 *deka*gram*	10 liters	=	1 *deka*liter*
		1 gram			1 liter
0.1 gram	=	1 *deci*gram*	0.1 liter	=	1 *deci*liter*
0.01 gram	=	1 *centi*gram*	0.01 liter	=	1 *centi*liter*
0.001 gram	=	1 *milli*gram	0.001 liter	=	1 *milli*liter
0.000001 gram	=	1 *micro*gram	0.000001 liter	=	1 *micro*liter*

*Units not commonly used.

Converting from the English System to the Metric System

Convert to Metric	When You Know	Multiply By	To Find
Weight	ounces (oz)	28	grams (g)
	pounds (lb)	0.45	kilograms (kg)
	teaspoons (tsp)	5	milliliters (ml)
	tablespoons (Tbsp)	15	milliliters
	fluid ounces (fl oz)	30	milliliters
	cups (c)	0.24	liters (l)
Volume	pints (pt)	0.47	liters
	quarts (qt)	0.95	liters
	gallons (gal)	3.8	liters
	cubic feet (ft^3)	0.03	cubic meters (m^3)
	cubic yards (yd^3)	0.76	cubic meters
Temperature	Fahrenheit (°F) temperature	5/9 (after subtracting 32)	Celsius (°C) temperature

Source: Adapted from "Some References on Metric Information" by U.S. Department of Commerce, National Bureau of Standards.

Converting from the Metric System to the English System

Convert to Metric	When You Know	Multiply By	To Find
Weight	grams (g)	0.035	ounces (oz)
	kilograms (kg)	2.2	pounds (lb)
	metric tons (1,000 kg)	1.1	short tons
	milliliters (ml)	0.03	fluid ounces (fl oz)
	liters (l)	2.1	pints (pt)
	liters	1.06	quarts (qt)
Volume	liters	0.26	gallons (gal)
	cubic meters (m^3)	35	cubic feet (ft^3)
	cubic meters	1.3	cubic yards (yd^3)
Temperature	Celsius (°C) temperature	9/5 (then add 32)	Fahrenheit (°F) temperature

Source: Adapted from "Some References on Metric Information" by U.S. Department of Commerce, National Bureau of Standards.

Weight Equivalents

	Milligram	Gram	Kilogram	Grain	Ounce	Pound
1 microgram (mg)	0.001	0.000001				
1 milligram (mg)	1.0	0.001		0.0154		
1 gram (g)	1,000.0	1.0	0.001	15.4	0.035	0.0022
1 kilogram (kg)	1,000,000.0	1,000.0	1.0	15,400.0	35.2	2.2
1 grain (gr)	64.8	0.065		1.0		
1 ounce (oz)		28.3		437.5	1.0	0.063
1 pound (lb)		453.6	0.454		16.0	1.0

Volume Equivalents

	Cubic Millimeter	Cubic Millimeter	Liter	Fluid Ounce	Pint	Quart
1 cubic millimeter (mm^3)	1.0	0.001				
1 cubic centimeter (cm^3)	1,000.0	1.0	0.001			
1 liter (l)	1,000,000.0	1,000.0	1.0	33.8	2.1	1.06
1 fluid ounce (fl oz)		30.(29.57)	0.03	1.0		
1 pint (pt)		473.0	0.473	16.0	1.0	
1 quart (qt)		946.0	0.946	32.0	2.0	1.0

Glossary

24-hour recall—listing the types, amounts, and preparation of all foods eaten in the past 24 hours

A

A1C—a blood test to determine how well blood glucose has been controlled for the last 3 months

absorption—taking up of nutrients in the intestines

abstinence—avoidance

acanthosis nigricans—dark velvety discoloration in body folds and creases often found in people with obesity-related insulin resistance

acid–base balance—the regulation of hydrogen ions in body fluids

acidosis—condition in which excess acids accumulate or there is a loss of base in the body

acquired immune deficiency syndrome (AIDS)—caused by the human immunodeficiency virus (HIV), which weakens the body's immune system, leaving it susceptible to fatal infections

acute renal failure (ARF)—suddenly occurring failure of the kidneys

adipose tissue—fatty tissue

adjustable gastric band—surgical reduction of stomach, but to lesser degree than bypass

adolescent—person between the ages of 13 and 20 years

aerobic metabolism—combining nutrients with oxygen within the cell; also called oxidation

albumin—protein that occurs in blood plasma

alcoholism—chronic and excessive use of alcohol

alkaline—base; capable of neutralizing acids

alkalosis—condition in which excess base accumulates in, or acids are lost from, the body

allergens—substance causing an allergic reaction

allergic reactions—adverse physical reactions to specific substances

allergy—sensitivity to specific substance(s)

amenorrhea—the stoppage of the monthly menstrual flow

amino acids—nitrogen-containing chemical compounds of which protein is composed

amniocentesis—a test to determine the status of the fetus in utero

amniotic fluid—fluid that surrounds fetus in the uterus

anabolism—the creation of new compounds during metabolism

anaerobic metabolism—reduces fats without the use of oxygen

anaphylaxis—serious allergic reaction that involves one or more body systems

anemia—condition caused by insufficient number of red blood cells, hemoglobin, or blood volume

anencephaly—absence of the brain

angina pectoris—pain in the heart muscle due to inadequate blood supply

anorexia—loss of appetite, especially as a result of disease

anorexia nervosa—psychologically induced lack of appetite

anthropometric measurements—measurements of height, weight, head, skinfold

antibodies—substances produced by the body in reaction to foreign substance; neutralize toxins from foreign bodies

antioxidant—substance preventing damage from oxygen

arteriosclerosis—generic term for thickened arteries

arthritis—chronic disease involving the joints

ascites—abnormal collection of fluid in the abdomen

ascorbic acid—vitamin C

aspirated—inhaled or suctioned

atherosclerosis—a form of arteriosclerosis affecting the intima (inner lining) of the artery walls

autoimmune disease—an illness that occurs when the body tissues are attacked by its own immune system

avitaminosis—without vitamins

B

balanced diet—one that includes all the essential nutrients in appropriate amounts

basal metabolism rate (BMR)—the rate at which energy is needed for body maintenance

beriberi—deficiency disease caused by the lack of vitamin B1 (thiamine)

bile—secretion of the liver, stored in the gallbladder, essential for the digestion of fats

bioavailable—ability of a nutrient to be readily absorbed and used by the body

biochemical tests—involving biology and chemistry

biotin—a B vitamin; necessary for metabolism

body mass index (BMI)—number calculated from a person's weight and height; fairly reliable indicator of body fatness for most people

bolus—food in the mouth that is ready to be swallowed

bomb calorimeter—device used to scientifically determine the caloric value of foods

bonding—emotional attachment

botulism—deadliest of food poisonings; caused by the bacteria *Clostridium botulinum*

bran—outer covering of grain kernels

buffer systems—protective systems regulating amounts of hydrogen ions in body fluids

built environment—man-made resources and infrastructure designed to support health and activity (parks, walking and bike paths, access to healthy foods, etc.)

bulimia—condition in which client alternately binges and purges

C

cachexia—severe malnutrition and body wasting caused by chronic disease

caliper—mechanical device used to measure percentage of body fat by skinfold measurement

calorie—also known as kcal or kilocalorie; represents the amount of heat needed to raise the temperature of one kilogram of water by 1 degree Celsius (C)

calorie requirements—number of calories required daily to meet energy needs

capillaries—tiny blood vessels connecting veins and arteries

carbohydrates (CHO)—the nutrient providing the major source of energy in the average diet

carboxypeptidase—pancreatic enzyme necessary for protein digestion

carcinogens—cancer-causing substances

cardiac sphincter—the muscle at the base of the esophagus that prevents gastric reflux from moving into the esophagus

cardiomyopathy—damage to the heart muscle caused by infection, alcohol, or drug abuse

cardiovascular—pertaining to the heart and entire circulatory system

cardiovascular disease (CVD)—disease affecting heart and blood vessels

carotenoids—plant pigments, some of which yield vitamin A

carriers—those who are capable of transmitting an infectious organism

catabolism—the breakdown of compounds during metabolism

catalyst—a substance that causes another substance to react

celiac disease—a disorder of the gastrointestinal tract characterized by malabsorption; also called gluten sensitivity

cellular edema—swelling of body cells caused by inadequate amount of sodium in extracellular fluid

cellulose—indigestible carbohydrate; provides fiber in the diet

cerebrovascular accident (CVA)—either a blockage or bursting of blood vessel leading to the brain

chemical digestion—chemical changes in foods during digestion caused by hydrolysis

chemotherapy—treatment of diseased tissue with chemicals

cholecystectomy—removal of the gallbladder

cholecystitis—inflammation of the gallbladder

cholecystokinin (CCK)—the hormone that triggers the gallbladder to release bile

cholelithiasis—gallstones

cholesterol—fat-like substance that is a constituent of body cells; is synthesized in the liver; also found in animal foods

chronic kidney disease—slow development of kidney failure

chylomicrons—the largest lipoprotein; transport lipids after digestion into the body

chyme—the food mass as it has been mixed with gastric juices

chymotrypsin—pancreatic enzyme necessary for the digestion of proteins

circulation—the body process whereby the blood is moved throughout the body

clinical examination—physical observation

coagulation—thickening

cobalamin—organic compound known as vitamin B12

coenzymes—an active part of an enzyme

collagen—protein substance that holds body cells together

colon—the large intestine

colostomy—opening from colon to abdomen surface

coma—state of unconsciousness

compensated heart disease—heart disease in which the heart is able to maintain circulation to all body parts

complementary proteins—incomplete proteins that when combined provide all nine essential amino acids

complete proteins—proteins that contain all nine essential amino acids

congestive heart failure (CHF)—a form of decompensated heart disease

coronary artery disease (CAD)—severe narrowing of the arteries that supply blood to the heart

creatinine—an end (waste) product of protein metabolism

Crohn's disease—a chronic progressive disorder that causes inflammation, ulcers, and thickening of intestinal walls, sometimes causing obstruction

cross contamination—unintentional transfer of harmful bacteria from one food or object to another

cumulative effects—results of something done repeatedly over many years

cystine—a nonessential amino acid

cysts—growths

D

daily values—represent percentage per serving of each nutritional item listed on new food labels based on daily intake of 2,000 calories

decompensated heart disease—heart disease in which the heart cannot maintain circulation to all body parts

deficiency diseases—disease caused by the lack of a specific nutrient

dehydrated—having lost large amounts of water

dehydration—loss of water

demineralization—loss of mineral or minerals

dentition—arrangement, type, and number of teeth

dermatitis—inflammation of the skin

descriptors—terms used to describe something

desensitized—having gradually reduced the body's sensitivity (allergic reaction) to specific items

diabetes mellitus—chronic disease in which the body lacks the normal ability to metabolize glucose

dialysis—mechanical filtration of the blood; used when the kidneys are no longer able to perform normally

diaphragm—thin membrane or partition

dietary fiber—indigestible parts of plants; absorbs water in large intestine, helping to create soft, bulky stool; some is believed to bind cholesterol in the colon, helping to rid cholesterol from the body; some is believed to lower blood glucose levels

Dietary Guidelines for Americans—national healthy eating guidelines for disease prevention and optimal health

dietary laws—rules to be followed in meal planning in some religions

Dietary Reference Intakes (DRIs)—combines the Recommended Dietary Allowances, Adequate Intake, Estimated Average Requirements, and Tolerable Upper Intake Levels for individuals into one value representative of the average daily nutrient intake of individuals over time

dietary-social history—evaluations of food habits, including client's ability to buy and prepare foods

dietitian—a professional trained to assess nutrition status and recommend appropriate diet therapy

digestion—breakdown of food in the body in preparation for absorption

disaccharides—double sugars that are reduced by hydrolysis to monosaccharides; examples are sucrose, maltose, and lactose

diuretics—substances used to increase the amount of urine excreted

diverticulitis—inflammation of the diverticula

diverticulosis—intestinal disorder characterized by little pockets forming in the sides of the intestines; pockets are called diverticula

dumping syndrome—nausea and diarrhea caused by food moving too quickly from the stomach to the small intestine

duodenal ulcer—ulcer occurring in the duodenum

duodenum—first (and smallest) section of the small intestine

dysentery—disease caused by microorganism; characterized by diarrhea

dyslipidemia—increased lipids in the blood

dyspepsia—gastrointestinal discomfort of vague origin

dysphagia—difficulty swallowing

E

eclamptic stage—convulsive stage of toxemia

edema—the abnormal retention of fluid by the body

electrolytes—chemical compounds that dissolve in water break up into electrically charged atoms called ions

elemental formulas—those formulas containing products of digestion of proteins, carbohydrates, and fats; also called hydrolyzed formulas

elimination—evacuation of wastes

elimination diet—limited diet in which only certain foods are allowed; intended to find the food allergen causing reaction

endocardium—lining of the heart

endogenous insulin—insulin produced within the body

endometrium—mucous membrane of the uterus

endosperm—the inner part of the kernel of grain; contains the carbohydrate

end-stage renal disease (ESRD)—the stage at which the kidneys have lost most or all of their ability to function

energy balance—occurs when the caloric value of food ingested equals the kilocalories expended

energy imbalance—eating either too much or too little for the amount of energy expended

energy requirement—number of calories required by the body each day

enriched foods—foods to which nutrients, usually B vitamins and iron, have been added to improve their nutritional value

enteral nutrition—feeding by tube directly into the client's digestive tract

enterotoxins—toxins affecting mucous membranes

enzymes—organic substances that cause changes in other substances

esophagitis—inflammation of mucosal lining of esophagus

esophagus—tube leading from the mouth to the stomach; part of the gastrointestinal system

essential hypertension—high blood pressure with unknown cause; also called primary hypertension

essential nutrients—nutrients found only in food

estrogen—hormone secreted by the ovaries

etiology—cause

exchange lists—lists of foods with interchangeable nutrient and kilocalorie contents; used in specific forms of diet therapy

exogenous insulin—insulin produced outside the body

extracellular—outside the cell

extracellular fluid (ECF)—water outside the cells; approximately 35% of total body fluid

F

fat cell theory—belief that fat cells have a natural drive to regain any weight lost

fats (lipids)—highest caloric-value nutrient

fat soluble—can be dissolved in fat

fatty acids—a component of fat that determines the classification of the fat

feces—solid waste from the large intestine

fermentation—changing of sugars and starches to alcohol

fetal alcohol syndrome (FAS)—subnormal physical and mental development caused by mother's excessive use of alcohol during pregnancy

fetal malformations—physical abnormalities of the fetus

fetus—infant in utero

fibrosis—development of tough, stringy tissue

flatulence—gas in the intestinal tract

flavonoids—naturally occurring water-soluble plant pigments that act as antioxidants

folate/folic acid—a form of vitamin B, also called folacin; essential for metabolism

food customs—food habits

food diary—written record of all food and drink ingested in a specified period

food faddists—people who have certain beliefs about particular foods or diets

food poisoning—foodborne illness

foodways—the food traditions or customs of a group of people

free radicals—atoms or groups of atoms with an odd (unpaired) number of electrons; can be formed when oxygen interacts with certain molecules

fructose—the simple sugar (monosaccharide) found in fruit and honey

fundus (of the stomach)—upper part of the stomach

fusion—a style of cooking that combines ingredients and techniques from different cultures or countries

G

galactose—the simple sugar (monosaccharide) to which lactose is broken down during digestion

galactosemia—inherited error in metabolism that prevents normal metabolism of galactose

galactosuria—galactose in the urine

gastric juices—the digestive secretions of the stomach

gastric ulcer—ulcer in the stomach

gastrin—hormone released by the stomach

gastroesophageal reflux disease (GERD)—backflow of stomach contents into the esophagus

gastrointestinal (GI) tract—pertaining to the stomach and intestines

gastrostomy—opening created by the surgeon directly into the stomach for enteral nutrition

genetic predisposition—inherited tendency

geriatrics—the branch of medicine involved with diseases of the elderly

germ—embryo or tiny life center of each kernel of grain

gerontology—the study of aging

gestational diabetes—diabetes occurring during pregnancy; usually disappears after delivery of the infant

ghrelin—a hormone from the stomach that signals the brain it's time to eat

glomerular filtration rate (GFR)—the rate at which the kidneys filter the blood

glomerulonephritis—inflammation of the glomeruli of the kidneys

glomerulus—filtering unit in the kidneys

glucagon—hormone from alpha cells of pancreas; helps cells release energy

glucose—the simple sugar to which carbohydrate must be broken down for absorption; also known as *dextrose*

gluten—protein found in grains

glycerol—a component of fat; derived from a water-soluble carbohydrate

glycogen—glucose as stored in the liver and muscles

glycogen loading (carb-loading)—process in which muscle's storage of glycogen is maximized; also called carb-loading

glycosuria—excess sugar in the urine

goiter—enlarged tissue of the thyroid gland due to a deficiency of iodine

growth spurt—significant rapid gain in size near the onset of adolescence

H

Hamwi method—a formula for estimating ideal body weight based on gender, height, and frame size

health disparities—a difference in health outcomes among subgroups often linked to social, economic, or environmental disadvantages

health literacy—the capacity to obtain, process, and understand basic health information needed to make appropriate health decisions

Helicobacter pylori—bacteria that can cause peptic ulcer

heme iron—part of hemoglobin molecule in animal foods

hemicellulose—dietary fiber found in whole grains

hemodialysis—cleansing the blood of wastes by circulating the blood through a machine that contains tubing of semipermeable membranes

hemolysis—the destruction of red blood cells

hemorrhage—unusually heavy bleeding

hepatitis—inflammation of the liver caused by viruses, drugs, and alcohol

hiatal hernia—condition wherein part of the stomach protrudes through the diaphragm into the chest cavity

high-density lipoproteins (HDLs)—lipoproteins that carry cholesterol from cells to the liver for eventual excretion

homeostasis—state of physical balance; stable condition

hormones—chemical messengers secreted by a variety of glands

human immunodeficiency virus (HIV)—a virus that weakens the body's immune system and ultimately leads to AIDS

hydrogenation—the combining of fat with hydrogen, thereby making it a saturated fat and solid at room temperature

hydrolysis—the addition of water resulting in the breakdown of the molecule

hydrolyzed formulas—contain products of digestion of proteins, carbohydrates, and fats; also called elemental formulas; used for clients who have difficulty digesting food

hypercholesterolemia—unusually high levels of cholesterol in blood; also known as high serum cholesterol

hyperemesis gravidarum—nausea so severe as to be life-threatening

hyperglycemia—excessive amount of sugar in the blood

hyperkalemia—excessive amount of potassium in the blood

hyperlipidemia—excessive amounts of fats in the blood

hypermetabolic—higher than normal rate of metabolism

hypersensitivity—abnormally strong sensitivity to certain substance(s)

hypertension—higher than normal blood pressure

hyperthyroidism—condition in which the thyroid gland secretes too much thyroxine and T3; the body's rate of metabolism is unusually high

hypervitaminosis—condition caused by excessive ingestion of one or more vitamins

hypoalbuminemia—abnormally low amounts of protein in the blood

hypoglycemia—subnormal levels of blood sugar

hypokalemia—low level of potassium in the blood

hypothalamus—area at base of brain that regulates appetite and thirst

hypothyroidism—condition in which the thyroid gland secretes too little thyroxine and T3; body metabolism is slower than normal

I

iatrogenic malnutrition—caused by treatment or diagnostic procedures

ileostomy—opening from ileum to abdomen surface

ileum—last part of the small intestine

immunity—ability to resist certain diseases

inborn errors of metabolism—congenital disabilities preventing normal metabolism

incomplete proteins—proteins that do not contain all of the nine essential amino acids

infarct—dead tissue resulting from blocked artery

inflammatory bowel diseases (IBDs)—chronic conditions causing inflammation in the gastrointestinal tract

insecticides—agents that destroy insects

insulin—secretion of the islets of Langerhans in the pancreas gland; essential for the proper metabolism of glucose

insulin reaction—hypoglycemia leading to insulin coma caused by too much insulin or too little food

intact grains—grains that contain all three layers intact—the bran, germ, and endosperm

internationals units (IUs)—unit of measurement of some vitamins; 5 mcg = 200 international units

interstitial fluid—fluid between cells

intracellular—within the cell

intracellular fluid (ICF)—water within cells; approximately 65% of total body fluid

intrinsic factor—secretion of stomach mucosa essential for B12 absorption

invisible fats—fats that are not immediately noticeable, such as those in egg yolk, cheese, cream, and salad dressings

iodized salt—salt that has the mineral iodine added for the prevention of goiter

ions—electrically charged atoms resulting from chemical reactions

iron deficiency—a condition in which the body does not have enough usable iron due to inadequate intake, bleeding, or absorption problems

iron-deficiency anemia—condition resulting from inadequate amount of iron in the diet, reducing the amount of oxygen carried by the blood to the cells

irritable bowel syndrome—functional gastrointestinal disorder

ischemia—reduced blood flow causing inadequate supply of nutrients and oxygen to, and wastes from, tissues

islets of Langerhans—part of the pancreas from which insulin is secreted

isoleucine—an amino acid

J

jaundice—yellow cast of the skin and eyes

jejunostomy—opening created by the surgeon in the intestine for enteral nutrition

jejunum—the middle section comprising about two-fifths of the small intestine

K

Kaposi's sarcoma—type of cancer common to individuals with AIDS

kcal—the unit used to measure the fuel value of foods

Keshan disease—condition causing abnormalities in the heart muscle

ketosis—condition in which ketones collect in the blood; caused by insufficient glucose available for energy

ketonemia—ketones collected in the blood

ketones—substances to which fatty acids are broken down in the liver

ketonuria—ketone bodies in the urine

kilocalorie—*see* kcal

Krebs cycle—a series of enzymatic reactions that serve as the main source of cellular energy

kwashiorkor—deficiency disease caused by extreme lack of protein

L

lactase—enzyme secreted by small intestine for the digestion of lactose

lactation—the period during which a mother is nursing her baby

lactation specialist—expert on breastfeeding

lacteals—lymphatic vessels in small intestine that absorb fatty acids and glycerol

lacto-ovo vegetarians—vegetarians who will eat dairy products and eggs but no meat, poultry, or fish

lactose—the sugar in milk; a disaccharide

lactose intolerance—inability to digest lactose because of a lack of the enzyme lactase; causes abdominal cramps and diarrhea

lacto-vegetarians—vegetarians who eat dairy products

lean body mass—mass percentage of muscle tissue

lecithin—fatty substance found in plant and animal foods; a natural emulsifier that helps transport fats in the bloodstream; used commercially to make food products smooth

legumes—plant food that is grown in a pod; for example, beans or peas

leptin—a belief that fat cells have a natural drive to regain any weight lost

leucine—an amino acid

lignins—dietary fiber found in the woody parts of vegetables

linoleic acid—fatty acid essential for humans; cannot be synthesized by the body

linolenic acid—one of three fatty acids needed by the body; cannot be synthesized by the body

lipids—fats

lipoproteins—carriers of fat in the blood

Lofenalac—commercial infant formula with 95% of phenylalanine removed

low-density lipoproteins (LDLs)—carry blood cholesterol to the cells

lumen—the hollow area in a tube

lymphatic system—transports fat-soluble substances from the small intestine to the vascular system

M

macrosomia—birth weight over 9 pounds

malignant—life-threatening

malnutrition—any nutrition imbalance

maltase—enzyme secreted by the small intestine essential for the digestion of maltose

maltose—the double sugar (disaccharide) occurring as a result of the digestion of grain

maple syrup urine disease (MSUD)—disease caused by an inborn error of metabolism in which the body cannot metabolize certain amino acids

marasmus—severe wasting caused by lack of protein and all nutrients or faulty absorption; PEM

masa harina—traditional flour made from field corn

mechanical digestion—the part of digestion that requires certain mechanical movement such as chewing, swallowing, and peristalsis

megadoses—extraordinarily large amount

megaloblastic anemia—anemia in which the red blood cells are unusually large and are not completely mature

menopause—the end of menstruation

menses—another term for menstruation

mental retardation—below-normal intellectual capacity

metabolic syndrome—a cluster of conditions that contribute to increased risk of heart disease, stroke, and diabetes

metabolism—the use of food by the body after digestion which results in energy

metastasize—spread of cancer cells from one organ to another

milliequivalents—concentrations of electrolytes in a solution

minerals—one of many inorganic substances essential to life and classified generally as minerals

mirin—rice wine with 40–50% sugar

miso—a thick fermented paste made from soy beans

modular formulas—made by combining specific nutrients

mold—a type of fungus

monosaccharides—simplest carbohydrates; sugars that cannot be further reduced by hydrolysis; examples are glucose, fructose, and galactose

monounsaturated fats—fats that are neither saturated nor polyunsaturated and are thought to play little part in atherosclerosis

morning sickness—early morning nausea common to some pregnancies

motivational interviewing—an evidence-based counseling approach designed to facilitate behavioral change by exploring and resolving ambivalence

mucilage—gel-forming dietary fiber

mutations—changes in the genes

myelin—lipoprotein essential for the protection of nerves

myocardial infarction (MI)—heart attack; caused by blockage of an artery leading to the heart

myocardium—heart muscle

myoglobin—protein compound in muscle that provides oxygen to cells

MyPlate—practical food guidance tool for consumers for making selections based on *Dietary Guidelines for Americans*, from the U.S. Department of Agriculture

N

nasogastric (NG) tube—the tube leading from the nose to the stomach for tube feeding

necrosis—tissue death due to lack of blood supply

negative nitrogen balance—more nitrogen lost than taken in

neophobic—a fear of new things or experiences

neoplasia—abnormal development of cells

neoplasm—abnormal growth of new tissue

nephritis—inflammatory disease of kidney

nephrolithiasis—kidney, or renal, stones

nephrons—unit of the kidney containing a glomerulus

nephropathy—damage to the kidneys

nephrosclerosis—hardening of renal arteries

neural tube defects (NTDs)—congenital malformation of brain and/or spinal column due to failure of neural tube to close during embryonic development

neuropathy—nerve damage

neurotoxins—toxins affecting the nervous system

niacin—a B vitamin

niacin equivalent (NE)—unit for measuring niacin; 1 NE equals 1 mg niacin or 60 mg tryptophan

nitrogen—chemical element found in protein; essential for life

nitrogen balance—when nitrogen intake equals nitrogen excreted

nonheme iron—iron from animal-derived foods that is not part of the hemoglobin molecule; and all iron from plant-derived foods

nutrients—chemical substance found in food that is necessary for good health

nutrient density—nutrient value of foods compared with number of calories

nutrient requirements—amount of specific nutrient needed by the body

nutrition—the result of those processes whereby the body takes in and uses food for growth, development, and the maintenance of health

nutritional status—one's physical condition as determined by diet

nutrition assessment—evaluation of nutritional status

nutritious—foods or beverages containing substantial amounts of essential nutrients

O

obesity—excessive body fat, BMI over 30

obstetricians—doctors who care for mothers during pregnancy and delivery

occlusions—blockages

oliguria—decreased output of urine to less than 500 mL a day

omega-3 fatty acids—polyunsaturated fatty acids found in fish oil; may contribute to the reduction of coronary artery disease

oncologist—doctor specializing in the study of cancer

oncology—study of cancer

on demand—feeding infants as they desire

opportunistic infections—caused by microorganisms that are present but that do not normally affect people with healthy immune systems

oral diabetes medications—oral hypoglycemic agents; medications that may be given to type 2 diabetics to lower blood glucose

osmolality—number of particles per kilogram of solution; solutions with high osmolality exert more pressure than those with fewer particles

osmosis—movement of a substance through a semipermeable membrane

osteomalacia—a condition in which bones become soft, usually in adult women, because of calcium loss

osteoporosis—condition in which bones become brittle because there have been insufficient mineral deposits, especially calcium

P

pancreas—gland that secretes enzymes essential for digestion, and insulin, which is essential for glucose metabolism

pancreatic amylase—the enzyme secreted by the pancreas that is essential for the digestion of starch

pancreatic lipase—the enzyme secreted by the pancreas that is essential for the digestion of fat

pancreatic proteases—enzymes secreted by the pancreas that are essential for the digestion of proteins

pancreatitis—inflammation of the pancreas

pantothenic acid—B vitamin

parenteral nutrition—nutrition provided via a vein

pathogens—disease-causing agents

pectin—edible thickening agent

peers—people who are approximately one's own age

pellagra—deficiency disease caused by the lack of niacin

pepsin—an enzyme secreted by the stomach that is essential for the digestion of proteins

peptic ulcers—ulcer of the stomach or duodenum

peptidases—enzymes secreted by the small intestine that are essential for the digestion of proteins

pericardium—outer covering of the heart

periodontal disease—disease of the mouth and gums

peripheral vascular disease (PVD)—narrowed arteries at some distance from the heart

peripheral vein—a vein that is near the surface of the skin

peristalsis—rhythmical movement of the intestinal tract; moves the chyme along

peritoneal dialysis—removal of waste products from the blood by injecting the flushing solution into the abdomen and using the client's peritoneum as the semipermeable membrane

pernicious anemia—severe, chronic anemia caused by the deficiency of vitamin B12; usually due to the body's inability to absorb B12

pH—symbol for the degree of acidity or alkalinity of a solution

phenylalanine—an amino acid

phenylalanine hydroxylase—liver enzyme necessary to metabolize the amino acid phenylalanine

phenylketonuria (PKU)—condition caused by an inborn error of metabolism in which an infant lacks an enzyme necessary to metabolize the amino acid phenylalanine

phlebitis—inflammation of a vein

physical trauma—extreme physical stress

physiological—relating to bodily functions

phytochemicals—substances occurring naturally in plant foods

pica—abnormal craving for nonfood substance

placenta—organ in the uterus that links blood supplies of mother and infant

plaque—fatty deposit on the interior of artery walls

plateau period—period in which there is no change

polycystic kidney disease—rare, hereditary kidney disease causing cysts or growths on the kidneys that can ultimately cause kidney failure in middle age

polydipsia—abnormal thirst

polymeric formulas—commercially prepared formulas for tube feedings that contain intact proteins, carbohydrates, and fats that require digestion

polypeptides—10 or more amino acids bonded together

polyphagia—excess hunger

polysaccharides—complex carbohydrates containing combinations of monosaccharides; examples include starch, dextrin, cellulose, and glycogen

polyunsaturated fats—fats whose carbon atoms contain only limited amounts of hydrogen

polyuria—excessive urination

positive nitrogen balance—nitrogen intake exceeds outgo

precursor—something that comes before something else; in vitamins it is also called a provitamin, something from which body can synthesize specific vitamin

pre-diabetes—a condition in which blood glucose is higher than normal but not high enough for a diabetes diagnosis

pregnancy-induced hypertension (PIH)—typically occurs during late pregnancy; characterized by high blood pressure, albumin in the urine, and edema

pressure ulcers—bedsores

primary hypertension—high blood pressure resulting from an unknown cause

prohormone—substance that precedes the hormone and from which the body can synthesize the hormone

proteins—the only one of six essential nutrients containing nitrogen

protein energy malnutrition (PEM)—marasmus and kwashiorkor

proteinuria—protein in the urine

provitamin—a precursor of a vitamin

psychosocial development—relating to both psychological and social development

purines—end products of nucleoprotein metabolism

pylorus—the end of the stomach nearest to the intestine

R

refined grains—grains that have had the bran and germ removed through grinding and sifting

regurgitation—vomiting

renal stones—kidney stones

renal threshold—kidneys' capacity

resection—reduction

respiration—breathing

resting energy expenditure (REE)—*see* basal metabolism rate

retardation—slowing

retinol—the preformed vitamin A

retinol equivalent (RE)—the equivalent of 3.33 IU of vitamin A

retinopathy—damage to small blood vessels in the eyes

riboflavin—vitamin B2

rickets—deficiency disease caused by the lack of vitamin D; causes malformed bones and pain in infants

S

saliva—secretion of the salivary glands

salivary amylase—also called ptyalin; the enzyme secreted by the salivary glands to act on starch

Salmonella—an infection caused by the *Salmonella* bacteria

satiety—feeling of satisfaction; fullness

saturated fats—fats whose carbon atoms contain all of the hydrogen atoms they can; considered a contributory factor in atherosclerosis

scurvy—a deficiency disease caused by the lack of vitamin C

secondary hypertension—high blood pressure caused by another condition such as kidney disease

secretin—the hormone that causes the pancreas to release sodium bicarbonate to neutralize acidity of the chyme

self-esteem—feelings of self-worth

sepsis—infection of the blood

serum cholesterol—cholesterol in the blood

set point theory—belief that everyone has a natural weight ("set point") at which the body is most comfortable

short bowel syndrome—malabsorption caused by surgical removal or dysfunction of part of the small intestine or colon

skeletal system—body's bone structure

skin tests—allergy tests using potential allergens on scratches on the skin

solute—the substance dissolved in a solution

solvent—liquid part of a solution

spina bifida—spinal cord or spinal fluid bulge through the back

spontaneous abortion—occurring naturally; miscarriage

Staphylococcus (staph)—genus of bacteria causing food poisoning called "staph" or "staphylococcal poisoning"

starch—polysaccharide found in grains and vegetables

stasis—stoppage or slowing

steatorrhea—abnormal amounts of fat in the feces

sterile—free of infectious organisms

stoma—surgically created opening in the abdominal wall

subcutaneous fat—fat stored directly under the skin

sucrase—enzyme secreted by the small intestine to aid in digestion of sucrose

sucrose—a double sugar or disaccharide; examples are granulated, powdered, and brown sugar

T

tetany—involuntary muscle movement

thiamine—vitamin B1

thrombosis—blockage, as a blood clot

thrombus—blood clot

thrush—a yeast infection of the mucus membrane lining the mouth and tongue

tocopherols—a form of vitamin E

tocotrienols—a form of vitamin E

total parenteral nutrition—*see* TPN

toxicity—state of being poisonous

TPN—total parenteral nutrition; process of providing all nutrients intravenously

trans-fatty acids (TFAs)—produced by adding hydrogen atoms to a liquid fat, making it a solid

transferase—a liver enzyme necessary for the metabolism of galactose

triglycerides—combinations of fatty acids and glycerol

trimester—3-month period; commonly used to denote periods of pregnancy

trypsin—pancreatic enzyme; helps digest proteins

tube feeding (TF)—feeding by tube directly into the stomach or intestine

type 1 diabetes—diabetes occurring suddenly between the ages of 1 and 40; clients secrete little, if any, insulin and require insulin injections and a carefully controlled diet

type 2 diabetes—diabetes occurring after age 40; onset is gradual, and production of insulin gradually diminishes; can usually be controlled by diet and exercise

U

ulcerative colitis—disease characterized by inflammation and ulceration of the colon, rectum, and sometimes entire large intestine

urea—chief nitrogenous waste product of protein metabolism

uremia—condition in which protein wastes are circulating in the blood

ureters—tubes leading from the kidneys to the bladder

uric acid—one of the nitrogenous waste products of protein metabolism

urticaria—hives; common allergic reaction

V

valine—an amino acid

vascular disease—disease of the blood vessels

vascular osmotic pressure—high concentration of electrolytes in the blood; low blood volume or blood pressure

vascular system—circulatory system

vegans—vegetarians who avoid all animal foods

very-low-density lipoproteins (VLDLs)—lipoproteins made by the liver to transport lipids throughout the body

villi—the tiny, hair-like structures in the small intestines through which nutrients are absorbed

visceral fat—fat stored within the abdominal cavity

visible fats—fats in foods that are purchased and used as fats, such as butter or margarine

vitamins—organic substances necessary for life although they do not, independently, provide energy

vitamin supplements—concentrated forms of vitamins; may be in tablet or liquid form

W

wasabi—Japanese horseradish

water—major constituent of all living cells; composed of hydrogen and oxygen

water soluble—can be dissolved in water

weaning—training an infant to drink from the cup instead of the nipple

wellness—a state of physical, mental, and social well-being

whey—the liquid part of milk that separates from the curd (solid part) during the making of hard cheese

X

xerophthalmia—serious eye disease characterized by dry mucous membranes of the eye, caused by the deficiency of vitamin A

xerostomia—sore, dry mouth caused by the reduction of salivary secretions; may be caused by radiation for treatment of cancer

Y

yo-yo effect—when a dieters' weight goes up and down over short periods due to swings in eating (from strict dieting to overconsumption)

References

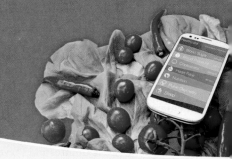

American Academy of Allergy, Asthma, and Immunology. *Anaphylaxis*. Retrieved October 2015 from https://www.aaaai.org/conditions-and-treatments/allergies/anaphylaxis.aspx

American Academy of Pediatrics. (2015, October 23). Lack of adequate food is ongoing health risk to US children: Nation's pediatricians release policy statement stressing the importance of federal, state and local nutrition programs to help combat the immediate and potentially lifelong impact of food insecurity. ScienceDaily. Retrieved from www.sciencedaily.com/releases/2015/10/151023083717.htm

American Diabetes Association. (2016). Standards of medical care in diabetes–2016. *Diabetes Care, 39* (Supp l 1). Retrieved from http://care.diabetesjournals.org/site/misc/2016-Standards-of-Care.pdf

American Institute for Cancer Research. (2013). Heal Well: A cancer nutrition guide. Retrieved from http://www.aicr.org/assets/docs/pdf/education/heal-well-guide.pdf

Apovian, C. M., Aronne, L. J., Bessesen, D. H., . . . Endocrine Society. (2015). Pharmacological management of obesity: An endocrine society clinical practice guideline. *Journal of Clinical Endocrinology and Metabolism, 100*(2), 342–362. Retrieved from http://press.endocrine.org/doi/pdf/10.1210/jc.2014-3415

American Cancer Society. (2015). *Does body weight affect cancer risk?* Retrieved from http://www.cancer.org/cancer/cancercauses/dietandphysicalactivity/body-weightandcancerrisk/body-weight-and-cancer-risk-effects

American Cancer Society. (2011). *Kaposi sarcoma*. Retrieved from http://www.cancer.org/cancer/kaposisarcoma

American Heart Association. *Conditions*. Retrieved from http://www.heart.org/HEARTORG/Conditions/Conditions_UCM_001087_SubHomePage.jsp

American Institute for Cancer Research. (2014). Recommendations for cancer prevention. Retrieved from http://www.aicr.org/reduce-your-cancer-risk/recommendations-for-cancer-prevention/?referrer=https://www.google.com

American Institute for Cancer Research, Savor Health, & Livestrong Foundation. (2013). *Heal well – A cancer nutrition guide*. Retrieved from http://www.aicr.org/assets/docs/pdf/education/heal-well-guide.pdf

American Society for Metabolic and Bariatric Surgery. *Bariatric surgery procedures*. Retrieved from https://asmbs.org/patients/bariatric-surgery-procedures

Baker, R. D., & Greer, F. R., & Committee on Nutrition American Academy of Pediatrics. (2010). Diagnosis and prevention of iron deficiency and iron-deficiency anemia in infants and young children (0–3 years of age). *Pediatrics, 126*(5), 1040–1050.

Binge Eating Disorder. The Nemours Foundation/Kids Health. (2015). Retrieved from http://kidshealth.org/en/parents/binge-eating.html

Brookes, L. (2006). Omni-heart - optimal macronutrient trial to prevent heart disease. *Medscape Medical News*. Retrieved from http://www.medscape.org/viewarticle/523041

Busko, M. (2015). Gastric balloon pill shows early promise in weight loss. *Medscape Medical News*. Retrieved from http://www.medscape.com/viewarticle/854287

Case Western University. *Center for evidenced based practice – motivational interviewing*. Retrieved January 2016 from https://www.centerforebp.case.edu/practices/mi

Carlson, J. J., Eisenmann, J. C., Norman, G. J., Ortiz, K. A., & Young, P. C. (2011). Dietary fiber and nutrient density are inversely associated with the metabolic syndrome in U.S. adolescents. *Journal of the American Dietetic Association, 111*, 1688–1695.

Castle, J. (2010). What's Your Feeding Style. *Just the Right Byte blog*. Retrieved from http://jillcastle.com/childhood-nutrition/whats-your-feeding-style

Centers for Disease Control and Prevention. Attention deficit/hyperactivity disorder data and statistics. (2011). Retrieved from http://www.cdc.gov/ncbddd/adhd/data.html

Centers for Disease Control and Prevention. (2013). *Strategies to prevent obesity and other chronic diseases: the CDC guide to strategies to support breastfeeding mothers and babies 2013*. Retrieved from http://www.cdc.gov/breastfeeding/pdf/BF-Guide-508.PDF

Centers for Disease Control and Prevention. (2013). Trends in the prevalence of alcohol use national YRBS: 1991–2013. Retrieved from http://www.cdc.gov/healthyyouth/data/yrbs/pdf/trends/us_alcohol_trend_yrbs.pdf

Centers for Disease Control and Prevention. (2013) Trends in the prevalence of marijuana, cocaine, and other illegal drug use, National YRBS: 1991–2013. Retrieved from http://www.cdc.gov/healthyyouth/data/yrbs/pdf/trends/us_drug_trend_yrbs.pdf

Centers for Disease Control and Prevention. (2014). Diabetes report card. Retrieved from http://www.cdc.gov/diabetes/pdfs/library/diabetesreportcard2014.pdf

Centers for Disease Control and Prevention. (2014). *Estimates of foodborne illness in the United States*. Retrieved from http://www.cdc.gov/foodborneburden/index.html

Centers for Disease Control and Prevention. (2014). National diabetes statistics report 2014. Retrieved from http://www.cdc.gov/diabetes/pubs/statsreport14/national-diabetes-report-web.pdf

Centers for Disease Control and Prevention. (2015). *Parasites: Crytosporidium*. Retrieved from http://www.cdc.gov/parasites/crypto/general.html

Centers for Disease Control and Prevention. (2014) *State Indicator Report on Physical Activity 2014*. Retrieved from http://www.cdc.gov/physicalactivity/downloads/pa_state_indicator_report_2014.pdf

Centers for Disease Control and Prevention. (2014). U.S. obesity prevalence maps 2014. Retrieved from http://www.cdc.gov/obesity/data/prevalence-maps.html

Centers for Disease Control and Prevention. (2015). *Youth and Tobacco Use*. Retrieved from http://www.cdc.gov/tobacco/data_statistics/fact_sheets/youth_data/tobacco_use/index.htm

Centers for Disease Control and Prevention, National Center for Chronic Disease Prevention and Health Promotion, Division for Heart Disease and Stroke Prevention. (2010). *Sodium: The facts*. Retrieved from www.cdc.gov/salt/pdfs/sodium_fact_sheet.pdf

Centers for Disease Control and Prevention, National Center for Health Statistics, in collaboration with the National Center for Chronic Disease Prevention and Health Promotion. (2000/2005/2009). *CDC growth charts: United States*. Retrieved from http://www.cdc.gov/growthcharts

Center for Science in the Public Interest. Nutrition Action Healthletter. (2014, October). *Sweet – Your guide to Sugar Substitutes*. Washington, DC.

Center for Celiac Research, Massachusetts General Hospital for Children. *Gluten Sensitivity Facts*. Retrieved November 2015 from http://www.massgeneral.org/children/services/celiac-disease/gluten-sensitivity-faq.aspx

Center for Medicare and Medicaid. *Decision Memo for Intensive Behavioral Therapy for Obesity*. Retrieved from https://www.cms.gov/medicare-coverage-database/details/nca-decision-memo.aspx?&NcaName=Intensive%20Behavioral%20Therapy%20for%20Obesity&bc=ACAAAAAAIAAA&NCAId=253&

Chen, J. (2015, October 21). Tasting flavor that doesn't exist. *The Atlantic*. Retrieved from http://www.theatlantic.com/health/archive/2015/10/tasting-a-flavor-that-doesnt-exist/411454

Choice of protein- and carbohydrate-rich foods may have big effects on long-term weight gain. (2015, April 9). *Science-Daily*. Tufts University. Retrieved from http://www.sciencedaily.com/releases/2015/04/150409133206.htm

Christensen, J. (2015). Sitting will kill you, even if you exercise. *CNN News*. Retrieved from http://www.cnn.com/2015/01/21/health/sitting-will-kill-you

Cleft Palate Foundation. *Feeding your baby*. Retrieved October 2015 from http://www.cleftline.org/who-we-are/what-we-do/feeding-your-baby

Clostridium Perfringens. Food Safety.gov. Retrieved September 2015 from http://www.foodsafety.gov/poisoning/causes/bacteriaviruses/cperfringens

Cost of obesity approaching $300 billion a year, Robert Preidt Health Day. (2011, January 21). *USA Today*. Retrieved from http://www.usatoday.om/yourlife/health/medical/2011-01-12-obesity-costs-300-bilion_N.htm

Crohn's and Colitis Foundation of America. (2013). *Short Bowel Syndrome and Crohn's Disease*. Retrieved from http://www.ccfa.org/assets/short-bowel-syndrome-and.pdf

DaVita. (2012). *Can children do peritoneal dialysis?* Retrieved from http://www.davita.com/treatment-options/home-peritoneal-dialysis/ what-is-peritoneal-disease-/can-children-do- peritoneal-dialysis?/t/5484

Daly, A., Franz, M., & Evert, A. (2008). *Choose Your Foods: Exchange Lists for Diabetes*. (6th ed.). Chicago, IL: American Dietetic Association and American Diabetes Association.

Department of Health and Human Services, Administration on Aging. (2011). *Aging statistics*. Retrieved from http://www.aoa.acl.gov/aging_statistics/index.aspx

Dinicolantonio, J., & Lucan, S. (2014, December 23). Sugar season. It's everywhere and addictive. *New York Times*. Retrieved from http://www.nytimes.com/2014/12/23/opinion/sugar-season-its-everywhere-and-addictive.html

Eckel, R. H., Jakicic, J. M., Ard, J. D., . . . Tomaselli, G. F. (2013). AHA/ACC guideline on lifestyle management to reduce cardiovascular risk: A report of the American College of Cardiology American/Heart Association Task Force on Practice Guidelines. *Circulation* 130, e278–e333.

Family Dinner Project. Retrieved November 2015 from http://thefamilydinnerproject.org/resources/faq

Federal Interagency Forum on Child and Family Statistics. America's Children: Key National Indicators of Well-Being, 2015. Washington, DC: U.S. Government Printing Office.

Fissell, W.H., & Shuvo, R. (2015). Bioartificial Kidney: The Next Frontier in ESRD Treatment? *The American Kidney Foundation*. Retrieved from http://www.kidneyfund.org/kidney-today/bioartificial-kidney.html?referrer=https://www.google.com/#.Vt6pvfkrLIU

Food Allergy Research and Education. *Food Allergy Facts and Statistics*. Retrieved October 2015 from http://www.food-allergy.org/file/facts-stats.pdf

Franks, P. W., Hanson, R. L., Knowler, W. C., Sievers, M. L., Bennett, P. H., & Looker, H. C. (2010). Childhood obesity, other cardiovascular risk factors, and premature death. *New England Journal of Medicine, 362*, 485–493.

Grant, M. L. (2015, April 29). U.S. Universities Offer International Students a Taste of Home. *U.S. News*. Retrieved from http://www.usnews.com/education/best-colleges/articles/2015/04/29/us-universities-offer-international-students-a-taste-of-home

Harris, J. H., & Benedict, F. (1919). *A biometric study of basal metabolism in man*. Washington, DC: Carnegie Institute of Washington.

Hayes, D. (2015). Feeding vegetarian and vegan infants and toddlers. Retrieved from http://www.eatright.org/resource/food/nutrition/vegetarian-and-special-diets/feeding-vegetarian-and-vegan-infants-and-toddlers

Home Food Safety. Four easy steps to reduce foodborne illness; keep it cool refrigerator/freezer storage chart; summer produce – what you can do to keep fruits and vegetables safe! (downloads). Retrieved September 2015 from http://www.eatright.org/resources/homefoodsafety

Institute of Medicine. Report Brief. (2010, November). *Dietary reference intakes for calcium and vitamin D*. Retrieved from https://iom.nationalacademies.org/Reports/2010/Dietary-Reference-Intakes-for-Calcium-and-Vitamin-D.aspx

Institute of Medicine. Report Brief. (2012, May). *Accelerating progress in obesity prevention*. Retrieved from https://iom.nationalacademies.org/~/media/Files/Report%20Files/2012/APOP/APOP_rb.pdf

Institute of Medicine. Report Brief. (2009, May). *Weight gain during pregnancy – reexamining the guidelines*. Retrieved from http://iom.nationalacademies.org/~/media/Files/Report%20Files/2009/Weight-Gain-During-Pregnancy-Reexamining-the-Guidelines/Report%20Brief%20-%20Weight%20Gain%20During%20Pregnancy.pdf

International Osteoporosis Foundation. (2011). *Facts and statistics about osteoporosis and its impact*. Retrieved from http://www.iofbonehealth.org/facts-and-statistics.html

Jing, Linyuan et al. Obese kids as young as age 8 show signs of heart disease. (2015, November). American Heart Association Meeting Report – Abstract 15439. Retrieved from http://newsroom.heart.org/news/obese-kids-young-as-age-8-show-signs-of-heart-disease

Johnston, L. D., O'Malley, P. M., Bachman, J. G., & Schulenberg, J. E. (2011). *Marijuana use continues to rise among U.S. teens, while alcohol use hits historic lows*. Ann Arbor, MI: University of Michigan News Service.

Jovanovic, L., Nathan, D., Greene, M., & Barss, V. (2011). *Glycemic control in women with type 1 and type 2 diabetes mellitus during pregnancy*. Retrieved from http://www.uptodate.com/contents/glycemic-control-in-women-with-type-1-and-type-2-diabetes-mellitus-during-pregnancy?source5search_result&search5 glycemic1control1in1women1with1type111and1 type121diabetes1mellitus1during1pregnancy& selectedTitle51%7E150

Karfonta, K. E., Lunn, W. R., Colletto, M. R., Anderson, J. M., & Rodriguez, N. R. (2010). Chocolate milk enhances glycogen replenishment after endurance exercise in moderately trained males. *Medicine & Science in Sports and Exercise, 42,* S64.

Keller, M. (2011). Food intolerances versus food allergies. *Today's Dietitian, 13*(10), 52. Retrieved from http://www.todaysdietitian.com/newarchives/100111p52.shtml

KidsHealth. (2012). *Kids and exercise*. Retrieved from http://kidshealth.org

Korioth, T. (2015). E-Cigarettes: dangerous, available, and addicting. *American Academy of Pediatrics*. Retrieved from http://www.healthychildren.org

Kulze, A. *Fast Food and Travel Eating*. Retrieved October 2015 from http://www.drannwellness.com/article162.cfmWwwdrannwellness.com

Landa, J. (2015, February 2). Ending the multivitamin debate: why taking one may actually save your life. *Fox News*. Retrieved from http://www.foxnews.com/health/2015/02/02/ending-multivitamin-debate-why-taking-one-may-actually-save-your-life

Li, J. (2014, October 10). What's the difference between a food intolerance and food allergy? *Mayo Clinic*. Retrieved from http://www.mayoclinic.org/diseases-conditions/food-allergy/expert-answers/food-allergy/faq-20058538

Lund, M. (2013). Intact grains. *Today's Dietitian, 15*(10), 38. Retrieved from http://www.todaysdietitian.com/newarchives/100713p38.shtml

Marniit, A. (2015, December 25). Apps to help you keep your new years resolutions: losing weight, quitting smoking and more. *Tech Times*. Retrieved from http://www.techtimes.com/articles/119286/20151225/best-apps-to-help-you-keep-your-new-years-resolutions-losing-weight-quitting-smoking-and-more.htm

May, A., Kuklina, E. V., Yoon, P. W. (2012). Prevalence of cardiovascular disease risk factors among U.S. adolescents 1999–2008. *Pediatrics, 129*(6), 1035–41.

Migala, J. (2015, May 11). 7 foods for your gut health. *ABC News*. Retrieved from http://abcnews.go.com/Health/foods-gut-health/story?id=30855530

Moore, L., & Thompson, F. (2015, July). Adults meeting fruit and vegetable intake recommendations – United States 2013. Centers for Disease Control and Prevention. *Mortality and Morbidity Weekly Report, 64(26),* 709–713. Retrieved from http://www.cdc.gov/mmwr/pdf/wk/mm6426.pdf

National Academy of Sciences. (2011). *Institute of medicine, food and nutrition board. dietary reference intakes: recommended intakes for individuals*. Retrieved from https://fnic.nal.usda.gov/sites/fnic.nal.usda.gov/files/uploads/recommended_intakes_individuals.pdf

National Cancer Institute. *Nutrition in cancer care-for health professionals*. Retrieved August 2015 from http://www.cancer.gov/about-cancer/treatment/side-effects/appetite-loss/nutrition-hp-pdq

National Center for Children in Poverty. (2015). *Child poverty*. Fact Sheets 2015. Retrieved from http://www.nccp.org/topics/childpoverty.html

National Diabetes Prevention Program, National Institutes of Health. Retrieved December 2015 from http://www.cdc.gov/diabetes/prevention/index.html

National Eating Disorders Association. *Get the facts on eating disorders*. Retrieved September 2015 from https://www.nationaleatingdisorders.org/get-facts-eating-disorders

National Heart Lung and Blood Institute, U.S. Department of Health and Human Services. (2014, March). *Who is at risk for iron-deficiency anemia?* Retrieved from http://www.nhlbi.nih.gov/health/health-topics/topics/ida/atrisk.html

National Institute of Arthritis and Musculoskeletal and Skin Diseases, National Institutes of Health. (2016). *Osteoporosis overview*. Retrieved from http://www.niams.nih.gov/Health_Info/Osteoporosis/default.asp

National Institute of Child Health and Human Development. (2012). *Why are tween and teen years so critical?* Retrieved from http://www.nichd.nih.gov/milk/prob/critical.cfm

National Institute of Health, National Institute of Diabetes and Digestive and Kidney Diseases. *Digestive diseases*

A-Z. Retrieved September 2016 from http://www.niddk. nih.gov/health-information/health-topics/digestive-diseases/Pages/default.aspx

National Institute of Health, National Institute of Diabetes and Digestive and Kidney Diseases. (2014, June). *Foodborne illnesses*. Retrieved from http://www.niddk.nih.gov/ health-information/health-topics/digestive-diseases/ foodborne-illnesses/Pages/facts.aspx

National Institute of Health. National Institute of Diabetes and Digestive and Kidney Diseases. (2013, September). *Irritable bowel syndrome*. Retrieved from http://www.niddk. nih.gov/health-information/health-topics/digestive-diseases/irritable-bowel-syndrome/Documents/ibs_508.pdf

National Institutes of Health, National Heart Lung and Blood Institute. *Classification of overweight and obesity by BMI, waist circumference, and associated disease risks*. Retrieved October 2015 from https://www.nhlbi.nih.gov/ health/educational/lose_wt/BMI/bmi_dis.htm

National Institutes of Health, U.S. National Library of Medicine, Medline Plus. (2014). *Aging changes in body shape*. Retrieved from https://www.nlm.nih.gov/medlineplus/ ency/article/003998.htm

National Institutes of Health, U.S. National Library of Medicine, Medline Plus. (2015, April). *Nutrition and Athletic Performance*. Retrieved from https://www.nlm.nih.gov/medlineplus/ency/article/002458.htm

National Institutes of Health, Office of Dietary Supplements. (2011, June). *Dietary supplements: what you need to know*. Retrieved from https://ods.od.nih.gov/Health Information/DS_WhatYouNeedToKnow.aspx

National Institutes of Health. The Office of Dietary Supplements. (2016, February). *Dietary supplement fact sheet: Vitamin D*. Retrieved from https://ods.od.nih.gov/ factsheets/VitaminD-HealthProfessional

National Institutes of Health. U.S. National Library of Medicine, Medline Plus. (2014, October). *Low- fiber diet*. Retrieved from http://www.nlm.nih.gov/medlineplus/ency/ patientinstructions/ 000200.htm

National Kidney Foundation. (2016). *Nutrition and chronic kidney disease (stages 1–4)*. Retrieved from https://www. kidney.org/nutrition

National Kidney Foundation. (2015). *Preventing diabetic kidney disease: 10 answers to questions*. Retrieved from https:// www.kidney.org/atoz/content/preventkiddisease

National Weight Control Registry. Brown Medical School/The Miriam Hospital Weight Control & Diabetes Research Center Retrieved November 2015 from http://www. nwcr.ws/Research/default.htm

Norwood, R. (2011, December 5). Young athletes and energy drink—A bad mix?. *USA Today/Sports*. Retrieved from http://www.usatoday.com

Nowson, C., & O'Connell, S. (2015). Protein requirements and recommendations for older people: a review. *Nutrients, 7*(8), 6874–99. Retrieved from http://www.ncbi.nlm.nih. gov/pubmed/26287239

NY Daily News. (2015, December 23). *Chipotle tweaks cooking methods after E. coli outbreak sickens more than 50 people*. Retrieved from http://www.nydailynews.com/life-style/health/chipotle-tweaks-cooking-methods-e-coli-outbreak-article-1.2475395

Nutrition 411. (2013). *Nutrition care for patients with chronic renal failure*. Retrieved from http://www.nutrition411.com/ content/nutrition-care-patients-chronic-renal-failure

Nutrition 411. (2009). *Estimating energy requirements for the obese patients*. Reviewed from http://www.nutrition411.com/content/estimating-energy-requirements-obese-patients

Nutrition Care Process. Retrieved August 2015 from http:// www.eatright.org/HealthProfessionals/content. aspx?id=7077

O'Connor, A. (2015, April 7). Study warns of diet supplement dangers. *New York Times*. Retrieved from http://well. blogs.nytimes.com/2015/04/07/study-warns-of-diet-supplement-dangers-kept-quiet-by-f-d-a/?_r=0

Office of Disease Prevention and Health Promotion. (2015, December). *Healthy people 2020*. Retrieved from http:// www.healthypeople.gov

Olantunbosun, S. T. (2015, January 30). Insulin resistance and differential diagnoses. *Medscape Reference*. Retrieved from http://emedicine.medscape.com/ article/122501-differential

Oldways Preservation Trust. *Mediterranean diet pyramid*. Retrieved February 2015 from http://oldwayspt.org/ traditional-diets/mediterranean-diet

Olson, K. L., & Emery, C. F. (2015). Mindfulness and weight loss: a systematic review. *Psychosomatic Medicine, 77*(1), 59–67. Retrieved from http://www.ncbi.nlm.nih.gov/ pubmed/25490697

Pappas, S. (2015, August 18). Weight loss drugs: pros and cons of 5 approved prescriptions. *Livescience*. Retrieved from http://www.livescience.com/51896-weight-loss-drugs-pros-cons.html

Parretti, H. M., Aveyard, P., Blannin, A., Clifford, S. J., Coleman, S. J., Roalfe, A., & Daley, A. J. (2015). Efficacy of water preloading before main meals as a strategy for weight loss in primary care patients with obesity. *Obesity (Silver Spring), 23*(9):1785-91. doi: 10.1002/oby.21167. Retrieved from http://www.ncbi.nlm.nih.gov/pubmed/26237305

Patenaude, J. (2011). Inflammation and food sensitivities – successful treatment begins with patient centered care. *Today's Dietitian, 13*(11), 18. Retrieved from http://www. todaysdietitian.com/newarchives/110211p18.shtml

Penner, E. (2015). *Is coconut water more hydrating?* Retrieved from http://www.huffingtonpost.com/elle-penner/is-coconut-water-more-hydrating_b_7882330.html

Preidt, R. (2015, October 2). For teens, late bedtime may lead to weight gain, health day. *US National Library of Medicine*. Retrieved from http://consumer.healthday.com/ kids-health-information-23/overweight-kids-health-news-517/for-teens-late-bedtime-may-lead-to-weight-gain-703835.html

Radlicz, C. (2015, October 8). Fish consumption during pregnancy: weighing the risk-benefit. *The American Society for Nutrition*. Retrieved from https://www.nutrition.org/asn-blog/2015/10/fish-consumption-during-pregnancy-weighing-the-risk-benefit

Reddy, S. (2015, April 20). A diet might cut the risk of developing alzheimer's. *The Wall Street Journal*. Retrieved from http://www.wsj.com/articles/a-diet-might-cut-the-risk-of-developing-alzheimers-1429569168

Reinberg, S. (2015, October 16). During menopause, "good" cholesterol may lose protective effect on heart. *Healthday*. Retrieved from http://consumer.healthday.com/women-s-health-information-34/menopause-and-post-menopause-news-472/during-menopause-good-choles-terol-may-lose-protective-effect-704232.html

Reinberg, S. (2015, August 11). Southern diet linked to big increase in heart disease. Healthday, *CBS News*. Retrieved from http://www.cbsnews.com/news/southern-diet-linked-to-big-increase-in-heart-disease

Saint Louis, C. (2014, September 2). Childhood diet habits set in infancy, studies suggest. *The New York Times*. Retrieved from http://www.nytimes.com/2014/09/02/health/childhood-diet-habits-set-in-infancy-studies-suggest.html?_r=0

Satter, E. (2013) Division of Responsibility in Feeding. Retrieved from http://ellynsatterinstitute.org/dor/divisionofre-sponsibilityinfeeding.php

Savoy, C. (2015, November). Dogs that smell cancer being tested in Britain in order to determine their effectiveness. *Inquisitr*. Retrieved from http://www.inquisitr.com/2582581/dogs-that-smell-cancer-being-tested-in-britain-in-order-to-determine-their-effectiveness

Schiavocampo, M. (2015, July 9). Affordable care act will cover weight loss medical services. *ABC News*. Retrieved from http://abcnews.go.com/Health/affordable-care-act-cover-weight-loss-medical-services/story?id=32317572

Science Daily. (2015). *Midnight munchies mangle memory*. Retrieved from https://www.sciencedaily.com/releases/2015/12/151223141445.

Scrivani, J. R. (2016). *The Importance of Stress Management for People with HIV/AIDS*. Retrieved from http://www.good-therapy.org/blog/importance-of-stress-management-for-people-with-hiv-aids-0107165

Seidenberg, C. (2015, September 23). Kids and protein powder: what you should know. *The Washington Post*. Retrieved from https://www.washingtonpost.com/lifestyle/wellness/say-nuts-to-protein-powders/2015/09/22/a5589dae-5e0c-11e5-9757-e49273f05f65_story.html

Singh, M. (2015, May 14). Why one grocery chain is thriving in Philadelphia's food deserts. *National Public Radio*. Retrieved from http://www.npr.org/sections/the-salt/2015/05/14/406476968/why-one-grocery-chain-is-thriving-in-philadelphias-food-deserts

State of obesity 2015: better policies for a healthier America. Robert Wood Johnson Foundation. Retrieved from http://stateofobesity.org/files/stateofobesity2015.pdf

Troiano, R. P., Berrigan, D., Dodd, K. W., Mâsse, L. C., Tilert, T., & McDowell, M. (2008). Physical activity in the United States measured by accelerometer. *Medicine & Science in Sports and Exercise 40*(1), 181–188.

Tufts Medical Center. (2011). *Guide for eating after bariatric surgery*. Retrieved from https://www.tuftsmedicalcenter.org/-/media/Brochures/TuftsMC/Patient%20Care%20Services/Departments%20and%20Services/Weight%20and%20Wellness%20Center/GBP%20Diet%20Man-ual12611.ashx

U.S. Department of Agriculture, Agricultural Research Service. (2015). *USDA national nutrient database for standard reference*. Retrieved November 2015 from https://ndb.nal.usda.gov/ndb/search

U.S. Department of Agriculture, Center for Nutrition Policy and Promotions. *MyPlate*. Retrieved August 2015 from http://www .choosemyplate.gov

U.S. Department of Agriculture, Center for Nutrition Policy and Promotions. *MyPlate Food Intake Patterns*. Retrieved August 2015 from http://www.choosemyplate.gov/profes-sionals/pdf_food_intake.html

U.S. Department of Agriculture, Center for Nutrition Policy and Promotions. (2010). *Healthy Eating Index*. Retrieved from http://www.cnpp.usda.gov/healthyeatingindex

U.S. Department of Agriculture, Food Safety and Inspection Service. (2013). *Foodborne illness: what consumers need to know*. Retrieved from http://www.fsis.usda.gov

U.S. Department of Agriculture. *Supertracker and BMI calculator*. Retrieved August 2015 from http://www.choosemy-plate.gov

U.S. Department of Agriculture Food and Nutrition Service, WIC. (2014). *WIC fact sheet*. Retrieved from http://www.fns.usda.gov/sites/default/files/WIC-Fact-Sheet.pdf

U.S. Department of Health and Human Services, National Institutes of Health, National Institutes of Child Health and Human Development. (2014). *Lactose intolerance*. Retrieved from http://www.niddk.nih.gov/health-infor-mation/health-topics/digestive-diseases/lactose-intoler-ance/Pages/facts.aspx

U.S. Department of Health and Human Services, National Institute of Diabetes and Digestive and Kidney Diseases, National Institute of Health. (2015). *Celiac disease*. Retrieved from http://www.niddk.nih.gov/health-information/health-topics/digestive-diseases/celiac-disease/Pages/facts.aspx

U.S. Department of Health and Human Services, National Heart, Lung and Blood Institute (2015). *DASH eating plan*. Retrieved from https://www.nhlbi.nih.gov/health/health-topics/topics/dash

U.S. Department of Health and Human Services, & U.S. Department of Agriculture. (2016). *Dietary guidelines for Americans, 2015–2020* (8th ed.). Retrieved from http://health.gov/dietaryguidelines/2015/guidelines

U.S. Department of Health and Human Services. (2008). *2008 physical activity guidelines for Americans*. Washington, DC: U.S. Department of Health and Human Services. ODPHP Publication No. U0036. Retrieved from http://www.health.gov/paguidelines

U.S. Food and Drug Administration. (2015). *Label claims*. Retrieved from http://www.fda.gov/Food/IngredientsPack-agingLabeling/LabelingNutrition/ucm2006873.htm

U.S. Food and Drug Administration. (2015). *Proposed changes to the nutrition facts label*. Retrieved from http://www.fda.gov/Food/GuidanceRegulation/GuidanceDoc-umentsRegulatoryInformation/LabelingNutrition/ucm385663.htm

U.S. Food and Drug Administration. *Refrigerator and freezer storage chart*. Retrieved November 2015 from http://www.fda.gov/downloads/Food/ResourcesForYou/HealthEducators/UCM109315.pdf

U.S. Food and Drug Administration. (2015). *Sodium in your diet: using the nutrition facts label to reduce your intake*.

Retrieved from http://www.fda.gov/Food/Resources ForYou/Consumers/ucm315393.htm

Webb, D. (2014). Athletes and protein intake. *Today's Dietitian, 16*(6), 22. Retrieved from http://www.todaysdietitian. com/newarchives/060114p22.shtml

Weisenberger, J. (2015). Fiber: fiber's link with satiety and weight control. *Today's Dietitian, 17*(2), 14. Retrieved from http://www.todaysdietitian.com/newarchives/ 021115p14.shtml

West, T. (2016, January). Diabetics soon to be free from insulin injections thanks to scientific breakthrough using patient's own skin cells. *Inquisitr*. Retrieved from http:// www.inquisitr.com/2691961/diabetics-soon-to-be-free-from-insulin-injections-thanks-to-scientific-breakthrough-using-patients-own-skin-cells

What to know about probiotics. (2015). *ABC News*. Retrieved August 2015 from http://abcnews.go.com/GMA/video/ probiotics--33008716

White, J., Guenter, P., Jensen, G., Malone, A., & Schofield M. (2012). Consensus statement of the academy of nutrition and dietetics/American society for parenteral and enteral nutrition: characteristics recommended for the identification and documentation of adult malnutrition (undernutrition). *Journal of the Academy of Nutrition and Dietetics, 112*(5), 730–738.

Youdim, A. (2013). *The merck manual, overview of nutrition.* Retrieved from http://www.merckmanuals.com/ professional/nutritional-disorders/nutrition,-c-, -general-considerations/overview-of-nutrition

Wing, R. R., & Phelan, S. (2005). Long term weight loss maintenance. *The American Journal of Clinical Nutrition, 82*(1), 222S–225S.

World Health Organization. (2013). *Botulism.* Retrieved from http://www.who.int/mediacentre/factsheets/fs270/en

Yale Rudd Center for Food Policy and Obesity. (2013). *Fast food facts 2013 – food advertising to children and teens score.* Retrieved from http://fastfoodmarketing.org/media/ FastFoodFACTS_Report_Summary.pdf

Yan, J., Liu, L., Zhu, Y., Huang, G., & Wang, PP. (2014). The association between breastfeeding and childhood obesity: A meta-analysis. *BMC Public Health, 14*, 1267. Retrieved from http://bmcpublichealth.biomedcentral.com/ articles/10.1186/1471-2458-14-1267

Zhu, W., Cai, D., Wang, Y., Lin, N., Hu, Q., Qi, Y., . . . Amarasekara, S. (2013). Calcium plus vitamin D3 supplementation facilitated fat loss in overweight and obese college students with very-low calcium consumption: a randomized trial. *Nutrition Journal, 12*, 43. Retrieved from http:// www.ncbi.nlm.nih.gov/pubmed/23297844

Bibliography

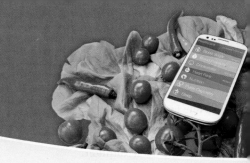

BOOKS

Castle, J., & Jacobsen, M. (2013). *Fearless feeding.* San Francisco, CA: Jossey-Bass and Wiley.

Clark, N. (2014). *Nancy clark's sports nutrition guidebook* (5th ed.). Champaign, IL: Human Kinetics.

Dietz, W. H., & Stern, L. (2012). *Nutrition: What every parent needs to know* (2nd ed.). Elk Grove Village, IL: American Academy of Pediatrics.

Duyff, R. L. (2012). *American dietetic association complete food and nutrition guide* (4th ed.). Hoboken, NJ: Wiley & Sons.

Grodner, M., Escott-Stump, S., & Dorner, S. (2016). *Nutritional foundations and clinical applications.* St. Louis, MO: Elsevier Mosby.

Katz, D. L., & Colino, S. (2013). *Disease proof.* New York: Hudson Street Press and Penguin Group.

Katz, D. L., Friedman, R., & Lucan, S. (2015). *Nutrition in clinical practice.* Philadephia, PA: Wolters Kluwer.

Kulze, A. (2014). *Weight less for life.* Nebraska: Wellness Council of America.

Moore, T. J., Murphy, M. C., & Jenkins, M. (2012). *The DASH diet for weight loss.* New York: Gallery Books, division of Simon & Schuster.

National Cancer Institute, National Institutes of Health, & U.S. Department of Health and Human Services. (2012). *Eating hints before, during, and after cancer treatment: Support for people with cancer.* Bethesda, MD: Author.

Nix, S. (2013). *Williams' basic nutrition and diet therapy* (14th ed.). St. Louis, MO: Elsevier Mosby.

Retelny, V. S., & Academy of Nutrition and Dietetics. (2016). *Total body diet for dummies.* Hoboken, NJ: Wiley and Sons, Inc.

Ross, T. A., & Geil, P. B. (2015). *What do I eat now? A step by step guide to eating right with type 2 diabetes* (2nd ed.). Alexandria, VA: American Diabetes Association, Inc.

Shapiro, A. N. (2013). *Lose it for the last time.* Smithtown, NY: Snewman Media.

Shield, J., & Mullen, M. C. (2012). *Healthy eating, healthy weight for kids and teens.* Chicago, IL: Academy of Nutrition and Dietetics.

Sizer, S., & Whitney, E. (2017). *Nutrition: Concepts and controversies* (14th ed.). Belmont, CA: Cengage Learning.

Smithson, T., & Rubin, A. (2014). *Diabetes meal planning and nutrition for dummies.* Hoboken, NJ: John Wiley and Sons, Inc.

Wansink, B. (2014). *Slim by design: Mindless eating solutions for everyday life.* New York: Harper Collins.

Warshaw, H. S. (2015). *Eat Out, Eat Well: The guide to eating healthy in any restaurant.* Alexandria, VA: American Diabetes Association.

Weisenberger, J. (2015). *21 Things you need to know about diabetes and your heart.* Alexandria, VA: American Diabetes Association.

Wright, H. (2013). *The prediabetes diet plan: How to reverse prediabetes and prevent diabetes through healthy eating and exercise.* New York: Ten Speed Press.

PERIODICALS

American Cancer Society, http://www.cancer.org

American Diabetes Association, http://www.diabetes.org

American Heart Association, http://www.americanheart.com

American Journal of Clinical Nutrition, The American Society for Nutrition.

American Journal of Public Health, American Public Health Association

American Obesity Association, http://www.obesity.org

American Society for Gastrointestinal Endoscopy, http://www.asge.org

American Society for Parenteral and Enteral Nutrition, http://www.clinnutr.org

Archives of Internal Medicine, American Medical Association

British Journal of Nutrition, Cambridge Journals

Circulation, American Heart Association

Diabetes/Metabolism Research and Reviews, John Wiley and Sons, Inc.

Family Economics and Nutrition Review, USDA, Center for Nutrition Policy and Promotion

Healthy Weight Journal, Healthy Weight Network

International Journal of Eating Disorders, John Wiley and Sons, Inc.

Journal of the Academy of Nutrition and Dietetics, Academy of Nutrition and Dietetics

Journal of the American College of Nutrition, American College of Nutrition

Journal of the American Medical Association, American Medical Association

Journal of Nutrition Education and Behavior, Elsevier; Society for Nutrition Education

Journal of Parenteral and Enteral Nutrition, American Society for Enteral and Parenteral Nutrition

New England Journal of Medicine, Massachusetts Medical Society

Nutrition in Clinical Practice, American Society for Enteral and Parenteral Nutrition

PUBLICATIONS

FDA Consumer, DHHS, Food and Drug Administration

Foundations of Wellness, University of California, Berkley

Food and Nutrition Research Briefs, USDA, Agriculture Research Service

Morbidity and Mortality Weekly Report, DHHS. Centers for Disease Control and Prevention

Nutrition Action Healthletter, Center for Science in the Public Interest

Team Nutrition E-Newsletter, USDA, Food and Nutrient Service, Team Nutrition

Today's Dietitian, Great Valley Publishing Co., Inc.

Tuft's University Health and Nutrition Newsletter, Tufts University, Friedman School of Nutrition Science and Policy

INTERNET SITES

Academy of Nutrition and Dietetics - http://www.eatright.org

Action for Healthy Kids - http://www.actionforhealthykids.org

Administration on Aging - http://www.aoa.gov

Alliance for a Healthier Generation - http://www.healthier generation.org

American Academy of Pediatrics - http://www.aap.org

Arthritis Foundation - http://www.arthritis.org

Center for Nutrition Policy and Promotion - http://www.cnpp.usda.gov

Centers for Disease Control and Prevention - http://www.cdc.gov

Food and Drug Administration - http://www.fda.gov

Dietary Guidelines for Americans - http://health.gov/dietaryguidelines/2015/guidelines

Food Allergy Research and Education - http://www.foodallergy.org

Food and Nutrition Information Center - https://fnic.nal.usda.gov

Healthfinder - http://healthfinder.gov

Healthy People - https://www.healthypeople.gov

Let's Move! - http://www.letsmove.gov

MyPlate - http://www.choosemyplate.gov

National Eating Disorder Association - http://www.nationaleatingdisorders.org

National Institute of Diabetes & Digestive & Kidney Diseases - http://www.niddk.nih.gov

National Institutes of Health - http://www.nih.gov

National Kidney Foundation - http://www.kidney.org

National Osteoporosis Foundation - http://www.nof.org

National Weight Control Registry, Brown Medical School/The Miriam Hospital Weight Control & Diabetes Research Center - http://www.nwcr.ws

Office of Disease Prevention and Health Promotion - http://health.gov

Pennington Biomedical Research Center - http://www.pbrc.edu

Physical Activity Guidelines for Americans - http://www.cdc.gov/physicalactivity/downloads/pa_fact_sheet_adults.pdf

President's Council on Fitness, Sports & Nutrition - http://www.fitness.gov

SuperTracker - http://www.choosemyplate.gov/tools-supertracker

U.S. Department of Health and Human Services - http://www.hhs.gov

World Health Organization - http://www.who.int

Index

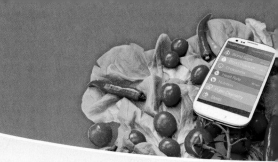